Contemporary Management of Motor Control Problems

Proceedings of the II STEP Conference

STEP

Sponsored by
Foundation for Physical Therapy
APTA's Neurology Section and Section on Pediatrics

First printing, 1991

Printed in the United States of America

Edited by Marilyn J. Lister, BS, PT

Designed and typeset by AAH Graphics, Seven Fountains, Virginia

Printed by Bookcrafters, Inc., Fredricksburg, Virginia

ISBN 0-9628807-0-1

Contents

Preface

Individuals with motor control problems, whether children or adults, represent a significant segment of physical therapy practice. Over the past several years, new information emanating from the sciences of motor control, motor learning, and motor development has begun to influence the thinking of physical therapists engaged in doctoral education. These therapists have begun to question traditional concepts of physical therapy and to provide new models for understanding motor control problems of our patients.

Members of the Section on Pediatrics and the Neurology Section of the American Physical Therapy Association recognized the need for a time to share this new information, discuss issues that arose as a result of our contemporary knowledge base in the sciences of motor behavior, and demonstrate how these new concepts could be incorporated into physical therapy education and practice.

This volume documents the proceedings of an 8-day conference entitled "II STEP: Contemporary Management of Motor Control Problems." The conference was held at Oklahoma University, in Norman, Okla, July 6 through 13, 1990; it attracted approximately 400 physical therapists, predominantly from the United States and Canada. A planning committee of physical therapists designed and organized the conference and oversaw activities during the meeting. Invited speakers presented original papers and participated in discussions of their work, prompted by questions from the audience. The speakers' prompt submission of their papers for publication has allowed this volume to appear in a timely manner.

The cost of the meeting was offset by matching funds from the Section on Pediatrics and the Neurology Section to the Foundation for Physical Therapy, Inc, and by the registration fees paid by participants. Proceeds from the conference and this volume go to the Foundation for Physical Therapy to support research and education related to pediatric and neurologic physical therapy.

The quality of this publication has been enhanced largely as a result of the excellent editorial guidance provided by Marilyn J. Lister, BS, PT. Her care and concern for the authors, their content, and the audience of physical therapists and physical therapy students who will use this volume is clearly evidenced in the final product.

These proceedings represent a truly worthy next step following II STEP. The II STEP conference will in large measure be considered a success if these proceedings serve as a reference in the search for new ways of thinking about motor control problems.

Ann F. VanSant, PhD, PT
Co-Chair, Conference Planning Committee
II STEP: Contemporary Management of Motor Problems

Introduction

The II STEP conference was originally conceived by physical therapists who were members of either the Neurology Section or the Section on Pediatrics of the American Physical Therapy Association. As members of the generation of therapists who benefited from the Northwestern University Special Therapeutic Exercise Project (NUSTEP), this group believed the time was ripe for a similar conference. The NUSTEP conference brought together a group of physical therapy educators during the summer of 1966 for 4 weeks "to be brought abreast, to analyze older and newer methods of therapeutic exercise and to search for ways to meet future needs of physical therapy students through reconsideration of objectives and of curriculum content."[1(p19)] Specifically, the content of NUSTEP included neurophysiology, motor development, motor behavior, and motor learning. The conference resulted in more widespread incorporation of these content areas within physical therapy curricula.

As a result of a meeting of the Neurology Section membership, a committee was appointed to investigate the feasibility of holding a conference that would be "a second NUSTEP." That committee, composed of Neurology Section and Section on Pediatrics members, met in conjunction with combined section meetings and annual conferences of the APTA. A major concern was the expense associated with a conference. The committee believed the cost of a meeting lasting as long as the original NUSTEP would be prohibitive. The committee asked a subcommittee to develop a plan for financing a conference of about 1 week in duration. The financial subcommittee was in many respects the key to the success of the conference. They prepared a plan that enlisted the financial support of the Neurology Section and Section on Pediatrics. Seed money was to be donated to the Foundation for Physical Therapy to cover the planning and initial expenses of the conference. Participants would pay registration fees. Income generated in excess of expenses would be donated to the Foundation for Physical Therapy to support research and scholarships related to neurologic and pediatric physical therapy.

With the support of the two sponsoring sections, the committee moved from studying the feasibility of the conference to the task of planning the conference. Committees were appointed to design the program, select the speakers, choose a conference site, and coordinate local arrangements; individuals on the planning committee assumed varied responsibilities to assure success of the conference. A great deal of support was offered to the planning committee by the Department of Education of the APTA. The director of APTA's Department of Education served as a member of the conference planning committee.

The purpose of the II STEP conference was to bring new theory and knowledge arising from the same content areas addressed at NUSTEP to an audience of physical therapy educators who work in both academic and clinical settings. The specific objectives of the program were that participants would be able to do the following:
1. Describe criteria for a theory.
2. Discuss how theories influence clinical practice.
3. Describe several types of theories.
4. Differentiate among motor learning, motor development, and motor control.
5. Outline stages of motor learning.
6. List issues in motor development across the life span.
7. Describe how current theories of practice relate to contemporary theories of motor control.
8. Describe quantitative and qualitative measures of motor performance.
9. Discuss how learning, perception, and motivation affect motor performance.
10. Describe clinical application of contemporary theories of motor control to individuals with developmental and neurologic deficits.
11. List specific assessment and treatment techniques for motor dysfunction in individuals with Parkinson's disease, cerebral palsy, hemiplegia resulting from cerebral vascular accident, spinal cord injury, spina bifida, Down syndrome, and brain trauma.

The Oklahoma Center for Continuing Education, at the University of Oklahoma in Norman, Okla, was selected as the conference site. The central location, excellent conference facilities for both plenary and small group sessions, and the economy of the room and board were primary considerations in selecting the host site. A local travel agency was selected to manage travel arrangement for participants.

PARTICIPANTS

A reduced registraton rate and a protected period of preregistration was offered to two individuals from each physical therapy education program in the United States and Canada. The educational program directors were asked to send individuals who would represent their clinical and academic faculty. Likewise, reduced rates were offered to sponsoring section members. Recognizing that many clinicians would be eager to attend, the planning committee decided that preference would be given to educators and members of the Neurology Section and Section on Pediatrics, but all physical therapists would be permitted to attend the conference. One hundred twenty-five individuals took advantage of the protected registration for educational program participants. When registration was opened to all physical therapists in February of 1990, the conference capacity was reached in a few short weeks, and many had to be turned away. At their request, a large number of individuals were placed on a waiting list to fill vacancies if cancellations were received. Some individuals were given notice they could attend the conference only days before it began. Faculty members from the University of Oklahoma, in return for staffing the speakers' lounge and trouble shooting day-to-day problems, were allowed to attend the conference sessions. They surely earned their registration.

SPEAKERS

In planning the program, the program committee suggested speakers who represented the areas of motor control, motor learning, and motor development. Their suggestions were circulated to members of the planning committee for feedback, and based on their input, speakers were invited to present at this conference. The planning committee was concerned with not only the speakers' knowledge base but also the ability of the individuals to present their ideas to a large group.

SUPPLEMENTARY MATERIALS AND PROGRAM AIDS

Several speakers provided handouts to the conference attenders. These handouts outlined their talks and provided references for further study of the topic presented. These materials have been incorporated into the proceedings as applicable. Only the videotaped presentation of patient problems presented on Day 4 of the conference could not be replicated for publication.

SESSIONS

The conference began on Friday July 6, 1990, and continued through the morning of Friday July 13, 1990. The proceedings began between 8 AM and 9 AM each day and concluded by 5 PM. The first 3 days addressed theory and its importance, followed by presentations of contemporary motor control, motor learning, and motor development theories. On the fourth day of the conference, traditional and contemporary theories were presented with an eye toward merging the concepts. Small group meetings were held on a daily basis to enable participants to become involved in the topics through discussion of issues that arose during each day's proceedings. On the fifth day, presentations on the measurement of motor performance and the abnormalities of motor behavior were followed by a presentation on recovery from brain damage. Cognitive and perceptual factors in motor control were the topics presented on the sixth conference day; the assessment and treatment of common neurologic disorders were the topics for the seventh day. The final day was devoted to a presentation on functional skills in context and to a discussion of action steps that should result from the conference. The proceedings were brought to an end by a summary address that put the conference in historical perspective.

SPECIAL EVENTS

Several social events highlighted the week. An opening reception, held in the lobby of the conference center, enabled participants and speakers to mingle on the evening before the program began. A special trip to the Cowboy Hall of Fame in Oklahoma City was arranged, with a buffet dinner served in the museum, for conference attenders. The exhibitors sponsored a reception at the end of the fifth day of the conference. The staff of the conference center hosted a barbecue at a nearby park one evening. Mealtimes were special events for the participants, with individuals lingering to discuss the day's events long into the evenings.

ASSESSMENT OF THE CONFERENCE

The conference topics were assessed with the assistance of APTA's Department of Education. The feedback from the conference attenders was overwhelmingly positive, with extremely high marks given to the topics covered in the program. Based on this input, the conference was judged to be an extraordinary success. The need to repeat the conference to enable additional persons to attend was taken under advisement. The lengthy planning process and the large numbers of individuals involved in planning and promoting the conference may interfere with repetition of a conference of similar quality in the near future.

PLAN OF THE PROCEEDINGS

The chapters in these proceedings follow in the order in which they were presented. Only one panel discussion and the small group discussions have not been included. The panel discussion was directed toward a patient problem that had been presented on videotape, which precluded meaningful communication of the panel discussion. Small group discussions were not recorded for publication.

For those who attended, we hope the proceedings will be useful in your teaching, practice, and research. For those who did not attend and for the students who may read these proceedings, we hope this publication will be of value as you seek further knowledge in the theory of physical therapy for persons with developmental and neurologic disorders.

Ann Van Sant and Ellen Spake
Co-Chairs, II STEP: Contemporary
Management of Motor Control Problems

Marilyn Lister
Editor

Reference

1. Wood EC, Voss DE, Bouman HD. Introduction. *Am J Phys Med*. 1967;46:19-24.

Chapter 1

Opening Remarks: A Generation Ago

Ann F. VanSant, PhD, PT
Co-Chair
II STEP Conference Planning Committee
Associate Professor
Department of Physical Therapy
College of Allied Health Professions
Temple University
Philadelphia, PA 19140

Welcome to the II STEP (Special Therapeutic Exercise Project) conference. The anticipation of this meeting has been great. It is a pleasure to be able to offer this survey of contemporary issues related to the treatment of children and adults with motor control disorders. We hope this will be a monumental conference in the tradition of the original NUSTEP (Northwestern University Special Therapeutic Exercise Project).

The NUSTEP conference served its purpose, because the written proceedings, published in the *American Journal of Physical Medicine,* served as a text for the next generation of students. But even more importantly, the neurosciences became an integral part of physical therapy curricula. In the one volume of NUSTEP proceedings,[1] students could read of all the neurophysiologic approaches and review the foundation sciences, including up-to-date information on the muscle spindle, motor development, cybernetics, and postural reflexes.

I was in that generation of students who benefited from NUSTEP. As a senior student I eagerly awaited the publication of the NUSTEP proceedings in February of 1967. By the time I headed off to my clinical affiliations—in my white uniform, white stockings, and white shoes and with my page-boy haircut, white headband, and Timex watch with a sweep-second hand—I was all set with my NUSTEP proceedings full of pages and pages of Rood, Bobath, proprioceptive neuromuscular facilitation (PNF), Brunnstrom, and Fay. And happily I went to a clinic in the summer of '67 where everyone of the staff therapists also had already purchased their copies of the NUSTEP proceedings. I remember the pride and excitement of learning the new culture of those neurophysiologic approaches, and it was a culture that left the next generation to ponder its archaeological artifacts such as brushes, vibrators, and giant inflatable balls.

Looking back after nearly 25 years, with the knowledge of what accomplishments our profession has made in that time period, I would like to share a perspective of NUSTEP that goes beyond the content of the conference.

At NUSTEP, physical therapists for the first time were presenting a group of theoretical approaches to patient care. This represented an important advance for the profession. Although Sister Kenny had devised an approach to poliomyelitis, she was a nurse, not a physical therapist. The NUSTEP conference demonstrated that physical therapists could read the scientific literature, interpret it, make hypotheses about their patients' movement disorders, and devise theory-based treatment procedures. Those NUSTEP therapists created a subculture of evaluation and treatment without prescription, because their theory-based evaluations and treatment plans were exclusively the work of physical therapists. Once we turned that corner, we have moved steadily forward.

In my mind, NUSTEP was a step toward independent practice. As a student affiliate I soon realized that the check mark on the physical therapy prescription form that requested therapeutic exercise meant "evaluate and treat as necessary," and I had clinical instructors who were dedicated to developing my ability to do just that using the newer neurophysiological treatment theories.

The idea that therapists as scientists are the featured speakers here at this II STEP conference is an indicator of the remarkable growth of our profession. Surely, those of us who eagerly awaited the proceedings of NUSTEP had little idea of where our profession might be in 20 years. At our national Association's annual conference last week, one of our well-known colleagues came up to me and asked why, when we planned II STEP, we did not consider having non-physical therapists as speakers. Well, we had considered that, and for the most part, e decided that we had the expertise within our profession to carry off this conference. I asked him if he could, just for a moment, step back and share the pride of what we are capable of doing. We need to set no bounds on the sharing of ideas, but we also have an increasingly rich source of expertise of doctoral-prepared scientists, many of whom are women, who are "moving and shaking" this aspect of our profession. The time is ripe to gather them together so that we all might benefit from their work.

I will return for a moment to the content of NUSTEP.

Those neurophysiologic approaches set the stage for neurologic and pediatric therapies for years to come because the educators of the profession incorporated the content into their curricula. Indeed, neurodevelopmental treatment (NDT) continues to be a predominant practice made in the clinical community. Yet the winds of change are blowing. The supporting basic and behavioral sciences of today are different than they were at the time of NUSTEP, and that change is precisely what has lead to this conference. Our colleagues are eager to share the new science that has altered their way of clinical practice.

I mentioned how sensitive I was as a student to the use of the term therapeutic exercise to denote "evaluate and treat as necessary." The term therapeutic exercise is also a symbol of the change we have undergone. Exercise was extended by the neurophysiologic approaches to include reflexive therapy, and it is only within the last several years that we are coming to realize that exercise and motor learning are not synonyms. So much of what we are about in neurologic and developmental therapy is the teaching and learning of motor skills; that thought is something we need to remember.

And one other instance of change should be noted. The profits from the published proceedings of this conference, unlike NUSTEP, will benefit physical therapy research and scholarship.

So we are proud to present II STEP. We are moving to the brink of new understanding. The planning is done, the speakers are ready, and we have just a few things left to do. A giant thank you to the entire memberships of the Pediatric and Neurology sections for their support of this conference and to the members of the original planning committee. Will each of you stand when I call your names: Susan Attermeier, Pam Duncan, Susan Harris, Carolyn Heriza, Becky Porter, Debra Shefrin, Darcy Umphred, and Carolee Winstein. I would also like to thank Steve Seater and the Foundation for Physical Therapy staff for their assistance. And to Rose Meyers and the staff of American Physical Therapy Association's Department of Education, a giant thank you. Rose has been at our planning meetings to offer all kinds of support, and we are grateful. Ellen Spake, my counterpart for this conference, from the Section on Pediatrics, and I would also like to recognize the following members of the financial planning committee and have each of them stand to be recognized: Suzann Campbell, Barbara Connolly, Susan Effgen, and

Patricia Montgomery. They willingly stepped forward to assist when the critical issue of funding was upon us. A special word about "Trish" Montgomery: when the funding was solidified, she offered to help with any other activities that needed her assistance. We took her up on her offer and she has done so many things. She started out as financial manager, but her duties were extended to include overseeing the brochure and registration, and she handled an inordinate number of phone calls since February regarding this conference. If there were an award for all this service, she would be our prime candidate. I am serious when I say that without Trish there would be no II STEP. She was there when we needed help, and she has not left our sides.

Finally, a very special recognition to Carolyn Heriza who so carefully put together this program. Her wisdom, diplomacy, and attention to detail are the keys to our success, and she has kept at it for nearly 4 years now. We all admire and respect her abilities, and we all know the quality of the program that she has put together. There is no one who could have done as well, and we are extremely glad and grateful that she is in charge of this program.

I would additionally like to extend a special recognition to the individuals who joined Carolyn, Trish, Ellen, and me, members of the planning committee. The individuals who have worked long and hard in the background to assure the success of our conference include Susan Attermeier, Martha Ferreti, Susan Harris, Rose Meyers, Roberta Newton, and Becky Porter. They are on duty here at this conference; if you need help just ask their assistance.

I want to give a very special recognition to Martha Ferreti who, as Chair of the Department of Physical Therapy here at Oklahoma University, has served as our local contact and local problem solver. She is a wonderwoman who identifies and solves problems quietly and effectively. We appreciate everything she has done for us.

And now Pam Duncan, who more than five years ago suggested this conference was long overdue, your dream has come true. Welcome to II STEP.

References

1. An exploratory and analytical survey of therapeutic exercise: proceedings of the Northwestern University Special Therapeutic Exercise Project. *Am J Phys Med*. 1967;46:9-1135.

Chapter 2

Opening Remarks: From Past to Present

Ellen Spake, MS, PT
Co-Chair
II STEP Conference Planning Committee
Chair and Assistant Professor
Physical Therapy Education
Rockhurst College
Kansas City, MO 64111

It is with great pleasure that I greet you this morning. The next 8 days are the culmination of the dreams, hard work, and visions of a group of people who have shared and planned for these days for the past 5 years. As I wandered through the crowd last night at the opening reception, speaking to some of you and catching just a bit of the conversation of other groups, I heard many different perspectives of what this conference is to be and what its impact will be on our profession. I thought it appropriate to give you a historical overview of how we all came to be here today and, in so doing, compare and contrast the original NUSTEP (Northwestern University Special Therapeutic Exercise Project) with today's II STEP.

The original NUSTEP was held at Northwestern University in Chicago for 4 weeks in the summer of 1966. The project was conceptualized to review what were then the new neurophysiologic approaches to therapeutic exercise. The conference was designed for faculty members in order that this new information could be incorporated into the curricula of physical therapy education programs. One hundred fourteen educators attended. The only clinicians who were allowed to participate were those physical therapists from institutions where physical therapy students at Northwestern University received their clinical experiences. Even then, clinicians were invited to attend only certain days of the 4-week conference and were not invited to be present for small group work. Thirty-five clinicians were in attendance across the 4 weeks.

In contrast, the planning committee for II STEP (Special Therapeutic Exercise Project) thought it important to bring together educators, clinicians, and researchers for this conference. Approximately 420 participants are registered. Ninety-nine percent of the registrants are physical therapists, with the other 1% representative of occupational therapy or medicine. Approximately 39% of the registrants are Academic Administrators, Academic Coordinators of Clinical Education, or faculty members, while 56% are either clinicians or clinical faculty members. Of the clinicians registered for this conference, 20% practice within a hospital setting, 6% are in a private practice, 2% work in the public schools, 19% practice in a rehabilitation center, and 5%

work within some other clinical setting. The median length of practice across all participants is 11 to 15 years.

Funding for planning of the NUSTEP conference was primarily through a 2-year planning grant from the Vocational Rehabilitation Administration. The Vocational Rehabilitation Administration and the Department of Health, Education and Welfare shared the cost of the meeting itself and the cost of publishing the proceedings. In contrast, funding for the II STEP conference came from seed monies donated by the Neurology Section and the Section on Pediatrics of the American Physical Therapy Association. The proceedings will be published by the Foundation for Physical Therapy, with all revenues from both the conference and the proceedings going to benefit research and education through the Foundation.

The Planning Committee for NUSTEP spent approximately 1-1/2 years in planning the conference. The committee came from very diversified backgrounds. Four were primarily physiologists. Several were members of physical therapy faculties, yet among these were an anatomist, a psychologist, a reflex physiologist, and one of the nation's outstanding experts in the teaching of massage. One member of the planning committee was a medical school dean. The presenters, while including a number of physical therapists, also included a large number of physicians and physiologists. In contrast, the planning committee for II STEP are all physical therapists who are representative of both academic and clinical programs. It has taken about 5 years to plan this conference, and the presenters, with only one exception, are all physical therapists.

Finally, we would be remiss not to note the goals, objectives, and purposes of the original NUSTEP conference. The NUSTEP Planning Committee considered four areas of knowledge to be of prime importance: neurophysiology, motor development, motor behavior, and motor learning. There were seven stated objectives of the conference, among them: 1) to explore the theses that an understanding of normal motor behavior is essential to optimum use of therapeutic exercise as a rehabilitative procedure and that exercise is bound inseparably to motor learning; 2) to analyze a large number of therapeutic exercise procedures, such as traditional ones and newer methods of treatment, in order to determine their influence on both normal and deviant, or distorted, motor behavior and motor learning; and 3) to identify common denominators among the many approaches to treatment.

As you look over the course description and objectives for II STEP you will note many similarities. Motor development, motor behavior, and motor learning and control continue to be a focus of our profession. We, too, intend to explore how motor behavior and motor learning affect therapeutic exercise. We, too, will look at traditional and newer methods of treatment and their influence on motor behavior, learning, and control. We, too, will identify common denominators among the many approaches to treatment. The question and issues are much the same as those facing our profession some 24 years ago. The answers may be a bit different as a result of the advances in our field over that time span.

On a final note, out of great respect for the historical NUSTEP conference we attempted to identify and locate as many former participants of NUSTEP as possible. We extended a special invitation to attend II STEP to those who were part of our profession's vision of the future. We would like to recognize two former NUSTEP participants who are in attendance at this conference: Martha Trotter from Seattle, Wash, and Edith Aston-McCrimmon from Montreal, Quebec.

And now, let us begin our exploration for answers to therapeutic exercise questions facing us today.

Chapter 3

Theory: Criteria, Importance, and Impact

Kay Shepard, PhD, PT, FAPTA
Associate Professor
Director of Advanced Graduate Studies in Physical Therapy
College of Allied Health Professions
Temple University
Philadelphia, PA 19140

In this opening paper for II STEP I will discuss theory: what theory is, why it is omnipresent and fascinating, and why theory is critical to the growth of practice and research in the care of patients with neurological problems. In the subsequent chapters in this volume the authors will be presenting theories specific to motor development, motor control, and motor learning. The purposes of this chapter are to present a format for how to think about theories and to encourage you to enjoy grappling with them.

I consider the readers of this book a perfect audience for this task. The primary reason is because so much of the physical therapy management of patients with motor control problems is elusive. From the very words you use to describe neurological conditions to the treatment plans you establish and the goals you predict for your patients, you function in a world of great ambiguity. It is a world that demands you remain open to your patient's responses from moment to moment, a world that has few machines or recording devices to assist you in evaluation or treatment, and a world that insists on your receptivity to new ways of making sense of the complexities of the healthy as well as the damaged nervous system.

So one thing you each have in common in attempting to harness the anxieties you sometimes feel in working in this patient care arena is the creation and use of theories. Simply, if you can say what you think is happening out loud, you feel more calm, more in control, more directed, and more empowered. If you do not have a place to start from, you have no direction—no place to go to. And your feelings about patient care alternate between boredom and helplessness. Therefore, during your treatment sessions, each of you think of an explanation or premise to guide your actions.

For an example, you may decide that the reason your pediatric patient is wailing is because he is having a thalamic attack. From this theoretical premise you choose to wait it out before beginning treatment. Or you decide the incessant crying is due to physical discomfort and thus begin a search to discover the offending source. Or you decide that the child is upset because it is summertime and all the other kids are at the swimming pool while he is in therapy; therefore, you set about to find ways to distract and amuse him so that you can get on with treatment. At a very basic level, these ideas about why the child is behaving as he is can be called theory.

WHAT IS THEORY?

Tammivaara and Shepard[1] write that "theory is a word encompassing two concepts: contemplation and observation. . . . Through contemplation and observation theories or ideas about how things relate together are developed."

Many definitions of theory exist, some of which are torturously complex. For your purposes at this conference, I will use the following most basic definition of theory: Theory is an abstract idea or collection of ideas used to explain physical or social phenomena (Fig. 3-1). The important words here are abstract and idea. Because theory is an idea that is abstract, it is particularly useful in its application to many different phenomena. Thus a theory of movement control transcends any one particular patient and allows us to

---

THEORY

Theory is an abstract idea or collection of ideas used to explain physical or social phenomenon.

* Evolves from experience or research

* Dynamic

* Not directly testable

* Requires Scope Conditions

* Requires Operational Definitions

Fig. 3-1. *Theory definition and basic tenets.*

consider treatment ideas for any number of patients with movement disorders.

Where does theory come from? It comes from our accumulated clinical observations and experiences, and it comes from the research literature on human movement. Theory is dynamic. As our experience, knowledge, and insight grow, so do our theories evolve and change. We chuckle at well known historical theories that have long since been proven false: The earth is flat, emotions are guided by four biles, or a child is just a miniature adult. You may remember with some embarrassment some of the theories you held about parenthood when you were teenagers. Theories that will profoundly be revolutionary at this conference may be in the rag bag in another 20 years. This dynamic nature of theories makes them fun. There is always more to discover, more to create, and different thought-provoking ways to interpret behavior.

Because theory is an idea and is abstract, it is not directly testable. We cannot hold a theory in our hands or hook it up to a measuring device to record its existence. To test theories, we usually set up hypotheses that are testable. Guided by these hypotheses, we gather and analyze information. If the information, or data, supports a hypothesis, we would suggest that the theory is true. I will return to hypothesis testing later in this paper and show you exactly how hypotheses are connected to theory.

Let me give you a simple example of the way we use theories in everyday life. Say you have an elderly Aunt Caroline that has begun to cry a lot in the last several months. Your theory is that she cries because she is depressed. Your cousin Matthew's theory is that Aunt Caroline cries because she wants attention. Your uncle Bernie postulates her crying is due to lack of vitamin B complex in her diet. Each of you are interacting with Aunt Caroline in a manner that is in concert with your theory. You suggest interesting day trips to bring her out of her depression. Cousin Matthew simply stays away because he is disgusted that anyone her age should behave in such an attention getting way. Uncle Bernie plies her with food rich in vitamin B complex.

Each of you could prove your theory by gathering and analyzing information that would support your theory. For your depression theory, you might have Aunt Caroline take the MMPI and look at the score she receives on the Depression scale. You might observe her physical appearance to see if she demonstrates the characteristic physical signs of depression such as poverty of movement, head down withdrawn posture, and lack of eye contact. You might also question her as to her sleeping and eating habits to find out if she demonstrates behaviors of the early morning waking and the eating disorders that are common in depressed people. Thus you would look at a number of factors in an attempt to build a strong case for your theory. Rarely is any theory proven by one piece of information. Commonly, information is gathered and correlated or triangulated to build a substantial case for the existence of theory. For your cousin Matthew to prove his theory that Aunt Caroline wants attention, he, likewise, would gather data on the cessation of crying whenever he visits Aunt Mary, whenever the family gathers for holidays, or whenever he observes her playing bridge with her friends. Uncle Bernie would set out to prove his vitamin B

theory by analysis of Aunt Caroline's diet before the crying began and now. He would bring evidence to bear from nutritional journals and would probably seek confirmation about his theory from an expert such as his geriatrician. Now it may turn out that the information gathered supports all three theories: the theories of depression, attention, and nutrition. Everyone is correct!

This would lead you to believe something else is operating, that is, another higher level or more all-encompassing theory accounts for Aunt Caroline's behavior. For example, perhaps in the course of your investigations you discover that Aunt Caroline has had several close friends stricken with cancer in the past 6 months. As you and Cousin Matthew and Uncle Bernie pool your information on depression—seeking solace in the company of others and disregarding self as manifested in poor eating habits—you come to the recognition that Aunt Caroline is exhibiting a typical grief reaction. Thus each of your individual theories is discarded. You accept the broadened theory that Aunt Caroline is experiencing a grief reaction. In accepting this alternative theory, you begin to apply more appropriate interventions to help her through this difficult time in her life.

Theory, therefore, typically gives us a starting place; it is a focal point for our thoughts and our observations, and it is a guide for action.

THEORY IN PRACTICE

We use theory everyday in clinical practice. Each of us evaluates and treats patients usually according to the implicit theories we hold about the cause and nature of function and dysfunction. As therapists we are often unaware of what theories we are using to guide our treatment interventions. The problem with our being unaware of theory is that our clinical skill levels will stagnate. Without theory there is no way to give coherence to what we are doing now and to view our patient-care outcomes in a way that transcends individuals.

For example, in the area of treatment for neurologically impaired patients many of us learned in school that movement was a matter of reflexes organized in a vertical hierarchy of control: spinal cord, brain stem, midbrain, and cortex. The theory espoused was that these reflexes resulted in movement patterns and that therapeutic interventions consisted of suppressing or facilitating certain reflexes to gain the desired functional movement pattern. This early theory has recently been replaced with a more complex dynamic systems theory in which the idea of reflexes has been replaced with pattern generators and the idea of hierarchical control has been replaced with multilevel, multisystem control. If one ascribed to the newer theory, one would begin to work with patterns of movement rather than with isolated reflexes.

If we view and contemplate about what we are doing, that is, explicate the theories we use, our theories of motor development, motor learning, and motor control will become increasingly rich in explaining the mysteries of movement science.

To use theory effectively we must be aware of the basic tenets of a theory. We have already touched on three of these tenets: A theory evolves from experience or a re-arch base; theory is dynamic, that is, it is open to constant change and refinement as our knowledge grows; and a theory is not directly testable. For any theory there are usually dozens of hypotheses that can be generated to prove or disprove the existence of the theory.

A fourth tenet is that of scope conditions. Scope conditions are the conditions or situations under which the theory will work. For example, take the theoretical concept that "Human beings are emotional." We can see right away that this theory is true under certain conditions. A human being may be emotional, for example, when she or he is experiencing loss or great joy. At other times, human beings are not what we would call emotional. Thus one of the things we attempt to determine with all theory is the scope of conditions under which the theory is operable. You, for example, may have a theory about what facilitates spasticity. Think about it. As part of your notions about this theory you can quickly list several common conditions under which spasticity will occur. These are the scope conditions of the theory.

We also need to be aware of differences in interpretations of the words used in a theory. To return to the theoretical concept that "Human beings are emotional," we might define emotional by certain observable behaviors that humans exhibit when they are emotional such as yelling or jumping up and down. For spasticity, if that word is still in use among the participants in this audience, I am sure there could be a dozen or more definitions. Do you see that theory cannot be shared unless the operational definitions of the major constructs in the theory can be defined?

When a theory does prove to be untrue, it may be that the theory itself is false. Or it may be that the scope conditions under which the theory was applied were incorrect. Or it may be that one or more operational definitions needed to be altered for the theory to hold. Or it may be that the hypotheses we set up and the information we gathered to prove the theory were invalid. Part of the fun of theory is the working back and forth between a theory and the testing of the theory to see what is true. Therefore, when you work with patients, if you constantly reflect on the theory you are using to guide yourtreatment you come closer and closer to what the "truth" is about the presentation of dysfunction and your ability to intervene effectively.

THEORY IN RESEARCH

Theory in research is imperative.[2,3] Without theory there is no context in which to have our questions and answers make sense. Without theory there is no way to build upon ideas, to determine conditions under which the theory is true (scope conditions), or to invent new theories to explain dissimilar phenomenon. Without theory there is no way to create the knowledge base of our profession; without an ever expanding knowledge base the future of our profession is indeed dim.

There are essentially two ways that theory can be used in research. The first way is to use theory to guide the development of a research project to answer a specific clinical question (and to confirm or disconfirm the theory). The second way is to gather field data about natural events that occur and then collate and scrutinize the data for emerging patterns that suggest theories.

Let me first guide you through a brief overview of two major research strategies. Then I will give an example of published research that has used each strategy. My focus will be on the place and significance of theory in the research process, not on the components of the research process.

Figure 3-2 depicts an overview of the research process. This figure is a modification of the original schema developed by Shepard et al.[4] One always begins with a research question. The research question comes from a problem or curiosity we have about our patient care activities, usually how or why something has happened. For example, how does one best facilitate a child's functional sitting balance or why does one patient who has experienced head trauma come from floor to standing easily while another patient who appears similar struggles.

Once we have our research question we can approach our research from one of two major philosophical perspectives. One of these perspectives is called *positivism* and one is called *phenomenological*.[5] Each perspective will guide our choice of research design, method, and data analysis.

The positivistic perspective leads us to seek the truth about a single objective reality. In this perspective the theoretical base is quite clear. The theory often suggests a cause and effect relationship between two or more variables. To test the relationship between variables, hypotheses are set up and data are gathered either in an experimental design format or in a descriptive correlational format. The resulting data, which are primarily quantitative, or numerical, prove

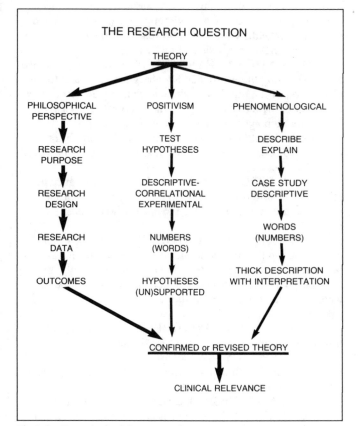

Fig 3-2. *Overview of the research process.*

or disprove the hypotheses. In turn, this proof either supports the original theory or suggests that the original theory should be revised (or discarded altogether).

The following is an example of how research is done from a positivistic perspective. This example is based on the research report entitled "Balance Performance, Force Production, and Activity Levels in Noninstitutionalized Men 60 to 90 Years of Age" by Iverson et al.[6]

RESEARCH QUESTION: What is the relationship between muscle weakness in old age and the ability to maintain equilibrium?

THEORY: One-third to one-half of the United States population 65 years and older have one or more falls a year (literature referenced). Decreased muscle mass, especially of the back extensors and proximal lower extremity muscles, is prevalent in the elderly population (literature referenced). Isometric and isokinetic force and torque measurements have been shown to decrease with increased age (literature referenced). Therefore, there is a relationship between muscle weakness in old age and maintenance of equilibrium.

PHILOSOPHICAL PERSPECTIVE: Positivism.

RESEARCH PURPOSE: To test a priori hypotheses.

CONCEPTUAL HYPOTHESIS 1. "Balance time and force production will have a positive correlation."[6(p349)] Note that this quoted hypothesis is in a format that is not directly testable and is therefore called a conceptual hypothesis. Out of any conceptual hypothesis, one or more operational hypotheses that are directly testable can be formed.

OPERATIONAL HYPOTHESIS 1a. Standing balance as measured by the one-legged stance test (OLST) and torque production of the hip flexor, abductor, and extensor muscles as measured by a dynamometer will be correlated positively in healthy men aged 60 years and over. (Note that this operational hypothesis is directly testable.)

OPERATIONAL HYPOTHESIS 1b. Standing balance as measured by the sharpened Romberg test (SR) and torque production of the hip flexor, abductor, and extensor muscles as measured by a dynamometer will be correlated positively in healthy men aged 60 years and over.

Note that if Operational Hypotheses 1a and 1b are proven to be correct, then Conceptual Hypothesis 1 is correct.

CONCEPTUAL HYPOTHESIS 2. "A difference in balance time and force production will exist between subjects who are active as opposed to those who are inactive."[6(p349)]

OPERATIONAL HYPOTHESIS 2a. Torque production of the hip flexor, abductor, and extensor muscles as measured by a dynamometer will be greater in healthy men aged 60 years and over who exercise five or more times a week compared with men of the same age who exercise less frequently or not at all.

OPERATIONAL HYPOTHESIS 2b. Standing balance time as measured by OLST and SR will increase in healthy men aged 60 and over who exercise five or more times a week compared with men of the same age who exercise less frequently or not at all.

RESEARCH DESIGN: Descriptive correlational.

RESEARCH DATA: Numerical (Pearson correlation coefficients and analysis of variance).

OUTCOMES:
Operational Hypothesis 1a confirmed.
Operational Hypothesis 1b confirmed.
Therefore, Conceptual Hypothesis 1 is confirmed.
Operational Hypothesis 2a confirmed.
Operational Hypothesis 2b confirmed.
Therefore, Conceptual Hypothesis 2 is confirmed.

THEORY: Confirmed for this sample (healthy men aged 60 years and over) on these measurements (standing balance as measured by sharpened Romberg test, one-legged stance test; muscle torque measured by a strain-gauge hand-held dynamometer) and using the authors' definitions of muscle weakness, old age, and upright equilibrium. Thus the theory under these scope conditions for sample and measurement and for these operational definitions is supported.

CLINICAL IMPLICATIONS: Increased strength in hip flexion, extension, and abduction and increased daily activity may improve balance in your elderly male patients.

See how neatly this all fits together? The data gathered support (or do not support) the accuracy of the operational hypotheses. The operational hypotheses, in turn, prove (or disprove) the conceptual hypotheses. In turn, the conceptual hypotheses confirm (or do not confirm) the theory. In turn, the theory helps to answer the original question.

Obviously, we could have generated many different conceptual and operational hypotheses to confirm the theory. In particular, think about how we might alter the scope conditions and gather different data on the same or a different sample to confirm the same conceptual hypotheses. And if we proceeded to do this and the many hypotheses we generated and tested were supported by our data, we would increasingly have convincing evidence that our theory was correct.

The sad fact is that not nearly enough incremental research is performed to support specific theories that undergird our practice. As long as we allow ourselves and our students to perform "shotgun" research we will never be able to establish the theoretical bases of our profession.

Now let us return to Figure 3-2 and follow the second philosophical approach to research, that is, phenomenology. If we chose a phenomenological approach, we approach the research question as if there were many possible realities. We do not know beforehand what really exists. In our search for what exists we will cast a wide net. We will not be constrained by a priori hypotheses. We will define only the field boundaries of our interest. Then we will enter this field to observe and gather all possible relevant data. From this data we will attempt to make sense of the field of observation and answer our question.

The following example of this approach is taken from an article entitled "Rising from a Supine Position to Erect Stance: Description of Adult Movement and a Developmental Hypothesis" by VanSant.[7]

RESEARCH QUESTION: Do functional movement patterns change with age?

THEORY: The developmental sequence for the task of coming from supine to standing is established in early childhood (literature referenced). The adult form of rising appears by the age of 4 to 5 years (literature referenced). Therefore, the specific movement patterns to be used in teaching adults to rise from a supine position are the same patterns used for children.

PHILOSOPHICAL PERSPECTIVE: Phenomenological.

RESEARCH PURPOSE: To observe and record the movement sequence of a group of adults coming from supine to standing and to determine if they are using the same developmental patterns as described for young children.

RESEARCH DESIGN: Descriptive.

RESEARCH DATA: Videotape content analysis of 10 trials for each of 32 subjects moving from the supine position to standing. Written descriptions prepared of movement in three components: head and trunk movement, upper extremity movements, and lower extremity movements. Movement descriptions refined until interrater observation classifications reached 90% or greater reliability. The number of different body action components computed.

OUTCOMES: Great variability exists in the patterns of movement used by adults in the supine-to-standing task.

REVISED THEORY: Developmental or age-related change in movement patterns (which are not attributable to learning) may occur throughout the life span. Therefore, the movement patterns to be used in teaching adults to rise from a supine position will vary.

CLINICAL APPLICATION: There is no one right way to teach the task of supine to standing in adults. Be aware of many possible factors that may influence the most functionally useful pattern for your patient. These factors may include but not be limited to age, body dimensions, and biomechanical constraints.

As with the positivistic approach, theory is again the beginning and end point of the phenomenological approach to research. Similarly, the scope conditions imposed include the sample type and the form of measurement. The primary terms that were operationally defined include development sequence, movement pattern, and body components. Thus the revised theory should hold true within the scope conditions of the original research if similar operational definitions are used.

As with all good applied theory, you will note that the endpoint theory in both approaches was immediately transferable into clinical usefulness. You will also note that the opportunity exists for many research studies to be performed to provide increased support for the theories as they now stand or to further define the scope conditions under which these theories would hold true.

THEORETICAL OR CONCEPTUAL FRAMEWORKS

I would be amiss in my discussion of theory if I did not mention a more elaborate theory format that will increasingly be used in the future. This more elaborate format is called a theoretical, or conceptual, framework.[8,9] A theoretical framework lays out all the possible influences that can be brought to bear relative to a research question. Some pieces of the framework contain theoretical components that have been verified. Other components yield or suggest theory that has yet to be "operationalized" and tested. This type of framework is commonly used by social scientists but is now beginning to appear in both basic biological and clinical research.

I would like to share briefly with you one example from my own research with Gail Jensen, Laurie Hack, and Jan Gwyer on what a theoretical framework is. In our work on the Master Clinician we first set out to define who the experienced clinician was and what distinguishes an experienced clinician from a novice clinician.[10] In building a theoretical framework we attempted to predict the most relevant practice environment variables that might distinguish between the experienced and novice clinician. These variables were identified from extensive reading of the literature about experts in many fields, from our own experiences, and from the experiences of our colleagues.

Figure 3-3 provides a graphic representation of our theoretical framework. The first level of the framework represents the components of a practice environment that at any point in time are "givens." We postulated that any one of these givens may influence patient outcomes. Physical therapist professional characteristics include age, gender, socioeconomic background, educational preparation, level of experience, interest in a clinical specialty area, personal traits including values and the ability to care, expectations regarding the course of the patient's disease, and expectations for therapeutic outcomes. Client characteristics include age, gender, socioeconomic background, education, expectations for therapy, and expectations regarding the course of disease or illness. Organizational factors that we proposed might influence patient outcomes include the type of clinical setting, payment system, geographic location of the clinic, other health care personnel involved in the patient's care, and time constraints on treatment.

In the second level of our theoretical framework we placed physical therapy tools used by the physical therapists including verbal and nonverbal communication techniques, manual skills, and modalities. The third level, the therapeutic intervention, was the one we considered the "black box." We called it a black box because so little is known about what actually happens between a physical therapist and a patient. All the elements of the preceding two levels are brought to bear on this third level. At the other side of the therapeutic intervention is the patient outcome.

Obviously, we can set up innumerable studies to find how these variables interface with each other to influence patient care outcomes, what significant variable differences exist between the experienced and novice clinician, and how one gets from novice to experienced (or expert) status. As with theory, the theoretical framework also is dynamic. As we proceed with our research we expect that some of these elements will be discarded and others may come into view. This theoretical framework provides us with a roadmap for guiding our research inquiries in a systematic and coherent way.

I would fully expect similar theoretical frameworks to be established to guide research into the areas of motor development, motor control, and motor learning. At the risk of seeming audacious I would like to share with you a possible theoretical framework for future motor control research (Fig. 3-4). As you can see, possible influencing variables within three environments are defined: biological, physical, and social. The framework suggests that the variables within these environments act and interact in such a way as to pro-

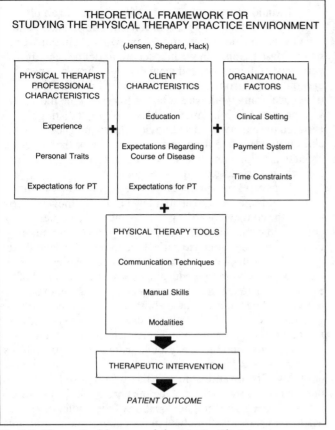

Fig 3-3. *Theoretical framework for Master Clinician.*

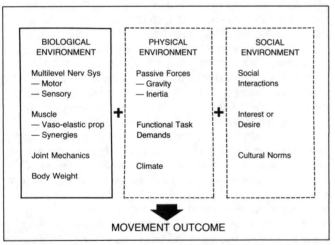

Fig 3-4. *Possible theoretical framework for dynamic action theory research.*

duce a unique motor outcome. If this framework is at all feasible, you certainly have your work cut out for you.

In closing I would like to say this. For those of you who treat neurologically impaired patients, the progression of your patients is not simple. Fractures and soft tissue injuries are simple; the organic pathology is clearly understood and the course of healing generally predictable. However, for your patients with neurological problems, the course and treatment of their pathology is complicated, progression is comparatively slow, and you as well as the patient and family are often frustrated. Thus you in this audience today, in particular, are open to new approaches, to new theories that could suggest more powerful treatment interventions and speedier recoveries. I am counting on your receptiveness to alternative ways of thinking about what you do and why you do it and on your acquired tolerance for proceeding despite unknowns to help make this II STEP conference a major milestone for the physical therapy profession in the 1990s and beyond.

References

1. Tammivaara J, Shepard K. Theory: the guide to clinical practice and research. *Phys Ther*. 1990;70:578-582.
2. Krebs D, Harris S. Elements of theory presentation in physical therapy. *Phys Ther*. 1988;68:690-693.
3. Payton O. The role of theory in research. In: *Research: The Validation of Clinical Practice*. 2nd ed. Philadelphia, Pa: F A Davis Co; 1986:chap 11.
4. Shepard K, Schmoll B, Jensen G, et al. A Model for Multiple Approaches to Clinical Research. Philadelphia Pa: Philadelphia Institute for Physical Therapy; 1989.
5. Jensen G. Qualitative methods in physical therapy research: a form of disciplined inquiry. *Phys Ther*. 1989;69:492-500.
6. Iverson G, Gossman M, Shaddeau S, et al: Balance performance, force production, and activity levels in noninstitutionalized men 60 to 90 years of age. *Phys Ther*. 1990;70:348-355.
7. VanSant A. Rising from a supine position to erect stance: description of adult movement and a developmental hypothesis. *Phys Ther*. 1988;68:185-192.
8. Fawcett J, Downs F. *The Relationship of Theory and Research*. Norwalk, Conn: Appleton-Century-Crofts; 1986.
9. Botha ME. Theory development in perspective: the role of conceptual frameworks and models in theory development. *J Adv Nurs*. 1989;14:49-55.
10. Jensen G, Shepard K, Hack L. The novice versus the experienced clinician: insights into the work of the physical therapist. *Phys Ther*. 1990;70:314-323.

Chapter 4

Assumptions Underlying Motor Control for Neurologic Rehabilitation

Fay B. Horak, PhD, PT
Associate Scientist
R.S. Dow Neurological Sciences Institute
Good Samaritan Hospital
Portland, OR 97209

How can I inhibit primitive tonic neck reflexes while facilitating normal equilibrium responses?

Will inhibitive casts reduce extensor muscle tone to allow normal gait patterns?

How can I teach my patient to develop movement strategies that are functional and adaptable to environmental changes?

The questions therapists ask of themselves in treating neurologically impaired patients reveal their underlying assumptions about how the brain controls movement. Similarly, the questions neuroscientists ask of themselves in designing and analyzing experiments in motor control reveal their underlying assumptions about how the brain controls movement. It is important for therapists to become aware of their own assumptions and the assumptions that neuroscientists hold about motor control because these assumptions shape, structure, and limit therapists' observations and treatment of their neurologically impaired patients. These sets of assumptions about how the brain controls movements, or models of motor control, are often held subconsciously or, at least, are unspoken. However, models of motor control are the basis for assumptions about physiologic process and therapeutic aims underlying neurologic rehabilitation.

Today, therapists are questioning their basic assumptions about how the brain controls movement because the models, based on scientific discoveries half a century ago, no longer fit the kinds of questions they are asking. Although many traditional assumptions remain useful for some aspects of neurological rehabilitation, others are not useful, and therapists are becoming dissatisfied with traditional models to help them resolve their patients' motor problems.[1] Therapists are looking for new rehabilitation models based on more recent discoveries and new understandings of motor control.

The theoretical models therapists use to design their therapeutic rehabilitation approaches are based on a cumulative history of clinical experience and scientific understanding. Figure 4-1 illustrates how motor control models and neurologic rehabilitation models are not generated spontaneously but rely on and incorporate earlier models.

For the sake of brevity, I have grouped sets of common assumptions from specific models into three general models of motor control and three general models of neurologic rehabilitation that form the basis for most of the common approaches to therapeutic intervention for neurologically impaired patients. There are thousands of documented models of motor control, each more or less useful for different purposes and each continually evolving in light of scientific findings. There are also many more models of neurologic rehabilitation than the three named in Figure 4-1, each more or less also useful for different clinical observations.

What realistic neurologic rehabilitation models are available to give therapists confidence that therapy advances, optimizes, or allows the miraculous natural processes for recovery and compensation from brain damage? What models of motor control can lead therapists to develop novel, effective therapeutic interventions? Therapists need to be familiar with the most fundamental assumptions of how the brain controls movement and how therapy can make a difference, because these assumptions form the bases of their understanding, their questions, and their hopes for therapeutic rehabilitation of the neurologically impaired patient.

This paper reviews the assumptions underlying the reflex, hierarchical, and systems models of motor control; the clinical implications of these models for neurological re-

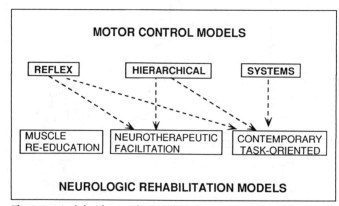

Fig 4-1. *Models of neurologic rehabilitation rely on different assumptions about how the brain controls movement inherent in models of motor control.*

habilitation; and their limitations in the light of experimental evidence that the models have difficulty accounting for. It reviews the general aims of the muscle re-education, neurotherapeutic facilitation (facilitation), and contemporary task-oriented (task-oriented) models of neurologic rehabilitation as based on the three motor control models; it also identifies the dissatisfaction with each rehabilitation model in light of clinical evidence that is difficult to account for. In addition, this paper summarizes critical neurophysiological concepts for an evolving contemporary view of therapeutic intervention. Finally, two neurologic rehabilitation models—facilitation and task-oriented—will be applied to balance and tone problems to demonstrate how motor control assumptions influence the assessment and treatment of neurologically impaired patients.

MOTOR CONTROL MODELS

An understanding of motor control implies an understanding of *what* is being controlled and *how* that process is organized.[2] Normal motor control implies the ability of the central nervous system to use current and previous information to coordinate effective and efficient functional movements by transforming neural energy into kinetic energy. This transformation is accomplished by activation of muscles that generate forces to affect their world. As Sherrington,[3] the founder of western motor physiology, so aptly stated: "To move is all mankind can do and for such, the sole executant is muscle, whether in whispering a syllable or in felling a forest."

Although muscles are the target of the final motor output from the nervous system, examination of models of motor control make it clear that there is no consensus on precisely *what* the nervous system is trying to control in organizing coordinated movements. Although models of motor con-

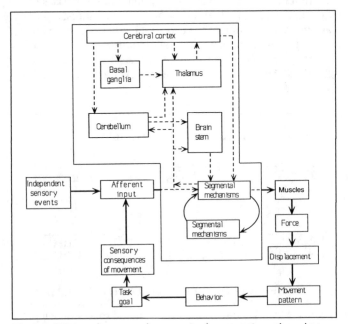

Fig 4-2. *Wiring diagram of anatomical connections thought to be important in motor control.*

trol should be constrained, or limited, by the basic anatomy of known synaptic connections among nervous system structures, physiologists have learned the hard way that these connections, or "wiring diagrams," do not lend automatic insight into what is being controlled or the processes whereby this control comes about. For example, Figure 4-2, adapted from a popular textbook on neurophysiology (Fig. 24-2 from Ghez[4]), illustrates known neural connections thought to be important in motor control. The nervous system delivers impulses to muscles and the muscles in turn develop contractile force to move (or to prevent movement of) the limbs in order to displace (or to prevent displacement of) joints. The nervous system almost always activates large groups of muscles that control displacements at many joints, and these movement patterns allow functional behaviors to accomplish task goals. These movement patterns may be represented back to the nervous system in different forms through sensory afferent signals that are, themselves, under neural control.

I have grouped particular assumptions from the motor control literature into three motor control models that are relevant to the development of three neurologic rehabilitation models. One issue distinguishing the motor control models is whether the nervous system "controls," "cares about," or "organizes its activity around" muscle activation, movement patterns, or behaviors and task goals.[5] In the reflex model the goal of the nervous system is to control muscle activation; in the hierarchical model the goal is to control movement patterns; and in the systems model the goal is to control motor performance in behavioral tasks.

The motor control models have their roots in the early 1900s from the writings of a particular, distinguished neuroscientist, but they have been modified and elaborated on over the last century. Each model reflects a set of common assumptions but does not represent any one individual's theory as originally presented. The limitations of each motor control model become apparent when they cannot account for new scientific results and clinical observations, and they restrict the development of promising hypotheses about motor control. These limitations eventually require a shift to new models in which different problems are considered important for the nervous system and for the neuroscientist and neurotherapist to solve.

The basic assumptions and limitations of the reflex, hierarchical, and systems models of motor control are summarized in Table 4-1.

Reflex Model of Motor Control

The reflex model of motor control has its roots in the classic experiments of Sir Charles Sherrington.[6] He regarded the nervous system as a "black box" in which control processes were implied by measuring motor outputs (muscle or motor nerve activation) in response to various types of sensory inputs imposed by the scientist on an unconscious, anesthetized animal. To simplify the control processes, Sherrington used "reduced" cat preparations by removing the neural structures above the midbrain. He found that he could stimulate specific sensory systems, such as muscle, joint, and pain receptors, and thus induce a variety of distinct, stereotyped movements in these animals. Similarly, Magnus used reduced rabbit preparations to stimulate stereotyped postural

Table 4-1. *Assumptions and Limitations of the Motor Control Models*

Assumptions

Reflex	Hierarchical	Systems
Sensory inputs control motor outputs	Central programs control muscle activation patterns	Interactive systems control behavior to achieve task goals
Movement is summation of reflexes	Organization is top-down	Adaptive, anticipatory mechanisms
Sensation is necessary for movement	Separation of voluntary and reflex	Normal strategies to limit degrees of freedom

Limitations

Reflex	Hierarchical	Systems
Deafferented animals show coordinated movements	Locomotion in spinal cats low level in control	Lack of consensus on terminology and definitions
Open-loop control demonstrated	Development not steplike	The basic set of motor problems and invariant control strategies have yet to be defined
Anticipatory, feedforward control	Blurred distinctions between voluntary and reflex	
	Similar kinematic coordination with alternative muscle activation patterns	Relation of neuroanatomy to systems unclear

responses.[7,8] These stereotyped responses to sensory inputs are called reflexes.

In the reflex model of motor control, reflexes are considered the basis for all movement.[9] "The unit reaction of nervous integration is the reflex, because every reflex is an integrative reaction, and no nervous action short of a reflex is a complete act of integration . . . . Coordination, therefore, is in part the compounding of reflexes."[6]

In the strictest sense, the reflex model assumes that chains of reflexes result in normal movement. Figure 4-3 shows chains of reflexes at spinal, brain stem, and cortical

areas. The reflex model and its derivative therapeutic approaches assume that afferent sensory inputs are a necessary prerequisite for efferent motor outputs: "for the execution of voluntary movements the entire sensory pathway from the periphery to the context must be functioning."[10] This view of motor control is "peripheralist" in that motor control comes from peripheral parts of the nervous system. The nervous system is a passive recipient of sensory stimuli that triggers, coordinates, and activates muscles that excite more sensory systems that in turn activate more muscles.

The "feedback" concept was applied to reflexes when engineers in the 1930s and 1940s began to develop electronic "closed-loop feedback systems." Figure 4-4 shows an engineering model applied to motor control. An engineering model of a feedback system is consistent with the neuroanatomy of the simplest and most studied reflex: the stretch reflex. In the stretch reflex, muscle stretch activates afferent sensory information from muscle spindle receptors. The sensory information feeds directly back to cause contraction of the muscles that hold the spindles, thus closing the loop and reducing the spindles' firing (see Fig. 2, p. 131 in Eldered[11]). The reduction of the sensory receptor's firing creates a negative feedback signal, as represented by the negative sign (-) in Figure 4-4. In this negative feedback model, the aim of the nervous system is to control the activation of sensory receptors that respond to external disturbances. From this engineering model comes very useful and popular motor control terminology, including "feedback," "gain," "phase," and "stability." Later versions of the reflex model include complex nested and hierarchically arranged reflex loops.[12,13]

What clinical implications can be drawn from the basic assumptions of the reflex model? One implication is that if therapists could identify the entire set of reflexes act-

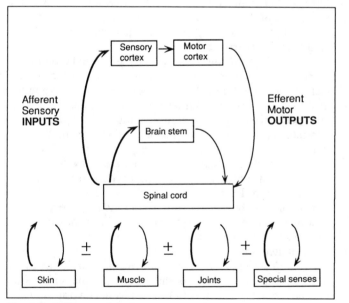

Fig. 4-3. *Reflex model of motor control.*

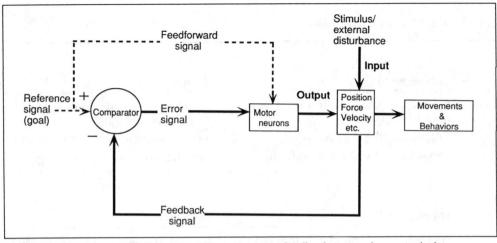

Fig. 4-4. *Engineering model of a closed-loop negative feedback system for control of movements (solid arrows). Addition of reference and feedforward signals allows movement in anticipation of sensory input (dashed arrows).*

ing in their patients, they would understand their patients' motor control and thus could predict the quality of motor function. In fact, the assumption that reflexes reflect motor control is used each time a therapist attempts to identify reflexes controlling movement in newborns and in brain-injured persons.[14,15] Another implication is that when therapists appropriately stimulate patients, they can elicit stereotyped reflex responses. This is apparent when therapists attempt to elicit righting reflexes by tipping a tilt board and eliciting neck reflex responses by turning the patient's head, as reflected in White's[16] description of a therapist's evaluation of a cerebral palsied child: "The therapist observes the child's response to sensory stimuli by moving him from one position to another . . . ."

Another implication of the reflex model, which is important for physical therapy intervention, is that therapists need to be skilled at stimulating "good" reflexes that cause normal movements and skilled at inhibiting "bad" reflexes that interfere with normal movement. For example, when tipping a prone child over a ball, a therapist looks for normal righting and equilibrium reflexes while inhibiting tonic extensor and neck reflexes.[17]

The limitations of the reflex model, summarized in the left column of Table 4-1, became apparent very early when Sherrington's colleague, T. Graham Brown, showed that movement was possible in deafferented animals without any sensory inputs to drive them.[18] Since then, Taub[19,20] has demonstrated that deafferented infant monkeys go through a normal motor developmental sequence in learning to crawl, walk, climb, and feed themselves without somatosensory feedback from the limbs. Polit and Bizzi[21] have quantitatively shown how monkeys, trained to make accurate arm movements to targets, maintain their accuracy following deafferentation, even without visual feedback. Also contrary to the assumption that sensation is necessary for movement is the observation that human fetuses make movements in the womb before making stimulus-induced responses.[22]

Other major limitations of the reflex model come from its inability to incorporate two important concepts: 1) centrally generated goals, or "open-loop" control, and 2) antici-

patory, or "feedforward," control. Figure 4-4 shows a simplified engineering model of how goals (reference signals) and anticipatory control (feedforward) can be added to the closed-loop control. The closed-loop reflex system is represented by the solid arrows showing how a stimulus to the system (an external disturbance) destabilizes the steady state position, force, and velocity of the output, which activates sensory systems. The responses to the stimulus feed signals back to the motor neurons that then restabilize body position, force, and velocity and deactivate the sensory systems. For a particular magnitude of sensory feedback, the gain of the system determines the magnitude of motor output, where gain is the ratio of output to input. A "high gain of the stretch reflex" is a popular model for spasticity (see Craik in this volume).

In the closed-loop model, if the feedback loop is interrupted, as by deafferentation described above, movements can only come about by internally generated open-loop control. In fact, because the feedback loop requires considerable time, many rapid movements are complete before sensory feedback can influence them.[23] Movements are generated centrally (reference signal), and this central command to move is then compared with sensory feedback signals recording the actual movement. Comparing desired and actual movement variables is thought to be an important role of the cerebellum.[24] Because not only centrally generated goals but also an external stimulus can influence motor output, this engineering model can, more easily than a strict feedback model, account for the functional adaptability seen in reflexes.[25] For example, Traub et al[26] describe a "sherry glass adaptation of the stretch reflex" as subjects respond differently to thumb displacements when the basic stretch reflex could break a sherry glass.

Feedforward control, in which the internal motor command initiates motor output in advance of sensory feedback, can help account for the fact that most movements are initiated *before* any sensory stimulus.[27] For example, before each heel strike in gait the gastrocnemius-soleus muscles contract in advance, in anticipation of their stretch. This anticipatory muscle activation accounts for "missteps" when stair height unpredictably changes, because slow feedback systems must substitute for the appropriately timed anticipatory activation. Even postural muscle activation, which was long thought to be due to equilibrium reflexes in response to vestibular and other sensory stimuli, has been shown to anticipate accurately upcoming sensory stimuli associated with self-initiated limb movements.[28-30]

Engineering models of feedforward control, however, are inadequate to account for the many ways the brain models and predicts characteristics of its physical world. For example, movement factors are tuned for efficiency by stored,

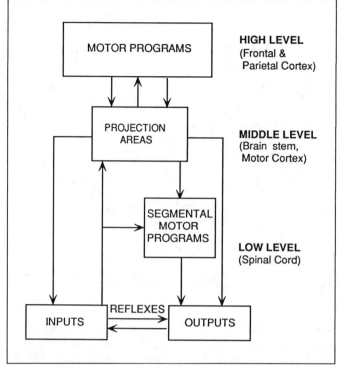

HIGH LEVEL
(Frontal &
Parietal Cortex)

MIDDLE LEVEL
(Brain stem,
Motor Cortex)

LOW LEVEL
(Spinal Cord)

Fig. 4-5. *Hierarchical model of motor control. (Adapted from Phillips and Porter,[35] Fig. 1.4.)*

prior experience with task performance; by initial biomechanical conditions; by cognitive information and expectations; and by intrinsic knowledge of body and environmental dynamics.[31]

Hierarchical Model of Motor Control

The hierarchical model of motor control was first articulated by the English neurologist, Sir Huglings Jackson, in 1932.[32,33] This model forms the basis of clinical neurology today. In the model, control of movement is organized hierarchically from lowest levels in the spinal cord, to intermediate levels in the brain stem, to highest levels in the cortex (Fig. 4-5). In contrast to the peripheralist view of the reflex model in which sensory stimuli drive movements, the hierarchical model holds a "centralist" view in which normal movements are driven by motor programs that specify muscle activation patterns issued from within the nervous system. Reflexive movements only dominate after injury to higher centers, as from stroke or cerebral palsy, as a result of lack of higher-level control onto lower-level, primitive reflexes.

The hierarchical model, which clearly separates high-level, voluntary control and low-level, reflexive control, has dominated western philosophy ever since Descartes.[34] Voluntary movements are initiated internally by the will, with specific goals in mind, and are manifested in an infinite

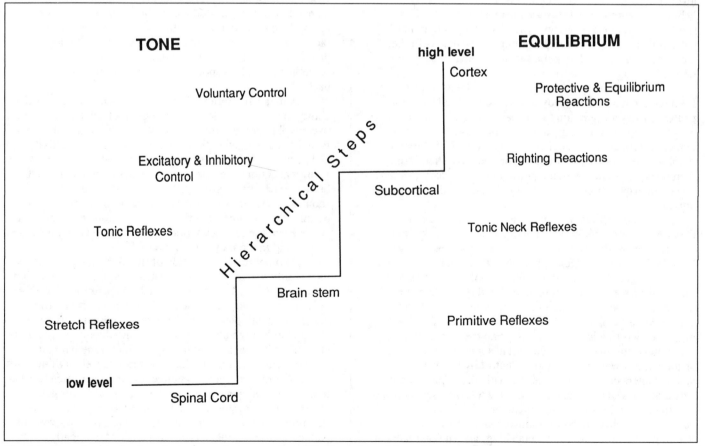

Fig. 4-6. *Stepwise levels of control of muscle tone and equilibrium using a hierarchical model of motor control.*

variety of forms, depending on the purpose of the movement. In contrast, reflex movements are initiated by sensory stimuli in a fixed relation between the intensity and form of the stimuli and the intensity and form of the response. More recent views of the hierarchical model allow for many levels of control from the "most automatic" at the lowest levels to the "least automatic" at the highest levels.[35] They also include complex control in which information from lower levels can affect higher levels.

The clinical implications of the hierarchical model of motor control are familiar to therapists today. Many nervous system lesions are considered to disrupt high-level control of lower level reflexes that then dominate movements. When lower-level, primitive reflexes are released, higher-level co-ordinated movement patterns are "blocked." "Reflexive reactions that are retained beyond the point at which they should have been integrated block the normal differentiation of movement."[36] Therefore, a reasonable goal for therapeutic intervention is to identify and to prevent primitive reflexes from taking over (eg, to eliminate dominance by tonic neck reflexes so that higher-level, equilibrium reactions can be in control) and to reduce hyperactive stretch reflexes so that higher-level, coordinated movements are allowed.[17]

The stepwise levels of control in a hierarchy imply a stepwise sequence of motor recovery and motor development from lower levels to higher levels (Fig. 4-6). The development of both muscle tone and postural equilibrium have been described as steplike stages from primitive, spinal level control to mature, cortical control as described by White.[16] "Primitive reflexes are the most immature responses; as maturation occurs, the infant begins to inhibit these reflexes and to develop righting reactions. As further maturation of the CNS occurs, the infant develops equilibrium reactions."[16]

Treatment progressions are often designed to progress from the most automatic, lower levels controlled by therapeutic sensory stimulation to the least automatic, higher levels voluntarily controlled, such as skilled tasks. A related clinical implication of the hierarchical model is that motor flexibility comes only from the highest levels. Therefore, therapists aim to help patients move out of low-level, stereotyped patterns to high-level control of individual joints and muscles.

The hierarchical model of motor control is useful in the clinic. For example, low-level reflexes are used to help identify the approximate location of neural lesions and to help predict to what extent a patient will recover from severe brain damage. However, the limitations of the hierarchical model of motor control, summarized in the middle column of Table 4-1, become apparent in attempting to explain recent and classic observations of motor behavior. For example, so-called low levels of control, like the spinal cord, appropriately dominate motor control in some situations, such as the withdrawal reflex to pain. Control by lower-level spinal centers can be seen most dramatically in paraplegic cats that can walk on treadmills despite total transections preventing any control from higher centers.[37-39] Very sophisticated, coordinated locomotor movement patterns, such as walking, trotting, galloping, scratching, and shaking, appear not to require control from the top down. In fact, responses

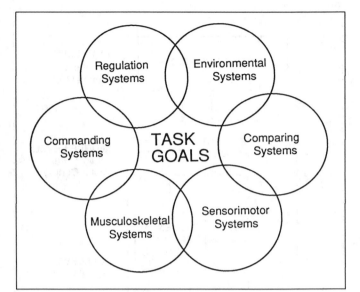

Fig. 4-7. *Systems model of motor control.*

to sensory stimuli vary functionally in response to paw perturbation in order to maintain gait.[25] These variations are flexible adaptations to phases of the step cycle, called phase dependent reflexes.

Another limitation of the hierarchical model is its assumption that motor development naturally follows a stepwise progression from reflexively driven to internally commanded movements. Studies, however, have shown that motor development does not follow such a progression. In fact, learning to reach, kick, and walk appears to begin with predictive, self-generated movements that eventually become increasingly responsive to ongoing sensory feedback.[40-42]

A major limitation of the hierarchical model is its inability to account for the increasingly blurred distinction between voluntary and reflex control. Every volitional movement has associated with it automatic synergistic activity and postural adjustments that subjects are unaware of. Many volitional actions are often adjusted automatically by sensory feedback. Likewise, volition can influence reflex responses to sensory stimuli. For example, responses to arm perturbations can be modified by instructions to let go or resist.[43] Even the monosynaptic stretch reflex can be modified by training in monkeys and humans.[44]

Another major limitation of the hierarchical model is its inability to handle the observation that muscle activation patterns and the characteristic kinematic patterns of movement are not always correlated. How can a person write his name on a small piece of paper using finger and wrist muscles and on a large blackboard using shoulder and trunk muscles and still have a recognizably distinct, kinematically unique signature? It is unlikely the brain has enough neurons to specify in the nervous system every unique muscle activation pattern for every movement a person will ever generate.[45] Thus the systems model evolved to account for the question of the potentially infinite generation of movement patterns: How can the nervous system systematically control so many degrees of freedom of motion without prescribing the details of muscle activation pattern?

Systems Model of Motor Control

The systems model of motor control was initiated as early as the reflex and hierarchical models, but it has its roots in the socialistic-heterarchical system of eastern Europe where it was first proposed in 1932 by a Russian neurologist, Nicoli Bernstein. Not until 1967 was Bernstein's theory translated into English.[45] According to the systems model, movements are not peripherally or centrally driven but emerge as a result of an interaction among many systems, each contributing to different aspects of control. As illustrated in the systems model in Figure 4-7, there are no higher and lower levels of control because there are many systems that distribute control at the same level. The control of movement includes neurologic systems for comparing, commanding, and recording motor control not only inside the nervous system but also in systems outside the nervous system, such as the musculoskeletal system and the environment. Thus motor control is achieved through functions regulating motor control for different types of movements in different environments.

As shown in the right-hand column of Table 4-1, a major assumption of the systems model is that the nervous system is organized to control the end points of motor behavior: the accomplishment of task goals. According to the systems model, normal movements are coordinated not because of muscle activation patterns prescribed by sensory pathways or by central programs but because strategies of motion *emerge* from interaction of the systems; they emerge to limit the degrees of freedom over which the nervous system exerts control. Therefore, control is not over muscles or sensory receptors, like in the reflex model, or over muscle activation patterns, like in the hierarchical model, but over abstract aspects of motor behavior, such as the relations among kinematic variables and the accomplishment of task goals. Many current studies of motor control are attempting to define the invariant relationships constraining kinematic and dynamic variables that may represent control strategies the nervous system uses to control the many degrees of freedom as hypothesized by Bernstein.[46-49]

Another assumption of the systems model is that the nervous system adapts to and predicts constraints placed on movement by the physical laws associated with the musculoskeletal system and its environment.[50] By continually comparing anticipated and actual interactions with the world, the nervous system constantly modifies its model to realize the most effective, kinematically efficient means to accomplish task goals.

Clinical implications of the systems model include the assumption that movements are organized around behavioral goals. Thus, it becomes critical to work on identifiable, functional tasks rather than on eliciting reflexes or motor patterns in isolation. Given the systems model assumption that normal movement strategies represent appropriate interaction with musculoskeletal and environmental constraints, therapists attempt to assess and manipulate those constraints, such as by having tasks practiced in a variety of postures and under varying surface, visual, and biomechanical condi-

tions.[51] Because many normal muscle activation patterns could accomplish one task goal, therapists who use a systems model are trying to help the nervous system learn to solve motor deficits in a variety of ways rather than activating a particular muscle activation pattern.[1] Motor deficits following brain damage are assumed not only to reflect lack of neural control but also to reflect the best attempt by remaining systems to accomplish task goals despite the injured systems. As Gordon[1] states, this is "looking at the deficit as a compensatory strategy . . . as a learned movement pattern . . . ."

A clinical advantage of the systems model is that it can account for the flexibility and adaptability of motor behavior in a variety of environmental conditions. In the systems model, both functional goals and environmental constraints are thought to play a major role in determining movement. Thus the same stimulus can result in very different movements and different stimuli can result in similar movements. For example, the same tap on the shoulder will elicit a different response if it is felt while anticipating arrival of a missed love one compared with feeling it while walking down a dark alley. The challenge for the therapist is to identify functional goals in motor tasks and to adapt environmental constraints to reduce the degrees of freedom that must be controlled by the nervous system.

Limitations of the systems model of motor control include 1) definitions and 2) testability of the model. There are many different models of motor control that include assumptions of the systems model, such as the dynamic action theory,[52] the ecological approach,[53] the neural network theory,[54] the task-oriented approach,[55] the action systems,[56,57] and the reafference principle.[58] However, there is no consensus on terminology and definitions of terms. Thus the evolution of the systems model and its clinical applications are hampered by researchers' and therapists' attempts to understand each other. For example, because words like "strategy" and "coordination" have different meanings to different scientists, it is difficult to compare results from scientific studies and clinical applications. Until a basic set of motor control terms and motor problems for the nervous system are defined and tentatively agreed on, the search for the underlying neural mechanisms remains problematic.

Another limitation of the systems model is that because the model is abstract and motor control is so distributed, it is difficult to relate individual theoretical component systems to neuroanatomy. Thus, it is difficult to test the model with the traditional approach of making nervous system lesions and determining which aspects of control are lacking.

NEUROLOGIC REHABILITATION MODELS

Physical therapy needs well-defined models of neurologic rehabilitation that outline the aims of the therapeutic intervention in physiologic and functional terms. These clinical models need to reflect the current state of scientific knowledge in many areas, including motor control, motor learning, recovery of function, nervous system plasticity, psychology, and sociology. The therapist's responsibility is to develop, modify, test, and determine the usefulness of these models. The usefulness of a therapeutic rehabilitation

Table 4-2. *General Aims and Dissatisfaction of Neurologic Rehabilitation Models*

Therapeutic Aims

Muscle Re-education	Neurotherapeutic Facilitation	Contemporary Task-oriented
Isolate muscle actions by focusing on individual muscles	Facilitate normal movement patterns with proprioceptive inputs	Practice ability to achieve task goals
Maximize strength and use of motor units remaining	Modify CNS from the experience of normal movement patterns	Teach motor problem solving (ie, adaptability to contexts)
Avoid secondary complications and compensatory patterns	Fractionalize movements by breaking up abnormal synergies	Learn strategies to coordinate efficient, effective behaviors
Teach functional activities	Inhibit abnormal tone and primitive reflexes	Develop effective compensations
Provide orthopedic support	Do not allow CNS to learn abnormal movement patterns	Use musculoskeletal and environmental constraints

Dissatisfaction

Muscle Re-education	Neurotherapeutic Facilitation	Contemporary Task-oriented
CNS plasticity not considered	No carryover to functional activities	Hard to quantify effective, efficient compensations
Cannot isolate muscle action in upper motor neuron lesions	Patients are passive recipients	Less "hands-on," too "cognitive"
Not lack of muscle activation but abnormal patterns often a problem	Does not take into account musculoskeletal and environmental effects	How to retrain anticipatory control and use of prior experience
	Inhibition of primative reflexes does not release normal movements	Hard to provide time-consuming practice of skills

model is defined by 1) practical outcomes, that is, the documentation of improvement from intervention and 2) how well it helps therapists to ask useful questions in their analyzing the motor deficiencies in neurologically impaired patients and developing effective therapeutic interventions. Assumptions underlying neurologic rehabilitation models provide therapists with physiologic and functional goals as they develop detailed treatment techniques.

Different neurotherapeutic techniques, such as neurodevelopment treatment,[59] proprioceptive neuromuscular facilitation,[60] and the motor learning approach,[61] are based on different motor control assumptions from the reflex, hierarchical, and systems models. However, the most common therapeutic techniques depend on one of three neurologic rehabilitation models: 1) the muscle re-education model; 2) the facilitation model; and 3) the task-oriented, or systems-based, model. (This contemporary task-oriented model of neurological rehabilitation has been called a motor-control or motor-learning model by some.[1,61,62]) Each model consists of a different set of assumptions about the general physiologic aims of therapy and the control of movement in neurologically impaired patients.

Each therapeutic rehabilitation model is useful in assessing aspects of neurologic damage and in developing specific therapeutic exercises. They are not completely independent of one another, but they build on and depend on one another. However, each therapeutic rehabilitation model influences how the therapist perceives the motor control problems in patients. The next section discusses the therapeutic

aims of each neurologic rehabilitation model and therapists' dissatisfaction with each model, as summarized in Table 4-2.

Muscle Re-education Model of Therapeutic Exercise

The muscle re-education model was advocated by Sister Kenny for the treatment of those suffering from poliomyelitis, during the 1940s and early 1950s. Before this time, neurologically impaired patients passively waited in bed for months to discover the permanent results of a nervous system injury. Sister Kenny believed that patients should actively participate in their own rehabilitation and would benefit more from activity than bed rest. The muscle re-education model was based not on a neurophysiological model of motor control but on knowledge of gross muscle anatomy and on faith in human willpower. Activity as the cornerstone of neurologic rehabilitation has scientifically been ratified many times since it was espoused.

In neurophysiologic terms, the muscle re-education model asserts that the nervous system's goal in motor control is to activate individual muscles and individual motor units. Not unlike in some technologically sophisticated biofeedback approaches today, therapists using the muscle re-education model assume that subjects can consciously channel their neural energy to activate individual muscles when provided appropriate feedback. Therefore, as summarized in the left-hand column of Table 4-2, one goal of therapy is to strengthen motor units remaining in muscles weakened by the disease. Another goal of therapy is to help the patient avoid secondary complications and ineffective, inefficient compensatory movement patterns. Movement, rather than bed rest, increases circulation and cardiac function, thus preventing unnecessary muscle wasting, joint contractures, and skin ulcers. Because muscles are often only temporarily weakened by the poliomyelitic virus, therapists teach patients to avoid compensatory movement patterns so that when the muscles regain strength, the compensatory movements are not retained. Once the acute phase of poliomyelitis passes, the basic assumption is that nothing more can be done to change the nervous system or muscles. As a result, patients are provided orthopedic supports, such as braces and crutches, to allow functional activities, such as independent ambulation.[63,64]

Dissatisfaction with the muscle re-education model grew when therapists tried to apply the model to a wide range of neurological disorders after the poliomyelitis epidemic was controlled in the mid-1950s. Therapists found it impossible to get patients with hemiplegia, cerebral palsy, and Parkinson's disease to isolate muscle activity. Therapists found these patients' lesions resulted in abnormal muscle activation patterns rather than muscle weakness. Finding muscle re-education less and less useful, therapists investigated the neurophysiological models of motor control and found hope that their therapeutic intervention could be aimed at the nervous system rather than at the final motor output: the muscles.

Facilitation Model of Therapeutic Rehabilitation

In the 1950s, the facilitation model of neurologic rehabilitation as developed by therapists and physicians, including Karl and Berta Bobath,[59,65] Kabat et al,[66] Knott and Voss,[60] Knott,[67] Stockmeyer,[68] and Brunnstrom.[10] They looked to the neurophysiological models of motor control available at the time (eg, Payton et al[69]) to develop therapeutic techniques aimed at affecting the nervous system itself rather than altering the secondary effects of nervous system damage on muscles, joints, skin, and behavior.

Based on the reflex and hierarchical models of motor control, facilitation approaches assume that nervous system lesions result in a lack of higher-level control over movements and a release of primitive and abnormal reflexes at lower levels. According to Bobath,[65] in cerebral palsy the lesion results in lack of inhibition, in primitive total patterns, and in insufficiently developed postural reflex mechanisms. Facilitation approaches also assume that abnormal movement patterns are the direct result of the neural lesions. They fail to consider the combined effects of neural, nonneural, and musculoskeletal limitations and of the patient's attempts to compensate for the lesion.

The primary neurophysiologic aims of the facilitation model are to 1) facilitate normal movement patterns and 2) inhibit abnormal tone and primitive reflexes. Therapists attempt this facilitation and inhibition by providing appropriate proprioceptive feedback with a hands-on approach of guiding movement patterns. Cutaneous, vestibular, muscle vibration, and temperature changes have also been advocated to recruit muscle activation.[70] Because the neurofacilitation model is based on the reflex and hierarchical models, therapeutic intervention starts at the lowest level by stimulating reflex responses and then progresses next to automatic responses and then to voluntary fractionalization of isolated movements.

The neurotherapeutic model assumes that the gradual progression from lower-level reflexes to higher-level voluntary movements, characteristic of motor development and of patients' recoveries from nervous system injuries, may be reversed in difficult or stressful situations. "Responses can spiral upward or downward depending on the ability to integrate sensory stimuli in a given situation. The normal adult may revert to more primitive responses in stress situations."[16] This model also assumes that the persistence of primitive reflexes at certain developmental ages or at certain stages of recovery blocks normal movement.

Clinicians generally accept that the motor deficit in cerebral palsy is characterized by persistence and dominance of primitive reflexes. [T]his state of affairs, in turn, interferes with the appearance and activity of more mature postural adjustment reactions, and hence, with the accomplishments of successive stages of motor development.[71]

A major but as yet untested assumption of the facilitation approach is that the nervous system can be modified to control movements more effectively if it experiences normal movement patterns guided by skilled therapists. Because the nervous system can learn abnormal as well as normal movement patterns, patients treated from the facilitation approach are not encouraged to begin functional activities, such as walking, too early in fear that abnormal, compensatory patterns may become ingrained.

Dissatisfaction with the facilitation model, as summarized in the middle column of Table 4-2, comes both from clinical frustrations and from lack of incorporation of new knowledge about neurophysiology into the reflex and hierarchical motor control models. Therapists express frustration with the lack of carryover of the facilitated normal movement patterns into functional activities of daily living. Therapists find that even when their efforts are successful in inhibiting a tonic neck reflex and facilitating a normal righting reaction in the prone position across a ball, there is no guarantee that this success will carry over to improved balance in walking or will improve the patient's ability to respond effectively to a stumble. Human beings are motivated by functional, task goals, such as "I want to walk" or "I want to be able to feed myself." It is difficult to convince patients to work on movement patterns isolated from the functional tasks. It is also getting more difficult to convince second party payers to finance therapy aimed at normalizing movement patterns, because it is more difficult to document changes in quality of movement than in functional behaviors.

A second dissatisfying feature of the facilitation model is that patients are often passive recipients of the therapy or are at least not encouraged to voluntarily assist in the process of recovery. Sensory stimuli, initiated by the therapist, is used to facilitate or inhibit responses from the patients. The model treats the nervous system as passively awaiting modification by the therapist rather than as actively working to determine its own perceptions and actions. It is critical to the recovery process for patients to become involved and feel in charge of their own rehabilitation and health. Neurophysiological studies have shown that passive experience is not equivalent to actively driven sensory experience for neural plasticity. For example, Hein and Held[73] showed that visual stimulation at a critical age of development of visual motor pathways in kittens is only effective if experienced during active locomotion, not during passive exposure while riding in a gondola. The motor learning literature also indicates that learning motor skills, such as a tennis serve, is better accomplished by practicing that very goal-directed task with regular, cognitive information regarding knowledge of results rather than by passively observing others or by practicing small components of the movement pattern in isolation from the task itself.[72] Although most therapists do not go to the extremes of Doman Delacatto's passive body manipulations, called patterning, the traditional facilitation approaches assume that therapeutic treatment starts only when the therapist uses his hands on the patient to facilitate movements.

A third dissatisfaction with the facilitation model is that it does not take into account the complex interactions of the musculoskeletal system and the environment. In an effort to free itself from the muscle re-education focus on the periphery, the facilitation model assumes that the nervous system lesion is responsible for abnormal movement patterns. Thus treatment is aimed almost solely at the nervous system. It is now known that prolonged activation of muscles in unusual or abnormal patterns causes profound changes in the muscle biochemistry and passive elastic elements. In addition, neurologically impaired patients often suffer orthopedic injuries as well as neural injuries or even exhibit a variety of a priori musculoskeletal conditions that necessarily influence their motor performance. Also, this model does not consider compensatory adjustments by the nervous system for joint range limitation, muscle strength, pain, and postural alignment.

Like the musculoskeletal limitations, the environment places limitations on what is possible in movement. For example, movement patterns that are grossly abnormal may look much more graceful in water because weakness prevents sufficient resistance to gravity.[74] Therapists need to consider the effects that support from their hands gives to their patients by providing external stability, realigning joints, and reducing the degree of freedom in the "normalization" of movement patterns. Some therapists using the facilitation model limit their clinical intervention to the hands-on approach. Patients, however, need to control normal movements ultimately in nonclinical environments without the therapists' guiding hands.

Another dissatisfaction with the facilitation model is that normal movement patterns are not automatically released, even when therapists feel successful at inhibiting abnormal tone and primitive reflexes that presumably "block" movement. In fact, patients who could accomplish a task such as locomotion or balancing on a tilt board using abnormal, low-level patterns may completely be unable to accomplish the task when these so-called primitive patterns are not allowed. There is no real evidence that inhibition of primitive reflex patterns promotes motor development or recovery. In fact, the research of Thelen and associates[75] has shown that promotion of primitive stepping in infants results in earlier independent locomotion. She has demonstrated

that disappearance of the so-called reflex stepping is not due to maturation of higher-level nervous system mechanisms but simply is due to a musculoskeletal limitation: increased weight of the infants' legs such that muscle strength is temporarily inadequate to lift the legs against gravity.[76]

Many therapists are frustrated with limitations on the types of questions they can ask of their patients' motor problems, given the facilitation model. They are reconsidering the impact of the periphery, such as the muscles, joints, and postural alignment, and the environment on the movement patterns that their patients demonstrate. They are becoming interested in defining success in therapy by accomplishing very practical task goals, not only improving movement patterns. They are looking to neurophysiological research from the more recent 40 years for new ways to ask questions about motor control and intervention.

Neuroscientists also are frustrated with the limitations placed on the types of questions they can ask of motor control given the reflex and hierarchical models. They also are reconsidering what limitations are placed on movement by the musculoskeletal system and how the nervous system becomes aware of and takes advantage of these limitations. They are becoming concerned about the nervous system's control of complex behaviors and the accomplishment of task goals, not only the control of isolated muscles and joints. While a new systems model of motor control is evolving from the new types of questions neuroscientists ask, a new task-oriented model of neurologic rehabilitation also is evolving.

Task-oriented Model of Neurologic Rehabilitation

A new model of neurologic rehabilitation is evolving, based on past models (reflex, hierarchical) as well as on more recent models (systems) of how the brain controls movement. It is applying some concepts of motor control so new that there is not yet a scientific consensus of their terminology, definitions, or usefulness. It is trying to incorporate concepts of motor control that have been well accepted in neuroscience but that have not yet been included in a model of neurologic rehabilitation. The task-oriented model incorporates current neurophysiological findings because many therapists who are developing the rehabilitation model are also neuroscientists specializing in motor control. And many of the neuroscientists are contributors to the II STEP conference. In fact, the conference itself is an important part of the development of the contemporary approaches to neurological rehabilitation.

Unlike the muscle re-education or the facilitation models, the task-oriented model does not assume that therapeutic influence on motor control should be aimed only peripherally at the musculoskeletal system and environment or only centrally at the nervous system. It targets both peripheral and central systems. From the systems model of motor control, the task-oriented model assumes that control of movement is organized around goal-directed, functional behaviors rather than on muscles or movement patterns (see the right-hand column in Table 4-2). As Carr and Shepard[77] state, in the treatment of the brain-damaged adult the major factor in this learning process is identification of the goal. Therefore, one of the major neurophysiological aims of the task-ori-

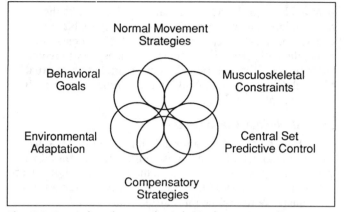

Fig. 4-8. *Examples of neurophysiological concepts of motor control yet to be applied adequately in clinical rehabilitation.*

ented model is to teach patients to accomplish goals for functional tasks, such as walking and rising from a chair. Because the same task may be accomplished effectively with a wide variety of movement patterns, therapists do not limit training to one "normal" movement pattern but allow patients to learn alternative movement strategies to coordinate motor behaviors as efficiently as possible. "Voluntary motion uses many different synergies and there may be a great variety of synergies in any one child for the same task. In time he chooses the most effective pattern."[78] Because the same task must be accomplished differently every time the environmental situation changes slightly (eg, the presence or absence of arm supports on a chair for arising to stand, the height of a step in stair climbing), therapists do not try to facilitate normal movement patterns for every possible situation but try to help teach the nervous system how to solve those types of motor problems by practicing tasks in a wide variety of environments.

Because the nervous system is not a passive recipient of sensory stimuli but actively seeks to control its own perceptions and actions, the patient must actively and voluntarily practice motor performance motivated by the goal of accomplishing specific tasks. Because the voluntary and automatic systems are thought to be very interrelated, patients are encouraged to assist voluntarily in accomplishing a motor behavior with the therapists' encouragement. Therapists can also provide verbal information to patients who are capable of using it, including information about results of their actions so they can improve performance. Because different sensory systems are not thought to be immutably connected to specific muscle patterns, sensory feedback and knowledge of results are provided to the patients by the therapists from every possible source including proprioceptive, cutaneous, auditory, and visual sources.

Because the nervous system is thought to be adapting continually dynamically to its environment and musculoskeletal constraints, therapists attempt to manipulate those environmental and musculoskeletal systems to allow efficient, purposeful motor behaviors. The nervous system will be exposed to its own bodily environment many more hours a day than the environment that includes therapists' hands; therefore, therapists must design intervention in which much of

the practice of new motor skills occurs outside of structured therapy sessions. Because the nervous system always seeks to accomplish important behavioral goals with whatever systems remain, important goals of the task-oriented approach are to identify and develop useful compensatory strategies and to help patients discard less useful, less efficient strategies.

Even while the task-oriented model of neurological rehabilitation evolves, several limitations to its clinical usefulness are becoming apparent. Although it is easier to quantify task accomplishment (how far the patient walks) than movement patterns, valid measures to quantify efficiency and effectiveness of motor behavior have yet to be developed. Another limitation for many therapists is the reduced emphasis on hands-on techniques and the increased emphasis on cognitive information provided to patients. Severely involved patients with neurological impairment will not be able to make good use of cognitive information regarding task goals and knowledge of results, and few of us can doubt the well-known power of a healer's touch on psychosocial aspects of behavior. A major but, hopefully, temporary limitation of the task-oriented approach to neurologic rehabilitation is that it has identified many more motor control problems than there are specific therapeutic exercises developed to treat those problems.

The next section summarizes some examples of important concepts of motor control that have inadequately been applied to rehabilitation of neurologically impaired patients.

CONCEPT OF MOTOR CONTROL INADEQUATELY APPLIED

Any models of neurologic rehabilitation that therapists adopt should allow them to solve problems of motor behavior deficits and to design effective therapeutic treatments. Many neurophysiological concepts of motor control are available that have yet to be adequately applied and tested in the clinical evaluation and treatment of neurologically impaired patients (Fig. 4-8). These concepts can be useful in allowing therapists to ask insightful questions about motor deficits in their patients.

Behavioral Goals

For what task-goals does the nervous system organize motor activity? Does the nervous system identify the critical goals needed to accomplish the task effectively and efficiently? Are the therapists' and patients' goals for the task the same? For example, if a therapist asks a patient to shift his center of mass to the limits of stability in order to reach for a distant object, the goal of the patient's nervous system may be to keep his center of mass far from the limits of stability. In that case, the therapist may not be able to elicit the desired movements, and the patient may not be able to accomplish the task.

The behavioral goals around which movements are organized are not often obvious or available to conscious awareness. Although we may be aware of the conscious goal to reach for a cup of coffee, we may be unaware of the powerful goals of our nervous system to "not fall down" and to "stabilize the cup with reference to gravity" to avoid spilling the coffee. Therapists need to appreciate the powerful organizing influence of goals that underlie behavioral tasks and need to use them to their therapeutic advantage. To work on successful reaching, for example, the therapist could first work on the goal of moving the center of mass near the limits of stability by making the patient consciously aware of this goal and by providing adequate information, such as verbally and proprioceptively with biofeedback, regarding the patient's success in realizing this goal.

Normal Movement Strategies

What are the primary organizing principles of a normal movement strategy? What are the critical constraints preventing normal movement strategies in the patient? Can therapists alter the constraints or help patients find an alternative movement strategy to accomplish a task?

A movement strategy is a large scale plan for how to accomplish a task goal artfully.[79] Normal movement patterns are beginning to be defined by their artful control of multiple degrees of freedom by keeping certain variable constants such as the ratio of multijoint forces[48,79,80] or the ratio of joint velocities[81]

The inability to execute a normal movement strategy may be due to a wide variety of neural and biomechanical constraints (see Horak et al for a review[82]). For example, the simple task of bending forward at the waist while standing involves smooth coordination between the hip and ankle joints in which a 4:1 ratio is maintained to keep the center of mass over the base of foot support.[49,83] If patients fall forward when attempting this task because they are not maintaining this hip-to-ankle ratio, 1) is it because of limited muscle strength or joint range at the ankles that could be altered by therapeutic intervention or 2) must a new movement strategy be found for accomplishing the task, such as flexion at the knees? By recognizing the critical elements the nervous system needs to control to accomplish a task and the types of constraints preventing this control, therapists can more easily decide whether and how to work for a normal movement strategy or an alternative movement strategy.

Compensatory Strategies

What aspects of the abnormal movement strategies used by neurologically impaired patients are due to the primary lesion in the nervous system? What aspects are due to the natural compensation processes that attempt to maintain behavioral functions despite the lesion? If therapists eliminate the secondary compensation for a lesion, will the need to accomplish task goals be served? Have neurologically impaired patients found the most appropriate, efficient, and effective compensatory strategy given constraints imposed by the damaged neural and musculoskeletal systems?

For example, some of the movement strategies used by spastic hemiplegics to walk independently may not be due to spasticity resulting from the neural lesion. They may be due to compensatory strategies the patients use to allow stance and swing requirements of gait, given their muscle weakness and poor multijoint coordination caused by the lesion.[84-86] If this is true, elimination of some of the abnormal movements, such as the stiff knee, toe support, and hip hiking, may result in a knee that buckles under their weight,

poor ankle control, and inadequate toe clearance to the extent that independent ambulation is now impossible. Of course, therapists must decide whether their patients have found the most effective, efficient compensatory movement strategies or if therapeutic intervention, including external biomechanical supports, could improve function and quality of movement.

Musculoskeletal Constraints

How much of the motor deficit in a neurological patient is due to deficits in the musculoskeletal system rather than to neural constraints? Should therapists substitute external biomechanical supports, such as braces or crutches, for inadequate control of the musculoskeletal system?

In the traditional facilitation approaches, therapy focuses on changing the nervous system, and motor deficits are seen to be due to lack of neural control. Because the therapists' goal is to normalize neural control of movement patterns rather than to maximize task accomplishment with compensatory strategies, biomechanical supports are withheld as long as there is hope of the return of normal neural control. In the task-oriented approach, the musculoskeletal system is considered a critical element of control in motor coordination. As a result, major effort must be placed, if possible, on identifying and correcting constraints placed on movement by deficits in the musculoskeletal system. For example, a therapist must determine whether excessive motion at the hips in stance and gait in a patient with hemiplegia is due to 1) "proximal instability" from poor neural control of the hip muscles or 2) a compensatory strategy in which the center of body mass is controlled by hip motions to compensate for reduced strength or range at the ankle joint. If the excessive hip motions are a compensation secondary to musculoskeletal constraints at the ankle, early bracing of the ankle should help reduce hip motions.

Environmental Adaptation

How must a movement strategy adapt to accomplish a task in a new environmental context? How can therapists teach their patients how to solve motor problems related to the adaptation of their movement strategies to new conditions?

The environment places severe constraints on movement strategies by determining the physical conditions under which movements are carried out and by limiting the availability of relevant sensory information for the task. The normal nervous system naturally adapts to sudden changes in conditions by gradually changing the movement strategy, taking into account prior experience with environmental conditions, and continuously evaluating the relative success of its actions.[49,87] Neurologically impaired patients may have lost the ability to adapt quickly to changes in environmental conditions.[82,88] For example, elderly subjects require more trials to adapt their postural responses to new surface and visual conditions.[89]

Because it is impossible to facilitate a normal movement pattern for every environmental condition neurologically impaired patients may ever encounter, new approaches must be developed to teach these patients the process of successful adaptation. Therapists need to determine whether par-

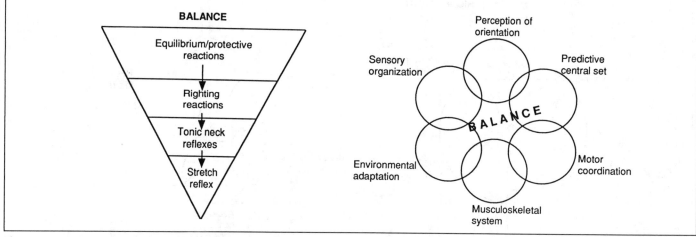

Fig. 4-9. *Assumptions underlying balance control based on the A. Neurotherapeutic Facilitation Model and the B. Contemporary Task-oriented Model of neurologic rehabilitation.*

ticular patients should avoid certain environments either because of their inability to adapt or because they lack adequate alternative resources given restricted physical conditions or limited sensory information. For example, if a patient lacks vestibular function, he will not be able to adapt to a situation in which there is inadequate information from vision and somatosensation for postural orientation, and he would do well to avoid those situations to prevent falling.[82,90]

Central Set and Predictive Control

Do neurologically impaired patients have an appropriate internal model of their body dynamics and the dynamics of their external world? Do patients accurately predict the sensory consequences of their actions and make appropriate movements in anticipation of those consequences? Are patients getting their movements into the "right ballpark"[55] based on prior experience?

Central set is the ability of the nervous system to prepare the motor system for upcoming sensory information and to prepare the sensory system for upcoming movements.[27] An inappropriate internal neural model of a patient's body and of the world can lead to poor predictions about the sensory consequences of situations and actions, resulting in anticipatory movements that are ineffective or destabilizing (ie, in the "wrong ballpark").[55] For example, postural adjustments have been shown to precede self-initiated arm, leg, and trunk movements to minimize postural instability that would have resulted.[91-93] Some patients with Parkinson's disease may lack appropriate anticipatory postural adjustments.[26]

Central set is used to predict the weight of an object and the dynamics of our limbs in complex, bilateral tasks like juggling.[94] Central set, based on prior experience, is also used to determine variables of movement upon initial encounter with a new situation during the time delay it takes

for sensory feedback to be used to update the system. For example, normal subjects but not cerebellar subjects scale the initial magnitude of their postural responses to expected displacement sizes.[31,95]

Therapeutic approaches to help neurologically impaired patients recover their ability to use predictive central set have yet to be developed. Therapists need to determine whether therapeutic intervention can be effective for patients who have lost the basic central set processes critical for motor learning.

BALANCE AND TONE MOTOR PROBLEMS

Models of neurologic rehabilitation necessarily affect the questions therapists ask in assessing motor problems and in designing interventions. Two of the most prominent and disabling effects of neural injury are problems in regulating muscle tone and balance. This section summarizes differences between how the facilitation model and the task-oriented model address these two motor problems.

Balance

The facilitation model assumes that postural equilibrium is maintained by reflex mechanisms organized hierarchically within the nervous system (Fig. 4-9A). Poor balance in neurologically impaired patients is thought to result from an abnormal "postural reflex mechanism" in which lower level, primitive postural reflexes, such as the stretch reflex and tonic neck reflexes, dominate and block higher-level equilibrium reactions. Thus therapists ask which postural reflexes are present or absent in their patients as they move them in order to stimulate each sensory system contributing to each reflex. If appropriate responses are not observed, therapists must try to determine whether their stimulus was inadequate, the sensory system insensitive, or the reflexes inappropriately integrated. Treatment is aimed at inhibiting in-

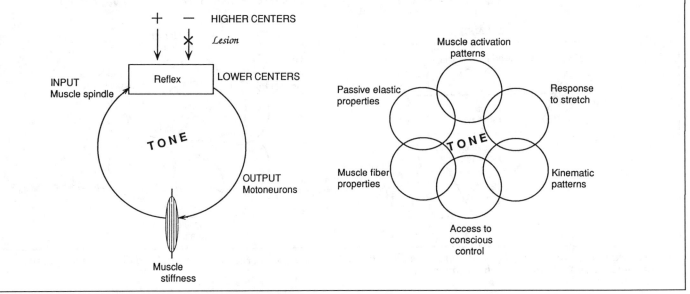

Fig. 4-10. *Assumptions underlying control of muscle tone based on the A. Neurotherapeutic Facilitation Model and the B. Contemporary Task-oriented Model of neurologic rehabilitation.*

appropriate, primitive postural reflexes and facilitating normal equilibrium reactions.

In contrast, the task-oriented approach assumes that normal postural motor behavior is the product of the interaction of many components organized around a fundamental behavioral goal to maintain equilibrium and orientation in the environment (Fig. 4-9B, Shumway-Cook and Horak,[96] Horak et al,[82] Horak[97]). In this approach, therapists ask, "What are the primary constraints limiting adequate control of balance?" Disorders of postural control are thought to result from constraints placed on the system from a multitude of sources, including the neural control of predictive central set, perception, and coordination and the physical limitations imposed by the musculoskeletal system and environment. After identifying the specific combination of constraints, therapists direct therapy at reducing or eliminating those constraints or helping patients find effective strategies for postural control given certain constraints that cannot be changed.

Tone

According to the facilitation model, excessive muscle tone, or spasticity, is due to lack of inhibition of higher centers on the now over-responsive stretch reflex (Fig. 4-10A). Because this approach assumes that this excessive tone blocks normal, coordinated movement, therapists ask, "How can I best reduce muscle tone in my neurologically impaired patients?" Once the pattern of abnormal tone is identified, therapeutic intervention involves using the proprioceptive system to reduce excessive tone and to facilitate normal movements.

The task-oriented model of neurologic rehabilitation views excessive muscle tone as a set of motor behaviors that

results as an emergent property of many interacting systems, any of which may be disordered (Fig. 4-10B). Therapists ask, "Which combination of systems, including muscle activation patterns, response to stretch, kinematic patterns, conscious control of muscle activation, muscle fiber properties, and passive elastic elements, are abnormal and limit optimal motor performance in the characteristic manner of 'spastic' patient?" Therapists may also ask if the spasticity is a primary result of the neural lesion or a secondary, compensatory strategy that allows certain functional behaviors. After this problem solving process, therapists determine which disordered components can be changed by therapeutic intervention and how they can help their patients find efficient, effective movement strategies given the limitations imposed by the systems.

CONCLUSION

Therapists use assumptions about motor control and neurologic rehabilitation in every aspect of their work. However, therapists need to concentrate more on testing the usefulness of their assumptions rather than on worrying about which particular assumptions of general models are "correct." We still have knowledge of only a minute fraction of the physical and chemical factors that mechanistically control the brain's output. Our current models of the brain, however, can allow us some predictive and some therapeutic power despite the incomplete data. "The predictive power of a model depends on its correct identification of the dominant controlling factors and their influence, not upon its completeness. An incomplete model can be more useful than an accurate one."[98]

Thus models are important for physical therapy. Models of neurologic rehabilitation are necessary to develop physical therapy from a practical *art* in which knowledge is used to a theoretical *science* in which knowledge is extended. Models will help change physical therapy from a *technology* of "skilled hands" to a *profession* of problem solvers. Even before the first NUSTEP conference on the physiologic basis of therapeutic exercise almost 25 years ago, physical therapists have recognized the need for development and change in neurologic rehabilitation. The future is here for those willing to ask new questions. As Hislop said:

Specializing in the techniques of physical therapy will not be enough—we will have to specialize in the *problems* of our patients . . . . The future cannot be planned by tired, rigid minds. Those who challenge the present system will bear the wounds of the challenge. But wounds heal and the scars that remain may serve as useful reminders that achievement is made only by those who are dissatisfied. Achievement is made only by those who are willing to advocate changes in institutions to keep pace with progress and enlightened thinking. We progress by difference. We regress by conformity. We advance by originality. We retreat by submission. We succeed by distinction. We fail by imitation. We achieve recognition through our maturity.[99]

References

1. Gordon J. Assumptions underlying physical therapy intervention: theoretical and historical perspectives. in: Car JH, Shepherd RB, Gordon J, et al, eds. *Movement Science: Foundations for Physical Therapy in Rehabilitation*. Rockville, Md: Aspen Publishers Inc; 1987:1-30.
2. Granit R. Comments on history of motor control. In: Brooks VB, ed. *Handbook of Physiology*. Baltimore, Md: Williams & Wilkins; 1981;2:1-16.
3. Sherrington CS. *The Integrative Action of the Nervous System*. New York, NY: Cambridge University Press; 1947.
4. Ghez C. Introduction to motor systems. In: Kandel E, Schwartz J, eds. *Principles of Neural Science*. New York, NY: Elsevier Science Publishing Co Inc; 1981:245; fig. 24-2.
5. Stein R. Peripheral control of movement. *Physiol Rev*. 1974;54:215-243.
6. Sherrington CS. *The Integrative Action of the Nervous System*. New Haven, Conn: Yale University Press; 1906:7.
7. Magnus R. Animal posture. *Proc R Soc Lond [Biol]*. 1925;98:339.
8. Magnus R. Some results of studies in the physiology of posture. *Lancet*. 1926;2:531, 585.
9. Easton T. On the normal use of reflexes. *American Scientist*. 1972;60:591-599.
10. Brunnstrom S. *Movement Theory in Hemiphegia: A Neurophysiological Approach*. New York, NY: Harper & Row, Publishers Inc; 1970.
11. Eldred E. Functional implications of dynamic and static components of the spindle response to stretch. *Am J Phys Med*. 1967;46:129-140.
12. Power W. *Behavior: The Control of Perception*. New York, NY: Aldine Publishing Co; 1973.
13. Desmedt JE. *Cerebral Motor Control in Man: Long Loop Mechanisms*. New York, NY: S Karger; 1978.
14. Jacobs MJ. Development of normal motor behavior. *Am J Phys Med*. 1967;46:41-51.
15. Fiorentino MR. *Reflex Testing Methods for Evaluating CNS Development*. Springfield, Ill: Charles C Thomas, Publisher; 1963.
16. White R. Sensory integrative therapy for the cerebral-palsied child. In: Scrutton D, ed. *Management of the Motor Disorders of Children with Cerebral Palsy*. Philadelphia, Pa: J B Lippincott Co; 1984:86-95.
17. Bobath K. The motor deficit in patients with cerebral palsy. In: *Clinics in Developmental Medicine, No. 23*. Lavenham, England: Lavenham Press; 1966:191-192.
18. Brown TG. On the nature of the fundamental activity of the nervous centres; together with an analysis of the conditioning of rhythmic activity in progression, and a theory of the evolution of function in the nervous system. *J Physiol*. 1914;48:18-46.
19. Taub E. Motor behavior following deafferentation in the developing and motorically mature monkey. *Advances in Behavioral Biology*. 1976;18:675-705.
20. Taub E, Goldberg I, Taub P. Deafferentiation in monkeys: pointing at a target without visual feedback. *Exp Neurol*. 1975;46:178-186.
21. Polit A, Bizzi E. Characteristics of motor programs underlying arm movements in monkeys. *J Neurophysiol*. 1979;42:183-194.
22. Hooker D. *The Prenatal Origin of Behavior*. Lawrence, Kan: University of Kansas Press; 1952.
23. Brooks V. Motor Control: how posture and movements are governed. *Phys Ther*. 1983;63:664-673.
24. Ito M. Control system model of the cerebellum. In: *The Cerebellum and Neural Control*. New York, NY: Raven Press; 1984:325-349.
25. Forssberg H, Grillner S, Rossignol S. Phasic gain control of reflexes from the dorsum of the paw during spinal locomotion. *Brain Res*. 1977;132:121-139.
26. Traub M, Rothwell JC, Marsden C. Anticipatory postural reflexes in Parkinson's disease and the alanetic-rigid syndromes and in cerebellar ataxia. *Brain*. 1980;103:393-412.
27. Evarts EV, Shinoda Y, Wise SP. *Neurophysiological Approaches to Higher Brain Function*. New York, NY: John Wiley & Sons Inc; 1984.
28. Belenkii V, Gurfinkel V, Paltsev Y. Elements of control of voluntary movements. *Biophysics*. 1967;12:135-141.
29. Horak FB, Anderson M, Esselman P, Lynch K. The effects of movement velocity, mass displaced and task certainty on associated postural adjustments made by normal and hemiplegic individuals. *J Neurol Neurosurg Psychiatry*. 1984;47:1020-1028.
30. Cordo P, Nashner LM. Properties of postural adjustments associated with rapid arm movements. *J Neurophysiol*. 1982;47:287-302.
31. Horak FB, Diener HC, Nashner LM. Influence of central set on human postural responses. *J Neurophysiol*. 1989;62:841-853.
32. Jackson JH; Taylor J, ed. *Selected Writings of John B. Hughlings, I and II*. London, England: Hodder & Stoughter; 1932.
33. Walsche FMP. Contribution of John Hughlings Jackson to neurology. *Arch Neurol*. 1961;5:99-133.
34. Reed ES. An outline of a theory of action systems. *Journal of Motor Behavior*. 1982;14:98-134.
35. Phillips CG, Porter R. *Corticospinal Neurones: Their Role in Movement*. New York, NY: Academic Press Inc; 1977.
36. Nelson CA. Cerebral palsy. In: Umphred D, ed. *Neurological Rehabilitation*. St. Louis, Mo: C V Mosby Co; 1985:171.

37. Grillner S. Locomotion in vertebrates: central mechanisms and reflex interactions. *Physiol Rev*. 1975;55:247-307.

38. Shik M, Orlovsky GM. Neurophysiology of locomotor automatism. *Physiol Rev*. 1976;56:465-501,

39. Smith J. Programming of stereotyped limb movements by spinal generators. In: Stelmach GE, Requin J, eds. *Tutorials in Motor Behavior*. Amsterdam, The Netherlands: North Holland; 1980.

40. von Hofsten C. Predictive reaching for moving objects by human infants. *J Exp Child Psychol*. 1980;30:383-388.

41. Bekoff A. Embryonic development of the neural circuitry underlying motor coordination. In: Crowan WM, ed. *Studies in Developmental Neurobiology*. New York, NY: Oxford University Press Inc; 1981:134-170.

42. Thelen E, Kelso JAS, Fogel A. Self-organizing systems and infant motor development. *Developmental Review*. 1987;7:39-65.

43. Hammond PH. The influence of prior instruction to the subject on an apparently involuntary neuromuscular response. *J Physiol (Lond)*. 1956;132:17-18.

44. Wolpow J. Adaptive plasticity in the spinal stretch reflex: an accessible substitute of memory? *Cell Mol Neurobiol*. 1985;5:147-165.

45. Bernstein N. *The Coordination and Regulation of Movement*. London, England: Pergamon Press Ltd; 1967.

46. Abbs JH, Cole KJ. Neural mechanisms of motor equivalence and goal achievement. In: Wise S, Evarts E. eds. *Higher Brain Function: Recent Exploration of the Brain's Emergent Properties*. New York, NY; John Wiley & Sons Inc; 1987.

47. Lacquaniti F, Soechting JF. EMG responses to load perturbations of the upper limb: effect of dynamic coupling between shoulder and elbow motion. *Exp Brain Res*. 1986;61:482-496.

48. Macpherson J. Strategies that simplify the control of quadrupedal stance: I. Forces at the ground. *J Neurophysiol*. 1988;60:204-217.

49. Horak FB, Nashner LM. Central programming of posture control: adaptation to altered support surface configurations. *J Neurophysiol*. 1986;55:1368-1381.

50. Turvey MT, Fitch HL, Tulley B. The Bernstein perspective in human motor behavior. In: Kelso JAS, ed. *Human Motor Behavior: An Introduction*. Hillsdale, NJ: Lawrence Erlbaum Associates Inc; 1982:239-283.

51. Duncan PW, Badke MB. Therapeutic strategies for rehabilitation of motor deficits. In: *Stroke Rehabilitation: The Recovery of Motor Control*. Chicago, Ill: Year Book Medical Publishers Inc; 1987:161.

52. Turvey MT. Preliminaries to a theory of action with reference to vision. In: Kelso JAS, ed. *Human Motor Behavior: An Introduction*. Hillsdale, NJ: Lawrence Erlbaum Associates Inc; 1982:211-265.

53. Gibson JJ. *The Senses Considered As Perceptual Systems*. Boston, Mass: Houghton Mifflin Co; 1966.

54. Arbib MA. Perceptual structures and distributed motor control. In: Brookhard JM, Mountcastle VB. Brooks VB, Geiger SR, eds. *Handbook of Physiology: The Nervous System, II*. Bethesda, Md: American Physiological Society; 1979:1440-1480.

55. Greene PH. Problems of organization of motor systems. In: Rosen R, Snell FM, eds. *Progress in Theoretical Biology*. San Diego, Calif: Academic Press Inc; 1972:304-338.

56. Gallistel CR. *The Organization of Action: A New Synthesis*. New York, NY: John Wiley & Sons Inc; 1980.

57. Reed ES. Applying the theory of action systems to the study of motor skills. In: Meijer OG, Roth K, eds. *Complex Movement Behavior: The Motor-Action Controversy*. Amsterdam, The Netherlands: North Holland Publishing Co; 1986.

58. von Holst E, Mittelstaedt H. The reafference principle. In: Gallistel CR, ed. *The Organization of Action: A New Synthesis*. Hillsdale, NJ: Lawrence Erlbaum Associates Inc; 1980.

59. Bobath K, Bobath B. The neuro-developmental treatment. In: Scrutton D, ed. *Management of the Motor Disorders of Children with Cerebral Palsy*. Philadelphia, Pa: J B Lippincott Co; 1984:6-17.

60. Knott M, Voss D. *Proprioceptive Neuromuscular Facilitation*. New York, NY: Harper & Row Publishers Inc; 1968.

61. Carr JH, Shepard RB, eds. *A Motor Relearning Programme for Stroke*. Rockville, Md: Aspen Publishers Inc; 1983.

62. Ostrosky K. Facilitation vs. motor control. *Clinical Management in Physical Therapy*. 1990;10:34-40.

53. Pohl JF. *The Kenny Concept of Infantile Paralysis and Its Treatment*. Minneapolis-St. Paul, Minn: Bruce; 1943:151-152.

64. Beard G. Foundation for growth; a review of the first forty years in terms of advocation, practice and research. *Phys Ther Rev*. 1961;41:843-861.

65. Bobath B. *Abnormal Postural Reflex Activity Caused by Brain Lesions*. Rockville, Md: Aspen Publishers Inc; 1985.

66. Kabat H, McLeod M, Holt C. Neuromuscular dysfunction and treatment of corticospinal lesions. *Physiotherapy*. 1959;45:251-257.

67. Knott M. Specialized neuromuscular techniques in the treatment of cerebral palsy. *Phys Ther Rev* 1952;32:73-75.

68. Stockmeyer SA. An interpretation of the approach of Rood to the treatment of neuromuscular dysfunction. *Am J Phys Med*. 1967;46:901-956.

69. Payton OD, Hirt S, Newton R. *Scientific Bases for Neurophysiologic Approaches to Therapeutic Exercise: An Anthology*. Philadelphia, Pa: F A Davis Co; 1977.

70. Flanagan EM. Methods for facilitation and inhibition of motor activity. *Am J Phys Med*. 1967;46:1006-1011.

71. Bobath B. Bobath K. *Motor Development in the Different Types of Cerebral Palsy*. London, England: William Heinemann Medical Books Ltd; 1975.

72. Schmidt RD, ed. *Motor Control and Learning: A Behavioral Emphasis*. Champaign, Ill: Human Kinetics Publishers Inc; 1982.

73. Hein A, Held R. Dissociation of the visual placing response into elicited and guided components. *Science*. 1967;158:390-392.

74. Thelen E, Fisher DM, Ridley-Johnson R. The relationship between physical growth and a newborn reflex. *Infant Behavior and Development*. 1984;17:79-83.

75. Thelen E, Whitley-Cooke D. Relationship between newborn stepping and later walking: a new interpretation. *Dev Med Child Neurol*. 1987;29:380-393.

76. Thelen E, Fisher DM. Newborn stepping: an explanation for a "disappearing" reflex. *Developmental Psychology*. 1982;18:760-775.

77. Carr JH, Shepard RB. *Physiotherapy in Disorders of the Brain*. Rockville, Md: Aspen Publishers Inc; 1980.

78. Levitt S. *Treatment of Cerebral Palsy and Motor Delay*. Boston, Mass: Blackwell Scientific Publications Inc; 1982.

79. Horak FB. Measurement of movement patterns to study postural coordination. Presented at 10th Annual Eugene Michels Researchers' Forum, Combined Sections Meeting, American Physical Therapy Association; February 2, 1990; New Orleans, La.

80. Johansson RS, Westling G. Programmed and triggered ac-

tions to rapid load changes during precision grip. *Exp Brain Res*. 1988;71:72-86.

81. Soechting JF, Lacquaniti F. Invariant characteristics of a pointing movement in man. *J Neurosci*. 1981;1:710-720.

82. Horak FB, Shupert CL, Mirka A. Components of postural control in the elderly: a review. *Neurobiol Aging*. 1989;10:727-738.

83. Horak FB, Shumway-Cook A. Clinical implications of posture control research. In: Duncan PW, ed. *Balance*. Alexandria, Va: American Physical Therapy Association; 1990:105-111.

84. Dietz V, Berger W. Normal and impaired regulation of muscle stiffnes in gait: a new hypothesis about muscle hypertonia. *Exp Neurol*. 1982;79:680-687.

85. Nashner LM, Shumway-Cook A, Marin O. Stance posture control in select groups of children with cerebral palsy: deficits in sensory organization and muscular coordination. *Exp Brain Res*. 1983;49:393-409.

86. Shumway-Cook A. Equilibrium deficits in children. In: Woollacott M, Shumway-Cook A, eds. *The Development of Posture and Gait Across the Lifespan*. Columbia, SC: University of South Carolina Press; 1989.

87. Nashner LM. Adapting reflexes controlling the human posture. *Exp Brain Res*. 1976;26:59-72.

88. Horak FB, Nashner LM, Nutt JG. Postural instability in Parkinson's disease: motor coordination and sensory organization. *Neurology Report*. 1988;12:54-55.

89. Woollacott M, Shumway-Cook A, eds. *Development of Posture and Gait Across the Lifespan*. Columbia, SC: University of South Carolina Press; 1989.

90. Horak FB, Shumway-Cook A, Crowe T, Black FO. Vestibular function and motor proficiency in children with hearing impairments and in learning disabled children with motor impairments. *Dev Med Child Neurol*. 1988;30:64-79.

91. Horak FB, Esselman P, Anderson ME, Lynch MK. The effects of movement velocity, mass displaced, and task certainty on associated postural adjustments made by normal and hemiplegic individuals. *J Neurol Neurosurg Psychiatry*. 1984;47:1020-1028.

92. Lee W. Anticipatory control of postural and task muscles during rapid arm flexion. *Journal of Motor Behavior*. 1980;12:185-196.

93. Frank JS, Earl M. Coordination of posture and movement. *Phys Ther*. In press.

94. Massion J, Hugon M, Wiesendanger M. Anticipatory postural changes induced by active unloading and comparison with passive unloading in man. *Pflugers Arch*. 1982;393:292-296.

95. Horak FB. Comparison of cerebellar and vestibular loss on scaling of postural responses. In: Brandt T, Paulus W, Bles W, et al, eds. *Disorders of Posture and Gait, 1990*. New York, NY: Georg Thieme Verlag: 1990:370-373.

96. Shumway-Cook A, Horak FB. Rehabilitation strategies for patients with vestibular deficits. *Neurol Clin*. 1990;8:441-457.

97. Horak FB. Clinical assessment of postural control in adults. *Phys Ther*. 1987:67:1881-1885.

98. Barlow H. The mechanical mind. *Annu Rev Neurosci*. 1990;13:15-24.

99. Hislop H. Today and beyond. *Phys Ther* 1966;46:584.

Chapter 5

Theories of Motor Control: New Concepts for Physical Therapy

Carol A. Giuliani, PhD, PT
Assistant Professor
Division of Physical Therapy
Department of Medical Allied Health
School of Medicine
University of North Carolina at Chapel Hill
Chapel Hill, NC 27599-7135

The purpose of this chapter is to present some of the current theoretical concepts of motor control related to physical therapy. In this chapter, I will discuss feedback and feedforward systems, motor programs, and dynamic systems theories of control. The reader should not be misled to believe that the theories discussed in this chapter are the only ones of merit or the most important. These theories are the ones that I believe are generating considerable research literature and are being applied to physical therapy. Other theories of motor control emphasize neural, behavioral, or mechanical concepts. The area of motor control is fairly new and is changing rapidly. I hope that the information presented here will stimulate you to question the assumptions of physical therapy treatment, to read and keep abreast of new concepts, and even to question what is presented in this document. Some day this information may be out of date.

MOVEMENT COORDINATION

How are movements coordinated? This important question for physical therapy has yet to be answered completely. Physical therapy practice has been guided by many assumptions about motor control that are based on anatomic, physiologic, and behavioral evidence. Several assumptions are listed for this discussion: 1) reflexes are the building blocks of movement, 2) motor control develops in a cephalocaudal direction, 3) movement skills are acquired in a predictable developmental sequence, and 4) sensory feedback is required for movement.

Studies of reflexes have dominated research in the neurophysiology of motor systems for most of this century. It is no wonder the sensory-motor input-output relationships formed the basis of neurotherapeutic exercise in physical therapy. Are reflexes the building blocks of movements? Yes and no. Yes, the neurons activated in reflex pathways may be used for other movements. In other words, neural circuitry may be reorganized for different types of movement. It is reasonable to assume that reflexes and purposeful movements share some of the same neurons and circuitry. However, all movement is not generated initially as a reflex and then later molded and refined under the influence of

supraspinal centers to become purposeful movement. In fact, evidence exists in many species including humans that first to develop is the motoneuron muscle connection, second is the supraspinal connection to the spinal circuitry, and last are the peripheral sensory connections to the central circuitry. It appears that supraspinal and spinal centers are developing at the same time.[1-3] Reports of early embryonic and fetal movement confirm that there is no fixed proximal-distal, or cephalocaudal, order to motor development.[4,5] Considerable evidence is available now that shows coordinated movement is not controlled by a series of integrated reflexes.[4,6-8]

Evidence also exists to support the hypothesis that sensory feedback is not necessary as was once thought for the production of accurate movement.[9-11] Animal studies confirm the ability to produce well-learned motor tasks without the presence of sensory information. Polit and Bizzi[11] reported that monkeys who had their upper limb deafferented were able to perform aiming, using an elbow flexion and extension task, without visual and sensory input from the upper limb. Any change in the orientation of the shoulder, however, produced an error that the monkey was unable to correct without sensory input. Apparently, although sensory information is not necessary for performing some movements, it is important for adjusting to environmental demand and for learning movement.

Feedback and Feedforward Control

Movement may be produced by two basic systems of control: feedback (closed-loop control) and feedforward (open-loop control).[12] Movements requiring feedback are usually complex and discrete movements requiring accuracy, such as a visual-motor tracking task. Feedback control is required during early skill acquisition and probably accounts for the slow movement execution during this stage.[12] Listening to a child practice the piano as he slowly locates each note can be an excruciatingly "painful" experience to the ear. However, even very complex accuracy movements such as playing a piano may not require feedback. Once the task is well learned, it can be performed accurately without sensory feedback. When the notes are played in rapid succession, you can actually recognize the melody.

The control of movement fluctuates between feedback and feedforward modes of control. Rapid movements and well-learned movements are performed with feedforward control.[12,13] Although the sensory information is available during rapid movements, it cannot be used to perform the movement because the movement proceeds faster than the nervous system can process and use the sensory information. Thus, it appears that well-learned, rapid, and automatic tasks may not require feedback for their execution. Feedback, or sensory information, is available and may be used before and after completing the movement, but it not required to produce accuracy during the movement.[12,13] Sensory information is necessary to modulate, adjust, and fine tune movement for adjusting to changes in the environment that are essential during activities such as walking, aiming, and precision tasks.

Motor Program Perspective

A motor program concept of motor control is based on an open-loop system of control. This perspective assumes that movements are preplanned and stored inmemory until called on for action. A *motor program* is defined as an abstract representation of a movement sequence that is stored in memory and contains certain variant and invariant features.[12] The invariant features of a motor program are those that remain fixed, whereas the variant features may be adjusted to produce variability of the motor task. Walking is used frequently as an example of a motor program. The sequence and relative timing of limb muscle activation are invariant for a range of walking speeds; however, the speed of walking and the direction may vary.[14] The invariances characterize a behavior so that we, for example, recognize one person's handwriting from another's. Handwriting is a good example of a well- practiced motor skill that may be controlled by a motor program. In this program, the shape of a letter may be constant (invariant), while the absolute size may be changed without changing the shape. (For complete discussion of motor programs, see Schmidt.[12])

The motor program model of motor control is based on the concept that the organization and maturational processes of the nervous system produce movement. Any change in motor output is a result of changes in the nervous system. Certainly, many physical therapy techniques for treating neurologically impaired patients are aimed at changing movement through the neuromuscular system. The neuromuscular system provides muscle forces that contribute to limb movement; however, inherent properties of the musculoskeletal system itself affect motor patterns.[15,16] Damage or normal changes in the musculoskeletal apparatus may produce abnormal movement even in the presence of a normal nervous system. For example, limb coordination changes when segment length changes. For a first hand experience of this concept, tape a tongue blade so it extends one-half inch from the end of your middle or index finger. Go about your routines for the day. How many times did you jam your hand into a wall or stick your finger in your face? How long did it take you to adjust? Your nervous system was still intact, yet this small change in the apparent length of your arm created

accuracy error in movement. Thus changes in the structure of the system alone can account for changes in movement patterns. Not all changes in motor coordination can be explained by maturation or by other changes in the nervous system.

DESCRIBING THE BEHAVIOR OF COMPLEX SYSTEMS

Much behavior in nature and in biological systems is chaotic but not without order. Studies of chaotic systems in nature provide an excellent example of the rich dynamics of complex systems.[17] Self-organizing and rapidly changing patterns of ocean currents and cloud formations emphasize the magnitude of complexity generated from relatively simple elements.[17] Those who study weather patterns and try to predict future events appreciate the difficulty of prediction, even when all the components of a system are known. With one small change in any component, the solution to the problem changes.[17] Gleick[17] and others believe that chaos, or chaotic states, are required for problem solving. Chaos provides an opportunity for optimization. *Optimization* is the search for the best possible solution to a problem. A certain amount of randomness is necessary to find the best solution to a problem as opposed to conducting a limited search that might lead to a suboptimal solution A nonlinear, dynamical systems approach provides an interesting theoretical perspective to investigate the behavior of complex systems. In this case, we want to understand the coordination of human movement.

Dynamical Systems Perspective

Dynamical systems theory, or systems theory, is a general terms that encompasses several theoretical approaches. Some are more well defined than others. In many instances, the term dynamical systems is used loosely and is poorly defined. This creates confusion to the student attempting to keep abreast of the latest theoretical concepts. Developmentalists applying a systems approach propose that the behavior of a child is the sum total of the interaction of various biological, cognitive, social, and environmental subsystems.[18] Special educators applying a systems approach stress the family-child interaction systems,[19] and developmental psychologists stress the interaction of cognitive, perceptual, and memory systems in the study of child development.[20] Although each discipline has a different perspective, the emphasis is on studying a complex system and acknowledging the importance of the interaction of many elements or subsystems in understanding behavior.

Dynamical systems theory is currently being applied to biological systems and to the study of motor control and the development of motor control. The basis of this theory, as related to motor control, has been attributed to concepts of von Holst[21] and Bernstein.[22] von Holst[21] emphasized the importance of studying limb coordination patterns and transitions in patterns for locomotion in quadrupeds and insects. Bernstein[22] suggested that the study of movement must include all the forces acting to move a limb, not just the forces provided by the nervous system. Consider the movement of the lower limb during the swing phase of locomotion. Very little muscle activity is present during the swing phase, yet there is a complex pattern of well- coordinated movement among all three joints. How is this possible? Movement of the limb is dependent on muscle tension in addition to gravity and other intersegmental forces acting on the limb. Some components of the trajectory and velocity of the segments are inherent in the structure of the limb, the properties of segmental linkages (joints), and the composition of the tissue that constitutes the joint. Dynamical systems theorists propose that movement and changes in movement patterns generated by a system are inherent in the structure itself, with the nervous system just one of the subsystems that contributes to movement.[23-25] Attributing movement patterns to the inherent structure of an organism is a new concept for therapists who have struggled for many years to understand the role of the neuromuscular system.

I am sure many of you have seen or owned a wooden puppet. Usually, the arms, legs, and trunk segments of these puppets are linked together, modelling the many limb and trunk segments of human limbs. A stick or handle is attached to the trunk segment by which the child or adult investigator can jiggle the puppet. A careful jiggler can make the wooden puppet jump, walk, and dance just by jiggling the handle at different frequencies. This puppet provides an excellent example of the variety of movement patterns possible independent of the discrete forces produced by the nervous system. In this case, the patterns of the organism (wooden puppet) were created by a person producing a driving force by jiggling the handle. New patterns emerged within the system by changing the frequency of the driving force. Consider that these complex patterns of limb movement were generated without a nervous system and muscles to produce forces at joints. How much human movement or change in human movement may be accounted for by the dynamics of the system alone? This is an interesting question to ponder.

Dynamical systems are complex in that they are composed of many elements, or, in the words of Bernstein,[15,24] many degrees of freedom. Degrees of freedom as used here is not limited to axes or planes of movement used for studying biomechanics. A degree of freedom may be any element of a system that can be altered or manipulated.[20-23] It is not reasonable to assume that each neural (neuron) and muscular component (motor unit) of the human body is controlled separately. Controlling this number of degrees of freedom would be a monumental task. How can the control of such a complex system composed of innumerable neurons, muscles, and muscle fibers be reduced so it can be controlled easily? Bernstein's[15,16] conception was that the multiple degrees of freedom for movement are constrained to act as a coordinative structure. He defined a *coordinative structure* as a functional group of muscles and joints that are constrained to act as a unit, thus reducing the number of degrees of freedom that need to be controlled.[15,16]

Important concepts of dynamic theory are that dynamical systems are complex, are composed of multiple elements or subsystems, and are self-organizing. Dynamical systems are high-dimensional systems (many elements) that are constrained or reduced to behave as low-dimensional systems. Self-organization is the ability of a system to produce new spatial or temporal patterns as the result of internal regulation in response to changing conditions.[18,23] Studying movement from this perspective provides a theoretical framework

for studying complex systems. Because the subsystems are interactive, there is an opportunity for multiple levels of movement analysis. The activity of a system may be described in behavioral, physiologic, neural, muscular, kinematic, or kinetic terms.

Studying individual elements of movement has increased our knowledge of the component parts of movement, but it has not improved our understanding of the function of the individual elements related to the behavior as a whole. There is still a void of understanding about how these elements function together or change with altered input. Using a dynamical systems approach to study behavior may help explain phenomena unaccounted for by other theoretical perspectives.

Researchers in motor control have been unable to explain satisfactorily the sudden appearance of new behaviors and the disappearance of acquired behaviors; the role of periods of instability, disorganization, and reorganization; or the fact that large changes in behavior can be produced by small perturbations or adjustments of the system.[18,24] Dynamical theory could provide some answers for us, because it already provides a rationale for the ability of simple systems to produce complex behavior and for very complex systems to produce well-coordinated behavior. Similarly, a neural maturation viewpoint leaves us with many unanswered questions about motor development. Acquisition of motor skills is certainly nonlinear and is characterized by periods of stability and instability in performance and by the inexplicable emergence of new motor abilities.[26,27] Some investigators propose applying a dynamical systems model to address questions and inconsistencies in development.[28-34] In this model, elements of movements can be assembled for function in a fluid task-specific manner determined by maturational state, experience, and current context of the movement. Within this framework, stability and change are fundamental characteristics of both developing biological systems and dynamical systems.[23,25,29]

As discussed above, dynamics is a relatively new perspective currently being explored and developed for studying movement. There is much that we do not know about the control of movement in normal systems. We know less about the control of movement in humans with motor dysfunction. Dynamical systems are being applied to the study of abnormal sleep patterns, heart and breathing rhythms, and other biological systems.[35,36] We are just beginning to examine the behavior of normal and abnormal systems, with the hope that this exploration will provide insights for improving motor control and for understanding how systems respond to sensory feedback, exercise practice, and external constraints.

Dynamic Pattern Theory

Building on the concepts of synergetics, several investigators are developing an operational approach to the study of coordinated movement: a dynamic pattern theory.[37-43] This new approach is an attempt to define terms and provide behavioral and mathematical predictions for the production of coordinated movement patterns.

The basic concepts of dynamic pattern theory are as follows: 1) the human system exhibits self-organizing behav-

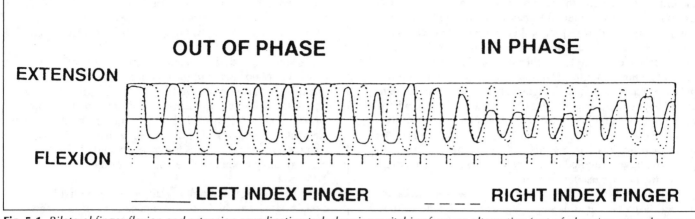

Fig. 5-1. *Bilateral finger flexion and extension coordination task showing switching from an alternating (out-of-phase) to a synchronous (in-phase) mode. The transition in phasing occurred at a critical frequency in finger movement. (Adapted from Scholtz and Keso.[40])*

iors and is a high-dimensional system that can be described by low-dimensional dynamics in terms of collective variables, 2) the relevant subsystems and their dynamics can be identified and characterized, 3) the identification of phase transitions in patterns is basic to understanding behavior, and 4) the study of the stability or instability of behavior about transition periods is a key factor for understanding pattern change in complex systems. Studying the phase transitions in patterned behavior and the relative stability and instability about the phase transition may provide considerable insight into the coordination of movement and may be applied to the study of other biological systems.

At this point, it may be enlightening to define some of the basic terms used in the discussion of dynamic pattern theory.[41,42] The language used to describe this theory can be cumbersome, and theorists have been criticized for the apparent use of neologisms that make understanding difficult for students of motor control.

1. *Self-organization.* Complex systems exhibit self-organized behavior, that is, patterns of movement are formed from the interaction of a large number of subsystems or elements. The patterns are not formed by external constraints per se but are the resulting behavior of the organism as a result of its intrinsic nature.

2. *Stability.* Stability may be measured by variability or the inherent noise in a system that produces perturbations. Standard deviation and the coefficient of variability are measures of stability. The stability of a pattern can also be measured by the time it takes to return from an unstable to a stable state. Just as the time to return to stability is important, the sensitivity to perturbation, or the ease of producing instability, is important.

3. *Collective variables.* These are sometimes referred to as "order parameters." These are the fewest number of variables that can most completely describe the behavior of interest.

4. *Phase transition.* Phase transitions are characterized by periods of increased variability, periods of slower restoration to a stable state, diminished restoration to the original state, and points at which new behaviors are observed.

5. *"Control parameters."* These are one or more parameters that act to reorganize the system. They do not encode change or represent change, and they may be nonspecific elements of movements such as temperature, frequency, pressure, or energy. Control parameters are those elements that can trigger a phase transition by a scalar change in one or more components or by contextual changes. As the system changes, so may the control parameters. Changes in control parameters are common during child development when rapid periods of growth and reorganization are occurring.

An example of applying dynamical systems theory to movement may help the reader understand the concepts as well as the terminology described here. When subjects were asked to move their index fingers rhythmically, one of two stable patterns was observed.[44,45] Subjects began the task by moving their index fingers, alternating finger flexion and extension in an out-of-phase mode, that is, as one finger flexed, the opposite finger extended. As subjects gradually increased the frequency of finger movement, they spontaneously switched to an in-phase mode with both hands moving in synchrony at a critical movement frequency (Fig. 5-1). If subjects started in the in-phase mode and gradually increased frequency, no switching was observed.[39-41] Scholz et al[39] and Scholz and Kelso[40,41] also observed that there was a critical slowing of responses and increased variability about the transition from out-of-phase to in-phase. Scholz[39] suggests that studying behaviors at the transition phase is the key to understanding the control of complex systems.

Phase transitions between limbs are commonly observed in quadrupedal locomotion with increased speed. As speed increases, the pattern switches from walk to trot, then to pace, and finally to a gallop.[46] Shapiro et al[14] showed that humans have critical frequencies for switching locomotion modes from walking to running. Disturbed interlimb phasing has been observed in spinal cats with sensory information reduced to one hindlimb (Fig. 5-2).[47] After one hind limb was deafferented, phase transitions in interlimb coordination occurred frequently. We observed periods of in-phase stepping, out-of phase stepping, and variable phase relationships

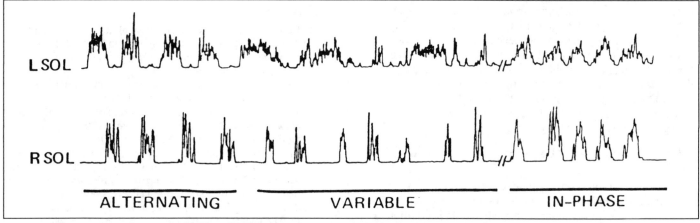

Fig. 5-2. *Electromyographic patterns of hindlimb stepping in a spinal cat that had the right hindlimb deafferented. Phase transitions occurred frequently between in-phase and out-of-phase modes. Many periods of activity had variable interlimb phasing.*

between the hindlimbs (Fig. 5-2). Controlling alternating lower-limb tasks appears to be disturbed in children with learning disabilities.[48] Normal children and children with diagnosed learning disability were asked to perform an alternating foot tapping task. Phase transitions occurred frequently with speed demands in the children with learning disability, while the normal children were able to maintain the speed and correct phase relationship. The sensitivity to speed and the frequency of transitions were not as common in the group of age-matched normal children (Fig. 5-3).[48]

Can these concepts of dynamic theory be useful to physical therapy? We observe the emergence of new patterns of movement in children and in adults. Does the concept of self-organization eliminate the therapist? If the system is capable of reorganization, how do we know we are affecting the system with extrinsic manipulations or perturbations? Maybe we can use these concepts to change the emphasis of our observations and assessment of movement. We may want to evaluate transition phases, behavioral stability, and periods of instability.

Although not identified as such, a dynamical systems approach is used frequently for examining the behavior of infants and neonates. Examining state and changes in states are a part of many standardized neonatal assessments.[49-51] Als et al[49] and Brazelton[50] assess neonates based on their ability to organize themselves and their ability to reorganize from a state of stress or disorganization. In these terms we interpret instability and disorganization as a sign of illness or of infants at risk for developing motor problems. We look for infants to achieve stability or organization as a sign of health. Generally, we do not think of adult motor behavior in terms of stability or instability, although we think of people as stable and unstable characters. For adults with neurologic disease, we are concerned with variable behavior or sterotypic behaviors as an indicator of motor control. Variability may not always be a sign of instability and is not necessarily a negative indicator.

Scholz[41] suggests that we can apply dynamic pattern analysis for understanding movement. The first step is to define the collective variables (order parameters), then to observe the behavior of the collective variable in different con-

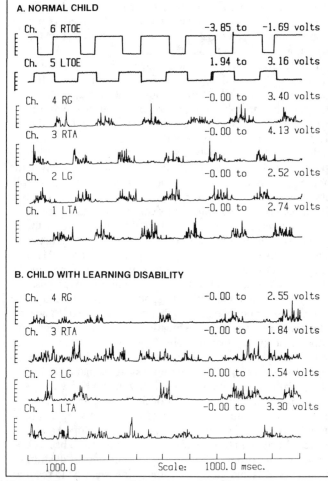

Fig. 5-3. *Electromyographic patterns of an alternating symmetrical foot tapping task for a normal child and a child with learning disability. The normal child (A) had a rhythmical pattern of alternating tibialis anterior (TA) and lateral gastrocnemius (G) muscle activity, for the right (R) and left (L) limbs. The child with diagnosed learning disability (B) had an irregular intralimb and interlimb pattern. His pattern was irregular and he tended to switch to a synchronous, or in-phase, mode of foot tapping.*

ditions (eg, time, speed, and response to perturbations). When observing the behavior, identify periods of stability and instability. As you examine periods of stability and instability, try to identify and characterize points of transition or change; propose potential control variables, that is, those variables that may be creating the transitions about instability points; and manipulate the variable to test that it really is a control variable. If it is, it should produce the change in the behavior that you hypothesize.

APPLYING DYNAMICAL SYSTEMS TO PHYSICAL THERAPY

Some therapists do examine transitional movement and apparently understand the value of a person's ability to change positions or behavior with relative ease in addition to his or her ability to maintain a position. What the dynamical systems theory suggests is that measurements of variability may be of more, if not equal, value to measurements of the average or best effort of a client. We might also try to identify exactly when movement performance breaks down. In others words, identify transition periods. Are there certain conditions that can create transitions, or periods of instability, or are there conditions that produce stability? We have all observed clients that produce two or three repetitions of a task very well and then their performance falls apart. It seems to take a while to get it back, or they may not pull their performance back together during that treatment session. Why does this happen? If we are observant, the dynamical systems theory may provide us with new clues. If a client's behavior is stable, we must decide when to try to produce periods of instability if this is how complex systems solve problems. From a motor learning perspective, instability should be important for the individual to learn new movement patterns. We *do* apply this concept to balance training when we perturb patients out of equilibrium and force them to adjust their own posture so they learn to produce the correct response. We *can* apply this concept to many other situations. Several researchers are identifying relative phasing and phase transitions for the study of human movement.

We are just beginning to apply concepts of dynamical systems and dynamic pattern theory to increase our understanding of normal and dysfunctional human movement. Although we know very little about the control of coordinated movement, we sometimes leap to apply new concepts developed from normal systems to those systems that produce dyscoordinated movement. We really do not know if these theories will apply to dysfunctional systems, and we can only test the assumptions and predictions and keep an open mind. Dynamical theory continues to be developed and tested. I urge you to keep abreast of this research because I believe it has promise for identifying elements of dysfunctional systems and guiding treatment intervention to resolve problems of control. Dynamical theory is only one of many approaches to the study of movement and is presented here for your consideration. As we continue our investigations, we must keep all new theoretical approaches in perspective. We would be remiss if we brought into play too haphazardly any one new approach, and we must refrain from shopping for the answer as we have done in the past.

References

1. Bekoff A. Embryonic development of the neural circuitry underlying motor coordination. In: Cowan WM, ed. *Studies in Developmental Neurobiology*. New York, NY: Oxford University Press Inc; 1981:134-170.
2. Okado N. Onset of synapse formation in the human spinal cord. *J Comp Neurol*. 1981;201:211-219.
3. Windle WF, Orr DW. The development of behavior in chick embryos: spinal cord structure correlated with early somatic motility. *J Comp Neurol*. 1934;60:287-308.
4. Bradley NS, Bekoff A. Development of locomotion: animal models. In: Wollacott M, Shumway-Cook A, eds. *The Development of Posture and Gait Across the Life Span*. Columbia, SC: University of South Carolina Press; 1989:48-73.
5. deVries JIP, Visser GHA, Prechtl HFR. The emergence of fetal behavior: I. Qualitative aspects. *Early Human Dev*. 1982;7:301-311.
6. Humphrey T. Some correlations between the appearance of human fetal reflexes and the development of the nervous system. *Prog Grain Res*. 1964;4:93-133.
7. Milani-Comparetti A. The neurophysiologic and clinical implications of studies on fetal motor behavior. *Seminars in Perinatology*. 1981;5:183-189.
8. Towen CL. Primitive reflexes-conceptual or semantic problem? *Clinics in Developmental Medicine*. 1984;94:115-125.
9. Lashley KS. The accuracy of movement in the absence of excitation from the moving organ. *Am J Physiol*. 1917;43:169-194.
10. Taub E. Movements in nonhuman primates deprived of sensory feedback. *Exerc Sport Sci Rev*. 1976;4:335-374.
11. Polit A, Bizzi E. Characteristics of motor programs underlying arm movements in monkeys. *J Neurophysiol*. 1979;42:183-194.
12. Schmidt P. *Motor Control and Learning*. 2nd ed. Champaign, Ill: Human Kinetics Publishers; 1989.
13. Marsden CD, Rothwell JC, Day BL. The use of pheripheral feedback in the control of movement In: Evarts EV, Wise SP, eds. *The Motor System in Neurobiology*. Amsterdam, The Netherlands: Elsevier Biomedical Press; 1985:215-222.
14. Shapiro DC, Zernicke RF, Gregor RJ, et al. Evidence for generalized motor programs using gait patterns analysis. *Journal of Motor Behavior*. 1981;13:33-47.
15. Turvey MT, Fitch H, Tuller B. The Bernstein perspective: I. The problem of degrees of freedom and context-conditioned variability. In: Kelso JAS, ed. *Human Motor Behavior*. Hillsdale, NJ: Lawrence Erlbaum Associates Inc; 1982:239-252.
16. Tuller B, Turvey MT, Fitch H. The Bernstein perspective: II. The concept of muscle linkage or coordinative structure. In: Kelso JAS, ed. *Human Motor Behavior*. Hillsdale, NJ: Lawrence Erlbaum Associates Inc; 1982:253-270.
17. Gleick J. *Chaos: Making a New Science*. New York, NY: Viking Penguin Inc; 1987.
18. Thelen E. Self-organization in developmental processes: can systems approaches work? In: Gunnar MR, Thelen E, eds. *Systems and Development. The Minnesota Symposia on Child Psychology*. Hillsdale, NJ: Lawrence Erlbaum Associates Inc; 1989:77-117.
19. Sparling JW, Seeds JW, Farran DC. The relationship of obstetrical ultrasound to parent and infant behavior. *Obst Gynecol*. 1988;72:902-907.
20. Fogel A, Thelen E. Development of early expressive and communicative action reinterpreting the evidence from a dy-

namic systems perspective. *Developmental Psychology.* 1987;23:747-761.

21. Gallistel CR. von Holst's coupled oscillators. In: Gallistel CR, ed. *The Organization of Action.* Hillsdale, NY: Lawrence Erlbaum Associates Inc; 1980:69-114.

22. Bernstein NA. *The Coordination and Regulation of Movements.* New York, NY: Pergamon Press Inc; 1967:104-113.

23. Haken H, Kelson JAS, Bunz H. A theoretical model of phase transitions in human hand movements. *Biol Cybern.* 1985;51:347-356.

24. Jerka JJ, Kelso JAS. The dynamic pattern approach to coordinated behavior: a tutorial review. In: Wallace SA, ed. *Perspectives on the Coordination of Movement.* New York, NY: Elsevier Science Publishing Co Inc; 1989:4-45.

25. Kelso JAS, Schoner G. Self-organization of coordinative movement patterns. *Human Movement Science.* 1988;7:27-46.

26. Sameroff AJ. Developmental systems: contexts and evolution. In: Mussen PH, ed. *Handbook of Child Psychology: History, Theory, and Methods.* 4th ed. New York, NY: John Wiley & Sons Inc; 1983;1:237-294.

27. Scott JP. Critical periods in organizational processes. In: Falkner F, Tanner JM, eds. *Human Growth: A Comprehensive Treatise. Developmental Biology: Prenatal Growth.* New York, NY: Plenum Publishing Corp; 1986;1:181-196.

28. Clark JE, Whithall J, Phillips SJ. Human interlimb coordination:the first 6 months of independent walking. *Dev Psychobiol.* 1988;21:445-456.

29. Fetters L. Motor development. In: Hanson MJ, ed. *Atypical Infant Development.* Baltimore, Md: University Park Press; 1984.

30. Heriza CB. Comparison of leg movements in preterm infants at term with healthy full term infants. *Phys Ther.* 1988;68:1687-1693.

31. Kugler PN, Kelso JAS, Turvey MT. On control and coordination of naturally developing systems. In: Kelso JAS, Clark JE, eds. *The Development of Movement Control and Coordination.* New York, NY: John Wiley & Sons Inc; 1982:5-78.

32. Newell KM. Constraints on the development of coordination. In: Wade MG, Whiting HTA, eds. *Motor Development in Children: Aspects of Coordination and Control.* Boston, Mass: Martinus Nijhoff; 1986:341-360.

33. Thelen E, Kelso JAS, Fogel A. Self-organizing systems and infant motor development. *Development Review.* 1987;7:39-65.

34. Ulrich BD. Development of stepping patterns in human infants: a dynamic systems perspective. *Journal of Motor Behavior.* 1980;21:392-408.

35. Tsonis PA, Tsonis AA. Chaos: principles and implications in biology. *Cabios.* 1989;5:27-32.

36. Glass L, Mackey MC. Pathological conditions resulting from instabilities in physiological control systems. *Ann NY Acad Sci.* 1979;316:214-234.

37. Kelso JAS, Tuller B. A dynamical basis for action systems. In: Gassaniga M, ed. *Handbook of Cognitive Neuroscience.* New York, NY: Plenum Publishing Corp; 1984:321-356.

38. Kelso JAS, Tuller B, Harris KS. A dynamic pattern perspective on the control and coordination of movement. In: Mac Neilage PF, ed. *Production of Speech.* New York, NY: Springer-Verlag New York Inc; 1987:137-173.

39. Scholz JP, Kelso JAS, Schoner G. Non-equilibrium phase transitions in coordinated biological motion: critical slowing down and switching time. *Physics Letters A.* 1987;123:390-394.

40. Scholz JP, Kelso JAS. Intentional switching between patterns of coordination depends on the intrinsic dynamics of the patterns. *Journal of Motor Behavior.* 1990;22:98-124.

41. Scholz JP, Kelso JAS. A quantitative approach to understanding the formation and change of coordinated movement patterns. *Journal of Motor Behavior.* 1989;21:122-144.

42. Schoner G, Kelso JAS. Dynamic pattern generation in behavioral and neural systems. *Science.* 1988;239:1513-1520.

43. Schoner G, Haken H, Kelso JAS. A stochastic theory of phase transitions in human hand movement. *Biological Cybern.* 1986;53:442-452.

44. Kelso JAS, Scholz JP. Cooperative phenomena in biological motion. In: Harken H, ed. *Complex Systems: Operational Approaches in Neurobiology, Physical Systems, and Computers.* New York, NY: Springer-Verlag New York Inc. 1985:124-149.

45. Kelso JAS, Scholz JP, Schoner G. Non-equilibrium phase transitions in coordinated biological motion: critical fluctuations. *Physics Letters A.* 1986;118:279-284.

46. Pearson KG. The control of walking. *Scientific American.* 1976;235:72-86.

47. Giuliani CA, Smith JL. Stepping behaviors in chronic spinal cats with one hindlimb deafferented. *J Neurosci.* 1987;7:2537-2546.

48. Stemmons VA, Wilhelm IJ. Electromyographic analysis of lower extremity motor coordination in children with learning disabilities. In: Sekerak D, ed. *Concepts in Motor Control, Motor Learning, and Exercise Physiology.* Chapel Hill, NC: Division of Physical Therapy, University of North Carolina at Chapel Hill; 1990;21-22.

49. Als H, Duffy F, McAnulty GB. The APIB: an assessment of functional competence in healthy preterm and fullterm infants regardless of gestational age at birth. *Infant Behavior and Development.* 1988;11:319-331.

50. Brazelton TB. *Neonatal Behavioral Assessment Scale.* 2nd ed. *Clinics in Developmental Medicine. No. 88.* Philadelphia, Pa: J B Lippincott Co; 1984.

51. Dubowitz LMS, Dubowitz V. *The Neurological Assessment of the Preterm and Fullterm Newborn Infant.* Philadelphia, Pa: J B Lippincott Co; 1981.

Chapter 6

How Theoretical Framework Biases Evaluation and Treatment

Emily A. Keshner, EdD, PT
Associate Professor
University of Illinois at Chicago
Chicago, IL 60612

Theory is most often considered the set of principles that guides and stimulates research.[1] On the basis of a theory, expectations are developed that can then be tested. But theories are not forged in concrete. Just the process of testing assumptions will generate results that will further refine the initial theory, making the underlying principles more accurate and effective.[1,2] Theory also underlies most of our clinical decision making. Consider the following situations:

1. A patient walks into your clinic holding his left arm in a flexed and pronated position. You discover that he has a history of transient ischemic attacks. You deduce that the position of the arm is indicative of a) a hyperactive flexor reflex, b) a biomechanical rearrangement of the center of mass in order to increase stability, or c) the substitution of brachialis and pronator teres muscles for a weakened biceps brachii muscle.
2. A patient with cerebral palsy has been walking within the parallel bars, and you decide that she is ready for a walker. She starts to ambulate across the gym floor. Just when she has to stop to let another patient pass her, she begins to fall. You deduce that a) she does not have enough lower extremity tone to support her during maintained stance, b) her postural reflexes are poorly developed, or c) the patient did not anticipate and plan for the change in the motor pattern.

There is no correct answer in the situations described above, but whichever option you would select is demonstrative of the theoretical framework under which you operate. By your following the definition of a theory as stated above, the next course of action would be to test your assumptions about the expected dysfunction. Clinical evaluation consists of a gross assessment of all systems, followed by definitive testing of areas of impairment.[3] Traditionally, this has included a separation of sensory and motor systems to assess strength, muscle resistance, and perception of specific sensory pathways. The process of evaluating these systems as separate entities is in itself an illustration of theoretical assumption. In other words, the assumption that the whole (ie, the functional or goal directed action) is simply a sum of the parts (ie, all of the participatory sensory and motor systems). Finally, the systems assessed as impaired are treated in a restorative fashion in an attempt to regain specific functions. A theoretical framework, therefore, sets up expectations to be tested that

govern the treatment approach to the extent that we only treat what has occurred to us to assess.

The history of neurotherapeutics in physical therapy is dominated by recipes for intervention stemming from the empirical observations of selected individuals. Although these treatments may have given some neurophysiological basis, this has usually occurred on a *post hoc* rather than a priori basis. Conclusions about the relationship between structure and function can change, and thus our treatment techniques must constantly be re-evaluated. Given new technology, new approaches, and new questions, we are constantly making new decisions about the operating characteristics of the system. Thus, it is preferable to understand why specific treatment techniques have been chosen rather than to learn a method of intervention for every symptom. Several papers have emerged in the recent past that elaborate on the changing concepts about central nervous processes and mechanisms and their relation to motor function but that do not attempt to address treatment technique.[4-6] Just incorporating changing neurophysiological concepts into previously established treatment techniques, however, implies a belief in 19th century localizationist theory that thought can be dissociated from action.[7] In this chapter, I will purport that the limiting factor in the growth and development of physical therapy as a valid clinical science is the theoretical framework that pervades both assessment and treatment. I have two specific goals for this paper. First, I plan to discuss the traditional and the current theoretical constructs that underlie neurotherapeutic techniques. I will use generic terms wherever possible to avoid any biases toward or against specific techniques. Second, I will demonstrate how traditional constructs have guided decision making processes in both assessment and treatment, and I will suggest how components that define central nervous system (CNS) motor disorders might change under a different conceptual approach. Through this, I hope to elucidate the importance of constantly testing and questioning the framework that guides clinical assessments and treatment.

BRIEF HISTORY OF NEUROTHERAPEUTIC THEORY

Most therapeutic interventions stem from beliefs about structure and function that emerged from developmental and clinical studies, but only some of the textbooks describing actual treatment techniques discussed the theoretical framework from which the treatment was developed.[3,8-10] Examination of primary sources and an overview of the theories permeating basic sciences at the time these treatments emerged does, however, present a comprehensive picture about how the CNS processes were viewed at that time. In the next two sections I will elaborate on these early ideas.

Structure of the Central Nervous System

The various neurotherapeutic approaches to CNS dysfunction are based on a unidirectional model of the CNS that derived from an evolutionary approach. Theories of CNS structure emerged from the maxim stating that phylogeny recapitulates ontogeny,[11] thereby suggesting that more complex nervoussystems were simply built in a vertical direction on the simpler systems found in less complex species. Simple functions translated into reflexes as the most basic unit of action to integrate the sensory stimulus and the motor response.[12] Complex functions were considered the most voluntary actions. The late development of cortex in the evolutionary scale supported the assumption that complex functions resided in higher levels of the nervous system. Thus the apparently stereotypical movement patterns seen early in child development (eg, tonic neck reflexes) were believed to be more primitive and eventually covered up or inhibited by the higher motor centers. Stereotypical movement patterns emerging later in motor development (eg, righting and equilibrium reactions) were considered indicative of adaptive functions of the higher motor centers.[13-14]

The 19th century neurologist, John Hughlings Jackson, was primarily responsible for expressing the concept of a brain responsible for movements and impressions rather than control of specific muscles. On the basis of clinical observation, Jackson originally described the CNS as a hierarchically functioning structure in which the normal, more complex patterns of behavior are, at a higher level of organization, combinations of the same movements that make up the abnormal, phylogenetically simpler behaviors (Fig.6-1).[15] The guiding principles of the hierarchical model were that the lowest motor and sensory centers (ie, spinal cord) were responsible for the simplest, most automatic, and least voluntary motor acts. The middle motor and sensory centers (ie, motor cortex) represent muscle combinations to produce movements that are less automatic and more voluntary. The highest motor centers (ie, frontal lobe) represent all of the body parts in a more complex fashion and constitute the anatomical basis for consciousness. Thus coordinated movement is generated by the compounding of simple reflexes.[12] A lesioned CNS is a system released from the inhibition of higher centers so that control of movement reverts to lower, more primitive motor centers. Thus the concept of abnormal "primitive" reflexes was developed.

A model such as this supported the use of the decerebrate animal to model CNS functions because separation of one level from another was believed simply to release lower motor centers from the inhibitory control of higher centers rather than to change the whole structure of CNS interaction. Later in this paper I will mention the ramifications of relying on the decerebrate model for making treatment decisions. A nervous system model that localized both specific physio-

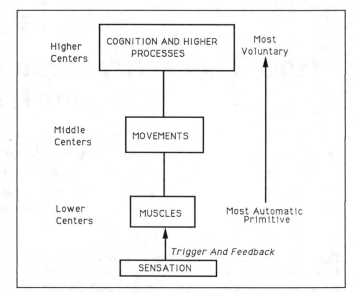

Fig. 6-1. *Hierarchical model of the central nervous system.*

logic and complex mental functions also emerged from clinical observations on the apparent loss of function with brain lesions and from electrical stimulation studies that elicited specified movements when exciting localized sites in cortex.[7,16] Localization of function implies that movements produced by a damaged CNS represent the loss of that specific function; therefore movement processes can be repaired by reinstating that function.

Although Jackson opposed narrow localizationist theory,[7] the existence of a somatotopic organization and modal specificity of primary projection areas in the brain cannot be denied. Purposive action, however is never elicited from stimulating a single pathway or locus of nervous tissue. In other words, the movement product or behavior is not localized in specific brain cell clusters. Functional, goal directed actions emerge instead from the process of transmission between overlapping networks (or subsystems) in the CNS that serve a particular function.[17] These actions are then shaped and modified to meet musculoskeletal dynamics and kinetic forces encounteredin the environment. As suggested by Weiss, "independent entities are interconnected by the common environmental matrix, in which they lie embedded, so that for every single one of the discrete items, every other item is part and parcel of the former's environment."[17(p6)] The establishment of interconnecting subsystems probably occurs during development, where connections between essential elements are formed.[7]

Developmental Principles

The belief that the developmental process reveals information about normal CNS processes also stems from a hierarchical model in which the establishment of skilled movement is reflective of an ontogenetic (ie, evolutionary) progression. Historically, theories of development have attempted to appoint a single locus of control over the developmental process (ie, evolution, genetics, or environment) and then to illustrate how all organismic behaviors emerge from that locus.[18] As any single locus has failed to account for the variations found in human behavior, an interactive theory between the three control mechanisms has emerged. Yet, as a result of hierarchical theory, two beliefs continue to dominate our approach to treatment of both children and adults with CNS damage. First, that stereotypic processes (ie, reflexes) dominate movement throughout early development, and second, that movements emerging from a damaged CNS represent a reversion to control by lower, more primitive motor centers.

A hierarchical framework would state that normal movement behavior is a developmental process of combining simpler reflexes, elicited by the appropriate stimuli from the environment or from the movement itself, into more complex behavior patterns of higher, later developing motor centers.[13,19] Early reflex patterns are believed to serve as building blocks, and normal movement is believed to occur as a highly automatic and consistent progression within the species from rolling to sitting, crawling, standing, and walking.[20] Because damage in the mature CNS represents a reversal to the early movement behaviors, adult patients with CNS damage have typically been treated by attempting to reinstate the childhood progression. Developmental assessment charts[21-22] and studies on the responsiveness of the fetal infant to sensory stimulation[23-24] support this consistent behavioral picture in posture and action throughout the period of gestation and on into the first years of life. The weakness in this belief is that it reflects a primacy of neural structure over function and fails to acknowledge the consistencies inherent in other aspects of development.

Alternative views of development, some emerging from basic research, do exist. Although Piaget[25] believed that the earliest patterns are genetically developed, he acknowledged that during movement the inherent behaviors are adapted to meet the environmental constraints: new patterns are assimilated to the old patterns while old patterns are accommodated to meet the new demands. Thus intercoordinated sensorimotor systems that subserve a structure-function relationship are developed. For example, a study of infant sucking behaviors in response to nutritive and nonnutritive stimuli revealed that children as young as 4 to 10 weeks old did not exhibit a specific response pattern but did learn adaptive strategies that varied across individuals.[26] Through histographic analyses of the structural maturation among feline litter mates, Scheibel and Scheibel[27] suggested that the uterine environment plays an active role in structural maturation and subsequent function. Environmental enrichment studies, using premature infants as subjects, have also found increased physiological growth rather than increased cognitive development.[28-29]

Maturational differences that correlate with consistent movement behaviors support the suggestion that, from conception, the dual influences of genetics and learning on the motor systems cannot be dichotomized. Although emergent movements appear as fixed behavior patterns, they should be viewed in the context of an adaptive species operating from a predetermined musculoskeletal system within the consistent forces encountered in the prenatal and postnatal environments.[30] Within this framework, it is unlikely that any two mature CNS and musculoskeletal systems, adapted to many years of individualized movement experiences, would produce exactly the same movement patterns or respond in exactly the same fashion to new stimuli. As will be discussed later in the paper, at some levels of analysis (ie, measurement of motor impulses or electromyographic responses) these differences can be revealed. Furthermore, within a theoretical framework that does not view movements exhibited by a damaged CNS as representative of a dissolution of the maturational process and release of primitive behaviors, using the developmental progression to assess and treat adult patients with CNS damage is inappropriate. One such framework, distributed control theory, will be expanded on in the next section.

CURRENT CONCEPTS OF CENTRAL NERVOUS SYSTEM ORGANIZATION

The discussion above suggests a CNS that controls movement from the highest cortical centers by inhibiting the output of lower motor centers and that relies on appropriate sensory inputs to produce behavior. Purposive movement is seen to develop from primitive, mass movement reflex patterns to voluntary motor patterns that are more precisely matched to the task only by the characteristics of the sensory inputs to which they are responsive.[19] Differentiation of function was thus considered to be dependent on further differentiation of the structures within the CNS.[16] This premise implies a system dependent on sensory inputs to initiate action, and it does not explain how new movements are incorporated into the system. In this section I will present an alternative view of the CNS in which structure and function are not inextricably linked, and complex movement patterns can be generated from within the central network. I will then explain how new definitions of certain motor mechanisms can affect therapeutic assessment and treatment within a model of central motor programs and overlapping networks.

Central Generation of Motor Patterns

Perhaps the single greatest conceptual change to the theory of central nervous function came with shifting the locus of motor control from the sensory stimuli that generated movement as part of the "black box," stimulus-response model, to central initiation of movements that can wholly be performed in the absence of sensory input.[31] Experimental evidence has consistently shown that complex, coordinated movement behaviors can be produced in the absence of sensory inputs.[32] Patterns of movement are neurally represented but not structurally imposed so that modifications can occur that successfully match the movement to changes in the task.

Clinical and experimental data supporting the concept of a central motor program is, perhaps, the strongest evidence against the hierarchical theory of complex, voluntary movements that are combinations of sensory dependent, simple reflexes.[32-33] The motor program is considered to be an abstract memory structure that is prepared or is present in the CNS in advance of the movement to be produced.[34] Rather than relying on sensory inputs to specify and trigger a movement pattern, the motor program is responsible for specifying which muscles are to participate, the order of contraction, the temporal phasing of muscle activation, and the relative force of contraction; sensory feedback is then used to correct errors in execution while the program is in operation.[34] Performers must actively process and make decisions about the information that is coming into the system, and the movement is more accurate when a performer is an active rather than passive participant.[35-36] In the information processing model, the responsibility of the sensory-motor system is to detect and correct errors of motor output rather than to initiate prepackaged movement patterns.

A central motor program, therefore, is a complex unit of behavior that is generated as a whole but that can be modified and varied by the sensory signals arising during execution. The effect of removing our reliance on specific sensory inputs to produce movement is to shift the locus of movement control from extrinsic to intrinsic factors, change the role of sensory signals in movement production, and consequently, affect the ways in which we facilitate movement behaviors during treatment. Shifting the focus of movement control away from sensory feedback could have major ramifications for both assessment and treatment methods in physical therapy. Reliance on a single modality of sensory input (eg, through tapping or stretching a muscle) becomes a questionable method of generating purposeful movement patterns within a framework in which the system has to set up a plan for movement to be matched against the movement generated feedback. Treatment concepts of facilitation and inhibition will be discussed further later in this paper.

Distributed Control Model

All of our popular treatment approaches for CNS dysfunction have been based on a unidirectional model of the CNS that ignores the multiple lines of communication at all levels. Although it is impossible to ignore the structural hierarchy that exists in the nervous system, the distributed control as opposed to the hierarchical model acknowledges that any behavior is subject to control by several different sites and that communication between sites can take place in an ascending, descending, and lateral fashion (Fig.6-2).[37] Analysis of the information received, in the form of synaptic processing, occurs at each juncture; thus the message transmitted is never exactly the same as the message received. The central hierarchy should not be perceived as a descending chain of command but as an overlapping circular network where each level can influence those both above and below.[38] By following this conceptualization, the role of a specific site in the CNS is no longer to produce a single product or outcome but to be part of the process underlying acquisition and control of skilled movement behaviors.[37]

A clear example of an overlapping network exists in the structural formation of the CNS. Every neuron receives convergent inputs that derive from both peripheral and central origins.[39] Neurons that have been converged on from many sources will then transmit to many other neurons that then transmit along their respective pathways (divergence). The final output of the network does not simply reflect a reflexive control over its own muscle's action, but it reflects a response calculated to achieve the overall goal of the system determined through the summation of both ascending and descending inputs. Convergence from many levels onto these interneurons, and their subsequent divergence of information distribution to more than one level of output, shifts the control over the final response. Rather than the control being

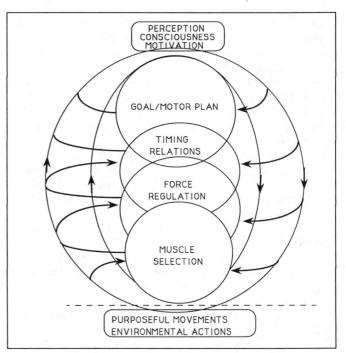

Fig 6-2. *Levels of the central nervous system hierachy illustrated as overlapping circular networks within a distributed control model (reprinted, by permission, from Evarts EV, Wise SP, Bousfield D, eds. The Motor System in Neurobiology. New York, NY: Elsevier Science Publishing Co Inc; 1985:104.)*

located either peripherally or centrally, a concept of distributed responsibility among all levels of the nervous system emerges.

Information flow in this theoretical framework carries import for error detection and correction as well as for generating a response. The process of error detection occurs as a comparison between the expected outcome and the actual outcome of our actions, and the process incorporates both the motor and sensory impulses. The motor program is an example of centrally initiated, motor impulses that are planned and available before the onset of the movement. On the sensory side, feedforward loops are indicative of central planning and anticipation of a movement behavior. Feedforward information prepares the system for the impending consequences of an activity, as observed through tuning or changing the threshold for activation of a pathway.[40-41] Mechanisms exist for detecting errors in movement production that are not dependent on sensory feedback to be triggered. For example, the gamma motoneurons produce an efference copy, or a copy of the motor command, to be sent to the comparison center in cerebellum.

Electrophysiological recordings have shown the existence of circular pathways between cerebellum and motor cortex[42] and between basal ganglia and association cortex[43] that could embody these feedforward loops for the purpose of error detection and correction (Fig.6-3). Rapid transmission between these sites would be indicative of a system that sends its intent or plan of action to another area for comparison. Comparators then match this information either with a previous plan of action (in the case of basal ganglia) or with

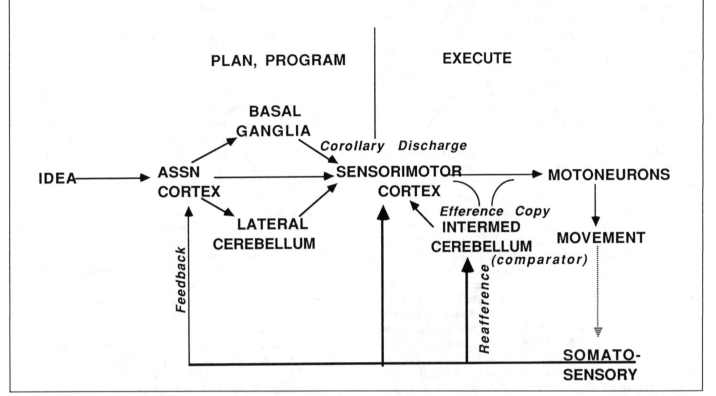

Fig 6-3. *Diagram of suggested directions of information flow in the central nervous system, for voluntary motor control (derived and reprinted from Brooks,[34] by permission of Oxford University Press.)*

the ongoing sensory-motor circumstances (in the case of cerebellum). Differences between the actual and intended plan can then be determined and actions adjusted or modified on the basis of both the previous movement experiences and the momentary demands of the task.

REDEFINING CRITERIA FOR ASSESSMENT AND TREATMENT

A comprehensive patient evaluation would usually include measures of range of motion (both passive and active), muscle strength, and independence in functional activities.[3] In the case of upper motor neuron disorders, muscle tone, reflex, and synergic patterns of movement would be examined. Treatments would then be instituted that attempted either to regain components that were lost or diminished or to lessen the influence of those components deemed "abnormal." Under the guise of a hierarchical system in which motor behaviors of a damaged nervous system are viewed as a loss of normal inhibitory controls, it makes sense to chart the "released" behaviors and to attempt either to inhibit[8] or to integrate[9] these behaviors into normal movements. With this approach, treatment concentrates on replacing specific movements and even specific muscle patterns rather than on enhancing or substituting functional behaviors. We seem to follow the thesis that "practice makes perfect" and continually elaborate on specific motor patterns that have been lost or changed by CNS lesion.

Under the theory of distributed control, functional behaviors are defined by an adaptive process with motor outputs that vary in accordance with the task constraints. There-

fore either assessing the presence of a single motor pattern or retraining a specified movement pattern does not incorporate the CNS mechanisms normally involved in the production of movement. Concepts of CNS organization emerging from the theoretical model of distributed control are as follows:
1. Multiple levels and mechanisms of control.
2. Central initiation of goal directed or purposive movements.
3. Preplanning or anticipation of environmental demands.
4. Modification of a response through sensory feedback.
5. Behaviors planned on the basis of sensory, biomechanical, *and* task outcome demands.

Research results evaluated on the basis of the distributed control model have produced new explanations for, and descriptions of, CNS processes. In the following sections, I will present the changing conceptualization of some symptoms, which are commonly associated with CNS disorders, in order to examine how assessment and treatment procedures are influenced by the theoretical framework.

Changing the Concepts Underlying Assessment

Spasticity and associated reactions. The widely accepted definition of spasticity is that of "a velocity dependent increase in tonic stretch reflexes (muscle tone), with exaggerated tendon jerks resulting from hyperexcitability of the stretch reflex."[44(p485)] The problem with this definition of hypertonicity is that it is derived from a decerebrate cat model. This model is not directly applicable to human cerebral spasticity because fusimotor drive in the decerebrate cat is abnormally high, whereas fusimotor drive in human upper motor neuron syndromes is normal.[45] Spasticity might be better thought of as the net result of supraspinal and spinal inputs rather than as a change in the spindle's response to stretch. The most likely cause is that the motoneuron pools are more depolarized as a result of a net increase in tonic excitatory synaptic inputs from descending pathways and local interneuron signals. If threshold is lowered, a smaller or slower motion than usual will result in a resistance to manual stretch and a muscle force that increases with an increased joint angle.

More important than the cause of apparent hypertonus is the finding that motor dysfunction in patients with CNS damage is not due just to changes in tonicity.[45] Both clinical and experimental investigations suggest that decreasing the level of hypertonicity will not enhance motor performance. Therefore assessment of tone and subsequently, concentration on its reduction through treatment will have doubtful impact on the ultimate improvement in motor control and production. Performance deficits that have been identified in patients include first, the *orderly recruitment* patterns within the motoneuron pool 'is lost' thereby producing inefficient muscle activation.[46] Second, the *timing* between agonist and antagonist actions is impaired, thereby producing ineffective muscle contractions.[47] Third, the *pattern* of muscles selected to perform the task is disturbed.[48] All of these are deficits in the basic characteristics of central motor programs; thus the motor effect of a CNS lesion is not a function of hyperexcitability but probably is a manifestation of a central motor program that has been altered to compensate for peripheral (ie, muscle weakness) and central changes.[48]

In patients with CNS lesions, weakness is compensated by the number of motor units recruited and the frequency of discharge.[49] A theoretical framework stating that biomechanical factors (eg, muscle strength) have a significant influence on the movement pattern would suggest that movements correlating with force production are indicative of muscle weakness. One such clinical behavior is associated reactions. Traditionally, these reactions have been attributed to a reflex tensing of muscle and involuntary limb movements that are associated with forceful movements in other parts of the body[9] resulting from tonic postural mechanisms released from voluntary control.[50] A study of patients with hemiplegia performing isometric contractions with controlled torque outputs demonstrated the effects of increasing force output during a directionally specific upper extremity task.[48] Performed on the uninvolved upper extremities of hemiparetic subjects, this investigation revealed an orderly spatial distribution in the normal limb, where each muscle could be activated over a broad range of motion and the EMG was scaled to force output.[14] The peak EMG value was at the angle of best mechanical advantage for that muscle. Muscles of the spastic limbs, however, exhibited severe disturbances both in the spatial orientation of their largest response output and in the linear scaling between muscle activation and force. Thus muscles that did not normally participate were recruited at forces that were unusually large for the task. These results suggest that associated reactions are a central reorganization of muscle activation patterns to compensate for musculoskeletal weakness rather than some postural reflex mechanism.

Reflexes. The concept of a primitive response pattern that must be inhibited by brain centers that developed later in evolution is an inefficient and unidirectional view of CNS processes. It is more economical for the CNS to use genetically predetermined movement patterns in support of complex movement than to devote precious space and attention toward masking undesirable responses. There is evidence suggesting that reflex patterns are either present in or supportive of normal movements. Hellebrandt[51] performed an often quoted study demonstrating that force at the wrist would increase when the subjects turned their heads, thereby eliciting the tonic neck reflex. The role of reflexes in normal movements has also been studied during locomotion where it was found that the placing reaction worked functionally to increase flexion during the swing phase in order to avoid stumbling.[52] When stimulated during the stance phase, however, the reflex did not exert an effect other than some slightly increased extension. Diminished reflex gains have also been found in the neck muscles of decerebate[53] and alert[54] cats; it was suggested that the cervicocollic reflex may be suppressed during active head movements to prevent its opposition to a desired head rotation. Spinal reflexes, therefore, may work as a simple motor set that either supports the ongoing movement or is called in to compensate for unexpected perturbations during movement.[55]

Evidence that invalidates the assumption that reflexes are building blocks of voluntary movement also exists. Movements generated in a particular direction by the voluntary motor system were found to use different muscle patterns than the same movements generated by the reflex system. Kinematic organization of motor commands acting on multiple neck muscles has been examined during the vestibulocollic reflex in decerebrate cats.[56] Each muscle was found to have a direction of whole body rotation in which it was maximally activated in a consistent pattern over time and across animals. The optimal response patterns of the muscles in a freely moving animal, however, were very different from the patterns elicited in decerebrate animals or in alert animals whose heads were stabilized (Fig.6-4).[57]

Increased complexity of sensory inputs might explain these kinematic differences. Unlike the vestibulocollic reflex, which occurs purely as a result of semicircular canal inputs, voluntary responses can be organized by retinal, somatosensory, vestibular, and descending inputs. Another explanation is that increased variability in vertebral joint motions alters muscle lever arms during active head movement. Consistent appearance of these movement patterns in a damaged CNS may reflect two possible modes of CNS reorganization. Either the EMG patterns in a disordered CNS are unrelated to any established normal pattern of motion (compensatory process) or the disruption of inputs to motor centers (ie, motor cortex, cerebellum, and basal ganglia) switches from control by the normally predominant pathways to control by alternative pathways (switching or plastic process). This would then modify the influence of specific inputs on the spinal motor servo.[47]

Given the above information, clinicians need to re-evaluate their belief that the simple, consistent motor patterns called primitive reflexes are truly interfering with the development of normal motor function. Instead of attempt-

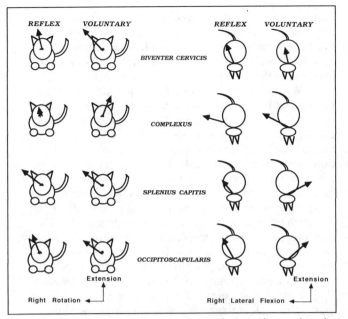

Fig. 6-4. *Electromyographic responses in four neck muscles of an alert cat during reflex and voluntary head movements. Direction and size of each arrow indicates relative direction and magnitude od activation. Arrows at bottom of figure indicate planes of head motion for the front facing and top down orientation of the cat.*

ing to inhibit what may very well be a compensatory response to a damaged CNS, we should concentrate more on the relevant inputs that elicit these stereotyped patterns of movement and on the client's ability to process and use the environmental information if we truly hope to influence motor output.

Synergies. Originally, the concept of a synergy was applied directly to muscles that supported the agonist muscle by preventing undesirable activity in other muscles.[58] Later, this concept was expanded to describe the stereotypical action of the limb in patients with hemiplegia.[9] Synergy then described a group of muscles that were activated consistently to produce a single limb motion. But that description assumes that movements are stored in the CNS, and it ignores the variability found in patterns of response to the same task. A study of upper extremity muscles during isometric contractions with controlled torque outputs has demonstrated that EMG activation of a muscle changes in relation to either the direction of motion or the bending of the joint.[59] Thus the synergic pattern appears to be highly situation-dependent rather than predetermined in the CNS.

Synergies are considered functionally essential because the brain could not possibly control all of the degrees of freedom and potential variables in any given movement.[60] These variables include the multiple muscle groups and mechanical couplings that occur. Another characteristic of a synergy is that the contraction of the muscles is spatially and temporally sequenced.[61] Thus the CNS relies on synergic mechanisms that are composed of a group of muscles that can span several joints and are constrained to act as a single unit. In the patient with CNS damage, the consistent response picture for single limb may be more representative of

a motor program attempting to compensate for muscle weakness (see discussion of associated reactions above) and being unable to process the regulatory sensory feedback than of a reversion to stereotyped movement patterns.

Recent experiments on other complex motor systems, including the oral-facial system[62] and the head and neck,[63] have demonstrated that the same action can be accomplished with a variety of different muscle patterns rather than a single muscular pattern or a synergy. Any movement behavior, therefore, cannot simply be described by the two-dimensional dichotomy of an agonist-antagonist. Instead, any single movement reflects the overall force summation of all the muscles around a joint and should be analyzed as a three-dimensional system where muscles act as linear force generators equally excitable under all conditions.[64] Redundancy exists in the CNS both in the potential control mechanisms (ie, sensory pathways, reflexes, and voluntary mechanisms) and in the response actuators (ie, muscles). Having more muscles than are necessary to control the musculoskeletal system provides the potential for multiple solutions to a single motor task. Finding that a single motor behavior can result from one of multiple muscle combinations (equifinality) is promising of a successful outcome with therapeutic intervention. This finding indicates that functional movement patterns can be under the control of different motor programs and can possibly use different control mechanisms, yet still attain the appropriate coordinated response.[62]

Postural control mechanisms. From the early studies of posture up to the present time, posture has variously been defined as 1) a component of movement, either the underlying tonus or the resultant position; 2) a process distinct from the movement it subserves; 3) a system of dynamic behaviors resulting from the summation of tonic reflexes; 4) a segmental reflex response; or 5) a behavioral adaptation developed through experience in a dynamic environment. Confusion exists about whether postural control is distinct from control of manipulation and translation and whether reflex production of static positioning of body segments is equivalent to control of posture. This confusion is reflected in our clinical assessments and treatment of balance. Traditionally, testing of dynamic postural reactions has relied on eliciting equilibrium responses by pushing on the trunk or perturbing the subject on a tiltboard.[65] We attempt to train balance by having patients maintain a static or dynamic standing position with a reduced base of support. Drawing functional conclusions from these procedures can be faulty because the characteristics of the stimulus and the task are unrelated to normal environmental constraints and the varied points of application of the disturbances will vary the importance of the sensory pathways conveying information about the perturbation. We do not replicate the forces that are imposed on the body when stumbling or being thrown in a moving vehicle, nor do we account for responses during functional tasks that require subtle postural adjustments during reaching or carrying a load.

When upright stance is disrupted, balance reactions could be generated by the peripheral nervous systems and the CNS in a number of ways. One extreme possibility is that the movement at each joint is solely dependent on local reflex responses to changes at that joint. The other extreme is to assume that both muscular activation and movement co-ordination are part of a centrally preprogrammed strategy triggered by the sensory inputs signalling the onset and direction of destabilizing forces. A centrally preprogrammed response would presumably involve coordinated patterns of muscle activity or synergies between and across joints.

Studies in which stimulus variables were controlled have shown that postural reactions occur at all segments of the body and that the final output may be organized by several different control mechanisms (eg, somatic, proprioceptive, and vestibular reflexes; voluntary processes; and body mechanics).[66] Stabilization studies on a posture platform have also shown a large amount of variability in the muscles selected to produce the postural strategy and in their spatial ordering.[67] The ultimate postural response is probably influenced by a variety of factors including initial joint position, site of perturbation, integrity of the musculoskeletal and neuromuscular systems, and functional constraints of the task. One primary function of postural reactions is to maintain axial support during limb movement. Posture is linked intrinsically with the use of the limbs; without the stability offered the limbs by the postural processes there can be no effective movement. The CNS must process the feedforward information related to the intended movement and the force characteristics encountered. A failure to compensate for imbalance could be indicative of an inability to produce the necessary muscle forces through weakness or lack of a preparatory set, improper information processing, impaired motor coordination, or a combination of these.

Re-examining Assessment and Treatment Procedures

Generally, the concepts above all share one single theme. Movement production is a process highly dependent on the integrity of the musculoskeletal system and the requirements of the immediate motor task. A corollary would be that movement responses are rarely simple flexor-extensor patterns that are replicable across all individuals. This variability causes difficulty for the clinician who is looking for well-defined motor deficits and who wants to teach a specific movement or muscle action to regain functional abilities. If the *process* of movement production rather than the movement itself becomes the goal of clinical intervention, then the definition of two predominant interventions, facilita-

tion and inhibition, are altered greatly. Facilitatory or inhibitory techniques would no longer be directed toward acquiring discrete muscle actions. Instead, the processing of relevant sensory information would be facilitated by augmenting sensory feedback (Fig.6-5).[68]

We have been following the assumption that enough practice will eventually lead to acquisition of a skill, although we know full well that this is not necessarily true in the presence of a sensorimotor deficit. Practicing a function that is impaired does not necessarily re-establish that function, nor does it automatically develop successful compensatory functions. Studies have been done, however, to determine how skilled movement is learned, and there are two basic concepts in motor learning that should facilitate the achievement of a successful treatment outcome.[68-69] First and foremost is feedback. Feedback can arrive along many routes and take many different forms including sensory inputs (visual, auditory, proprioceptive), cognitive processing (discussion and planning), and movement-related signals (kinesthetic inputs, successful attainment of a movement goal). During learning, it is helpful to supply two kinds of feedback: knowledge about the movement process and knowledge about the result of the movement. This means communicating with your patient on some level (either verbally or by augmenting feedback during the performance of a task) about the treatment goals and how they are to be attained. Adaptation is another concept important to motor relearning, particularly because the mechanisms usually responsible for setting up, triggering, or performing the correct motor program are disordered. Because there is little evidence that learning a response to meet the task demands in one situation will necessarily carry over when the constraints of the task have changed, it is important to practice the desired movement under as many sensory and environmental conditions as possible. Conditions for motor relearning should most closely resemble the environmental context encountered during the patient's daily activities, but overlearning can inhibit adaptation. Do not make the patient so comfortable with a single response pattern that he or she will attempt to use that response even when it interferes with the generation of a more appropriate response.

It is tempting to believe that we can teach a specific pattern of movement that will resolve all of the motor disor-

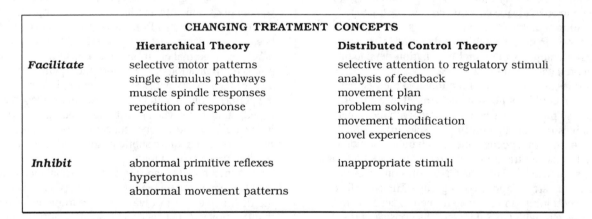

CHANGING TREATMENT CONCEPTS		
	Hierarchical Theory	**Distributed Control Theory**
Facilitate	selective motor patterns	selective attention to regulatory stimuli
	single stimulus pathways	analysis of feedback
	muscle spindle responses	movement plan
	repetition of response	problem solving
		movement modification
		novel experiences
Inhibit	abnormal primitive reflexes	inappropriate stimuli
	hypertonus	
	abnormal movement patterns	

Fig. 6-5. *Effects of two different theoretical frameworks on the treatment concepts of facilitation and inhibition.*

ders found in our patients. In the context of a distributed control framework, however, functional movements cannot be taught. But the process of identifying relevant stimuli, recognizing movement goals, analyzing feedback, and modifying the movement to match the demands of the task may be taught.[68-69] The assessment process in which the clinician must engage requires that the area of dyscontrol be identified (eg, information processing, feedforward, feedback, motor coordination). Then therapeutic conditions need to be controlled. These conditions would include testing responses to novel versus predictable events, controlling stimulus characteristics (direction, velocity, intensity, duration), and controlling the nonregulatory events in the environment to which we do not wish the patient to respond.

CONCLUSIONS

Treatment planning traditionally depends on the assessment tools. To that end, assessments have been devised that examine multiple components of movement. Components deemed important to assess, however, have been derived from the existing model of the CNS. Any information garnered about the CNS disorder is totally dependent on assessment procedures. Criteria for assessment are based on the underlying theoretical framework and subsequently, determine the criteria for treatment. Regrettably, choices about assessment are often made without consideration of any other possible criteria. Also, evaluation techniques are often used as the treatment itself. For example, the motor disorder of the first patient presented at the beginning of this paper is expressed in the position of the left upper extremity. Adherence to the hierarchical model would lead you to suspect hyperactive stretch reflexes as the cause of the postural arrangement; thus you would assess and treat the patient for hypertonicity and stereotypical behaviors. If you believed that developmental principles override all normal movement organization and that elevated upper extremities represent a reversion to a more immature locomotor pattern as a result of CNS lesion, then the developmental reflexes would be tested and the patient taken through the developmental progression as a standard for treatment. The last selection might stem from a belief in a theoretical model in which muscle activation patterns were organized to adapt to changes in the musculoskeletal system, thereby requiring that muscle weakness and modified recruitment patterns be assessed and treated.

In the second case study, choices "a" and "b" can be explained, respectively, by the hierarchical framework in which an inability to support stance is due either to abnormal tonus or to an inability of the postural reflexes to provide stability. In either case, this patient would probably receive treatment protocols very similar to that of the first patient. Yet option "c" implies that the performer's ability to process and plan for changing environmental stimuli will have significant effects on the movement outcome. In this case, it might be as important to train the patient to anticipate changes in the movement pattern as it is to teach the pattern itself; thus the patient with cerebral palsy would receive an individualized and very different protocol than the patient with transient ischemic attacks.

We need to become more creative in identifying the underlying causes of a movement problem and in finding alternative routes to compensate for the absent or impaired function. For this reason, it is essential that clinicians continually keep abreast of current research findings and operational theories. New theories of CNS organization should be viewed with optimism. A CNS that does not follow specific labelled lines between anatomy, physiology, and function presents more opportunity for external intervention and re-education than does a system in which loss of structural integrity means the loss of any opportunity to restore function. Most importantly, clinicians need to be continually aware of the concepts governing their assessment and treatment choices and to incorporate new research and information that has an impact on their own clinical decision making.

Acknowledgment

I thank Dr. Judith Stoecker for her insightful comments and stimulating discussions about the topics presented in this paper.

References

1. Cox RC, West WL. *Fundamentals of Research for Health Professionals*. Rockville, Md: RAMSCO Publishing Co; 1982.
2. Payton OD. *Research: The Validation of Clinical Practice*. Philadelphia, Pa: F A Davis Co; 1979.
3. Sullivan PE, Markos PD, Minor MAD. *An Integrated Approach to Therapeutic Exercise: Theory and Clinical Application*. Reston, Va: Reston Publishing Co; 1982.
4. Keshner EA. Reevaluating the theoretical model underlying the neurodevelopmental treatment approach. *Phys Ther*. 1981;61:1035-1040.
5. Gordon JH. Assumptions underlying physical therapy intervention: theoretical and historical perspectives. In: Carr JH, Shepherd RB, Gordon J, et al, eds. *Movement Science: Foundations for Physical Therapy in Rehabilitation*. Rockville, Md: Aspen Publishers Inc; 1987:1-30
6. Keshner EA. Can changing concepts enhance efficacy in physical therapy? *Pediatric Physical Therapy*.1990. In press.
7. Luria AR. *The Working Brain: An Introduction to Neuropsychology*. New York,NY: Basic Books Inc; 1973.
8. Bobath K. The normal postural reflex mechanism and its deviation in children with cerebral palsy. *Physiotherapy*. 1971;57:515-525.
9. Brunnstrom S. *Movement Therapy in Hemiplegia: A Neurophysiological Approach*. New York, NY: Harper & Row Publishers Inc; 1970.
10. Knott M, Voss DE. *Proprioceptive Neuromuscular Facilitation*. 2nd ed. New York, NY: Harper & Row Publishers Inc; 1968.
11. Fay T. The origin of human movement. *Am J Psychiatry*. 1955;11:644-652.
12. Gallistel CR. *The Organization of Action: A New Synthesis*. Hillsdale, NJ: Lawrence Erlbaum Associates Inc; 1980.
13. Roberts TDM. Reflex balance. *Nature*. 1973;244:156-158.
14. Weisz S. Studies in equilibrium reactions. *J Nervous Ment Dis*. 1938;88:150-162.
15. Foerster O. The motor cortex in man in light of Hughlings Jackson's doctrines. In: Payton OD, Hirt S, Newton RA, eds. *Scientific Bases for Neurophysiologic Approaches to Therapeutic Exercise: An Anthology*. Philadelphia, Pa: F A Davis Co; 1977:13-18.

16. Penfield W. Mechanisms of voluntary movement. In: Payton OD, Hirt S, Newton RA, eds. *Scientific Bases for Neurophysiologic Approaches to Therapeutic Exercise: An Anthology*. Philadelphia, Pa: F A Davis Co; 1977:19-31.

17. Weiss PA. The living system: determinism stratified. In: Koestler A, Smythies JR, eds. *Beyond Reductionism: New Perspectives in the Life Sciences*. New York, NY: Macmillan Publishing Co; 1969:3-42.

18. McGraw M. Maturation of behavior. In: Carmichael L, ed. *Manual of Child Psychology*. New York, NY: John Wiley & Sons Inc; 1946.

19. Twitchell TE. Reflex mechanisms and the development of prehension. In: Connolly K, ed. *Mechanisms of Motor Skill Development*. New York, NY: Academic Press Inc; 1970:25-37.

20. Jacobs MJ. Development of normal motor behavior. *Am J Phys Med*. 1967;46:41-51.

21. Amiel-Tison C. Neurological evaluation of the maturity of new- born infants. *Arch Dis Childhood*. 1968;43:89-93.

22. Dargassies St.A. *Neurological Development in the Fullterm and Premature Neonate*. New York. NY: Elsevier Science Publishing Co Inc; 1977.

23. Hooker D. Development reaction to environment. *Yale J Bio Med*. 1960;32:431-440.

24. Humphrey T. Embryology of the central nervous system: with some correlations with functional development. *Embryology*. 1964;1:60-64.

25. Piaget J, Inhelder B. The gaps in empiricism. In: Koestler A, Smythies JR, eds. *Beyond Reductionism: New Perspectives in the Life Sciences*. New York, NY: Macmillan Publishing Co; 1969:118-148.

26. Bruner JS. On voluntary action and its hierarchical structure. In: Koestler A, Smythies JR, eds. *Beyond Reductionism: New Perspectives in the Life Sciences*. New York, NY: Macmillan Publishing Co; 1969:161-179.

27. Schiebel M, Schiebel A. Some structural and functional substrates of development in young cats. *Prog Br Res*. 1964;9:6-25.

28. Powell LF. The effect of extra stimulation and maternal involvement on the development of low birth weight infants and on maternal behavior. *Child Dev*. 1974;45:106-113.

29. White JL, Labarba RC. The effects of tactile and kinesthetic stimulation of neonatal development in the premature infant. *Dev Psych*. 1976;9:569-577.

30. Anokhin PK. Systemogenesis as a general regulator of brain development. *Prog Br Res*. 1964;9:54-86.

31. Keele SW. Learning and control of coordinated motor patterns: the programming perspective. In: Kelso JAS, ed. *Human Motor Behavior: An Introduction*. Hillsdale, NJ: Lawrence Erlbaum Associates Inc; 1982:161-186.

32. Taub E, Berman AJ. Movement and learning in the absence of sensory feedback. In: Freedman SJ, ed. *The Neuropsychology of Spatially Oriented Behavior*. Homewood, Ill: Dorsey Press; 1968:173-192.

33. Lashley KS. The accuracy of movement in the absence of excitation from the moving organ. *Am J Physiol*. 1917;43:169-194.

34. Schmidt RA. More on motor programs. In: Kelso JAS, ed. *Human Motor Behavior: An Introduction*. Hillsdale, NJ: Lawrence Erlbaum Associates Inc; 1982:189-218.

35. Goodwin GM, McCloskey DI, Matthews PBC. The contribution of muscle afferents to kinesthesia shown by vibration induced illusions of movement and by the effects of paralyzing joint afferents. *Brain*. 1972;95:705-748.

36. Held R. Plasticity in sensory-motor systems. *Sci Am*. 1967;213:84-94.

37. Brooks VB. *The Neural Basis of Motor Control*. New York, NY: Oxford University Press Inc; 1986.

38. MacKay WA. The motor program: back to the computer. In: Evarts EV, Wise SP, Bousfield D, eds. *The Motor System in Neurobiology*. New York NY: Elsevier Science Publishing Co Inc; 1985:101-105.

39. Baldissera F, Hultborn H, Illert M. Integration in spinal neuronal systems. In: Brooks VB, ed. *Handbook of Physiology. The Nervous System—Motor Control*. Bethesda, MD: American Physiological Society; 1981;2 (pt 1):509-595.

40. Kelso JAS. Concepts and issues in human motor behavior: coming to grips with the jargon. In: Kelso JAS, ed. *Human Motor Behavior: An Introduction*. Hillsdale, NJ: Lawrence Erlbaum Associates Inc; 1982:21-58.

41. Gelfand IM, Gurfinkel VS, Fomin SV, et al. *Models of the Structural-Functional Organization of Certain Biological Systems*. Massachusetts, Mass: The MIT Press; 1971.

42. Allen GI, Tsukahara N. Cerebrocerebellar communications systems. *Physiol Rev*. 1974;54:957-1006.

43. Delong MR, Georgopoulos AP, Crutcher MD. Cortico-basal ganglia relations and coding of motor performance. In: Massion J, Paillard J, Schultz W, Wiesendanger M, eds. *Neural Coding of Motor Performance*. New York, NY: Springer-Verlag New York Inc; 1983:30-40.

44. Lance JW. Symposium synopsis. In: Feldman RG, Young RR, Koella WP, eds. *Spasticity: Disordered Motor Control*. Chicago, Ill: Year Book Medical Publishers Inc; 1980:485-494.

45. Katz RT, Rymer WZ. Spastic hypertonia: mechanisms and measurement. *Arch Phys Med Rehabil*. 1989;70:144-155.

46. Dietz V, Ketelsen UP, Berger W, et al. Motor unit involvement in spastic paresis: relationship between leg muscle activation and histochemistry. *J Neurol Sci*. 1986;75:89-103.

47. McLellan DL, Hasan N, Hodgson JA. Tracking tasks in assessment and spasticity. In: Delwaide PJ, Young RR, eds. *Clinical Neurophysiology in Spasticity: Contribution to Assessment and Pathophysiology*. New York, NY: Elsevier Science Publishing Co Inc; 1985:131-139.

48. Bourbonnais D, Vanden Noven S, Carey K, et al. Abnormal spatial patterns of elbow muscle activation in hemiparetic human subjects. *Brain*. 1989;112:85-102.

49. Duncan PW, Badke MB. Determinants of abnormal motor control. In: Duncan PW, Badke MB, eds. *Stroke Rehabilitation: The Recovery of Motor Control*. Chicago, Ill: Year Book Medical Publishers Inc; 1987:135-160.

50. Walshe FMR. On certain tonic or postural reflexes in hemiplegia, with special reference to the so-called "associated movements." In: Payton OD, Hirt S, Newton RA, eds. *Scientific Basis for Neurophysiologic Approaches to Therapeutic Exercise: An Anthology*. Philadelphia, Pa: F A Davis Co; 1977:155-166.

51. Hellebrandt FA, Schade M, Carns ML. Methods of evoking the tonic neck reflexes in normal human subjects. *Am J Phys Med*. 1962;41:90-139.

52. Forssberg H, Grillner S, Rosignol S. Phase dependent reflex reversal during walking in chronic spinal cats. *Brain Res*. 1975;85:103- 107.

53. Peterson BW, Boldberg J, Bilotto G, et al. The cervicocollic reflex: its dynamic properties and interaction with vestibular reflexes. *J Neurophysiol*. 1985;54:90-109.

54. Banovetz JM, Rude SA, Perlmutter SI, et al. A comparison

of neck reflexes in alert and decerebrate cats. *Society for Neuroscience Abstracts*. 1987;13:1312.

55. Grillner S. Locomotion in vertebrates: central mechanisms and reflex interaction. *Physiol Rev*. 1975;55:247-304.

56. Baker J, Goldberg J, Peterson B. Spatial and temporal response properties of the vestibulocollic reflex in decerebrate cats. *J Neurophysiol*. 1985;54:735-756.

57. Keshner EA, Peterson BW. Motor control strategies underlying head stabilization and voluntary head movements in humans and cats. In: Pompeiano O, Allum JHJ, eds. *Vestibulospinal Control of Posture and Movement: Progress in Brain Research*. New York, NY: Elsevier Science Publishing Co Inc; 1988:329-339.

58. Beevor CE. The Croonian lectures on muscular movements and their representation in the central nervous system. In: Payton OD, Hirt S, Newton RA, eds. *Scientific Bases for Neurophysiologic Approaches to Therapeutic Exercise: An Anthology*. Philadelphia, Pa: F A Davis Co; 1977:5-12.

59. Buchanan TS, Rovai GP, Rymer WZ. Strategies for muscle activation during isometric torque generation at the human elbow. *J Neurophysiol*. 1989;62:1201-1212.

60. Tuller B, Turvey MT, Fitch HL. The Bernstein perspective: II. The concept of muscle linkage or coordinative structure. In: Kelso JAS id. *Human Motor Behavior: An Introduction*. Hillsdale, NJ: Lawrence Erlbaum Associates Inc; 1982:253-270.

61. Horak RB, Esselman P, Anderson ME, et al. The effects of movement velocity, mass displaced, and task certainty on associated postural adjustments made by normal and hemiplegic individuals. *J Neurol Neurosurg Psychiatry*. 1984;47:1020-1028.

62. Abbs JH, Cole KJ. Neural mechanisms of motor equivalence and goal achievement. In: Wise SP, ed. *Higher Brain Functions: Recent Explorations of the Brain's Emergent Properties*. New York, NY: John Wiley & Sons Inc; 1988:15-43.

63. Keshner EA, Campbell D, Katz R, et al. Neck muscle activation patterns in humans during isometric head stabilization. *Exp Brain Res*. 1989;75:335-364.

64. Peterson BW, Pellionisz AJ, Baker JF, et al. Functional morphology and neural control of neck muscles in mammals. *American Zoologist*. 1989;29:139-149.

65. Martin JP. Tilting reactions and disorders of the basal ganglia. *Brain*. 1965;88:855-877.

66. Keshner EA, Allum JHJ. Muscle activation patterns coordinating postural stability from head to foot. In: Winters J, Woo S, eds. *Multiple Muscle Movement Systems: Biomechanics and Movement Organization*. New York, NY: Springer-Verlag New York Inc; Chapt 29. In press.

67. Keshner EA, Woollacott MH, Debu B. Neck and trunk muscle responses during postural perturbations in humans. *Exp Brain Res*. 1988;71:455-466.

68. Winstein CJ. Motor learning considerations in stroke rehabilitation. In: Duncan PW, Badke MB, eds. *Stroke Rehabilitation: The Recovery of Motor Control*. Chicago, Ill: Year Book Medical Publishers Inc; 1987:109-134.

69. Schmidt RA. *Motor Control and Learning: A Behavioral Emphasis*. Champaign, Ill: Human Kinetics Publishers Inc; 1982.

Chapter 7

Motor Learning Principles for Physical Therapy

Richard A. Schmidt, PhD
Motor Control Laboratory
Department of Psychology
University of California, Los Angeles
Los Angeles, CA 90024-1563

Up until a few years ago, I considered the field of physical therapy to be quite distinct from, and essentially irrelevant to, my own area of research concerned with the acquisition of skill—frequently termed *motor learning*. Much of this came from my lack of familiarity with physical therapy. I had a very sketchy understanding about what kinds of activities comprised the practice of physical therapy and how therapists were educated; so I naturally harbored many false assumptions about the nature of the problems that were to be addressed and the methods that were used to treat them. But the fundamental problem was that I viewed physical therapy from the wrong perspective. For me, the problem for physical therapy was an *organic* one, for want of a better term; this was due, I suppose, to the fact that many of the patients had real, quantifiable injuries that could be "seen" quite clearly with various diagnostic procedures. These were problems such as spinal cord injuries from a motorcycle accident, head injuries from a blow to the skull, or strokes. To use computer terminology, physical therapy seemed to be involved with "hardware" problems, analogous in a way to malfunctions in the physical structure of the machine.

Motor learning, on the other hand, has always been concerned mainly with the acquisition of new skills with practice. This emphasis has been blended somewhat with the field of motor control, so that the ideas about how skills are learned and particularly how they are performed differently after practice were an important emphasis. Usually, the focus has been on learners engaging in meaningful practice, such as an athlete perfecting a pole-vaulting performance, a musician practicing at the piano, or the industrial worker learning to operate a computer keyboard. The learner was typically uninjured, usually "normal" by various criteria (although one branch of motor learning has dealt with handicapped populations). The concern has been to understand the principles by which these new skills were acquired and to develop theories that would account for them. Thus the problem was concerned with how the motor system is organized differently after practice so as to allow high-level skills to be performed, whether it be the more effective analysis and use of feedback for action or the "construction" of larger and better motor programs. To me, these issues were essentially "software" problems, analogous to understanding the programs that control the hardware's activities, and they had little in common with the hardware problems of physical therapy.

These two fields were easily segregated on these kinds of grounds. Almost no mention was made of physical therapy in textbooks on motor learning because therapy was not seen as relevant to the problems of skills or their modification. Similarly, only a few universities providing training in physical therapy emphasized motor learning, and many programs did not even have a course in motor learning in the curriculum (Carolee Winstein, PhD; personal communication; May 1990); principles of learning were apparently not seen as relevant to therapist's activities. (Some of the reasons for this thinking have also been discussed elsewhere. [1]) Therapists and motor learning specialists attended difference conferences, published their data in different journals, and maintained a nearly complete separation between each other.

COMMONALITIES BETWEEN MOTOR LEARNING AND PHYSICAL THERAPY

Recently, I have begun to see the relationship between the fields of physical therapy and motor learning somewhat differently, joined (or perhaps led) by numerous others in both fields. The new perspective is this: In a physical therapy session, many different things happen, of course, but one of these things can be regarded as *practice*. That is, patients are engaged in repeated attempts to produce motor behaviors that are beyond their present capabilities, analogous to a person learning to play the trumpet, for example. In physical therapy, though, the behaviors are not exactly new as they are in motor learning settings, but they can be considered as new in the sense that they have been lost as a result of an injury (eg, loss of gait in stroke). In this way, at least part of the product of physical therapy seems to be the acquisition of the capabilities to use the existing (albeit damaged) motor system. The patient seems to be *learning* to use the damaged motor system in a new way to accomplish an environmental goal that may have been achieved earlier—but perhaps in a different way—before the system was damaged. In this process, the therapist acts as a facilitator-instructor, using many of the same kinds of techniques that have been emphasized (although often under different names) in motor learning, such as providing instructions, physical or verbal guidance, feedback about errors, suggestions for modifications, and encouragement, just as a teacher or coach in motor learning would do. How the therapy session is structured and what activities are to be done, in what order, and in what relative amounts are all problems that face both the therapist and the traditional instructor in planning their respective sessions.

This blended view of physical therapy and motor learning has been reinforced for me by several events, such as my invitation to speak about motor learning at several recent conferences, short-courses, and workshops in physical therapy and rehabilitation medicine. In these settings, the ideas about the role of motor learning in physical therapy has been received with great interest, although not always without a great deal of controversy (which is as it should be). This meeting is one more example of the interest in this fusion on the part of therapists. The time seems right for these fields to move closer to each other as the similarities between them are begun to be recognized.

This chapter is written in this spirit of cooperation. Beginning with this new perspective about the learning aspects of physical therapy, I have thought about the various experimental methods, principles, and theoretical ideas from my own field of motor learning that would have the most relevance for people in physical therapy. I begin with some fundamental notions about the nature of learning and how it is conceptualized and measured in the laboratory (or hospital). Then, I discuss some earlier, almost classical notions about how practice has been considered over the past few decades, where repetition and the production of "correct" actions in practice has been emphasized. I then argue that there is much more to understanding practice than this, and I provide several lines of evidence that seem to shake our earlier understanding about how practice and learning are accomplished. Finally, this evidence about the nature of practice not only contributes to the development of theory, but it also has several practical implications that should be of use in designing effective activities in physical therapy.

LEARNING: SOME FUNDAMENTAL CONCEPTS

In my own field, I believe that until recently progress has been slowed somewhat by a general lack of agreement about the nature of the learning process and how its products should be evaluated. I present a view of learning here that is becoming reasonably well accepted and that provides a basis for understanding a number of diverse findings about the role of various experimental variables in practice. Beginning with some definitional issues, I will then turn to some questions of methodology and measurement.

Earlier Viewpoints about Learning

An earlier, more or less traditional perspective (and definition) regarded learning as being related to processes n-derlying changes in behavior (or performance). The focus was on the changes in performance seen during practice. It was argued that variables in practice that increased the rate of improvement or that enhanced performance were factors that influenced learning. In this way, the changes in performance charted by learning curves and the differences in those curves as a function of experimental variables were taken to be literal measures of the products of learning, almost as if learning *were* these changes in performance. This way of thinking about learning has, in my view, retarded our understanding of the learning process; it forced investigators (and practitioners) to focus on the "wrong" effects of experimental variables, namely those effects that occurred during practice itself. As we shall see in the next sections, there is much more to the learning process than effects during practice; the recognition of this notion has led to the general rejection of these earlier perspectives about learning.

Modern Perspectives on Learning

Two fundamental difficulties exist with the earlier perspectives on learning mentioned in the last section. First, this view did not consider the different kinds of effects that experimental variables can have during practice, with some of the effects being transient and easily lost with time and with others becoming almost perfectly permanent. Second, this view did not consider the various criteria, or what could be termed *goals,* of the learning process whose achievement is seldom captured by an analysis of the relative proficiency during practice. Both of these notions have strong implications for theory in learning and for practical applications to physical therapy and other areas; they are treated in the next sections.

Learning performance distinction. The first problem mentioned above was that experimental variables can have several different kinds of effects on performance. For our purposes here, let us segregate these effects into two broad categories: those effects on performance that are transitory, momentary, and temporary and those effects that are lasting and permanent, becoming a part of the learner's repertoire. This is an old idea, fostered by Guthrie,[2] Hull,[3] and Tolman,[4] and adopted by several others, subsequently (eg, Adams and Reynolds,[5] Schmidt,[6] Stelmach,[7] and Schmidt[8(chap 11)]). For them, learning was something "relatively permanent" that was the product of practice. Therefore, just because some variable influenced performance during the practice phase was not necessarily evidence that this variable had influenced learning because it had to be demonstrated that the relative gains in proficiency would survive various layoffs, shifts in conditions, or other such changes. This led to the notion that learning should not be evaluated during practice (where temporary and permanent effects of the variables were hopelessly intermixed) but rather on some kind of retention or transfer tests.

This thinking has led to the adoption of a particular brand of experimental design for evaluating motor learning in the laboratory (and, I argue, in practical settings as well), which are generally termed *transfer* (or *retention*) *designs* (Schmidt[8]). First, two experimental groups are treated differently during practice, and their performances as a function of this manipulation are plotted in performance curves. Any differences between conditions in this *acquisition phase* are viewed with caution because we have no way of knowing whether they are temporary or relatively permanent. Then, learners are given various kinds of retention, or transfer, tests in what is called a *transfer phase.* This phase has two primary defining characteristics: 1) the test is given with sufficient rest or layoff from the tasks so that any temporary effects of the variables have been allowed to dissipate and 2) the groups are treated identically so that no differential temporary influences will arise with further practice on the test. In this way, the transfer test is thought to be an index of the relative strengths of the permanent effects of the variable, with the transient or temporary effects having been removed. A strict view of this method would essentially ignore any differential effects on performance during the acquisition phase and would focus entirely on the performance difference in the retention or transfer phase. We will see several examples in the later sections here where this method has been used to great advantage.

Criteria for learning. A second problem for the earlier conceptualization of learning is the realization that there are, in addition to effective performance during practice, several goals (or criteria) against which improvements in performance from practice can be measured. These criteria can be thought of as the therapist's (or instructor's) goal for what the learners are supposed to be able to do as a result of training. In what sense does training make the performers better, when, and under what conditions? Some of these goals are discussed next.

Performance during practice. Of course, one goal of practice (the major goal for the earlier perspectives on learning) is the improvement of performance during the practice session itself. But, as we have just discussed, it is not necessarily the case that factors improving performancein practice will have effects that carry over into retention or transfer tests; therefore this goal of practice is a relatively unimportant one for most researchers in this area. As a more serious concern, later I will provide several lines of evidence that, relative to more or less "standard" practice methods, certain variables that enhance performance during practice actually provide worse performance in a retention test or transfer test. It is clear that performance during practice is not a particularly useful criterion for learning, especially as compared with the others listed below.

Retention. As implied earlier, a very important goal of practice is the capability to do what has been acquired in a later test, away from practice. Of course, this is important because it provides evidence of the relatively permanent nature of the changes. But practically speaking, when we train people to do skills we are seldom interested in performance at the time but rather in how they will do these skills at some time in the future. Practice at the piano must transfer to the recital this Saturday, and therapy concerning weight shifting in gait must carry over to walking behaviors when the patient has left the hospital. In other words, a major goal of practice is the capability to retain what has been learned, and it makes little sense to be able to perform skills in the hospital if they cannot be performed when the patient returns to his home or job tomorrow. In terms of research, this criterion might be evaluated by testing two groups of subjects in an acquisition phase, but the group that has "learned more" by this criterion is the one that performs best on the retention test one week later. Various alternative therapies could be evaluated in the same way, by asking which group of patients performs best at retention.

Very long-term retention. Although this criterion is not so critical for physical therapy, one can imagine settings where the training I receive today will not be applied for months or even years. Training for soldiers, police, fire fighters, medical personnel, and life guards, for example, is like this, where the skills that are learned must be placed "on hold" indefinitely until they are needed in an emergency,

and then they must be performed effectively on demand. Thus, if this is the criterion for learning, procedures in training must be used that ensure very long-term retention. This also brings in the question related to refresher training: How much and how often should it be provided to maximize long-term retention? As before, the condition in practice that is best according to this criterion is the one that generates the most effective performance at a long-term retention test.

Generalizability. In many (if not most) real-world skills, the version of the skills experienced in practice is different in various ways from the version(s) that face the learner when training is over. The grade that a patient must negotiate from his porch to the garage is different from that practiced on the treadmill at the hospital. Gait training must be sensitive to the facts that the patient will probably be wearing different shoes at home than she is at the hospital and that the surfaces will also be different. This is the critical problem of generalizability, where the skills that are actually practiced must transfer to, or generalize to, other similar activities that are the actual goal of learning. Here the laboratory test of generalizability concerns which conditions in practice produce the most effective performance on tasks that are different, or in some sense novel, as compared with the practice activities. The condition that produces the most effective transfer to some new task will have generalized best. There are many complexities with this idea, such as what kinds of transfer tasks to use for evaluation and how different they should be from the practice task. But ingeneral, the therapist's goal would seem to be strongly aligned with the ideas of generalization; training should be adjusted so that this criterion is achieved. There is good evidence that conditions enhancing long-term retention do not necessarily enhance generalizability, and vice versa (Wulf and Schmidt[9] and T.D. Lee, G. Wulf, and R.A. Schmidt; unpublished data; 1990), which seems to demand that the therapist be sensitive to which of the criteria are most critical for a given skill or type of patient.

Altered contexts. This criterion is related closely to that of generalizability just discussed, but here the goal is to be able to perform the same skill in a different context. For example, athletes training in practice must be able to perform their skills in environments filled with crowd noise; patients must be able to perform their learned activities in the presence of their family and friends, whether fatigued or sleepy, and often in the dark as well as in the light. In a way, one can say that the skill is different in the light than in the dark because certain feedback channels become nearly useless (vision) and others become relatively more important (proprioception) as the lighting conditions change. Such altered contexts would seem to be an important goal for therapy, and training needs to be adjusted to accommodate it.

Modern Definitions of Learning

We are now in a position to consider definitions of learning that are sensitive to these arguments about the learning-performance distinction and the various criteria for learning. Here is one that I use: Motor learning is a set of processes associated with practice or experience leading to relatively permanent changes in the capability for responding.[8(p346)] The focus here is on the *capability* for responding, a quantity that is not directly observable, but whose effects can be observed by examining various performance tests. Such capabilities may well be relatively specific to the particular kinds of tests for learning that will be used, so that we could say that practice leading to the capability for long-term retention may not lead at the same time to the capability for generalization.

SOME RECENT PRINCIPLES OF MOTOR LEARNING

Armed now with the notions of learning discussed in the earlier sections, we can turn to the evaluation of several experimental variations of practice that seem most important in the present context. First, they are important because they cause serious doubts on earlier theories and frameworks of the learning process; indeed, they cast doubts on the entire set of processes thought to be involved in practice. These findings are destined to become important because they seem to require adjustments to theory in order to accommodate them. Second, almost by coincidence, these findings have strong practical implications. They tend to deal with variables that are under the control of teachers and therapists, and unlike many other variables that could have been named here, they can be implemented with minimal difficulties into the procedures currently used in training and therapy. Finally, these results are interesting for practical settings because they seem to contradict much of what we have taken for granted about the role of practice and the variables that determine its effectiveness.

In the sections that follow, I deal with two major classes of variations of practice. One deals with the overall organization of practice; it has to do with how the teacher or therapist structures the activities that are to be used in a training session. The second deals with issues about the role of information feedback from an instructor to the student-patient: how this information is involved in the learning process and how the therapist can optimize it for various learning criteria.

Scheduling and Organization of Practice

One of the first questions that any practitioner must answer when designing practice concerns the overall organization of the practice session. What activities are to be taught, how much time is to be devoted to each, and in what order should learners experience the various tasks to be learned? It turns out that investigators dealing with these relatively simple sounding questions have discovered some very important principles of practice. These answers have been relatively shocking to those who felt that they understood how to specify effective practice.

Blocked versus random practice. Suppose that you have an hour with a patient and you decide there are three activities (call them A, B, and C) that should be practiced in that period of time. Further, suppose that these activities are quite different from each other: one activity cannot simply be seen as a parametric (scaled) variation of another one. How should one distribute these three tasks across the practice session?

Shea and Morgan[10] examined this question in a pioneering experiment on practice. They studied two practice schedules that they termed *Blocked* and *Random* practice. In Blocked practice, all of the practice at Task A was com-

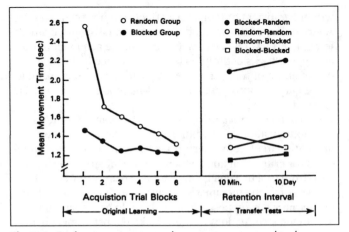

Fig. 7-1. *Performance on complex movement speed tasks under random and blocked presentations (redrawn from Shea and Morgan[10]).*

pleted before the learner switched to Task B, and so on. This is more or less the standard way that practice would be scheduled, where the learner can concentrate on the errors and strategies for mastering Task A before switching to other activities. Blocked practice is also closely related to what has been called "drill," where many repetitions of a given activity are given to facilitate learning. The second schedule they used was Random practice, where trials of Tasks A, B, and C were intermixed randomly, so that no task would be repeated on two consecutive trials. In their experiment, there were the same number of trials of Tasks A, B, and C (18 of each) for both groups, the only difference being the ordering of these experiences across the practice period. The tasks to be learned all involved rapid arm movements to knock over small barriers. The tasks differed in terms of the distances and directions between the barriers; that is, the patterns of arm movement were different from task to task, even though the tasks all involved knocking over the barriers.

The results from the Shea-Morgan[10] experiment are shown in Figure 7-1. In the acquisition session graphed at the left, we can see that the Blocked condition produced much better performance than the Random condition did, where all of the tasks' performances within each condition are averaged together. The Blocked group improved much more quickly in the first block of trials and continued to perform more effectively even by the end of practice. Which group learned more? Without a doubt, Blocked practice is to be preferred to Random if the criterion is related to the level of proficiency during practice. It is not clear, however, that these differences are learning differences because the benefits for the Blocked condition could be temporary. What is needed is a transfer or retention design to separate the temporary and permanent effects of these variables.

Shea and Morgan[10] used a version of the transfer design described in an earlier section, where half of each group was tested under the same conditions as in acquisition, and the other half tested under the opposite conditions. This actually resulted in two mini-experiments: the effect of Blocked versus Random conditions in acquisition on retention of 1) the task under Blocked conditions and 2) the task under Random conditions. (This was actually a 2 × 2 design, where the factors were conditions in acquisition [Blocked versus Random] and conditions in retention [Blocked versus Random].) At the right of the figure are the performances shown separately for two retention tests, one done after 10 minutes and another after 10 days. Consider the performance of the groups tested under Blocked conditions, shown as the squares in the figure. Here, there is a small advantage for the group that practiced under the Random conditions in the acquisition session, present at both of the retention intervals. Next, examine the groups shown as circles in the figure, which were tested under the Random conditions in the retention test. In this case, there is a very large advantage for the groups that had received acquisition practice under the Random conditions. Notice that regardless of the conditions under which the subjects were tested (Blocked or Random) there was always an advantage for the groups that had practiced under Random conditions in acquisition. If the criterion for learning is the capability for retention, then we must conclude that Random conditions in practice are more beneficial for learning than are blocked conditions. This finding provided quite a shock to researchers in the field, because Random practice was a variable that degraded practice in acquisition (relative to Blocked practice), yet it facilitated learning.

These results argue against a relatively well-accepted viewpoint about learning termed the *specificity of learning* hypothesis (Henry[11]). This general view, which stems from the ideas that motor skills are very specific (ie, uncorrelated with each other) and therefore dependent on fundamentally different abilities, argues that the conditions under which the performances are practiced results in memory representations that are specific to those conditions. A similar viewpoint is the encoding-specificity view of Tulving and Thomson.[12] This view comes from the literature on contextual effects in verbal learning where, for example, a retention test in a given room is performed better if the practice was also received there (as opposed to having practiced it in a different room). Both these views predict that if a given task is to be performed under Blocked conditions, for example, the best way to learn it would be under Blocked practice. We see from Figure 7-1 that this is certainly not the case. Even for the group that had a Blocked retention test (the squares in the figure), it was still slightly better to have learned the task under Random conditions.

There is a small advantage, however, for practicing under the same conditions in acquisition as in retention, as the specificity view might expect, but this difference is not very large compared with the effect of Blocked versus Random conditions in acquisition. This is evident by the fact that the effect of Random practice is far larger if the Random conditions are also used at test (circles) than if the blocked conditions are used at test (squares), as if the similarity in acquisition and test conditions made a small difference. So there are actually two effects here, whose effects are more or less additive: Random practice is better for retention than Blocked practice, and there is a small advantage for practicing under the same conditions in acquisition as in test. Clearly, the worst condition for learning was the group

shown as filled circles: Blocked conditions in acquisition, with a switch to Random conditions on the retention test.

Generality and limits of the blocked-random effect. These effects of blocked versus random practice have been studied considerably since the original Shea-Morgan[10] experiment, and it is fair to say that the effects are remarkably robust across several different kinds of laboratory tasks and testing situations. The benefits for random practice hold for physical education activities such as badminton serves (Goode and Magill[13]) and for learning to recognize patterns in industrial tasks that involve wiring diagrams (Schneider[14]). The benefits are also akin to the results from the so-called spaced-repetitions effect in verbal learning, where increasing the number of intervening items between repetitions of a given item degrades performance of the item during practice but enhances retention (Landauer and Bjork[15] and R.A. Schmidt and R.A. Bjork; unpublished data; 1990).

There are probably limits on the effectiveness of random practice; one of these seems to be the level of proficiency of the learning. Shea et al[16] gave different amounts of blocked or random practice to different groups before switching them to a retention test. For the lowest level of practice, the blocked conditions in acquisition was slightly superior to random. But as the amount of practice was increased, an advantage for random practice in acquisition emerged that was essentially like that seen in Figure 7-1. These various effects are discussed by Magill and Hall[17] in a recent review of the blocked-random experiments.

Understanding the random practice superiority. How can we understand the findings that random practice produces more effective retention performance, even though it degrades performance during practice? There are several interrelated viewpoints about it, all of which focus on the processes that are generated when subjects are engaged in random practice.

Depth of processing. Shea and Morgan[10] originally interpreted their findings in terms of a depth-of-processing notion suggested by Craik and Lockhart.[18] In this view, factors in practice that cause the learner to process information more "deeply," connecting it to other previously learned materials (elaboration) or creating ways to make the different tasks distinguishable (distinctiveness), are thought to require deeper processing and provide more effective retention as a result. In a later study, Shea and Zimny[19] reported that random subjects provided descriptions of the tasks indicating that they had processed them relatively meaningfully, such as statements like "Task A is like an upside-down Z" (elaboration) and "Task A is just like B, except that the first part is reversed" (distinctiveness). Blocked subjects, on the other hand, seemed to produce the movements more or less automatically, without having to engage in processes that would make them distinct. Thus this view holds that random practice required subjects to engage effortful, meaningful processing during practice to keep the tasks separated; this requirement was detrimental to performance in practice, but it provided benefits at retention.

Regeneration. Lee and Magill[20] disagreed with Shea and Morgan's view and argued that random practice provides a different kind of advantage. In the Lee-Magill view, random practice requires learners to abandon, or forget, the solution to the motor problem just produced so they can generate the solution to the task on the next trial. It is this regeneration, according to their view, that is beneficial for learning. Blocked practice, on the other hand, allows learners to use the same solution on each of a long string of trials, which effectively blocks the regeneration processes (except for the first trial in the block) because the solution had already been generated earlier. In this view, blocked practice makes it too easy for learners because they do not have to engage in effortful processing activities that will benefit them later.

Cuddy and Jacoby[21] provide a nice analogy to this process, which makes it easier to understand. Say I am a sixth grader, and you are trying to teach me to do long division "in my head." You give me problems, and I respond with the answers if I can. In blocked practice, the first problem is 21/3, and I struggle to determine that the answer is 7. Then, the next trial is 21/3, and I remember that the solution was 7, so I just give the answer without doing any of the processing necessary to figure it out. On the next trial it is even easier to remember the answer 7, and so on. With random practice, however, my first problem is 21/3, and I generate the answer; then my next problem might be 12/4, and I have to generate its answer too. After a few other trials, you return to 21/3. By now, I have forgotten the solution and must regenerate it again. In this view, random practice causes the learners to forget the solutions so that they have to be regenerated later on when that item is repeated again. This is the basis for the seemingly curious title of the Cuddy-Jacoby[21] paper, "When forgetting helps memory." Forgetting the solution to the problem facilitates memory in the long term, because it forces the subject to generate it later on, facilitating the capabilities at recall.

Retrieval practice. The Lee-Magill[20] view is similar to notions in verbal learning called *retrieval practice.* Here, random practice requires the subject to regenerate the answer to the problem (ie, to *retrieve* it from memory) on each trial, which provides practice at retrieving. Retrieving is seen as a kind of skill much like any other, so that providing practice at retrieving makes one more effective at retrieving information in the future on the retention test. Blocked practice does not require this retrieval practice, and the retention performance suffers as a result. (See Bjork[22,23] and Landauer and Bjork[15] for more details about this viewpoint.)

Transfer-appropriate processing. All of these views share common features that are central to an interesting perspective about learning proposed by Morris,[24] termed *transfer-appropriate processing.* This view stresses the idea that at transfer (or in this case, at a retention test) certain processes are required in order that the learner perform effectively. Performance in transfer will be facilitated if the activities in acquisition also require practice at the same processes. That is, to the extent that processes that are appropriate for transfer or retention are practiced in acquisition, then performance in transfer will be maximized. In the blocked-random example, such a view would probably hold that random practice requires regeneration (Lee-Magill) or deeper processing (Shea-Morgan) in acquisition, that blocked practice prevents them, and that these processes are necessary for effective performance at retention. Thus random practice requires processes that are appropriate for the retention test; blocked practice does not.

This perspective forces the therapist-instructor to consider what kinds of processes are going to be required at the retention test, so that the practice activities can be adjusted to exercise the processes that are eventually going to be needed. Also, at first glance, this view seems just to be a specificity view in which the superficial features of the practice activities should match the features of the test environment (as with identically colored rooms, for example). But note that the transfer-appropriate processing view requires that the underlying processes be appropriate, not just the superficial features. This is why random practice is more effective for retention on a blocked retention test than blocked practice: random practice requires the important processes that are needed at retention. So here is a good example where the equality of the superficial conditions is not sufficient to ensure that the underlying processes are appropriate.

This general view of transfer-appropriate processing is one that has applications to many different kinds of practice phenomena, as we will see later on when we turn to feedback for learning. It has proved useful as an effective way to think about the processes involved in effective practice.

Implications for physical therapy. Several important and counter intuitive implications emerge from this literature on blocked and random practice. As I advocated in my text on teaching skills (Schmidt[25]), blocked practice and drill are highly ineffective ways to generate learning and should almost never be used. Once the learner can perform the actions at all, the evidence is very clear that practice should be randomized and repetitions avoided. Make people do different tasks on each trial; rotate among the tasks to be learned; intersperse other activities that cause the learners to forget the solutions so that they must regenerate them when the task is tried again.

The exception to this rule might involve very early practice where the learner is just acquiring the basic pattern, where blocked practice might be slightly more effective. It is difficult to know where this line between early and later practice might fall for tasks involved in physical therapy. Many of the activities have been practiced before, but the capabilities to perform may have been lost through the injury, making the performance almost like that of a beginner. My guess would be that if the movements can be performed at all, begin randomizing practice and avoid drills.

Related to this point is the notion that practice, if it is to be effective, needs to be somewhat difficult and effortful: practice should not be so difficult that the learners simply cannot function, of course, but also not so easy that important information processing activities are avoided. This strategy for structuring practice is often contrary to the personal need and goals of the therapist, who after all is strongly motivated to make things better for the patients. Here is the problem. If the goal is to make things better during therapy, then one way this can be accomplished is to provide blocked practice; the difficulty is that blocked practice will not provide the long-term capabilities that are also important. Making things better in the short term is, as we have argued here, actually detrimental to the therapist's main goal of making the patient better in the long term, such as when the patient is away from the hospital or out of the therapist's hands or when tomorrow or next week comes.

Feedback for Skill Acquisition

Another area of research with important practical applications to teaching and physical therapy settings involves the ways that feedback that can be provided by the instructor-therapist. It has long been recognized that the information about the success of the movement in meeting the environmental goal is a critical ingredient in motor learning (for reviews see Bilodeau[26] and Salmoni et al[27]). In tasks where the learners cannot attain this information for themselves, the evidence is clear that learning is markedly impaired or even eliminated altogether unless feedback about success is given by some alternative means (eg, from a teacher or therapist).

Classifications of feedback. In the research literature, the study of feedback for learning has generally focused on what has been termed *knowledge of results* (KR): augmented, postresponse, "verbalizable" information about success in meeting the environmental goal. This is extrinsic information, over and above that provided by the task itself, and it may or may not be redundant with the intrinsic information the learner receives during of after the action (eg, the patient sees the movements of his feet). The tasks that have been used have generally been simple, laboratory actions, structured so that the learner could not use the intrinsic feedback to determine the outcome (eg, blindfolded positioning tasks). Then, the experimenter has added feedback in the form of KR and has studied numerous variations in the scheduling and content of this information in determining learning.

A form of feedback potentially more useful for practical settings is *kinematic feedback*, or what was termed *knowledge of performance* by Gentile.[28] This is also augmented, postresponse, verbalizable information, but it is about the pattern of actions that led to the acheivement (or not) of the environmental goal, such as information that the elbow was not straight in a golf backswing or that the weight was not distributed equally between the two feet in a patient with gait difficulties. Because it is usually less redundant with the intrinsic feedback than KR, kinematic feedback is extensively used in practical settings by instructors and therapists. The difficulty is that this form of feedback has not been studied as extensively as KR has (see Schmidt and Young[29] for discussion), so we are not in a position to be as clear about its principles as we would be with KR. There are strong hints that the principles for KR and kinematic feedback may be very similar (Young[30]; D.E. Young and R.A. Schmidt, unpublished data, 1990), at least within limits.

Earlier principles of feedback for learning. I think it is fair to say that before about 1982 the principles of feedback could be summarized fairly easily. Most of the research on feedback for learning pointed to the generalization that any variation in feedback that makes the information more frequent, more immediate, more accurate, more "useful," or more informationally "rich," was beneficial for learning (Adams,[31] Bilodeau,[26] and see Salmoni et al[27] for a review). This generalization was consistent with Thorndike's[32] tradition that emphasized feedback's role in the strengthening of

"bonds" between stimuli and responses. According to this view, which dominated thinking in this area for decades, more and better information about errors facilitated these links; failure to provide any feedback would leave the bonds unaffected, producing no learning. Therefore, it was not surprising when most of the research in this period supported this general view. As a result, the principles that found their way into the textbooks generally advocated frequent, immediate, informationally rich feedback information for maximizing learning. As Winstein discusses in this volume, procedures for physical therapy also generally followed this idea, advocating feedback that would bring the learner to the target and allow relatively errorless repetitions of behavior.

But there were difficulties with these principles, as pointed out by Salmoni et al[27] in their review of the research on feedback. The most important problem was that the effects of the variations in feedback were nearly always evaluated on performance during the acquisition session, where the feedback was present and under manipulation. As we have discussed earlier in this chapter, the difficulty with this procedure is that we cannot be sure whether any variation of feedback has influenced performance in a relatively permanent way or has simply altered performance temporarily. There is ample reason to suspect that feedback would have very strong temporary effects, such as motivation or "energizing" effects in boring tasks, and such influences have been demonstrated several times many years ago (eg, Arps,[33] Crawley,[34] Elwell and Grindley[35]). More recently, it has been recognized that feedback's strong informational effects might act in a temporary way, facilitating performance while the information is present but allowing performance to regress when the information is removed (Salmoni et al[27]). Even more importantly, I provide evidence later that feedback conditions during practice that facilitate performance might actually interfere with learning. Although the learning-performance distinction was clearly recognized throughout this period, feedback was treated as if it were a very special variable that was somehow immune from these effects. Writers (myself included) confidently ignored the possibility that any gains in performance from variations in feedback could be anything other than permanent effects that were due to learning. We were wrong.

Several lines of research on feedback—some very old and largely ignored, and others done recently—point to the inadequacy in this earlier line of thinking about the role of feedback for learning. In the sections that follow, I mention several of these experiments and point out how these have led to the beginnings of a new conceptualization about feedback. As with the new ideas about practice discussed in the previous section, these issues on feedback have strong implications for practical application to teaching and physical therapy.

Modern principles of feedback for learning. In the next sections, I focus on two different variables that have had a marked effect on our conceptualizations of feedback. One deals with a method of giving information called *summary feedback*, where feedback is given in summary form after a series of no-feedback trials. The second variable concerns manipulations of feedback frequency, where feedback is intentionally withheld on certain trials in the acquisition phase.

Summary feedback. Almost three decades ago, Lavery[36] published the results of a series of experiments on feedback that have had a strong influence on our thinking about this variable. He used three different conditions for feedback presentation for learning simple motor tasks. One of these was termed *immediate feedback*, where the information about errors was given after each trial in a more or less traditional way (Immediate group). A second condition received *summary feedback*, where feedback was withheld for a set of trials (20, in this case), and then a graph was provided showing the learner's scores on each of the 20 trials in the set (Summary group). Thus feedback was given about each trial, but the learner had to wait for as many as 20 trials to receive it. Finally, Lavery used a Both condition, where both immediate feedback was given after each trial and summary feedback was given after each 20-trial set (Both group). From an earlier perspective about feedback, we would suspect that summary feedback would not be effective for learning because subjects can not use feedback after each trial to modify the behavior on the next trial; errors would seem to be perpetuated, and performance should be degraded relative to the every-trial feedback with the Immediate group.

Lavery's results are shown in Figure 7-2, with the three groups plotted over the 6 days of practice in the acquisition phase. It is clear that the Summary group performed less well than either the Immediate or Both groups, with a slower rate of improvement and a poorer level of proficiency by the end of acquisition. But these performance differences in acquisition could merely be temporary effects, and a proper test of learning would provide some sort of retention or transfer test. In an unusual method for that period, Lavery also provided no-feedback retention tests on the next 4 days and at 37 and 93 days later. These retention tests

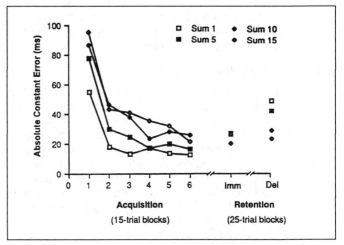

Fig. 7-3. *Mean errors in a movement-patterning task for four different summary-KR lengths in acquisition and on no-KR retention tests given after 10 min (Imm) or 2 days (Del) (redrawn from Schmidt et al[37]).*

are the evidence about the learning effects of the conditions in acquisition. What is surprising is that the Summary group was far more proficient than the other two groups. This effect continued throughout Days 7 to 10, was somewhat diminished by Day 37, and was essentially absent by Day 93. These retention data force us to the conclusion that even though the summary condition produced poorer performance than the immediate and both conditions in the acquisition phase, it generated more learning as measured on retention tests.

In our own research program at UCLA, we have extended these findings from Lavery to somewhat more complicated tasks, searching for an optimal number of trials to be included in the summary feedback (termed summary *lengths*). We had the idea (discussed later here) that frequent feedback produced two kinds of effects: a temporary guiding effect that improved performance in acquisition and a "dependency"-like effect that caused learners to regress when the feedback was removed. If the summary lengths were too short, the informational properties of the feedback would tend to create a dependency on it; on the other hand, if summary lengths were too long, there would not be sufficient guidance for effective learning. This general view predicted an inverted-U effect between summary length and retention performance, with optimum learning being generated when these two kinds of effects were in proper balance.

In one study using a three-directional arm movement task (Schmidt et al[37]), summary feedback lengths of either 1 (essentially immediate feedback), 5, 10, or 15 trials were examined, where a summary report about the trials in the set was given after the number of trials indicated throughout practice. These results are in Figure 7-3. In the acquisition phase, when feedback was present and being manipulated, there was a clear tendency for the groups with the largest summary lengths to have the poorest performance. This tendency was seen as a very slow rate of approach to the asymptote as compared with the groups with 1-trial summary feedback. In the retention tests, however, given without any feedback after 10 minutes and after 2 days, the ordering of

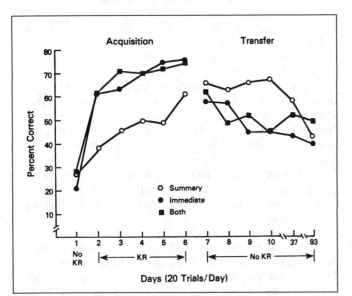

Fig. 7-2. *Percentage of responses from various summary-KR conditions in acquisition and in no-KR retention tests (redrawn from Lavery[36]).*

Contemporary Management of Motor Problems

the groups was reversed. The most effective group was the 15-trial summary condition, and the least effective was the 1-trial summary condition. Again, relative to every-trial feedback, summary feedback degraded performance in the acquisition phase, but it facilitated learning as measured by performance at retention. But there was no clear optimum summary length here, with any optimum lying beyond the 15-trial summary length used in the experiment.

In other work, we extended these findings to a more complicated task, with the idea that the optimal summary length should be shorter as task complexity increases and that any such optimum would then lie within the range of 1 to 15 trials that we were studying (Schmidt et al[38]). We used a laboratory simulation of hitting a moving object with a lever (analogous in some ways to hitting a ball with a bat), again studying summary lengths of 1, 5, 10, and 15, trials. With this more complex action to be learned, we found an inverted-U relationship between the length of the summary in the acquisition and performance at retention, with the optimal summary length being 5 trials. The suspicion is that the optimal summary length will generally be shorter for more complex tasks, because more guidance from trial to trial is needed in acquisition and there is less opportunity for dependency-producing effects. With very simple tasks, on the other hand, summary feedback lengths can be relatively large and still produce effective learning, probably because of the strong tendency for feedback to generate a kind of dependency when it is provided too frequently. We will return to this general idea later in the chapter.

A seemingly good question to ask is why summary feedback is so good for learning. Actually, if we examine more closely Lavery's effects in Figure 7-2, we will discover that this is not such a good question after all. If summary feedback were so good for learning, it should also have been good for the Both group that had the summary feedback in addition to feedback after each trial. But it was not, because we see that the Both group performed essentially like the Immediate group during the acquisition phase and very poorly during the retention tests. This leads to the almost unavoidable conclusion that it was not the summary condition that was so good for learning but rather the feedback after each trial (present for the Immediate and Both groups) that was detrimental for learning. What a conclusion to make in view of the earlier principles of feedback! Saying that frequent feedback is detrimental to learning contradicts this view directly. We will turn to this idea later, but for now let it be left that, relative to summary feedback, frequent feedback seems to generate strong guiding or motivational effects during the acquisition phase (enhancing performance there), but it produces dependency-like effects that block or degrade learning (as measured at retention). In this view, summary feedback is only "good" for learning in that it prevents the detrimental effects of every-trial feedback.

Frequency of feedback presentations. According to the earlier perspectives on feedback based on Thorndike's notions, if the learner did not know the results of his or her action on a given practice trial, this attempt was thought to be "neutral" with respect to learning, neither contributing to nor detracting from the learner's capabilities to perform. Such notions were supported at various times in the literature,

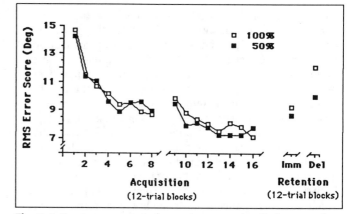

Fig. 7-4. *Root mean squared error in a complex limb patterning task as a function of relative frequency of feedback in the acquisition phase (redrawn from Winstein and Schmidt[42]).*

where it was shown that frequent (every-trial) feedback produced much more accurate responding than schedules where the feedback was given only occasionally (eg, Bilodeau and Bilodeau,[39] see Bilodeau[26] for a review). The difficulty with this research, pointed out by Salmoni et al,[27] was that the temporary versus permanent effects of these variations in feedback were confounded in this research. On the other hand, subsequent work by Ho and Shea[40] and R.W. Johnson et al (R.W. Johnson, G.G. Wicks, and D. Ben-Sira; unpublished data; 1981) used retention tests without feedback to evaluate differential learning effects. They produced results pointing to the possibility that reducing the frequency of feedback may be a potent variable for enhancing learning, contrary to the earlier viewpoints.

Carolee Winstein, a physical therapist working on motor learning in our laboratory several years ago, and I followed the lead of these authors, contrasting 100% feedback conditions with 50% feedback conditions (with total number of trials being constant) during acquisition phase of a relatively complex movement patterning task (Winstein[41] and Winstein and Schmidt[42]). Feedback was given in the form of a position-time trace on a computer terminal in addition to the root-mean-squared (RMS) error in reproducing the pattern. The results are shown in Figure 7-4. During two days of practice where feedback was provided, there was a slight advantage for the group with 100% feedback over the 50% feedback condition. But in the 10-minute and especially the 2-day retention tests (given without feedback), there was an advantage for the group that had received feedback only 50% of the time in acquisition. Contrary to the existing viewpoint about feedback frequency, reducing feedback (trials constant) facilitated learning as measured on a retention test, even though it tended to degrade performance in practice. (See Winstein's chapter in this volume for additional details and insights concerning these effects.)

The alert reader will already have noted that these results could have been due to a kind of specificity (or similarity) effect, as mentioned in the previous section on practice scheduling. That is, the 50% feedback condition in practice was more like the no-feedback retention test than was the 100% feedback condition; this similarity could be the (uninteresting) reason that the 50% condition was more effective in retention. Winstein and Schmidt[42] tested this possibility in another, essentially identical experiment, but where all subjects transferred instead to a 100% feedback retention test. In this case, any benefits that were due to the similarity of the acquisition and test conditions would benefit the 50% group, and the results at retention should be reversed. In fact, the differences between conditions in the 2-day retention test were very similar to those in Figure 7-4, with the 50% condition in acquisition again having more effective retention performance. Thus these benefits are not due to any similarity of conditions between acquisition and test. Rather, the reduction of feedback frequency in practice provided additional gains in the capability to perform, revealed mainly as a benefit at retention, independent of the retention conditions.

In terms of not only the criteria for learning discussed earlier but also the need for physical therapists to maximize long-term retention, these findings have very strong implications for practical application. Systematic attempts to reduce the amount of feedback information provided to learners, provided the learners have enough to correct the important errors, seem to be an effective way to enhance long-term retention of the activities practiced in the hospital.

Faded feedback. In the work just discussed, we had the general idea (described in the previous section on summary feedback) that frequent feedback generated a kind of learner-dependency that the summary feedback in some way avoided. Therefore, in the experiments just described, we used a faded-feedback schedule in an attempt to reduce these dependency effects. In this schedule, a 50% condition received feedback on every trial in the earlier stages of practice when it was presumably needed for correcting the largest performance errors; then feedback was reduced gradually as practice progressed, so that it was provided relatively infrequently in later practice, presumably reducing the possibility for dependency-producing effects. This schedule was created so that the relative frequency of feedback was 50% when all trials were considered. Unfortunately, the Winstein-Schmidt[42] experiments therefore confounded the relative frequency of feedback (100% versus 50%) with the fading schedule that was given only in the 50% condition. We do not know if these effects were due to the reduced feedback, the fading schedule, or some combination of the two.

Another physical therapist with us at UCLA, Diane Nicholson, worked on several experiments to unravel these effects (D.E. Nicholson and R.A Schmidt, unpublished data, 1990). In one experiment, three 50% feedback schedules were contrasted with an every-trial (100% feedback) schedule. We used a 50%-faded schedule essentially as in the Winstein experiments, a 50% schedule where the feedback and no-feedback trials were alternated throughout practice, and a third 50% schedule where feedback and no-feedback trials were alternated in blocks of five trials. The main result was that all three 50% conditions produced better retention performance than the 100% condition, but there were essentially no differences among the various 50% schedules. This experiment cast some doubt on our ideas that scheduling (in particular, fading) was an important vari-

able for learning, at least in the ways we were thinking of it in terms of avoiding dependencies, and suggested that the most powerful influence was actually the reduced frequency of feedback.

An additional experiment suggested that there was a role of scheduling after all. Here, we used a uniform 50% feedback condition and contrasted it with the 50%-faded condition (slightly modified from that used in the earlier experiments) and with a "reversed" 50%-faded condition, where the frequency of feedback was low in early practice and gradually increased as practice continued. With all groups receiving a 50% feedback schedule, if there were any additional effect of the distribution of these no-feedback trials across practice, we should find that the 50%-faded condition would be best for learning and that the reversed-50%-faded condition would be worst for learning. This is what happened. There was a small advantage for the 50%-faded condition over the uniform-50% condition, but the reversed-50% condition was reliably poorer in retention performance than was the uniform condition. This experiment supported our notion that fading feedback is an effective factor in practice, probably because it reduces dependency-like effects of frequent feedback in later practice. These data generally indicated that the scheduling of feedback is a variable that deserves attention in the design of many real-world practice settings, including physical or occupational therapy.

Bandwidth feedback. This work on faded feedback has strong ties to other experiments using so-called bandwidth feedback. In this method, the experimenter, or instructor, gives error information to the learner in the usual way only if the movement is outside a predetermined band of correctness. If the error is small, however, falling within this band, no information is given. Here, of course, the learner understands that no information means that the error was acceptably small, and thus this report is more or less like saying "correct." Several experimenters have shown that, relative to every-trial feedback, bandwidth feedback produces benefits in long-term retention (Sherwood[43]; T.D. Lee et al, unpublished data, 1990).

These bandwidth procedures have a number of interesting features. First of all, they reduce the amount of feedback provided during practice, because many of the trials will have scores that fall within the band and thus receive no error information. But second, they provide a kind of automatic fading schedule. Early in practice, where most of the movements have errors that are outside the band, feedback is frequent; but later in practice, when performances have stabilized and errors are within the band, feedback is far less frequent, which could (if the band is set appropriately) provide a pattern of feedback and no-feedback trials that strongly resembles faded feedback. Further, as Lee et al have shown, there is more to bandwidth feedback's advantage over every-trial feedback than just fading or reduced relative frequency (although these are part of the benefit), but it remains unclear as to how these advantages should be characterized. But whatever the processes involved, in terms of practical applications to training and therapy, this bandwidth-feedback method has many advantages because it produces strong gains in retention performance and is easily implemented in real-world settings.

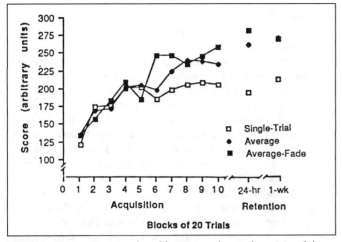

Fig. 7-5. *Score on a simulated batting task as a function of the presentation of kinematic feedback in the acquisition phase (from D.E. Young and R.A. Schmidt, unpublished data, 1990).*

Kinematic feedback. A criticism of much of the work on KR is that this form of feedback may not be very relevant to practical situations. This is so because KR by definition is about movement outcomes, which are often obvious in most real-world situations (the batter knows where the ball went, and the patient knows if she has lost balance). An important question, therefore, is whether these variations of feedback discussed in the earlier sections also apply to kinematic feedback about the patterns of actions, which are more typical of the information provided in physical therapy. One of the major goals in our group in the past several years has been to establish a suitable laboratory paradigm for studying kinematic feedback and to examine the role of various scheduling variables analogous to those in the previous sections.

Schmidt and Young[29] developed a new paradigm that separates the goal of the movement from the pattern of action that produces it. The task is a laboratory analog of hitting a moving ball with a bat, produced with a backswing followed by a forward swing, with the goal to make the imaginary object go as far as possible on each trial. The learner's goal is to maximize the *score* (the outcome of the action), which is sensitive to both 1) how fast the bat was going when it "struck" the object and 2) how accurately the object was struck; thus, both factors define the distance that the object would have traveled. From pilot experiments, we know several things about the optimal patterns for maximizing the task score, one of which is that the optimum backswing position is about 165° from the subject's frontal plane, where the object is to be struck when the limb is a 90°. Thus we have a basis for providing kinematic feedback about the pattern of themovement (the maximum backswing position) independent of the score that the subject received. In our view, this is analogous to giving a patient information about symmetry in weight transfer patterns (which may not be very obvious to the patient otherwise) independent of information about whether the locomotion was successful in behavioral terms (eg, five consecutive steps were taken).

In one experiment using this task, Young (Young[30];

D.E. Young and R.A. Schmidt, unpublished data, 1990) examined what was called *average feedback*, similar to the summary feedback discussed earlier except that the learner receives the average backswing position after a block of trials (5 trials in this case) rather than information about each of them as with the summary feedback. This was contrasted with an every-trial kinematic feedback condition that received feedback after each trial and with another group that received a faded presentation of average feedback. Information about the goal of the action (ie, KR), on the other hand, was given after every trial in the experiment. The results are shown in Figure 7-5, where the average and average-fade groups performed more effectively than the every-trial condition in acquisition and in 24-hour and 1-week retention tests without feedback. To the extent that average feedback and summary feedback can be considered as similar (in that they summarize a set of trials just performed, albeit in different ways), these results both suggest that reduced feedback provided after a set of trials benefits learning. This provides some encouragement to the idea that knowledge of results (about movement outcome) and kinematic feedback (about movement patterning) may follow the same laws.

The underlying notion is that average feedback in this experiment, like summary feedback in Figure 7-2, prevents the use of every-trial feedback that is detrimental to learning. In keeping with this viewpoint, Proteau et al (L. Proteau, T.D. Lee, and R.A. Schmidt; unpublished data; 1990) have evidence that kinematic information (about backswing position) given only about the last trial in the set is just as effective for learning as information about all of the trials given as average feedback; both of these conditions were better than every-trial information for learning. This finding bolsters the idea that the major effect of average feedback is the blockage of detrimental effects of every-trial feedback, rather than some benefit on the additional information provided in the summary or average feedback reports themselves.

Overall, there is much more research to be done to come to an effective understanding of kinematic feedback for learning. But several lines of evidence provide encouragement that we may not need separate laws for outcome feedback (KR) versus kinematic feedback; all forms of feedback may ultimately follow the same principles. I take this position here, suggesting that the principles discussed can be applied to therapeutic sessions regardless of whether the feedback is classed as kinematic feedback or outcome feedback. In the last sections, I turn to some preliminary theoretical ideas about how these various forms of feedback seem to operate to contribute to learning.

Preliminaries to a guidance theory of feedback. We can summarize in a general way all of the effects of feedback discussed in this section by saying that reducing, in one way or another, the amount or "usefulness" of feedback information during practice seems to facilitate learning relative to providing feedback in a "standard," every-trial way. This general result occurred for the reduced capability to use information when presented in a summary formatand when actually withholding information in the study of feedback frequency. First, this contradicts directly the earlier traditions and beliefs about the role of feedback in learning, based primarily on Thorndike's notions, which held that trials without feedback should not contribute to learning. Second, it is challenging to understand how this infrequent feedback can operate in facilitating learning, because it provides a relatively poor link between the trial that was in error and the information given about it, often allowing separations of several minutes of time and other trials. Traditionally, researchers emphasized that the connection between the performance and the feedback information needed to be direct, immediate, and clear in order for learning to be maximized; the forms of feedback discussed here (summary, average, bandwidth, and infrequent feedback) have none of these features. Third, it is difficult to understand on traditional grounds how, relative to every-trial feedback, a variation of feedback that makes performance poorer during practice can result in enhanced retention capabilities. Clearly, existing theoretical ideas about the role of feedback are inadequate to account for these newer effects. These problems are addressed below, and the answers provided form the preliminaries to a new theory of feedback that might serve as a replacement for the earlier ones.

Feedback seems to have at least two distinct roles during practice. First, it has a "positive" role, which during practice guides the learner away from errors and toward the correct response patterning. Second, feedback seems to have several "negative" roles in learning, which detract from the capabilities to perform on a retention test.

Positive roles of feedback. The beneficial aspects of feedback have been recognized for many decades (eg, see Bilodeau[26] for a review). Certainly, feedback has an informational role in that it tells the learner what went wrong and indicates how the movement should be corrected the next time. This "prescriptive" aspect of feedback provides very strong guidance for the performer, reporting on errors when they arise and motivating corrections on subsequent trials to keep the performer on target. Feedback also has an "energizing" function that keeps the subject alert and motivated, particularly in boring tasks or long practice periods. This is particularly important for physical therapy because feedback can make extended, difficult practice periods more interesting and can result in the patient trying harder and longer. People are also motivated by feedback in that they seem to want to know how they are doing and are pleased when they know the results of their efforts.

These various effects of feedback would seem, on the surface at least, to be effective for learning. They certainly are effective for performance during practice. The difficulty is that their effects may be temporary, or transient, in nature, so that benefits received during practice either may not survive until a retention test is given or may not survive the withdrawal of the information in a later situation. More importantly, these effects of frequent feedback may actually detract from the learning processes, by providing one or more "side effects" that interfere with information-processing activities necessary for effective long-term retention capabilities.

Negative roles of feedback. In what ways could frequent feedback provide negative effects on learning? We are not certain of the answers at the present time because rese-

arch into these questions has just begun; however, below are several possibilities that are currently under study in various laboratories.

One possibility is that frequent feedback interferes with the capability of the learners to acquire error-detection capabilities that could be used later (eg, in a retention test) to correct their own errors and even to improve performance. The notion is that when feedback is provided frequently, the information-processing activities are diverted from the analyses of response-produced intrinsic feedback to the information provided by the experimenter or teacher. Failure to process intrinsic feedback, it is argued, then prevents the learner from becoming sensitive to the patterns in it that signal performance errors. The result is effective performance in acquisition, because feedback holds behavior on target, but poor performance in retention, which is a pattern seen in many of the experiments mentioned in the previous sections. Schmidt et al[37] have shown that relative to every-trial feedback, summary feedback not only produces more effective retention performance but also more effective capabilities to estimate their own scores in a retention test. This latter capability is what one would expect if error detection capabilities were implicated here.

A second possibility is that frequent feedback produces what have been termed "maladaptive short-term corrections." The idea is that feedback encourages or even forces the learner to make a compensation on the next trial, even though the amount of error is otherwise acceptably small. These compensations provide relatively good performance because errors are never very large, but they seem to prevent the learner from being stable. This hypothesis holds that in encouraging such instability, the learner does not acquire the stable, enduring patterns necessary for effective long-term retention.

A version of this view is that when the errors are very small, particularly in tasks where the subject attempts to repeat the same response from trial to trial, a relatively large part of the reported error is due to random, neuromuscular noise (Schmidt et al[44]). This noise is systematic but small, and it is thought to be smaller than the subject is capable of controlling. Therefore, when performance is relatively near the goal, the noise component will be a relatively large part of the reported error, and attempts to correct for this source of variability will produce maladaptive corrections and considerable variability driven only by random processes. In either of these two situations involving maladaptive corrections, the learner is thought to be too influenced by the error information and makes changes from trial to trial that are actually counterproductive in terms of learning stable, long-term learning capabilities.

Finally, it is even possible that these reduced-feedback effects have the same basis as the random-practice effects discussed earlier in this chapter (Fig. 7-1). One view in that work was that blocked practice made the performance on the next trial too easy in that the solution of the motor problem was already generated and only had to be repeated on the next trial to produce an effective performance. Frequent feedback could operate in much the same way because of its capability to guide the learner in the correction of errors. Every-trial feedback thus facilitates performance on the next trial by allowing directed modifications to the movement produced on the previous trial, which might block or prevent the learner from certain retrieval operations, more or less like blocked practice is thought to interfere with retrieval practice.

SUMMARY AND IMPLICATIONS

For essentially two reasons, in this chapter I have focused on two major lines of research in the motor learning area: practice scheduling and feedback. First, these areas of research, more than most others, have revealed the shortcomings in our existing theories and understanding about motor learning. Both of these lines of work show that the practice variables that can generate large improvements in performance during practice may not be all that effective for learning as it is measured on various retention tests. How a variable can provide benefits for practice, yet degrade learning, has represented a challenge to our earlier understanding about how learning progresses: we have been taught to think that factors improving performance in practice or therapy are necessarily benefiting learning. In trying to understand these effects, I am forced to reaffirm the usefulness of the old learning-performance distinction (Guthrie,[2] Hull,[3] Tolman[4]), because it provides an effective way to think about how a variation in practice can influence performance in one way and yet influence learning in another. It also reminds us that the principles of performance on the one hand and the principles of learning on the other are necessarily different.

Along similar lines, these results enforce the idea that learning is not a unitary concept, but rather it should be thought of as a set of capabilities that are more or less applicable depending on the conditions at test. In this case, then, learning seems to be evaluated differently depending on whether the criterion involves long-term retention or generalizability or if it requires shifts to altered contexts. Without such a notion about learning to unify our thinking, we would have no effective way to understand the results seen in the experiments presented here. This notion is also consistent with the ideas of transfer-appropriate processing (see Winstein in this volume), where the goal of the instructor-therapist is to provide activities in practice that will exercise the processes that will have to be used in the criterion test. This goal forces us to determine what these criterion processes are and to be ingenious in organizing therapy so that these processes cannot be avoided or bypassed.

Second, the results described here were chosen in part because they have such strong implications for practice in real-world setting such as teaching, coaching, and of course, physical therapy. Each of these variations in practice consists of a behavioral manipulation that could easily be implemented in almost any real-world setting. Randomizing practice among several tasks to be taught in a therapy session is accomplished easily with a little planning. Providing feedback less frequently or in a summary or averaged form can be done by altering the ways the therapist reports errors in performance to the patients. Further, each of these manipulations seems to produce relatively large differences in learning, and such effects are some of the more potent in the literature. And these variations in practice have their effects on a criterion for learning that most of us would recognize as

a critical one for physical therapy: the capability to produce the behavior on a retention test, especially when the therapist and the intervention provided have been removed. This is what we want patients to be able to do as a result of our efforts, and these variables seem to provide strong benefits for this kind of learning goal.

The usefulness of these variables in practice seem to require some re-evaluation of the therapist's role in the practice session. First of all, as I have emphasized several times here, the goal is not necessarily to provide the most effective performance during therapy. This would at first seem strange to the therapist, I imagine, because major motivations for being a therapist are to help people improve, to watch people perform effectively in therapy and take pride in their accomplishments (and yours), and to receive at least their implicit appreciation for doing so. What the literature seems to suggest, though, is that the goal is not to facilitate performance in practice, but to organize practice in a way that proficiency in retention (or generalization) is maximized. This means that the therapist must make things somewhat difficult for the patient in practice and that the patient will not be so pleased with you as a result. Scheduling of tasks should apparently be randomized, which will degrade performance in practice relative to drill-like blocked practice. Feedback should probably be provided infrequently or in a summary form, which also will degrade performance in practice relative to the use of every-trial information that is not so effective for retention. There are many other examples not discussed here, such as considerations of the use of physical or verbal guidance to improve performance in practice and the use of concurrent, continuous feedback (eg, from a goniometer) while the patient is performing; these variables provide remarkable gains in performance while they are present, but they do not achieve the goal of enhancing learning as measured on retention tests (Schmidt[8,25]). If these goals are to be accepted, the dilemma is that the therapist probably should avoid using many of the procedures that seem so natural and so rewarding during the therapy session. On the other hand, we need to consider the possibility that patients need to be educated about these principles so they can appreciate that this difficult practice is the most effective way to achieve their own long-term goals.

We are a long way, of course, from understanding the processes involved in the acquisition of skills in normal, intact humans. But the principles described here are bringing us along toward this end relatively well, primarily because they are leading to the overthrow of existing theory and to the understanding about the learning process, which ultimately leads to the establishment of more effective theories that can encompass the new data. We are even further from understanding how learning processes might operate in therapy sessions with patients who are learning skills with various neurological impairments or relearning skills lost from an accident. Thinking about the processes in therapy in terms of the newer concepts in motor learning may lead to considerable insight. Although the links between motor learning and physical therapy may seem logical and promising, much research is still needed to test these ideas in physical therapy sessions with patient populations to be certain of the connections. This is an exciting prospect, though, because it will serve to bring together these two areas of inquiry that have not communicated very well with each other in the past.

References

1. Schmidt RA. Toward a better understanding of the acquisition of skill: theoretical and practical contributions of the task approach. In: Skinner JS, Corbin CB, Landers DM, et al, eds. *Future Directions inExercise and Sport Science Research*. Champaign, Ill: Human Kinetics Publishers Inc; 1989:395-410.
2. Guthrie ER. *The Psychology of Learning*. New York, NY: Harper & Row, Publishers Inc; 1952.
3. Hull CL. *Principles of behavior*. New York, NY: Appleton-Century-Crofts; 1943.
4. Tolman EC. *Purposive Behavior of Animals and Men*. New York, NY: Century; 1932.
5. Adams JA, Reynolds B. Effect of shift in distribution of practice conditions following interpolated rest. *J Exp Psychol*. 1954;47:32-36.
6. Schmidt RA. A schema theory of discrete motor skill learning. *Psychol Rev (Washington)*. 1975;82:225-260.
7. Stelmach BE. Efficiency of motor learning as a function of intertrial rest. *Research Quarterly*. 1969;40:198-202.
8. Schmidt RA. *Motor Control and Learning: A Behavioral Emphasis*. 2nd ed. Champaign, Ill: Human Kinetics Publishers Inc; 1988.
9. Wulf G, Schmidt RA. The learning of generalized motor programs: reducing the relative frequency of knowledge of results enhances memory. *J Exp Psychol [Learn Mem Cog]*. 1989;15:748-757.
10. Shea JB, Morgan RL. Contextual interference effects on the acquisition, retention, and transfer of a motor skill. *J Exp Psychol [Hum Learn Mem]*. 1979;5:179-187.
11. Henry FM. Specificity vs. generality in learning motor skill. In: Brown RC, Kenyon GS, eds. *Classical Studies on Physical Activity*. Englewood Cliffs, NJ: Prentice Hall Inc; 1968:331-340.
12. Tulving E, Thomson DM. Encoding specificity and retrieval processes in episodic memory. *Psychological Review*. 1973;80:352-373.
13. Goode S, Magill RA. The contextual interference effects in learning three badminton serves. *Research Quarterly for Exercise and Sport*. 1986;57:308-314.
14. Schneider W. Training high-performance skills: fallacies and guidelines. *Hum Factors (Baltimore)*. 1985;27:285-300.
15. Landauer TK, Bjork RA. Optimum rehearsal patterns and name learning. In: Gruneberg MM, Morris PE, Sykes RN, eds. *Practical Aspects of Memory*. San Diego, Calif: Academic Press Inc; 1978:625-632.
16. Shea CH, Kohl R, Indermill C. Contextual interference: contributions of practice. *Acta Psychol (Amst)*. 1990;73:145-157.
17. Magill RA, Hall KG. A review of the contextual interference effect in motor skill acquisition. *Human Movement Science*. In Press.
18. Craik FIM, Lockhart RS. Levels of processing: a framework for memory research. *Journal of Verbal Learning and Verbal Behavior*. 1972;11:671-684.
19. Shea JB, Zimny ST. Context effects in memory and learning movement information. In: Magill RA, ed. *Memory and Control of Action*. Amsterdam, The Netherlands: North-Holland; 1983:345-366.
20. Lee TD, Magill RA. The locus of contextual interference in motor-skill acquisition. *J Exp Psychol [Learn Mem Cogn]*. 1983;9:730-746.
21. Cuddy LJ, Jacoby LL. When forgetting helps memory: analysis of repetition effects. *Journal of Verbal Learning and Verbal Behavior*. 1982;21:451-467.
22. Bjork RA. Retrieval as a memory modifier. In: Solso R, ed. *Information Processing and Cognition: The Loyola Symposium*. Hillsdale, NJ: Lawrence Erlbaum Associates Inc; 1975:123-144.
23. Bjork RA. Retrieval practice and the maintenance of knowledge. In: Gruneberg MM, Morris PE, Sykes RN, eds. *Practical Aspects of Memory, II*. New York, NY: John Wiley & Sons Inc; 1988:396-401.
24. Moriss CD, Branford JD, Franks JJ. Levels of processing versus transfer appropriate processing. *Journal of Verbal Learning and Verbal Behavior*. 1977;16:519-533.
25. Schmidt RA. *Motor Performance and Learning: Principles for Practitioners*. Champaign, Ill: Human Kinetics Publishers Inc. In press.
26. Bilodeau IM. Information feedback. In: Bilodeau EA, ed. *Acquisition of Skill*. San Diego, Calif: Academic Press Inc; 1966:255- 296.
27. Salmoni AW, Schmidt RA, Walter CB. Knowledge of results and motor learning: a review and critical reappraisal. *Psychol Bull (Washington)*. 1984;95:355-386.
28. Gentile AM. A working model of skill acquisition with application to teaching. *Quest*. 1972;17:3-23.
29. Schmidt RA, Young DE. Augmented kinematic information feedback for skill learning: a new research paradigm. *Journal of Motor Behavior*. In press.
30. Young DE. *Knowledge of Performance and Motor Learning*. Los Angeles, Calif: University of California, Los Angeles; 1988. Dissertation.
31. Adams JA. A closed-loop theory of motor learning. *Journal of Motor Behavior*. 1971;3:111-150.
32. Thorndike EL. The law of effect. *Am J Psychol*. 1929;39:212-222.
33. Arps GF. Work with KR versus work without KR. *Psychological Monographs, 28*. 1928. Monograph 125.
34. Crawley SL. An experimental investigation of recovery from work. *Arch Psych*. 1926;13:26.
35. Elwell JL, Grindley GS. The effect of knowledge of results on learning and performance. *Br J Psych*. 1938;29:39-53.
36. Lavery JJ. Retention of simple motor skills as a function of type of knowledge of results. *Can J Psychol*. 1962;16:300-311.
37. Schmidt RA, Swinnen S, Young DE, Shapiro DC. Summary knowledge of results for skill acquisition: support for the guidance hypotheses. *J Exp Psychol [Learn Mem Cogn]*. 1989;15:352-359.
38. Schmidt RA, Lange C, Young DE. Optimizing summary knowledge of results for skill learning. *Human Movement Science*. In press.
39. Bilodeau EA, Bilodeau IM. Variable frequency knowledge of results and the learning of simple skill. *J Exp Psych*. 1958;55:379-383.
40. Ho L, Shea JB. Effects of relative frequency of knowledge of results on retention of a motor skill. *Percept Mot Skills*. 1978;46:859- 866.
41. Winstein CJ. *Relative Frequency of Information Feedback in Motor Performance and Learning*. Los Angeles, Calif: University of California, Los Angeles; 1988. Dissertation.
42. Winstein CJ, Schmidt RA. Reduced frequency of knowledge

of results enhances motor skill learning. *J Exp Psychol [Learn Mem Cog]*. 1990;16:677-691.

43. Sherwood DE. Effect of bandwidth knowledge of results on movement consistency. *Percept Mot Skills*. 1988;66:535-542.

44. Schmidt RA, Zelaznik HN, Hawkins B, et al. Motor-output variability: a theory for the accuracy of rapid motor acts. *Psychol Rev (Washington)*. 1979;86:415-451.

Suggested Reading

Bjork RA, Allen TW. The spacing effects: consolidation or differential encoding? *Journal of Verbal Learning and Verbal Behavior*. 1970;9:567-572.

Bransford JD, Franks JJ, Morris CD, Stein BS. Some general constraints on learning and memory research. In: Cermack LS, Craik FIM, eds. *Levels of Processing in Human Memory*. Hillsdale, NJ: Lawrence Erlbaum Associates Inc; 1979:396-401.

Lee TD. Transfer-aplpropriate processing: a framework for conceptualizing practice effects in motor learning. In: Meijer DG, Roth K, eds. *Complex Motor Behavior: The Motor-Action Controversy*. New York, NY: Elsevier Science Publishing Co Inc; 1988:201-215.

Lee TD, Carnahan H. Bandwidth knowledge of results and motor learning: more than just a relative frequency effect. *Q J Exp Psychol [A]*. In press.

Melton AW. Repetition and retrieval from memory. *Science*. 1967;158:532.

Schmidt RA. A schema theory of discrete motor skill learning. *Psychol Rev (Washington)*. 1975;82:225-260.

Chapter 8

Designing Practice for Motor Learning: Clinical Implications

Carolee J. Winstein, PhD, PT
Assistant Professor
Department of Physical Therapy
University of Southern California
Los Angeles, CA 90033

In general, the therapeutic approaches used in neurorehabilitation are based on a set of implicit and explicit assumptions about motor control and skill acquisition.[1] These operating assumptions, derived primarily from a neurophysiological knowledge base, characterize neuromotor control on the basis of reflexes within a hierarchically organized nervous system (see Horak in this volume for a discussion). Over the last two decades, since the original NUSTEP conference, the relevant knowledge base has evolved considerably, with new developments in the neurosciences and a merging of ideas and approaches from such fields as cognitive psychology, motor behavior, kinesiology, and biomechanics (eg, Churchland[2]). This evolution in turn has had and will continue to have important clinical implications, some of which have only begun to be considered (see Winstein and Knecht[3] for further discussion).

Therapeutic techniques derived from the older models of motor control have begun to be replaced. Before information-processing models of motor planning[4] evolved, skill acquisition was viewed primarily as a passive stimulus-response bonding process with little cognitive or perceptual motor involvement.[5] Neurotherapeutic intervention strategies that developed from this primarily "reflex" view were not concerned with the "processing operations" brought about by certain practice conditions. Such active processing was simply not part of the reflex view. Instead, any repetition of a motor act (eg, passive, active, guided, unguided) was thought to be beneficial to learning, especially if it was followed by some form of reward (ie, reinforcement). Repetition was viewed as a means for the passive "stamping in" of the desired response. Practice as defined by English and English[6] was "performance of an act one or more times, with a view to its fixation or improvement." In fact, Cross[7] in his chapter entitled "The role of practice in perceptual-motor learning," in the 1967 NUSTEP volume, used English and Englishs'[6] definition of practice as a reasonable starting point for his review.

More practically, remnants of this passive view of learning are reflected in such techniques as reflex-inhibiting postures (RIPs). These RIPs were presumed to provide for more normal movement patterns.[8] More recently, stimulated by years of experience and a reappraisal of treatment approaches in the semblance of efficacy concerns, the developers and practitioners of the RIP approach have begun to de-emphasize such passive techniques. Instead, more active goal-directed functional actions are encouraged in therapy.[9]

A Changing Perspective: The Way it Is

Present research pertaining to movement with respect to motor learning draws on a diverse set of theoretical models that use constructs such as perceptual traces,[10] coordinative structures or synergies,[11] distributed schemata,[12] engrams,[13] two-stage organism-environment action plans,[14] and motor programs.[15] Each of these constructs has its own set of theoretical underpinnings and associated predictions related to motor learning. Despite the diversity, one common thread that appears either implicitly or explicitly within each of these theoretical models is that the organism is viewed as an active participant in the learning process. This participation takes many forms including interacting with the environment, comparing intrinsic and extrinsic error information, solving problems, and processing relevant sensory cues.

Learning Versus Performance and Neurotherapeutic Exercise

The process of motor learning has been described at the neuronal level (eg, with the vestibuloocular reflex being involved in "long-term negative feedback"[17]) and at the behavioral level (eg, with motor skills having "a relatively permanent change in the capability for responding"[17]). Regardless of the level of analysis (neural or behavioral), motor learning researchers are interested in determining those conditions that lead to the kind of intrinsic processes associated with relatively permanent changes in the capability to produce a given response.[16-18]

Likewise, in the context of neurorehabilitation techniques it is of both theoretical and practical importance to determine those processes critical for learning in the form of retention and transfer of motor skills. Although this issue is of fundamental importance to the motor behaviorist,[19-21] little if any direct consideration of the practice conditions that maximally facilitate these relatively long-term functional changes is apparent in the neurorehabilitation literature (see Gentile[22] for an exception). Instead, most of the currently used techniques emphasize the importance of performance changes regardless of learning and transfer.

This critical omission undoubtedly stems from some confusion with respect to the differences between performance and learning. As emphasized by Schmidt (see Schmidt in this volume for details), a change in performance does not necessarily imply that learning has occurred.[23,24] In this chapter, the learning-performance distinction provides the basis from which several commonly used practice regimens will be evaluated.

Designing Practice to Optimize Learning

Descriptions of most neurotherapeutic approaches generally emphasize the specifics of treatment such as the particular hand placements or the magnitude and form of assistance or cueing one should provide (eg, verbal, tactile). It is assumed that these specifics of treatment are predicted on a desire to achieve some degree of neuromuscular learning or relearning. Equally apparent is that the majority of these approaches hold that practice, or repetition, is one of the most important criteria for motor learning to occur.[25,26] Yet, specific information related to the principles governing the overall organization of that practice is in most cases based on immediate performance effects rather than on learning and transfer-appropriateness.

Transfer-Appropriate Processing

Based on the earlier work of Bransford et al,[27] Lee,[28] has proposed a "transfer-appropriate processing" framework for considering the effects of certain motor skill practice methods on motor learning. In Lee's[28] framework, an effective training condition is one that puts the learner into a problem-solving mode most appropriate for later (transfer) performance. If later performance relies on the retrieval of certain motor sequences, then a practice condition that requires retrieval processes (see Bjork[29,30] for further discussions) would be most appropriate, even if this condition is more detrimental to immediate performance than a condition with less retrieval practice. Similarly, if later performance of a particular action will be required in various environmental contexts, practice conditions that require problem solving within differing task contexts will be most appropriate, again, even if it is detrimental to immediate performance (ie, contextual-interference effect; see Schmidt in this volume for a discussion). Finally, if later performance requires an anticipatory mode of motor control in contrast to a reactive mode, practice conditions that require feedforward processing will be most appropriate, even if this is more detrimental to immediate performance than practice of feedback processing.

For clarification, it is important to note that when considering the conditions of practice that are transfer appropriate, a distinction is made between a similarity of practice and transfer in terms of the processing operations and a similarity of the superficial conditions of practice and transfer. Lee[28] suggests that it is the similarity in active processing operations that is the critical element underlying the beneficial effects of various practice conditions on transfer and retention performance. "The concept of transfer-appropriateness emphasizes that practice conditions that promote a particular type of processing during acquisition trials will facilitate transfer to the extent that these processing activities are also encouraged during the transfer trials."[28(p203)]

The purpose of this chapter is to review the empirical evidence from several commonly used conditions of practice for which controlled experiments exist. The first of these concerns the frequency, scheduling, and type of information feedback presented during practice. The second concerns two different instructional practice strategies termed *adaptive* and *part-task training*. Evidence from each practice condition will be considered with respect to its transfer-appropriateness and its clinical implications. These topics were chosen because they have a relatively strong empirical base in the motor skills literature, they are currently used in some form in the majority of the so-called neurotherapeutic techniques, and they show promise with respect to clinical research.

AUGMENTED ERROR INFORMATION FEEDBACK

Aside from practice itself, augmented error information provided to the performer about goal achievement is considered to be one of the most critical variables affecting skill acquisition.[31-33] This kind of feedback has been referred to variously in the literature as knowledge of results (KR), knowledge of performance, verbal feedback, information feedback, and augmented feedback. *Knowledge of results* is operationally defined as augmented, verbal (or verbalizable), postresponse information about the movement outcome in terms of the environmental goal (see Winstein[34,35] for recent discussions of KR in physical therapy). Knowledge of results has been the focus of a large body of research in motor learning (see Salmoni et al[20] for a recent review) and has assumed an important role in motor skill acquisition. Bilodeau and Bilodeau[36] stated in a review of KR and motor learning that KR is "the strongest, most important variable controlling performance and learning." Likewise, Adams,[10] in his well-known theory of motor learning, stated that "performance improvement in acquisition depends on knowledge of results."

Similarly, in the clinical rehabilitation literature, the importance of augmented feedback for movement re-education is also emphasized. It is generally accepted in rehabilitation that information feedback variations that tend to increase the immediacy, amount, or usefulness of the information are more beneficial than those that provide less information and allow movement errors to occur. For example, Carr and Shepherd[26] suggested that the therapist should relay to the patient "information about muscle contraction immediately as it occurs." Herman[37] emphasized that the brain-damaged person would relearn more effective motor control if he were given continuous accurate feedback.

These commonly held views about the frequency and scheduling of augmented information feedback are primarily based on the well-known detrimental effects on immediate performance from conditions, or situations, with less frequent, less immediate, less precise, or less useful error information. In other words, performance looks better when error information is provided and looks worse when error information is removed. Thus conditions where error information is provided must be beneficial. What evidence is there to support this view? In particular, we may ask about the relatively permanent effects from these practice conditions. We know that KR has both temporary and relatively permanent effects on performance.[17] Are conditions with less frequent, less immediate, less useful error information also detrimental to learning? From a motor learning perspective, recent empirical evidence provides some serious challenges to the traditionally accepted principle of KR that more is better for learning.[20] The evidence from these studies will be highlighted next.

Knowledge of Results Relative Frequency

Operationally, the *relative frequency* of KR is the proportion of practice trials for which KR is provided, while *absolute frequency* refers to the total number of KR trials in a practice session. These KR frequency variables are relevant to structuring the learning environment and, as such, have received considerable attention.[20] One of the earliest and most influential studies of KR relative frequency was done over 30 years ago by Bilodeau and Bilodeau[38] using a simple lever-pulling task. By holding the number of KR trials constant (absolute frequency was 10) and varying the number of interpolated no-KR practice trials between KR presentations, they produced four different relative frequency practice conditions with values of 10%, 25%, 33%, and 100%. Blindfolded subjects pulled a vertically extended hand lever to a goal position. The KR about the direction and amount of position error was presented in accord with the particular relative frequency schedule.

Comparison of the four groups on the trials after each KR presentation (KR + 1 trial) revealed no differences that were due to relative frequency (Fig. 8-1). This suggested that the no-KR trials interspersed between the KR presentations were not particularly useful. In fact, the 10% group's performance deteriorated on the sets of nine intervening no-KR trials (Fig. 8- 2). Bilodeau and Bilodeau[38] concluded that "learning is related to the absolute frequency, and not the relative frequency of KR . . . ." As summarized by Salmoni et al,[20] the Bilodeau and Bilodeau[38] study was

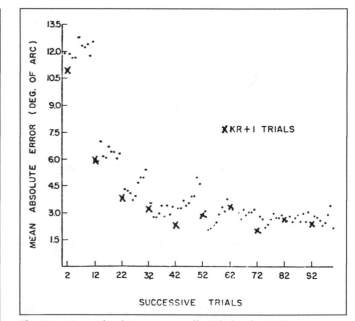

Fig. 8-2. *Mean absolute error on all trials for the 10% group. Performance on trials following KR are designated with an x. (Adapted from Bilodeau and Bilodeau.[38])*

flawed. With the omission of a proper transfer or retention test, Bilodeau and Bilodeau failed to consider the important learning-performance distinction long known to learning psychologists.[24] Thus their experiment provides no evidence with regard to learning.

Fortunately, later experiments extended the work of Bilodeau and Bilodeau[38] by using no-KR retention tests and similarly simple motor tasks. These studies demonstrated similar performance and in some cases superior performance on a no-KR retention test for groups having practiced in the low KR relative-frequency conditions (Ho and Shea[39]; R.W. Johnson, G.G. Wichs, and D. Ben-Sira; unpublished data; 1981). These results suggested that KR relative frequency was perhaps an important variable for learning. More importantly, these results suggested that conditions with less frequent KR, though detrimental to immediate performance during practice, were beneficial to learning as measured on a no-KR retention test. Unfortunately, these and several other KR relative frequency experiments are difficult to interpret because KR relative frequency and the total number of trials were confounded by holding the KR absolute frequency constant. With this experimental confound, the presumed beneficial effects from practice in low relative frequency conditions may have simply been due to the amount of practice and not the relative frequency manipulation.

Recently, with a more complex spatial-temporal movement task, an attempt was made to optimize the beneficial learning effects attributed to practice in reduced relative frequency conditions by directly manipulating the schedule of KR and no-KR trials within the practice session.[40] Two groups of subjects practiced a discrete arm movement task over a 2-day period under either high (100%) or moderate (50%) KR relative frequency conditions. In this experiment, trials were held constant across groups, thus allowing rela-

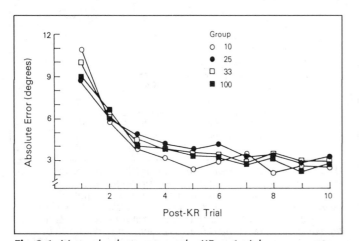

Fig. 8-1. *Mean absolute error on the KR + 1 trial across practice for the four KR relative frequency groups. (Adapted from Bilodeau and Bilodeau.[38])*

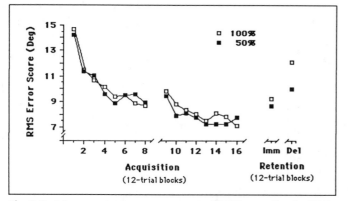

Fig. 8-3. *Mean root-mean-square error (RMS) score for the 50% and 100% KR relative frequency groups during acquisition (Blocks 1-16) and retention (immediate and delayed). (Reprinted from Winstein and Schmidt[40] by permission of the publisher; Copyright 1990 by the American Psychological Association.)*

tive and absolute frequency to covary. A faded KR schedule was used in the 50% condition so that on each day the proportion of KR trials was relatively high early in practice (100%) but was gradually reduced toward the end of practice (25%). After the 2-day practice session, each group was given an immediate (5 minute) and delayed (1 day) no-KR retention test. Group mean error scores are displayed in Figure 8-3 for both the acquisition and the transfer phases.

Although no group differences were found during the acquisition phase across the two practice days, performance of the 50% group was slightly better than the 100% group on the immediate no-KR retention test and considerably better (35%) on the delayed retention test (Fig. 8-3). Performance for both groups deteriorated over the retention interval, but the 100% KR group showed a much greater degree of deterioration compared with that of the 50% group. These results have implications for both theory and practice. First, these findings run counter to most traditional viewpoints about how KR works for learning.[5,10,15] With these traditional views, less frequent KR should degrade learning. Instead, a condition with less frequent KR was shown to enhance learning, at least as measured on a no-KR retention test. Second, from a practical standpoint, conditions that provide KR more frequently may be appealing because of their temporary effects on performance, but these effects may not be beneficial to learning in the form of retention performance when compared with conditions with less frequent KR. In fact, on closer examination, the subjects in the 50% condition did perform worse than subjects in the 100% condition on trials for which KR was not provided (compare similar results in Fig. 8-2 from Bilodeau and Bilodeau[38] with those in Fig. 8-4 from Winstein and Schmidt[40]). Interestingly, this relationship was reversed when examined in a delayed retention test.

These results were replicated in a second experiment[40] in which a delayed KR retention test was used. In this experiment, the same KR schedule as in the previous experiment was used during the 2-day practice period. However, a 12-trial delayed retention test (1 day) was administered with KR provided after each trial. Surprisingly, the 50% group per-

formed significantly better than the 100% group even on this KR retention test. These results run counter to those expected from a specificity of training view, which would predict superior retention performance for subjects in the 100% condition who practiced in a condition exactly the same as the retention test. In contrast to a specificity of practice viewpoint, the faded 50% KR relative frequency schedule seemed to facilitate the development of a capability for responding that appeared immune to the particular superficial characteristics of the practice and retention conditions. Although a superficial similarity between low relative frequency practice and retention conditions does not appear to account for these findings, it may be that a similarity in processing requirements as suggested by Lee's[28] transfer-appropriateness would account for these results. Later, an examination of some of the possible processing operations facilitated by reduced KR relative frequency practice will be provided. For now, I turn to issues related to the precise schedule of KR presentations.

Scheduling of Knowledge of Results

In the experiments discussed thus far, a faded KR schedule proved to be better than one with 100% KR. However, it was not clear whether other schedules would be as effective. Nicholson and Schmidt[41] extended the results of Winstein and Schmidt,[40] using the same experimental task with three 50% KR relative frequency conditions and one 100% condition. Two of the 50% conditions had uniformly distributed KR trials: one alternated single KR trials and the other alternated 5-trial KR and no-KR blocks. The third 50% group used a faded KR schedule similar to the original Winstein and Schmidt[40] faded schedule. On a 1-day delayed no-KR retention test, nodifferences were found among the three 50% groups, all of which performed better than the 100% group. This finding suggests that the beneficial effects of a reduced KR relative frequency were due to relative fre-

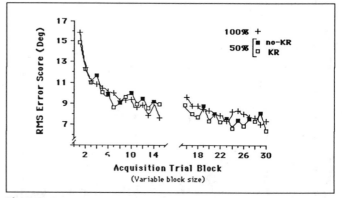

Fig. 8-4. *Mean root-mean-square error (RMS) for KR and no-KR blocks across the acquisition phase for the 50% KR relative frequency group. Trials are similarly blocked for the 100% group, but all blocks are composed of KR trials. Block size varies across the abscissa but is constant for any given block across groups. (Reprinted from Winstein and Schmidt[40] by permission of the publisher; Copyright 1990 by the American Psychological Association.)*

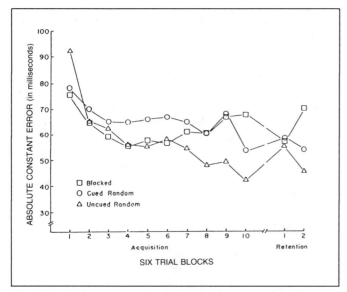

Fig. 8-5. *Absolute constant error for the three KR scheduling groups across acquisition (Block 1-10) and retention (Block 1-2). (Adapted from Lee and Carnahan.[43])*

quency and not the particular schedule used. However, in a second experiment[42] in which an expanding 50% KR schedule (reverse faded) was used, they found worse performance for the expanded group on a delayed no-KR retention test compared with the 50% faded and the alternating groups that were not different from each other. These findings suggest that to some degree the schedule of KR is important because some schedules of reduced KR relative frequency are more detrimental to learning than others.

Using a different experimental design, Lee and Carnahan[43] asked about the scheduling of KR for a multigoal timing task. In their task, the subject began the movement at a start button and then moved consecutively to knock down three wooden barriers located at varying distances in a left, right, left direction, away from the body. The task was to accomplish each of the three segments with specific movement times (160, 380, and 250 ms). In the first experiment, KR was scheduled for the blocked group such that KR for one of the three segments was presented in a blocked fashion for the first 20 trials, followed by that for another segment for 20 trials, and finally the last segment for 20 trials. Two random groups received segmental KR across six- trial sets in a random fashion such that for every six trials each segment had received KR two times. One random group was cued about which segment would receive KR before the trial, the other random group (uncued) was not provided with any information before the trial.

The results of this first experiment showed that the randomly scheduled KR was in general better for both acquisition and retention performance than a blocked schedule (Fig. 8-5). Although there was an advantage for the uncued over the cued random group in acquisition, this advantage did not persist for the retention test. It is interesting that when performance for the blocked group was examined by segment, performance for the particular segment for which KR was provided was quite good during acquisition. However, performance of that segment deteriorated progressively dur-

ing the block of trials for which KR was provided for another segment (Fig. 8-6). The authors suggest that the blocked schedule produced an attentional focus that benefited one segment at the expense of the others. "By varying the attention to segments across trials, attention would be distributed more evenly to the deficiencies of all three segments, without one particular segment benefiting at the cost of the other two, as in the blocked schedule."[43]

In a second experiment, the authors[43] customized the random KR schedule by providing KR for the segment that had been performed with the largest timing error. They contrasted this custom-random group with a "yoked" control group for which the KR schedule was the same, but obviously, it was not customized to the performance of that group. Finally, a standard blocked KR group was used as in the first experiment.

The results of this second experiment replicated those of the first in suggesting rather counterintuitively that working on one part of a complex task by giving KR about that part across a number of trials in *not* the most beneficial for the learner. Instead, a KR schedule that forces the learner to focus on different parts of the task in a nonrepetitive manner by scheduling KR in a random fashion was more beneficial for learning. The secondcounterintuitive finding was that customizing the provision of KR based on performance was no more beneficial for learning than simply providing a nonrepetitive feedback schedule.[43] This scheduling variation of KR, a "performance sensitive" manipulation, did not enhance learning. Previous work with a KR variation known as bandwidth KR has shown beneficial effects from at least one form of performance sensitive KR.

Bandwidth Knowledge of Results

In bandwidth KR, feedback is given only if the response is outside a given error range. This procedure is quite different from the other KR variations thus far considered; here, the absence of KR actually informs the subject that the previous response was acceptable. This variation provides two kinds of feedback: that which is motivating for trials falling inside the bandwidth (eg, "good, do that again") and that

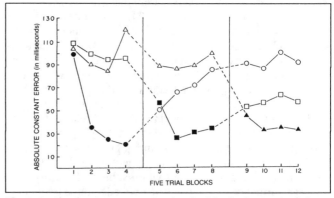

Fig. 8-6. *Absolute constant error for the blocked KR schedule. Each symbol represents a different segment of the task. The filled symbols indicate when KR was provided for each segment. (Adapted from Lee and Carnahan.[43])*

which is informative with respect to errors for trials falling outside the bandwidth.

Sherwood[44] investigated the effects of bandwidth KR with a ballistic timing task in which a lever was to be moved through a target amplitude in 200 ms. He used two (5% and 10%) bandwidth-KR conditions and one control condition for which KR was provided on every trial (0% bandwidth). In the 5% bandwidth condition, subjects received movement time KR only if their absolute error was greater than 10 ms. Likewise, the 10% group received KR if their movement time error was greater than 20 ms. His results showed no differences among groups neither during acquisition for accuracy or consistency nor during retention for accuracy. However, the 10% bandwidth group performed more consistently (ie, lower variable error) and with higher overall accuracy (a mathematical combination of constant error and variable error) on the retention test than either the 5% bandwidth or the control groups.

These retention-test results with bandwidth KR are consistent with those for KR relative frequency in that overall accuracy was highest for those subjects having practiced in conditions with less frequent KR trials. On the average, in Sherwood's[44] study the 5% bandwidth group received KR on 31% of the trials while the 10% group received it on 54% of trials. Because larger bandwidth KR conditions result in reduced KR relative frequencies compared with smaller bandwidth conditions, it is unclear how much of the beneficial effects from larger bandwidths are due simply to the reduced relative frequency. To answer this question, Lee and Carnahan[45] attempted to unravel the contribution of KR relative frequency from the bandwidth-KR variation by using a yoking procedure.

Using a timing task with a 500 ms goal, Lee and Carnahan[45] compared the performance of subjects in four KR conditions. Two of the groups were the same as those used by Sherwood,[44] namely a 5% and 10% bandwidth KR that received verbal KR about their timing error from the goal according to the prescribed bandwidths. The other two conditions designated the yoked-5% and yoked-10% conditions were created by pairing each of the bandwidth subjects with a yoked counterpart with respect to the frequency of KR. Thus subjects in the yoked conditions received KR (about their own performance) on precisely the same trials as the bandwidth subjects; however, the KR was not customized to their performance, and the absence of KR was not indicative of "good" performance as it was in the bandwidth conditions.

The results of this experiment indicated that the beneficial effects of a bandwidth condition on learning were not due simply to a KR relative frequency effect. During acquisition, the bandwidth condition seemed to enhance accuracy and stability over that achieved in the yoked relative frequency conditions. Further, during retention, although there were no significant differences among groups with respect to accuracy (ie, constant error), the subjects in the bandwidth conditions were less variable (within-subject variability) in their performance than those in the yoked relative frequency conditions. Thus the beneficial learning effects of the bandwidth KR variation over a pure relative frequency condition appear to be in terms of movement consistency. In that skilled performances are characterized as having both accuracy and stability, feedback variations that enhance performance consistency are equally important as those that pertain to accuracy.

Theoretical and Practical Implications

In the relative frequency and scheduling variations previously discussed, it is counter to intuitive practices that those conditions in which KR was provided less frequently or more randomly seemed to be more beneficial for motor learning than conditions in which KR was provided more frequently or scheduled in a more regular fashion. Lee's[28] transfer-appropriate processing framework suggests that these beneficial KR practice conditions evoke certain processes that are beneficial for learning. The following discussion highlights some of the current hypotheses regarding what these beneficial processes might be.

One view termed the *guidance hypothesis* (Schmidt et al[46] and Schmidt in this volume) holds that when KR is provided frequently the subject begins to rely on its guiding properties. The KR is said to act like a crutch that is not needed to the degree to which it is used. This overdependence on KR may actually prevent the processing of important task-related information (eg, response-produced feedback) and thus block the development of important relationships needed at the time of retention and transfer.

Another view termed the *consistency hypothesis*, supported by a number of other studies as well as the bandwidth KR work, suggests that frequent KR induces frequent response modifications, or "maladaptive short-term corrections."[40] These frequent response modifications make performance inconsistent from trial to trial.[47-49] In turn, this induced response variability interferes with the establishment of a stable action plan necessary for later response production.

Finally, it has been suggested that a schedule with intermittent KR allows for a more obvious contrast between performance driven by the KR and that which is independent of the KR (ie, during no-KR trials). It is evident that performance errors are greatest during no-KR trials.[40,43,45,50] Further, the nature and awareness of those errors may only become apparent to the subject after the next KR trial. In other words, in contrast to a schedule with frequent KR, an intermittent KR schedule provides an opportunity for the subject to obtain information about performance errors (eg, drift from the target pattern) occurring when KR is not directly driving the response. This process of comparison, in turn, may be beneficial for learning. Thus, although trials for which KR is not provided appear by immediate performance standards to be detrimental (ie, less accurate, though they may be more consistent, especially with the bandwidth KR variation), the processing operations that are suggested to occur during this period seem to be beneficial to learning in the long run.

In general, the KR research presented suggests a re-examination of the documented neurotreatment techniques demanding performance accuracy; requiring strong guidance, either manual, tactual, or verbal; advocating frequent and continuous feedback: and not permitting performance of "abnormal" movements. It may be that a page out of the motor learning literature would provide a potential explanation for the often-cited less-than-expected "carry-over" and the limited retention of motor skills retraining when such documented practices are used.

Undoubtedly, highly skilled and experienced therapists intuitively use techniques analogous to the faded, intermittent, and bandwidth KR conditions; however, the rationale has not been well articulated nor understood from the standpoint of motor learning principles. Of course, direct application of the KR research to the practice of neurotherapeutic techniques should be done cautiously until the proper clinical studies have been performed. The reader, therefore, is advisedly warned of the need for further confirmatory data from which exacting recommendations can be made in the therapeutic domain. In the next section I discuss another relevant issue in motor learning concerned with practice procedures requiring a transfer of learning from one task variation to another.

TRANSFER OF TRAINING

Transfer of learning has been defined in the literature as the influence that experience or practice of one task has on some other subsequent task.[51] This influence may be positive in that performance on one task may facilitate performance on another task. It may be negative in that performance on one task may actually interfere with or inhibit subsequent performance on a second task. Finally, transfer may be neutral in that performance on one task may have no effect whatsoever on performance of another task. From a therapeutic standpoint, we are particularly interested in those conditions that facilitate positive transfer; obviously, we would prefer to avoid those that produce negative transfer.

Two commonly used transfer of training methods in motor skills are presented. The first of these, termed *adaptive training* (AT), is a method that is performance sensitive. Basically, the difficulty of the task is adjusted through feedback from performance. The three primary elements in adaptive training regimens consist of the following: 1) a task variable (eg, some measure of performance) that reflects performance of the trainee, 2) an adaptive variable that is some dimension of the task along which difficulty is regulated (eg, precision, speed), and 3) adaptive logic that prescribes the relationship between the adaptive variable and the performance measure.[52]

The second transfer method, termed *part-task training* (PT), is generally defined as practice on some components of the whole task as a pretraining for performance of the whole task. A number of variations of part practice relate to the manner of task partitioning such as pure part, progressive part, repetitive part, retrogressive part, and isolated part.[53,54]

Although not specified as such, these two training methods are advocated and used extensively in neurorehabilitation techniques. For example, a form of adaptive training is when exercises are performed first in modified positions, such as standing with support, and then as performance improves, the task is gradually made more difficult by decreasing the amount of support. This approach is thought to facilitate later performance of the more difficult criterion task of standing independently (see Sullivan et al Fig. 8- 32[55] for an example). Another example of adaptive training is when a particular movement task is practiced more slowly initially

and, as performance improves, is practiced gradually at faster and faster rates.

Examples of part practice also are numerous in neurotherapeutic intervention. In the treatment of locomotor deficits in patients after cerebrovascular accidents, Bobath[9] advocates prone lying (especially for the younger patient). "The therapist bends the patient's knee until there is no resistance to flexion, he is then asked to hold it flexed and to maintain various degrees of flexion when the leg is gradually extended."[9] In this way, practice of a critical part of the locomotor pattern is meant to facilitate performance of the whole task of walking. Recently, Carr and Shepherd[26] advocated part, or "component," practice particularly if the component is difficult for the patient.

> Using the example of standing up, the patient may need to practise [sic] inclining his extended trunk forward at his hips and pushing down through his feet in order to get his center of gravity appropriately placed for standing up. This constitutes practise of a component. He must then practise standing up from the chair, concentrating on the component he has just practised.[26(p173)]

Although it is intuitively appealing to assume that adaptive and part-task training methods are beneficial to the learning of motor skills, the evidence in support of these approaches is not overwhelming. In the following two sections, some of this evidence will be reviewed and an explanation for the lack of clear support for these approaches will be offered in the context of transfer appropriate processing and motor learning.

Adaptive Training

Two main hypotheses are behind the adaptive training approach. First, learning a complex skill will be better if the learner starts with a less difficult version of the task and makes a gradual transition to the more difficult version. Second, learning is presumed to be better if the transitions in difficulty are performance-based rather than fixed externally by the trainer. The level of task difficulty can be adjusted during performance so an optimal level of difficulty is maintained throughout practice.[52]

In a recent study that was part of a larger multicenter learning strategies project funded by the US Defense Advances Research Projects Agency, Man et al[56] used a complex perceptual-motor task and compared adaptive and part task training methods. Briefly, the task consisted of playing a microprocessor based video game entitled "Space Fortress" (see Donchin[57] for a complete description of the project and the task). Performance of the game demanded manual control of a lever and two buttons; visual monitoring and scanning capabilities; and memory requirements, both short- and long-term. The game was complex, was interesting (ie, intrinsically motivating), and allowed independent manipulation of different components for experimentation and analysis.

The experimental design consisted of four groups: two adaptive groups (AT 5, AT 10); one part-task group (PT); and one control group (FT) that practiced the full game each session. The AT 5 group practiced a slowed down version of

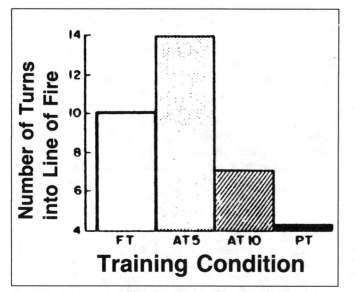

Fig. 8-7. *Average number of times that the subject's space ship crossed the fortress line of fire for the four practice conditions. FT=full task training, AT5=adaptive training at one-fifth speed, AT10=adaptive training at one-half speed, PT=part-task training. (Reprinted from Mané et al[56] by permission of Elsevier Science Publishing Corp Inc.)*

the game such that initially the speed of the "hostile" elements (eg, enemy fortress) on the screen were reduced to one fifth of the original speed. During practice, the speed was adjusted based on performance such that it was incremented by one unit after destruction of two "foe" mines, incremented by two units after destruction of one fort, or decremented by two units after the subject's ship was destroyed. There was a limit on the amount of decrement, and once the real game speed was achieved, the practice was continued at this fixed level. The AT 10 group started with a slowed down version that was reduced to one half of the original speed initially, and the same adaptive algorithm was used to adjust the speed as used for the AT 5 group.

The PT group practiced three drills, each related to different skill components. Part-task training occurred before the first real practice session. The three drills focused separately on an isolated motor component, an appraisal component, and a perceptual-motor component.

All groups practiced for a total of 20 five-minute blocks over three sessions (total 100 minutes). The PT group had an additional 14 minutes of practice on the component tasks before their first whole task practice session. In addition, to facilitate a comparison of performance across groups, a transfer test was conducted on blocks 5, 12, and 20 in which the criterion task (ie, full game) was performed regardless of training condition.

A number of interesting findings came from this experiment; however, only a few will be highlighted here. First, the PT practice condition was better thanall other conditions. However, when the PT and FT conditions were compared while controlling for actual time on the machine, no differences were found between them. Second, the AT-5 group performed better than the other three groups early in

practice. However, this simply reflects that as a result of the adaptive manipulation the task was easier. Additional measures of performance on the last block of practice revealed that the AT-5 group was significantly worse than any of the other groups. Specifically, the number of times the AT-5 subjects' space ships crossed the "line of fire" of the enemy fortress was considerably higher than that for any of the other conditions (Fig. 8-7). Because flying into the line of fire increased the chances of getting hit, the action clearly corresponded to the poor overall performance score for the AT-5 group at the end of practice.

Why was the AT-5 group so poor on this measure? A closer analysis of the response patterns of the AT-5 subjects revealed that the concept of line of fire was considerably altered when the game was played at the slower speed. Essentially, the slowed down version of the game allowed the subject to control the movements of the space ship in such a way as to wait for the enemy fortress to fire and then to *react* to the firing by changing the direction of the ship's flight. This reactive mode of control, though adequate for the slowed variation of the game, not only was inadequate but also was detrimental to performance in the normal speed of the game. In fact, during normal game speed once a shell was shot it was too late to react by moving the ship. Instead, for successful performance at the normal speed the subject needed to *anticipate* a shot from the enemy fortress and control the ship by staying away from the line of fire. Thus, although the practice of the slowed down version of the task was beneficial to immediate performance, the practice resulted in negative transfer to the criterion task. It is worth noting that the performance of the AT-10 group did not show the same negative transfer effects as that of the AT-5 group, suggesting that moderate slowing of the task allowed the development of control strategies that were appropriate for the criterion task.

From the perspective of motor learning and transfer-appropriate practice, the results of this study and others (see Lintern and Gopher[58] for a review) provide little support for the adaptive training approach in the motor skills domain. Reducing the difficulty of the task most certainly will bring about an improvement in performance. Improved performance, however, does not necessarily mean improved learning (Gutherie[24] and Schmidt in this volume). More importantly, practice of some less difficult variations of the to-be-learned task, although intuitively appealing, may facilitate control strategies that not only are inappropriate for performance of the transfer task but also interfere with that performance. This negative aspect was exemplified here in the acquisition of a feedback rather than a feedforward control strategy. From a neurotherapeutic standpoint, one potentially important principle to keep in mind is that practice of any variation of a task that considerably changes the nature of that task (ie, underlying control structure) could be detrimental to transfer and learning. This perspective will be considered in the next section where the efficacy of part-task practice is reviewed.

Part-Task Training

A practical research question that has received considerable attention, in the past but not so much recently, deals with whether it is preferable for thelearner to practice the whole task from the initial stages or for the task to be broken down into parts that are practiced separately.[8,51,54] The basic question is under what conditions is part practice more beneficial than whole practice. In general, previous research in part practice has been mixed with results suggesting that the effectiveness of this technique depends to a large extent on the type of task examined.[59-63]

In this area, Schmidt and Young[61] recently suggested that the effectiveness of transfer of training methods such as part practice should be considered with respect to the underlying control structure of the criterion task. They contend that in rapid, discrete (so-called programmed) actions, the designated parts that the instructor defines are really not separated naturally with respect to the motor control representation. Practice of these unnatural parts in isolation, therefore, does not represent practice of the same action as that embedded in the criterion task. In Lee's[28] terms, such practice is transfer inappropriate in that the processes involved in constructing the action plan for the part in isolation are not those needed to perform the whole action. In contrast, a discrete and natural subaction, or a "small whole,"[53] contained in a long-duration sequential or continuous task is quite similar to the same subaction performed in isolation; in this case, part practice would be beneficial and transfer appropriate to whole task learning. An example of each of these cases will be summarized next.

Part-task training for locomotion. Recently, we conducted a clinical study with postacute hemiparetic subjects to determine if part-task practice of dynamic weight-shifting would transfer to locomotor performance.[64] There were two groups of matched subjects in this study. One group received standing weight-shifting PT with a specially designed video feedback device that provided dynamic visual information about relative weight distribution over the paretic and nonparetic limbs. In addition to the PT, this group also received standard gait training. The other group received no

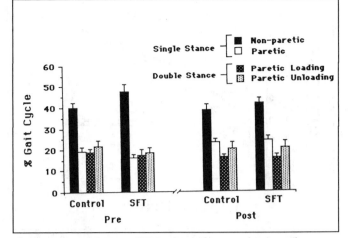

Fig. 8-9. *Group means (SEM) of percentage of gait cycle duration attributed to paretic limb single stance, nonparetic limb single stance, double-limb stance with respect to paretic limb loading, and unloading at before and after training. (Reprinted from Winstein et al[64] by permission of the publisher.)*

such PT, but did receive standard gait training (whole-task practice). Both groups were treated for a 3 to 4 week period. After the training period, both groups were tested on standing weight-shifting and locomotor performance. Our hypothesis was that if part-task standing weight-shifting training transferred positively to locomotion, then the locomotor performance of the part-task group would be significantly better than that for the whole-task group. Our results indicated that subjects trained with the feedback device showed significantly better standing weight-shift symmetry than did subjects who did not receive augmented feedback training (Fig.8-8). More importantly, although the PT subjects demonstrated a more symmetrical standing posture after treatment than did the whole-task trained group, a correspondingly greater improvement in locomotor performance was not obtained (Fig. 8-9). Indeed, in this study part- task training was as effective for locomotor performance as whole-task training.

One interpretation of these results in terms of the nature of the underlying control structure of locomotion suggests that the weight-shifting component (ie, loading phase) of the locomotor cycle is not a natural subtask of locomotion. Examination of the kinematics of the center of mass during locomotion does not provide evidence for a discrete subtask during weight transfer from one limb to another. In fact, the progression from one limb to the other appears continuous as would be expected for a smooth, programmed action. This suggests that the individual parts or phases of a locomotion cycle may represent relatively inseparable portions of a rapid, short- duration, centrally generated action. Thus the partitioned weight-shiftingcomponent, when practiced separately, seems to facilitate a form of control that is not the same as that which is needed as an integrated portion of the entire locomotor cycle. Thus, consideration of the underlying control structure of the criterion task should provide some guidance to the therapist with regard to the efficacy of a part- versus whole-task training approach.

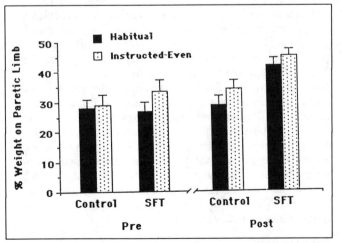

Fig. 8-8. *Mean (SEM) percentage of body weight borne by the paretic limb during habitual and instructed-even standing conditions for the control and the part-task trained groups. (Reprinted from Winstein et al[64] by permission of the publisher.)*

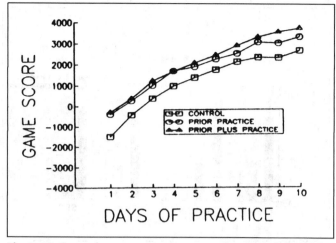

Fig. 8-10. *Space fortress game scores as a function of part-task training condition across days of practice. (Reprinted from Newell et al[65] by permission of Elsevier Science Publishing Corp Inc.)*

Part-task training for a complex perceptual-motor task. In a recent study performed with the same Space Fortress task discussed earlier for adaptive training, Newell et al[65] demonstrated that the PT was an effective training method when small wholes were used as part tasks. In contrast to Man et al,[56] Newell et al[65] used a part-practice regimen in which smaller coordinated "natural" subunits of the game were practiced rather than the "isolated" subunits used previously. They argued that the more natural subcomponents represented integrated parts within the total task context.

There were three practice groups in this experiment. The prior-practice group received 25 minutes of total practice on four subtasks before beginning formal practice on the whole game. The subtasks consisted of the following drills: linear ship control, curvilinear ship control while firing on the fortress, ship and fortress interaction, and ship and mine interaction. The second group (prior plus part) had the same prior part practice as the first group, but they also continued to have part practice along with the formal full-game practice. In addition, the level of difficulty of the continued part practice was increased. Finally, the control group had no part practice but did participate in full-game practice. All three groups practiced the game for 10 days and progressed to 40 minutes a day over the last 8 days.

The results showed a clear advantage for the two part-practice groups over the control group, both in total-game score and in measures of response dynamics of joystick and ship motion (Fig. 8-10). The prior-plus-part group also showed considerably better response dynamics for joystick control (position and acceleration) and ship velocity control than even the prior group, suggesting some beneficial effects from the continuation of part practice during the whole task training period. The effects were not evident in the total-game score.

These results suggest that prior part practice can be beneficial to learning as long as the subtasks designated as parts are natural subunits rather than isolated parts of the whole task. Although there is no formal method for designat-

ing natural subunits of a complex motor skill, some guidance may be provided by examination of the kinematics.[66,67] Natural breaks in the resultant velocity profile of a multisegment movement could reflect the end of one subunit and the beginning of the next. Specific measures of variability and correlation have been used in the past to suggest the end of one programmed unit and the beginning of the next unit.[67-68]

Theoretical and Practical Implications

The transfer-appropriate processing view holds that regimens such as adaptive and part-task practice are effective only to the extent that the processing operations practiced during acquisition are similar to those required at the time of the transfer test (ie, performance of the criterion task). As noted by Bransford et al,[27] one problem with this view is that it suffers from a circularity of logic. Until the critical processing operations can be identified a priori, the transfer appropriateness of a particular practice regimen can only be inferred based on transfer or retention performance or both. However, as noted by Lee,[28] this framework "constrains researchers to consider the processing activities promoted by the transfer test as an aspect of the experimental design that is equally important as the acquisition processing activities."[28(p212)]

This same constraint could be applied to the neurotherapeutic physical therapy practitioner in the context of designing practice to optimize the performance of functional tasks. An appreciation for the possible processing operations required for performance of the criterion functional task will most certainly influence how practice regimens are designed and implemented. For example, consider the criterion task of sit-to-stand. A transfer appropriate processing view would predict that prior practice of a natural subunit of the criterion task such as forward lean in combination with a properly timed activation of lower limb extension would be more beneficial (appropriate) for whole-task transfer than practice of forward lean in isolation.

Implicit in most of the neurorehabilitation techniques is the notion that complex (and even not so complex) actions should be decomposed into parts or made less difficult and that practice of those manageable parts or less difficult variations is advocated before actual criterion task performance is attempted. It is also generally suggested that after part practice or adaptive practice, the parts should be integrated back into the whole by practice of the whole action when possible. Certainly, from an intuitive standpoint, it would seem reasonable that practice of a part or a less difficult variation of a skill should enhance performance of the criterion skill more than simply practicing the criterion task itself. From the foregoing discussion of the success and failure of PT and AT regimens, one could argue that an appreciation for the learner as an active processor of information will help to promote the reasoned design of neurotherapeutic procedures geared not simply to enhance motor performance but also to enhance motor learning.

References

1. Gordon J. Assumptions underlying physical therapy intervention: theoretical and historical perspectives. In: Carr J, Shepherd RB, Gordon J, et al, eds. *Movement Science: Founda-*

tions for Physical Therapy in Rehabilitation. Rockville, Md: Aspen Publishers Inc; 1987:3-30.

2. Churchland P. Cognition and the brain. *TINS*. 1988;11:304-307.

3. Winstein C, Knecht HG. Movement science and its relevance to physical therapy. *Phys Ther*. In press.

4. Posner MI. *Chronometric Explorations of Mind*. Hillsdale, NJ: Erlbaum Associates Inc; 1978.

5. Thorndike EL. The law of effect. *Am J Psychol*. 1927;39:212-222.

6. English HB, English AC. *A Comprehensive Dictionary of Psychological and Psychoanalytical Terms*. New York, NY: Longmans, Green & Co; 1958.

7. Cross KW. Role of practice in perceptual-motor learning. *Am J Phys Med*. 1967;46:487-510.

8. Bobath B. *Abnormal Postural Reflex Activity Caused by Brain Lesions*. London, England: William Heinemann Medical Books Ltd; 1971.

9. Bobath B. *Adult Hemiplegia: Evaluation and Treatment*. 2nd ed. London, England: William Heinemann Medical Books Ltd; 1978.

10. Adams JA. A closed-loop theory of motor learning. *Journal of Motor Behavior*. 1971;3:111-149.

11. Tuller B, Fitch H, Turvey MT. The Bernstein perspective: II. The concept of muscle linkage or coordinative structure. In: Kelso JAS, ed. *Human Motor Behavior: An Introduction*. Hillsdale, NJ: Erlbaum Associates Inc; 1982:253-270.

12. Arbib MA. Perceptual structures and distributed motor control. In: Brooks VB, ed. *Handbook of Physiology. The Nervous System—Motor Control*. Bethesda, Md: American Physiological Society; 1981;2(pt2):1449-1480.

13. Bernstein N. *The Coordination and Regulation of Movements*. New York, NY: Pergamon Press Inc; 1967.

14. Gentile AM. A working model of skill acquisition with application to teaching. *Quest*. 1972;17:3-23.

15. Schmidt RA. A schema theory of discrete motor skill learning. *Psychol Rev*. 1975;82:225-260.

16. Lisberger SG. The neural basis for learning of simple motor skills. *Science*. 1988;242:728-735.

17. Schmidt RA. *Motor Control and Learning: A Behavioral Emphasis*. Champaign, Ill: Human Kinetics Publishers Inc; 1988.

18. Alkon DL. *Memory Traces in the Brain*. New York, NY: Cambridge University Press; 1988.

19. Adams JA. Historical review and appraisal of research on the learning, retention, and transfer of human motor skills. *Psychol Bull*. 1987;101:41-74.

20. Salmoni AW, Schmidt RA, Walter CB. Knowledge of results and motor learning: review and critical reappraisal. *Psychol Bull*. 1984;3:355-386.

21. Fischman MG, Christina RW, Vercruysen MJ. Retention and transfer of motor skills: review for the practitioner. *Quest*. 1982;33:181-194.

22. Gentile AM. Skill acquisition: action, movement, and neuromotor processes. In: Carr J, Shepherd RB, Gordon J, et al, eds. *Movement Science: Foundations for Physical Therapy in Rehabilitation*. Rockville, Md: Aspen Publishers Inc; 1987;93-154.

23. Adams JA, Reynolds B. Effect of shift in distribution of practice conditions following an interpolated rest. *J Exp Psychol* 1954;47:32-36.

24. Guthrie ER. *The Psychology of Learning*. Rev ed. New York, NY: Harper & Row, Publishers Inc; 1952.

25. Moore J. Neuroanatomical considerations relating to recovery of function following brain injury. In: Bach-y-Rita P, ed. *Recovery of Function: Theoretical Considerations for Brain Injury Rehabilitation*. Baltimore, Md: University Press; 1980:9-90.

26. Carr JH, Shepherd RB. *A Motor Relearning Program for Stroke*. 2nd ed. Rockville, Md: Aspen Publishers Inc; 1987.

27. Bransford JD, Franks JJ, Morris CD, et al. Some general constraints on learning and memory research. In: Cermak LS, Craik FM, eds. *Levels of Processing in Human Memory*. Hillsdale, NJ: Erlbaum Associates Inc; 1979:331-354.

28. Lee TD. Transfer-appropriate processing: a framework for conceptualizing practice effects in motor learning. In: Meijer OG, Roth K, eds. *Complex Movement Behavior: The Motor-Action Controversy*. Amsterdam, The Netherlands: North-Holland; 1988:201-215.

29. Bjork RA. Retrieval as a memory modifier. In: Solso R, ed. *Information Processing and Cognition: The Loyola Symposium*. Hillsdale, NJ: Erlbaum Associates Inc; 1975:123-144.

30. Bjork RA. Retrieval practice and the maintenance of knowledge. In: Gruneberg MM, Morris PE, Sykes RN, eds. *Practical Aspects of Memory, II*. New York, NY: John Wiley & Sons Inc;1988:396-401.

31. Bilodeau IM. Information feedback. In: Bilodeau EA, ed. *Acquisition of Skill*. San Diego, Calif: Academic Press Inc; 1966:255-296.

32. Newell KM. Knowledge of results and motor learning. In: Keogh J, Hutton RS, eds. *Exercise and Sport Sciences Reviews*. Santa Barbara, Calif: Journal Publisher Affiliates; 1976;4:195-228.

33. Magill RA. *Motor Learning Concepts and Application*. 2nd ed. Dubuque, Iowa: C Brown Group; 1989.

34. Winstein CJ. Motor learning considerations in stroke rehabilitation. In: Duncan PW, Badke MB, eds. *Stroke Rehabilitation: The Recovery of Motor Control*. Chicago, Ill: Year Book Medical Publishers Inc; 1987:109-133.

35. Winstein CJ. Knowledge of results and motor learning: implications for physical therapy. *Phys Ther*. In press.

36. Bilodeau EA, Bilodeau IM. Motor-skills learning. In: Farnsworth PR, et al, eds. *Annual Review of Psychology*. Palo Alto, Calif: Annual reviews; 1961;12:243-280.

37. Herman R. Augmented sensory feedback in the control of limb movement. In: Field WS, ed. *Neural Organization and its relevance to Prosthetics*. New York, NY: Intercontinental Medical Book Corp; 1973:197-212.

38. Bilodeau EA, Bilodeau IM. Variable frequency knowledge of results and the learning of a simple skill. *J Exp Psychol*. 1958;55:379-383.

39. Ho L, Shea JB. Effects of relative frequency of knowledge of results on retention of a motor skill. *Percept Mot Skills*. 1978;46:859-866.

40. Winstein CJ, Schmidt RA. Reduced frequency of knowledge of results enhances motor skill learning. *J Exp Psychol [Learn Mem Cogn]*. 1990;16:677-691.

41. Nicholson DE, Schmidt RA. Scheduling information feedback: fading, spacing, and relative frequency of knowledge of results. In: Proceedings of the North American Society for the Psychology of Sport and Physical Activity; June 1-4, 1989; Kent State University, Ohio. Page 47.

42. Nicholson DE, Schmidt RA. Scheduling information feedback: gradually increasing the frequency of knowledge of results across practice degrades skill learning. In: Proceedings of the North American Society for the Psychology of Sport and Physical Activity; May 17-20, 1990; Houston, Tex. Page 11.

43. Lee TD, Carnahan H. When to provide knowledge of results during motor learning: scheduling effects. *Human Performance*. In press.

44. Sherwood DE. Effect of bandwidth knowledge of results on movement consistency. *Percept Mot Skills*. 1988;66:535-542.

45. Lee TD, Carnahan H. Bandwidth knowledge of results and motor learning: more than just a relative frequency effect. *Q J Exp Psychol [A]*. In press.

46. Schmidt RA, Young DE, Swinnen S, et al. Summary knowledge of results for skill acquisition: support for the guidance hypothesis. *J Exp Psychol [Learn Mem Cogn]*. 1989;15:352-359.

47. Bilodeau IM, Jones MB. Information feedback in positioning problems and progress. In: Smith LE, ed. *Psychology of Motor Learning*. Chicago, Ill: The Athletic Institute; 1970:1-23.

48. Lee TD, White MA, Carnahan H. On the role of knowledge of results in motor learning: exploring the guidance hypothesis. *Journal of Motor Behavior*. 1990;22:191-208.

49. Rubin WM. Application of signal detection theory to error detection in ballistic motor skills. *J Exp Psychol [Hum Percept]*. 1978;4:311-320.

50. Hagman JD. Presentation- and test-trial effects on acquisition and retention of distance and location. *J Exp Psychol [Learn Mem Cogn]*. 1983;9:334-345.

51. Ellis HC. *The Transfer of Learning*. New York, NY: Macmillan Publishing Co; 1965.

52. Kelly CR. What is adaptive training? *Human Factors*. 1969;11:547-556.

53. Stammers R, Patrick J. *The Psychology of Training*. London, England: Muthuen; 1976.

54. Holding DH. *Principles of Training*. New York, NY: Pergamon Press Inc: 1965.

55. Sullivan PE, Markos PD, Minor MA. *An Integrated Approach to Therapeutic Exercise: Theroy and Clinical Application*. Reston, Va: Reston Publishing Co; 1982.

56. Man AM, Adams JA, Donchin E. Adaptive and part-whole training in the acquisition of a complex perceptual-motor skill. *Acta Psychol (Amst)*. 1989;71:179-196.

57. Donchin E. The learning strategies project. *Acta Psychol (Amst)*. 1989;71:1-15.

58. Lintern G, Gopher D. Adaptive training of perceptual motor skills: issues results and future directions. *International Journal of Man-Machine Studies*. 1978;10:521-551.

59. Annett J, Kay H. Skilled performance. *Occupational Psychology*. 1956;30:112-117.

60. Blum ML, Naylor JC. *Industrial Psychology*. New York, NY: Harper & Row, Publishers Inc; 1968.

61. Schmidt RA, Young DE. Transfer of movement control in motor skill learning. In: Cormier SM, Hagman JD, eds. *Transfer of Learning*. Orlando, Fla: Academic Press Inc; 1987:47-79.

62. Wightman DC, Lintern G. Part-task training for tracking and manual control. *Human Factors*. 1985;27:267-283.

63. Stammers RB. Part and whole practice in training for procedural tasks. *Human Learning*. 1982;1:185-207.

64. Winstein CJ, Gardner ER, McNeal DR, et al. Standing balance training: effect on balance and locomotion in hemiparetic adults. *Arch Phys Med Rehabil*. 1989;70:755-762.

65. Newell KM, Carlton MJ, Fisher AT, et al. Whole-part training strategies for learning the response dynamics of microprocessor driven simulator. *Acta Psychol (Amst)*. 1989;71:197-216.

66. Newell KM, McGinnis PM. Kinematic information feedback for skilled performance. *Human Learning*. 1985;4:36-56.

67. Young DE, Schmidt RA. Units of motor behavior: modifications with practice and feedback. In: Jeannerod M, ed. *Attention and Performance, XIII. Motor Representation and Control*. Hillsdale, NJ: Erlbaum Associates Inc; 1990:763-795.

68. Weiss P. Self-differentiation of the basic patterns of coordination. *Comparative Psychology Monographs*. 1941;17:Whole No. 4.

Chapter 9

Life-Span Motor Development

Ann F. VanSant, PhD, PT
Associate Professor
Department of Physical Therapy
College of Allied Health Professions
Temple University
Philadelphia, PA 19140

The purpose of this chapter is to present a life-span concept of motor development. I will also share with you some research data on which this life-span concept is being built. Before beginning the discussion, I will take an opportunity to discriminate among the terms *motor control, motor learning,* and *motor development.* Newer theories of motor control, motor learning, and motor development are a primary focus of this conference. Definitions of these three key terms are an appropriate beginning. Brooks,[1] a well-known neurophysiologist, has defined motor control in his text as "the study of posture and movements that are controlled by central commands and spinal reflexes, and also to the functions of mind and body that govern posture and movement." Although motor control is now an area of multidisciplinary study, as therapists we associate motor control theories with the study of neurophysiology. According to Richard Schmidt,[2] a psychologist and eminent motor learning researcher, motor learning is a set of processes associated with practice or experience that lead to relatively permanent changes in the capability for producing skilled action. And finally, I regard motor development as the set of age-related processes of change in motor behavior.

DISCRIMINATING AMONG TERMS

Obviously, motor learning, control, and development are concerned with motor behavior. A relatively simple method of discriminating among the three areas is by reference to the time scale over which the processes of control, learning, and development take place. When Brooks[1] referred to central commands and spinal reflexes, he implied a time frame of milliseconds or seconds in which such neural control processes occur. For Schmidt,[2] skill acquisition associated with practice or experience is usually denoted in terms of trials or blocks of trials that imply minutes, hours, and sometimes days as the time frame for change. In some less common instances, motor learning is studied across weeks and months. For the developmentalist, time is usually measured in years. Yet for the very young, developmental time may be more aptly expressed in weeks or months; for adults, decades are more often the scale over which changes are measured.

My reference to the time frame among these three areas is not necessarily the only way to discriminate. Theo-

ries of change also differ across the three areas. But ideas originating in each of these fields are often incorporatedinto the thinking of theorists and researchers in the other areas. This overlapping and sharing of ideas makes reconsideration of what one means by the terms motor control, motor learning, and motor development worthy of continued consideration.

As physical therapists, one of our unifying foundation sciences is kinesiology. We are interested in understanding human movement in order to be able to describe our patients' deficits and plan programs to assist those with movement disorders. There are multiple approaches to the study of human movement, which would fall under the general heading of kinesiology, and these approaches can include motor control, learning, and development. Probably the most familiar approach to kinesiology is biomechanical. In the field of biomechanics, the principles of mechanics are applied to description and explain human movement. A critical assumption of biomechanics is that the body can be modeled as a series of rigid links, with joints serving as pivots between the rigid segments. From this assumption, the description of limb or body displacements, velocities, and accelerations are generated. One can move from this descriptive kinesiologic method, called kinematics, to the realm of kinetics that incorporates the notion of forces as the cause movements. The two forces of greatest interest in the modeling of human movement are gravity and muscles. Although the biomechanical model has much to offer to the description and explanation of human movement, it also has limitations as an explanatory model. For example, the model does not help us understand why an individual capable of generating sufficient force to move a limb segment against the force of gravity cannot generate sufficient force to move the limb when the force of gravity is eliminated. Simply put, the biomechanical model does not portray gravity as a stimulus or facilitator of action through the structures of the nervous system. Rather, the biomechanical model portrays gravity as a constant physical force that either assists or resists limb movement dependent on the limb's relationship to the direction of the pull of gravity. Now we can switch, at will, from the biomechanical model to the model that defines gravity as a stimulus. We know that when one theoretical framework does not work, we are at liberty to adopt another. Sometimes we do this so quickly and intuitively that we forget we have switched.

Some approaches to the understanding of human movement are grounded in biological sciences, some in the physical sciences, and some in the behavioral sciences. Each brings to the understanding of human movement a different perspective. None of these are right or wrong. They are just more or less useful. Theories and models are inventions created to help further our understanding.

Neurophysiology extends our understanding of the cause of human movement to stimuli, the environmental agents that cause motor behavior. Understanding gravity as both a constant physical force from a biomechanical perspective and as a stimulus for movement from a neurophysiological viewpoint enables an alternative explanation when one model inadequately explains our observations. Both biomechanics and neurophysiology have served us well. They have given us language through which we can describe action and communicate with one another and can measure change in our patients. We use the neurophysiological model, derived from study of the function of the nervous system, to describe action in terms of phasic or tonic reflexes; or we may use the biomechanical model to describe accelerations and decelerations accompanying the stance and swing phase of gait. Neither the biomechanical nor the neurophysiological approach is right or wrong; they both are just more or less useful.

WHY STUDY MOTOR DEVELOPMENT?

So, why study motor development? Developmental science provides us with yet another approach to the understanding of human movement. Most specifically, developmental science provides us with a model that expands the time gradients over which movement is studied. The millisecond to hour block time intervals meaningful for the study of motor control and motor learning are extended to intervals of months, years, and decades by the developmentalist. The change processes that act over weeks, months, years, decades, and a lifetime bring understanding of other types of change requiring longer periods for their expression. Developmental change would be missed on the relatively microscopic time scales of the neurophysiologist or motor learning researcher.

A developmental perspective can be adopted within just about any of the major approaches to kinesiology; therefore, saying that one is a developmentalist only identifies one as being interested in age-related change. One could study the biomechanics of developmental change, the neurophysiology of developmental change, or the age-related change in motor learning processes.

The term age-related change is used here to indicate specifically that age alone causes nothing. Age is just a marker variable, a measure of time. It is not uncommon to see the term *the effects of age* as though age was a causative agent. Time measured in years, decades, or age is the fabric on which developmental change is painted. But age alone causes nothing. When one discusses the effect of age, one is pleading ignorance of the cause of the change.

The expanded time scale of the developmentalist is an appropriate backdrop for studying change in our patients.

We do follow our patients over long-term time courses: beyond infancy, when the early signs of conditions such as cerebral palsy are identified, into early childhood; beyond childhood, when a scoliosis may appear, and into the teen and early adult years, when growth of the spine normally terminates; beyond the period in young adulthood, when a catastrophic event such as spinal cord or brain injury occurs or when a chronic debilitating disease process such as multiple sclerosis is identified, into the adult years; and beyond the late middle adulthood, when a stroke could occur, into old age. The study of age-related change in motor behavior forces a long-term look at motor behavior. And this perspective is important to put physical therapy interventions into a meaningful context within a patient's life course.

Developmental science has provided a base for the traditional neurophysiologic approaches.[3-5] Each has incorporated developmental concepts and principles as a framework for describing abnormalities of motor behavior and as a guide for assessing patients and planning therapeutic interventions. We understand disorders of motor control in children as expressions of abnormal motor development, evidenced by a failure of righting and equilibrium reactions to evolve fully.[6] We also understand these disorders with reference to the development and interweaving of mobility and stability functions.[4] Evaluations of children with motor control problems traditionally leads to an assessment of motor abilities from a developmental framework. Treatment plans routinely take into account the child's developmental status.

Our models of development have been extended to describe adult motor pathology and, further, the assessment and treatment of motor control problems in adults. The application of ideas generated from the study of infant and child motor development to the description, assessment, and treatment of adults' motor disorders, however, has not always been easy. Specifically, the question arises "To what extent do developmental theories formed to explain age-related change in infant's and children's motor behavior explain age-related change in adults?"

LIMITATIONS OF CHILD-ORIENTED THEORIES OF MOTOR DEVELOPMENT

The first problem with using child motor development theories to explain age- related change in adults is that child-oriented theories stop short of explaining life-span change in motor behavior. The theories were conceived to explain progressive and cumulative change leading to an ideal end state that we term maturity. In that sense, motor development theories are idealistic: maturity represents the ideal. As a consequence, if development is viewed solely as a progressive process of growth, regression and losses are viewed as abnormalities.

The first step in moving toward a life-span model of development is to accept aging as a complimentary process of traditional concepts of growth. But aging is not the same process as the process of growth. The recognition of growth and decline as complimentary but different processes is a well-accepted premise in contemporary thought concerning motor development.[7-9] Assuming that both growth and decline are legitimate developmental processes, a life-span theory of development must be able to explain change in two directions. A life-span concept of development must account for both progressive and regressive processes. By having to explain the characteristics of both progressive and regressive processes, one is obliged to step back and take broader perspective of motor development. Initially, one might envision what is termed the *inverted U* model of development and aging: the early years being characterized by gains and progress leading toward maturity, and the later years characterized by decline and regression. But life-span motor development is not that simple. Once recognized as tenable developmental processes, growth and decline are found to be characteristic of all phases of the life span.

Developmental neurobiologists, such as Oppenheim,[10] have pointed to the proliferation and subsequent reduction in neuronal numbers as characteristic of the fetal period of development. Neurons that do not make connections with their target cells die. Postnatally, progressive and regressive change in axonal and dendritic neuronal processes are typical. In fact, neural remodeling is typical of the entire life span. Neuronal cell processes such as axons and dendrites, which early in life are prolific, allowing for many synaptic connections, are reduced in number through neuronal remodeling. This process seems to be associated with more efficient functioning, and it is considered by Oppenheim[10] as an adaptive regulatory mechanism.Overgrowth followed by selective attrition is believed to stabilize a predominant function. In the later years, such neural remodeling continues, although the process seems to affect different brain regions selectively. There is even evidence that neuronal growth to produce new synapses continues in the human life span well into later periods of the life span. Growth and decline are both integral developmental processes throughout the life span.

Another problem arises with child-oriented theories when it comes time to explain motor development across the life span. Having maturity defined as the ideal end state, the direction of the steps leading to maturity then appear to become predetermined. Early behaviors and processes seem to be prerequisites for latter behaviors and functional processes. This mode of thinking is easy to slip into. Variation from such predetermined courses are then believed to represent errors, or abnormalities. These variations are often the result of environmental and cultural differences in child rearing. We are well aware of the need to normalize tests of developmental milestones for infants and young children on the populations of children who will be tested. When these tests are given to children in cultures other than the one on which the test was standardized, we might inappropriately identify precocity or developmental delay.

Finally, I would suggest that traditional models of development are a breeding ground for ageism. The mature young adult is the standard against which all performance is judged. This standard is used often as a prejudice against those older or younger who are judged less than the ideal by either being immature or past their prime. I would suggest that each period of the life span is important within itself and should not be judged against the standard of a single period such as young adulthood. Furthermore, each period has something rich to teach the life-span developmentalist.

CHARACTERISTICS AND CAUSES OF LIFE-SPAN MOTOR DEVELOPMENT

Both the gains and losses of motor development are characterized by periods of reformative reorganization of motor behavior. In those reformative and reorganizational processes, some motor behaviors become predominant and others may be lost. The processes of reorganization and reformation that underlie motor development across the life span are the result of complex systems within the body interacting with complex environmental systems. Whether the level of analysis for understanding motor development is focus on microscopic cellular changes in the neurons or on the macroscopic changes in an individual's motor behavior as a part of a social function, such as dancing or participating in a team sport, many internal and external agents are interacting to produce change. And these internal and external factors are undergoing constant change. For example, the nervous system is constantly remodeling, the musculoskeletal system grows and transforms the body shape from infant to adult to aged adult, and the environments external to the individual change systematically. Social forces dictate that specific skills are expected of individuals during specific periods of the life span. By a year or so of age, an infant should accomplish upright locomotion. The physical skills required to accomplish primary self-care tasks are expected by the time a child enters school. Fundamental motor skills needed to participate in sports are important during childhood and adolescence. Skills for work and labor are important during later adolescence and young adulthood. Therefore, each period of the life span has different expectations for motor behaviors.

During a recent conversation I had with a colleague (J. Walker, PhD; Physical Therapy Program Director; Dalhousie University, Halifax, Nova Scotia), we were discussing the notion of efficiency and energy cost and how this theoretical construct of efficiency might be related to performance in the task that I have been studying of rising from the floor. I described to her how smoothly the young adults performed, moving from lying directly through sitting, transferring their weight from buttocks to feet in squatting, and then moving on up to standing. Older adults tend to break the task down into a series of steps through progressively less stable transitional postures: rolling up and over to get on hands and knees; walking the hands back toward the knees; and moving to kneeling, then to half-kneeling, and then up to standing. I asked her if she thought the older adults are demonstrating a balance control problem, which requires that a stable posture be regained periodically. When viewed in slow motion, the elderly individuals almost stop at each transitional posture before moving on the next. I would think older adults would choose the most efficient way of performing, which is to move directly forward. Walker remarked that efficiency means different things to younger and older adults. The older adults are efficient if you put them in a proper context. They are concerned with conserving energy. Energy conservation is not a concern of the young. Their energy stores are relatively boundless. They do not have to plan their day so that they can take in active events after four o'clock in the afternoon; they can generate large bursts of energy to complete tasks rapidly. Older adults tend to use strategies that will enable them to maintain performance over the course of a day.

Does this mean that balance and flexibility do not also influence motor performance in this task? No, developmental change is multifactorial. The point is that in multifactorial change we must remember to choose appropriate contextual frameworks in which to judge performance and not to hunt for the easy answer—the single variable that accounts for change. Although we may come to understand and appreciate those elements that influence change from one behavior to another, constant reorganization and reformation of motor behavior is a complex process of many different systems interacting. It is important to remember that these systems and processes of change may well be different at different periods within the life span.

No period is more or less important than another. Rather, each period is different and must be judged within the framework of both a changing body and a changing environment. Different periods are characterized by different modes of functioning and in different contexts.

The philosophical base for this life span theory may be found in Ecclesiastes 3:1-8 (KJV).

To every thing there is a season, and a time to every purpose under the heaven:

A time to be born, and a time to die; a time to plant, and a time to pluck up that which is planted;

A time to kill, and a time to heal; a time to break down, and a time to build up;

A time to weep, and a time to laugh; a time to mourn, and a time to dance;

A time to cast away stones, and a time to gather stones together; a time to embrace, and a time to refrain from embracing;

A time to get, and a time to lose; a time to keep, and a time to cast away;

A time to rend, and a time to sew; a time to keep silence, and a time to speak;

A time to love, and a time to hate; a time of war, and a time of peace.

LIFE-SPAN PERSPECTIVE OF RIGHTING ABILITIES

With this theoretical perspective as a backdrop, I will use the research data from my studies of righting to illustrate how I have come to this understanding of life-span motor development.

Righting tasks involve those bodily movements that enable one to assume upright posture. A major developmental accomplishment in infancy is the capability of rising to erect stance. Over the course of the first year of life, infants gradually acquire the ability to move from one stable body posture to another, progressively elevating the center of gravity above the support surface. Ultimately, these postural transi-

tion skills of infancy are incorporated into the action of rising from recumbency to erect stance. According to Bayley's schedules, the average age of accomplishment of the first form of rising from recumbency (Aufstehn I) is 14.0 months.[11]

Righting tasks are particularly well suited for life-span motor development study. These abilities are acquired early in the life span and, barring catastrophic events, remain until death. For this reason, righting tasks provide an excellent vehicle for study of life-span change in motor behavior.

Movement patterns used to right the body comprise a developmental dimension,[12] that is, the movement patterns are an aspect of motor behavior that varies with age. Having been studied in infants, the form of the movements used to attain erect stance were found to change over time.[11,13] Yet, righting movements had not been studied systematically beyond early childhood.

I will restrict discussion here to our studies of the task of rising from a supine position lying on the floor. As with most worthwhile endeavors, this research program is the result of teamwork. The graduate students who have participated in this research are the greatest measure of its success. They include Randy Richter,[14] Sandra Sarnacki,[15] Elizabeth Francis,[16] Annabel Lewis,[17] Jeanne Boucher,[18] Paul Sabourin,[19,20] Shari Luehring,[21] Jeanne O'Neil McCoy,[20,22] Cheryl Ford-Smith,[20,23] Susan Cromwell,[20] and Archana Deo.[20]

My studies of righting began with a study of young adults performing the task of rising from a supine position.[24] That study involved a bit of risk taking. First and foremost, it involved studying a single age group of young adults from a developmental perspective. Developmental studies are most typically designed either as cross-sectional surveys of different age groupsor as longitudinal studies of a single group at different times. This first study of young adults included just one age group, studied at a single point in time. Further, although it is common to study infants and children from a developmental perspective, it is most uncommon to study young adults without a younger or older comparison group. My initial study[24] can be considered a legitimate approach to begin to identify a developmental dimension question if the assumptions of that original study are understood. First, I assumed that motor development is a life long process. From that assumption it logically holds that any age group represents a legitimate group for developmental study. Second, I assumed, following Robertson's lead,[25] that sequences of motor development are universal and invariant. As an extension of this assumption, I thought if individuals are moving through a developmental sequence of behaviors, at any point in time behavior should be reflective of one's developmental stage. If the individual is in transition between two developmental stages, their behavior should be reflective of those neighboring stages. Variability in performance across several trials of a task should reflect neighboring stages in a developmental sequence.[26]

In my study of rising from the floor,[24] the subjects performed 10 trials in succession. All were recorded on videotape. Movement patterns of three body regions—the upper extremities, the axial region, and the lower extremities—were described in writing, and movement pattern categories

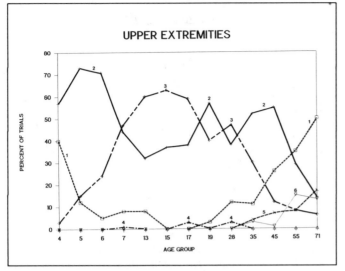

UPPER EXTREMITIES

Fig. 9-1. *Incidence of upper extremity region movement patterns in each age group. Step 1, Push and Reach to Bilateral Push; Step 2, Push and Reach; Step 3, Symmetrical Push; Step 4, Bilateral Reach; Step 5, Push and Reach with Thigh Push; and Step 6, Push and Reach to Bilateral Push with Thigh Push.*

of action were formed. These categories were then used to classify the individual's rising movement across all 10 trials. I then analyzed the variability of each subject, seeking to identify a developmental sequence of movement patterns for each body region. The sequence that resulted was then verified in a study of young children. There were 30 boys and girls in each of four age groups in the second study. Each child performed the same task of rising under the same conditions that were used with the adults.[27] As a result of that study of children, I confirmed the developmental order of the movement patterns hypothesized in the adult study. Although the youngest children demonstrated movement patterns that had not been observed in adults, those patterns seen in adults had been placed in correct developmental order as a result of analyzing subjects across trial variability. The new patterns identified in children were predicted to be earlier appearing than those demonstrated by adults, and they were placed as beginning steps in the developmental sequences. Luehring[21] studied older adults performing this task, Sabourin[19] extended this work to teenagers, and we[20] have gone on to study additional age groups of adults performing the same task under the same conditions. With the exception of Luehring's[21] study of older adults, each age group was composed of about 30 subjects, and each subject performed 10 trials. There were 60 older subjects who each performed 5 successive trials.

Figure 9-1 illustrates the age differences in incidence of each upper extremity pattern across the age groups ranging from 4 years into the seventies. One should note that the *x* axis for this graph (and for the other two graphs presented) is not a chronological time scale. Rather, the age groups studied are placed in chronological order with equal intervals between each group. The age groups reflect what we thought were meaningful intervals of developmental change for this task: years for young children, 2-year intervals for teen-aged

subjects, and decades for adults. The movement pattern hypothesized to represent Step 1 of a developmental sequence for arm action in the rising task is labeled 1 in Figure 9-1. That pattern, termed *Push and Reach to Bilateral Push,* demonstrates a decreasing incidence with respect to age up to the teen years. It was not observed in 15- or 17-year-old subjects, but then was observed to demonstrate a steadily increasing incidence with increasing age beginning in the late teen years. This step predominates in the older adults.

Step 2 is relatively common at all ages. This pattern is termed *Push and Reach.* It predominates in young children, in 19-year-olds, and in those in their thirties and forties; however, it is replaced by Step 1 as the most common pattern in those in their fifties and in older adults who were in their early seventies. Step 3, termed the *Symmetrical Push* pattern, was the predominant pattern of teens and young adults. Although, interestingly, in 19-year-old subjects, Step 2 (Push and Reach pattern) predominated. The *Symmetrical Reach* pattern, labeled 4 in Figure 9-1, was seen with very low incidence in three subjects: a 7 year old, a 17 year old, and a young adult. The low incidence of this pattern causes me to conclude that it is not a developmental step for this task. Step 5 (termed *Push and Reach with Thigh Push*) involves a push and reach pattern followed by pushing on one or both thighs. This pattern was observed initially by Luehring[21] in her older-adult subjects, and it has subsequently been seen in subjects in their thirties, forties, and fifties, with an increasing incidence with respect to age. A similar upper extremity-thigh push was observed in adults who demonstrated an initial Push and Reach to Bilateral Push pattern. After pushing with both hands against the floor, one or both hands then pushed against the thigh. It appears that the subjects are assisting the action of trunk extension or knee extension when they push against their thighs in the process of rising. Thus new patterns of action appear in adults who are over 30 years, patterns that are not seen in younger subjects. Figure 9-1 confirms the age-related variability in the incidence of upper extremity movement patterns across a wide range of the human life span. If it were not for these two new patterns appearing in older subjects, a simple progressive and regressive process could have been hypothesized to account for these data. But the different patterns observed in those over 30 years cannot be ignored. A simple progression and regression hypothesis will not account for these data.

Figure 9-2 illustrates age-related variability in the incidence of axial region movement patterns for this task. In this component, Step 1 (*Full Rotation Abdomen Down*), involving full rotation with the abdomen in contact with the support surface, was seen in only one 4-year-old subject. I continue to regard this as a developmental step because of the reports of both McGraw[13] and Schaltenbrand[28] that indicate the first form of rising involves rolling into the prone position before elevating the trunk in the all-fours posture. I would predict that a study of children under the age of 4 years performing this task would demonstrate a grater incidence of this pattern. The pattern labeled 2, the *Full Rotation Abdomen Up pattern,* was relatively common in young children, and it also predominated in the oldest group of adults. This full rotation pattern was not seen in 15 and 17 year olds. *Partial Rotation,* Step 3 of the developmental se-

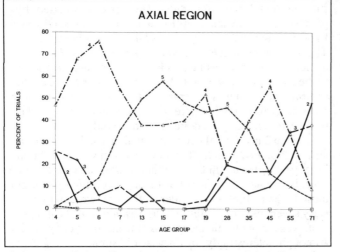

Fig. 9-2. *Incidence of axial region movement patterns in each age group. Step 1, Full Rotation Abdomen Down; Step 2, Full Rotation Abdomen Up; Step 3, Partial Rotation; Step 4, Forward with Rotation; and Step 5, Symmetrical.*

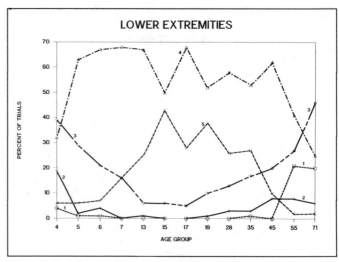

Fig. 9-3. *Incidence of lower extremity movement patterns in each age group. Step 1, Kneel; Step 2, Jump to Squat; Step 3, Half Kneel, Step 4, Asymmetrical Squat; and Step 5, Symmetrical Squat.*

quence, was like Step 2, relatively common in the youngest children and in the oldest subjects. The Partial Rotation pattern predominated only in those in their fifties and was seen least frequently in the teens and youngest adult subjects. The pattern labeled 4 (*Forward with Rotation*), involving a predominantly forward trunk pattern with some rotation, was most common in the children, the 19 year olds, and those in their thirties and forties. The other teen and young-adult subjects predominantly demonstrated Step 5 (*Symmetrical*) of the sequence: a symmetrical pattern of trunk flexion followed by extension to the vertical, with the earlier steps of the sequence seen with greatly decreased frequencies.

Figure 9-3 illustrates the varying incidence of patterns for the lower extremities. Again, as in the other two body regions, patterns hypothesized torepresent earlier appearing steps (Steps 1, 2, and 3) are more common in the youngest and oldest subjects. The latest appearing steps tend to be most common in the teen and young-adult years. For the lower extremities, an interesting relationship exists between patterns labelled 4 and 5 across the teen and young-adult groups. Their incidence appears to vary reciprocally: when pattern 4 demonstrates an increased incidence, then pattern 5 shows a decreased incidence, and visa versa. These two patterns represent symmetry and asymmetry in squatting patterns used in the process of rising. The asymmetrical pattern is predicted to develop in advance of the symmetrical pattern. At the time when the symmetrical pattern is most common, between the ages of 13 and 30 years, it appears as if subjects sometimes rise symmetrically and sometimes asymmetrically. Symmetrical performance seems to require careful control of force production and balance. Variations in force production between the legs result in asymmetrical lower extremity patterns. In many respects, patterns 4 and 5 could represent a discrimination of the degree of motor control exhibited in the performance of the symmetrical pattern across these age groups.

IMPLICATIONS OF THE RIGHTING STUDIES

As a result of these studies, I am now confident of my initial assumption that movement patterns vary with age across the human life span. We have extended this work to the tasks of rolling from supine to prone,[11,14,15] rising from a bed,[12,19,20] and rising from a chair.[13] As additional data are gathered from a variety of tasks and age groups, the complexity of the developmental processes underlying age related differences in movement patterns becomes increasingly apparent.

The correlates of gender and body dimensions[29] and of activity level are being examined.[21,30] Although it is easy to understand how the movement patterns used to rise from a bed and chair might be sensitive to differences in body dimensions, the task of rising from the floor may at first glance appear to be less influenced by body size. We have found correlations between body dimensions and movement patterns in the latter task.[29] These relationships are particularly strong in adult women. As a follow-up to these findings, we are currently studying the effects of various levels of weight on the performance of the task in young-adult subjects, and I am studying a small group of pregnant women across the period of pregnancy.

The righting tasks also appear to be affected differentially by the activity level of the individual.[21] Experience with the task may also affect performance. One subject, who was 19 years old, remarked during the study of rising from the floor that she was not sure how long it had been since she had laid down on the floor.

I am also beginning to notice differences in the movements of individuals of different ages who perform the same developmental pattern. Young subjects are smoother in transition from one posture to another, while older subjects seem to pause in each stable posture. The squat pattern of young children performing the supine-to-stand task is accomplished more commonly with medial rotation of the hips, while the squat of young adults involves more lateral rotation. These differences will likely require a more detailed kinematic analysis.

SUMMARY

In summary, my concept of life-span motor development is growing richer day by day. Simple notions of progression and regression have been replaced by a concept of many dynamic systems, both within and surrounding the individual, collectively determining age-related change in motor behavior. These systems include, of course, the musculoskeletal and nervous systems that also undergo constant change across the life span. The changes in these systems are reflected in physical growth and decline and in reformation and reorganization of neural processes. The environmental milieu and the social contexts in which we function also change systematically, placing various changing demands on individuals across their lives. The research program we have started is leading in many interesting directions, and along the way we are learning more and more about the whys of age-related change in motor behavior across the human life span.

References

1. Brooks VB. *The Neural Basis of Motor Control*. New York, NY: Oxford University Press Inc; 1986:5, 129-150.
2. Schmidt RA. *Motor Control and Learning: A Behavioral Emphasis*. 2nd ed. Champaign, Ill: Human Kinetics Publishers Inc; 1988:195, 227-298, 346.
3. Bobath K, Bobath B. Cerebral palsy: Part 1: Diagnosis and assessment of cerebrl palsy. Part 2: The neurodevelopmental approach to treatment. In: Pearson PH, Williams CE, eds. *Physical Therapy Services in the Developmental Disabilities*. Springfield, Ill: Charles C Thomas, Publishers; 1972:31-185.
4. Stockmeyer SA. A Sensorimotor approach to treatment. In: Pearson PH, Williams CE, eds: *Physical Therapy Services in the Developmental Disabilities*. Springfield, Ill: Charles C Thomas, Publishers; 1972:186-222.
5. Voss DE. Proprioceptive neuromuscular facilitation: the PNF method. In: Pearson PH, Williams CE, eds. *Physical Therapy Services in the Developmental Disabilities*. Springfield, Ill: Charles C Thomas, Publishers; 1972:223-282.
6. Bobath K. *The Motor Deficits in Patients with Cerebral Palsy. Clinics in Developmental Medicine. No. 23*. London, England: William Heinemann Medical Books Ltd; 1966.
7. Eckert HM. *Motor Development*. 3rd ed. Indianapolis, Ind: Benchmark Press; 1987.
8. Payne VG, Isaacs LD. *Human Motor Development: A Lifespan Approach*. Mountain View, Calif: Mayfield Publishing Co; 1987.
9. Haywood KM. *Life Span Motor Development*. Champaign, Ill: Human Kinetics Publishers Inc; 1986.
10. Oppenheim RW. Ontogenetic adaptions and retrogressive processes in the development of the nervous system and behavior: a neuroembryological perspective. In: Connolly KJ, Prechtl HFR, eds. *Maturation and Development: Biological and Psychological Perspectives: Clinics in Developmental Medicine. No. 77/78*. Philadelphia, Pa: J B Lippincott Co; 1981:73-109.
11. Bayley N. The development of motor abilities during the first three years. *Monograph of the Society for Research in Child Development*. 1935;1:1-26.
12. Wohlwill JF. *The Study of Behavioral Development*. New York, NY: Academic Press Inc; 1973.
13. McGraw MB. *The Neuromuscular Maturation of the Human Infant*. New York, NY: Hafner Publishing Co; 1945.
14. Richter RR, VanSant AF, Newton RA. Description of adult rolling movements and hypothesis of developmental sequences. *Phys Ther*. 1989;69:63-71.
15. Sarnacki SJ. *Rising from Supine on a Bed: A Description of Adult Movement and Hypothesis of Developmental Sequences*. Richmond, Va: Virginia Commonwealth University; 1985. Thesis.
16. Francis ED. *Description of the Sit-to-Stand Motion in Children and Young Adults: Hypothesis of Developmental Sequences*. Richmond, Va: Virginia Commonwealth University; 1987. Unpublished thesis.
17. Lewis AM. *Age-related Differences in Rolling Movements in Children*. Richmond, Va: Virginia Commonwealth University; 1987. Unpublished thesis.
18. Boucher JS. *Age-related Differences in Adolescent Movement Patterns During Rolling from Supine to Prone*. Richmond, Va: Virginia Commonwealth University; 1988. Unpublished thesis.
19. Sabourin P. *Rising from Supine to Standing: A Study of Adolescents*. Richmond, Va: Virginia Commonwealth University; 1989. Unpublished thesis.
20. VanSant AF, Cromwell S, Deo A, et al. Rising to standing from supine: a study of middle adulthood. *Phys Ther*. 1988;68:830. Abstract.
21. Luehring S. *Component Movement Patterns of Two Groups of Older Adults in the Task of Rising from Standing from the Floor*. Richmond, Va: Virginia Commonwealth University; 1989. Unpublished thesis.
22. McCoy JO. *Age-related Differences in the Movement Patterns of Adolescents 11, 14, and 17 Years of Age Rising to Standing from Supine on the Bed*. Richmond, Va: Virginia Commonwealth University; 1989. Unpublished thesis.
23. Ford-Smith C. *Age Differences in Movement Patterns Used to Rise from a Bed: A Study of Middle Adulthood*. Richmond, Va: Virginia Commonwealth University; 1989. Unpublished thesis.
24. VanSant AF. Rising from a supine position to erect stance: description of adult movement and a developmental hypothesis. *Phys Ther*. 1988;68:185-192.
25. Roberton MA. Stability of stage categorizatins across trials: implications for the "stage theory" of overarm throw development. *Journal of Human Movement Studies*. 1977;3:49-59.
26. Roberton MA, Williams K, Langendorfer S. Pre-longitudinal screening of motor development sequences. *Research Quarterly for Exercise and Sport*. 1980;51:724-731.
27. VanSant AF. Age differences in movement patterns used by children to rise from a supine position to erect stance. *Phys Ther*. 1988;68:1130-1138.
28. Schaltenbrand G. The development of human motility and motor disturbances. *Archives of Neurology and Psychiatry*. 1928;20:720-730.
29. VanSant AF, Cromwell S, Deo A, et al. Relationships among body dimensions, age, gender, and movement patterns in a righting task. Poster Presentation at the 64th Annual Conference of the American Physical Therapy Association; June 12, 1989; Nashville, Tenn.
30. Green LN. The relationship between activity level and the movement patterns of supine to standing. Manhattan, Kan: Kansas State University; 1989. Thesis.

Chapter 10

Should the Normal Motor Developmental Sequence Be Used as a Theoretical Model in Patient Treatment?

Susan Attermeier, MA, PT
Assistant Clinical Professor
Division of Physical Therapy
Department of Medical Allied Health Professions
School of Medicine
University of North Carolina at Chapel Hill
Chapel Hill, NC 27514
Section Head, Physical Therapy
Center for Development and Learning
University of North Carolina at Chapel Hill

Before the development of the neurotherapeutic approaches, normal developmental sequences were not used as a framework for treatment with neurologically involved patients; instead, the emphasis was on teaching of functional activities. With the advent of the new approaches, however, the notion of recapitulation of ontogenetic development, combined with the reflex-hierarchical model of the central nervous system, resulted in specific application of developmental sequencing. Although the developers of the different techniques produced different versions of sequences, the notion of using developmental sequences was specified as a common denominator at the NUSTEP conference.[1] Margaret Rood, in an early writing, summed up their philosophy as follows:

> It seemed to me that if it were possible to apply the proper sensory stimuli to the appropriate receptor as it is utilized in normal sequential development, it might be possible to elicit the motor responses reflexly, and by following neurophysiological principles establish proper engrams. The movement which results in response to a summation of reflexes is "boosted" up to higher centers for final reception at the sensory cortical level.[2]

Clearly, the idea was to emulate the natural course of things as a way of bringing the abnormal back to or at least closer to normal. We still operate on the assumption that following normal development as a model in treatment can make sense, but we are developing much more complex notions about how and why the normal child changes over time. The current emphasis on functional positions and activities need not be viewed as reversionary, provided we clarify what we mean by development. The suitability of using developmental sequencing for treatment, thus, needs to be considered in light of several issues, none of which are currently resolved.

SEQUENTIAL DEVELOPMENT VERSUS FUNCTION

Some motor skills, specifically the ability to roll, sit, stand, and walk, are included in any list of developmental skills, but they are also fundamental to daily living and therefore are part of any sound therapy program. In addition, the normally developing infant generally displays additional capabilities such as prone-on-elbows, prone-on-hands, creeping, and kneeling. The strict developmentalist would hold that these skills should be taught to a patient in the same sequence as they would appear in a normal healthy child; to skip a step would be detrimental to the performance of the next one. Likewise, the practice of a "lower level" skill such as rolling would be considered at least beneficial and perhaps necessary for performance of a "higher level" skill such as standing. This notion has resulted in the use of extensive regimens of mat activities for adult and pediatric patients. In the absence of research data either supporting or refuting this practice, the best course would be to devise clinical measures for individual patients that would allow the therapist to judge whether practice of a particular activity has a beneficial effect on performance of another. False dichotomies should also be avoided. Rolling, for example, is not a low level skill if the task is getting out of bed.

LEVELS OF ANALYSIS

Many of our current problems with describing abnormal motor development-behavior stem from gaps in our knowledge of normal motor development-behavior. It may be helpful to discuss this with respect to the different levels of analysis that can be used when dealing with motor activity.[3,4]

Behavioral (Functional) Level

We have many tests and checklists available that describe the emergence of "normal" motor behaviors. These address the questions of *what* should occur and *when* it should occur. Just what the items are, however, will depend entirely on the theoretical stance of the investigator. An instrument developed on the basis of observation of spontaneous movement patterns will be very different from one developed by studying responses to preset situations or handling maneuvers. Examples of the former can be found in the work of Pikler[5] and Milani-Comparetti.[6] The latter approach is exemplified in much of Gesell's[7] work and in reflex testing of any sort. An investigator such as Wolanski,[8] who is looking for parallel strands of behaviors related to a particular ability, will produce a different instrument from someone such as Bayley,[9] who is observing sequential emergence of various motor abilities. There is no single test that provides up-to-date and complete norms on the full range of motor behaviors seen in the normally developing child. Furthermore, information on the evolution of motor patterns in disabled children and adults is very sparse, leaving the clinician to decide whether or not the normal abilities should be practiced.

Kinesiological-Biomechanical Level

At this level of analysis, we are concerned about the properties of the musculoskeletal system at rest and during movement, and we are asking questions about *how* movement is occurring. It is here that we, as therapists, focus much of our attention, attempting to change features of movement, such as alignment, synergistic combinations, and temporal characteristics. We have been lumping this information into a category of "quality," but in fact much of it can be quantified. Descriptions of the evolution of posture and movement that are currently being generated[10-12] have the potential for providing the "gold standard" by which we assess the effect of treatment.

Neurophysiological Level

At this level of analysis, we are asking *why* external events are occurring, in terms of internal processes. In the past, we have used the hierarchical-reflex model to explain observable events and have, for example, referred to integration of primitive reflexes and to improvement of vestibular function, even though there was no way of documenting that any changes in the nervous system had occurred. With our current state of knowledge, we realize that we are far from being able to describe behaviors at this level. For clinical purposes and for professional credibility, the first two levels of analysis mentioned are far superior.

INTRINSIC PROBLEMS OF SEQUENCING

Regardless of which level of analysis we are using, if we want to entertain the notion of developmental sequencing there are certain fundamental issues that need to be addressed.[13] We define a sequence strictly as A→B. This means A always comes first and produces B. It also means that without A, B will not occur.

The observed sequence, however, is usually A→B but sometimes B→A, then it is not a strict sequence and cannot be relied on as a guide in therapy. For example, most chil-

dren show equilibrium capability in prone position before they do in sitting or standing, but is this a strict sequence? We know that it is not because some children who are placed in baby walkers for large parts of the day gain control in upright before doing so in prone position. We could conclude from this common clinical finding and from published evidence of cross-cultural variation[14] that capabilities may be developed on the basis of demand rather than on the basis of some inherent order.

Another issue in developmental sequences has to do with the search for the very first item in a sequence. If we believe that motor development is a process of building one skill on another, then we want to know what the first skill is in the series. This is an admittedly linear mode of thinking that may not be congruent with an overall systems approach to motor function. Nevertheless, there may be subsystems within an organism that are organized in linear fashion, and these may be relevant to therapy.

We must also determine, in any given set of events, whether A is necessary or merely sufficient to produce B. There may in fact be different paths to the same endpoint, and this concept has great implications for planning therapy programs. Furthermore, there is evidence that parallel or overlapping sequences exist in motor development and that their courses may be asynchronous. There may be components from different strands in the motor domain that must co-occur before a particular ability can emerge. Finally, and most interestingly, as we consider the implications of the dynamical action model, we are challenged to look beyond the intrinsic characteristics of the child and study the environment, the interactions with parents, and the social milieu to explain the emergence of motor ability.

Clearly then, the issue of developmental sequencing has taken on extraordinary complexity, leading us to question its utility for patients of any age. The next two chapters discuss the use of developmental sequences with pediatric and adult patients.

Acknowledgment

This work was supported by the Bureau of Maternal and Child Health Resources Development, Office of Maternal and Child Health, Grant #MCJ000916-25.

References

1. Proceedings: An Exploratory and Analytical Survey of Therapeutic Exercise. Northwestern University Special Therapeutic Exercise Project (NUSTEP). *Am J Phys Med.* 1967;46:1037-1047.
2. Rood M. Neurophysiological reactions as a basis for physical therapy. *Phys Ther Rev.* 1954;43:444-449.
3. Schmidt RA. *Motor Control and Motor Learning: A Behavioral Emphasis.* Champaign, Ill: Human Kinetics Publishers Inc; 1988:4-5.
4. Carr JH, Shepherd RB, Gordon J, et al. *Movement Science: Foundations for Physical Therapy in Rehabilitation.* Rockville, Md: Aspen Publishers Inc; 1987:24-26.
5. Pikler E. Learning of motor skills on the basis of self-induced movements. In: Helmuth J, ed. *Exceptional Infant: Studies in Abnormalities.* New York, NY: Brunner/Mazel Inc; 1971;2:51-89.
6. Milani-Comparetti A. Pattern analysis of normal and

abnormal development: the fetus, the newborn, the child. In: Slaton DS, ed. *Development of Movement in Infancy*. Chapel Hill, NC: Division of Physical Therapy, University of North Carolina at Chapel Hill; 1980.

7. Knobeloch H, Pasamanick B, eds. *Gesell and Amatruda's Developmental Diagnosis: The Evaluation and Management of Normal and Abnormal Neuropsychologic Development in Infancy and Early Childhood*. 3rd ed. New York, NY: Harper & Row, Publishers Inc; 1974.

8. Wolansky N. A new method for the evaluation of motor development in infants. *Polish Psychological Bulletin*. 1973;4:43-53.

9. Bayley N. *Bayley Scales of Infant Development*. New York, NY: The Psychological Corp; 1969.

10. Thelan E, Fisher DM. The organization of spontaneous leg movements in newborn infants. *Journal of Motor Behavior*. 1983:15:353- 377.

11. Heriza CB. Comparison of leg movements in preterm infants at term with healthy fullterm infants. *Phys Ther*. 1988;68:1687-1693.

12. Woolacott M, Shumway-Cook A, Williams H. The development of posture and balance control in children. In: Woollacott M, Shumway-Cook A, eds. *Development of Posture and Gait Across the Life Span*. Columbia, SC: University of South Carolina Press; 1989:77-96.

13. Campbell RL, Richie DM. Problems in the theory of developmental sequences: prerequisites and precursors. *Human Development*. 1983;26:156- 172.

14. Cintas H. Cross cultural variation in motor development. *Physical & Occupational Therapy in Pediatrics*. April 1988;8:1-20.

Chapter 11

Should the Normal Motor Developmental Sequence Be Used As a Theoretical Model in Pediatric Physical Therapy?

Sarah W. Atwater, MPT, PT
Acting Instructor
Division of Physical Therapy
Department of Rehabilitation Medicine
University of Washington
Seattle, WA 98195

Normal development is a broad term that may be defined differently by any two given physical therapists. It can be thought of in different frames of reference such as when functional milestones are reached, when specific developmental milestones are accomplished, when the components of those specific milestones occur, or when the neurophysiological entities that make up the components are completed. Development can also be broken down into the different psychomotor domains such as cognitive, social, motor, and language. For the purposes of this discussion, the one area of motor development will be considered in light of each of the above mentioned frames of reference and in relationship to development in the other domains. This chapter will focus on how and when the different theoretical models of normal motor development can be applied to physical therapy programs for children.

All of the major neurophysiological treatment approaches developed from the 1950s to the early 1970s (neurodevelopmental treatment, Rood techniques, sensory integration, Domain-Delacato patterning, and proprioceptive neuromuscular facilitation) are based theoretically on the use of a normal motor developmental sequence.[1-5] This concept has influenced when we introduce and how we plan treatment of motor delay and pathological conditions for an extended time. The underlying theory of motor control to support these approaches is a hierarchical model, which states essentially that the higher brain structures gradually exert control over the lower brain and spinal cord structures.[6,7] It was thought that motor development proceeded in a hierarchical fashion from head to toe, from proximal to distal structures, and from gross movements to fine movements.[8] Some approaches were insistent that therapy programs follow a progression of motor activities sequenced according to the normal development of motor milestones,[5] whereas others expressed normal development in terms of the components of the motor milestones (mobility, stability, righting and equilibrium reactions) and espoused that these components needed to be introduced and mastered in a developmental sequence.[1-4]

A recent survey of pediatric occupational therapists' clinical practice patterns found that therapists reported a developmental sequence as the most common frame of reference that was important to their practice.[9] (A neurodevelopmental sequence was the second most common frame of reference reported.) A survey of pediatric physical therapists would likely find similar results. The major neurophysiological therapies supporting the use of a developmental sequence are the most popular therapies used with children inthe United States.[6] However, efficacy research studies on these developmental treatment approaches have yet to provide definite support for these therapies.[6,10-15]

Because of these widespread beliefs and practices, it is important to review our understanding of developmental issues. New alternative ideas on motor development and motor control are being formulated. The theories presented in the original writings regarding these neurophysiological treatment approaches[1-5] need to be reviewed and updated to foster improvement of our treatment techniques and to better analyze treatment efficacy.

DISCUSSION

Recent Developmental Research Findings

Current research has shown that some of our ideas regarding a normal motor development sequence have been incomplete. For example, Case-Smith et al[16] have found that the theory of proximal to distal development may be an oversimplification. Although they found that proximal and distal control are correlated, each seems to follow a separate developmental sequence and to have its own documented separate motor control pathways.[16,17] Shumway- Cook and Woollacott[18] have shown that young children have a motor strategy, the ankle strategy, for maintenance of balance in standing; it is completed by muscle activation beginning from distal musculature and progressing to proximal musculature. Thus our use of treatment procedures that call for facilitating the development of proximal control before distal control may need to be modified.

Thelan[19] has examined the development of the human gait pattern in great detail and found that infants' kicking patterns are orderly and resemble later gait pattern movements in timing and synchrony. She advocates, from a dynamical theory of motor control, that the central nervous system uses preprogrammed motor programs to decrease the degrees of freedom inherent in our musculoskeletal system. She hypothesizes that the gait pattern of muscle activation is present from birth. Heriza's[20] studies suggest that this may occur even earlier. Other dynamics, such as body mass and dimensions, relative muscle tone, and muscle strength, must mature for the gait pattern to be expressed as upright independent walking.[19] These factors mature to the necessary extent around one year of age, which is when children who are developing motor skills in a typical fashion take their first independent steps.

Shumway-Cook and Woollacott[18] have found similar developmental progressions in the motor reactions that occur when a child's center of gravity moves out of his or her base of support. They state that both the motor patterns of an ankle and the hip strategy for maintenance of standing balance are basically present at age 15 months to 3 years, but they undergo some disorganization between the ages of 4 to 6 years. The motor patterns of standing balance become mature and adult-like at age 7 to 10 years. Shumway-Cook and Woollacott[18] postulate that this disorganization, at 4 to 6 years of age, is due to the major growth spurt that children undergo with changes in body proportions and strength. Fetters[21] also notes that directed arm movements at a fixated target, the prereaching of a newborn, disappears at around 6 weeks age, only to reappear at 3 to 4 months age. Based on these studies, the idea of cephalocaudal development must be reconsidered.

Bly,[22] in an analysis of the development of the components of proximal movements and balance reactions, presents the unfolding of our movements in a cephalocaudal fashion but in a series of complicated circular progressions. According to Bly,[22] infant motor development starts with physiological flexion, which is due to the infant's position in the small intrauterine environment. The infant moves then to antigravity extension and then to antigravity flexion. Cocontraction of both flexors and extensors produces antigravity lateral flexion, and last, coordination of both flexors and extensors produces rotational movements. This process occurs around the neck, the shoulders, the trunk, and the pelvis, with the infant working on many of these behaviors in overlapping sequences in the different body sites.

Gilfoyle and Grady[23] also describe the motor development process as occurring in a circular pattern. They illustrate the progression of development as an "ever-widening and upward continuum of a spiral."[23(p49)] The spiraling continuum reflects the ongoing upward process of development, with the spiral-effect emphasizing the integration of old and new motor behaviors. This spiraling process is influenced by environmental experiences and changes in the child's neuromuscular system. Fetters[21] carries the idea of environmental influence further, stating that development is always changing based not only on the experiences of the child but also on those of the family and the therapist. She describes a transactional model of development that is dependent on the environment. For the infant, that environment includes all the players involved in interactions with the child as well as the child himself.

The Bobaths,[24] in their most recent writings on neurodevelopmental treatment, state that it may not be appropriate to follow a normal motor developmental sequence too closely. They state, "Contrary to the impression that could be gained from the charts of development such as Gesell (1947), Griffiths (1954) and Illingworth (1960), development often does not proceed in a definite sequence, in which 'milestones' follow each other."[24(p9)] These sequences of motor milestones as presented in standardized tests are useful only in detecting an abnormality but should not be used to plan a treatment program. Instead, they think that in normal development many motor activities are developed simultaneously to culminate in a milestone.

A normal motor developmental progression seems not only to move in overlapping sequences but also to demonstrate great variability in the age that a motor milestone emerges. Examination of any of the developmental motor scales reveals this.[25-27] The specific quality of the movements can also vary a great deal. For example, Bottos et al,[28] in a prospective study of locomotor strategies that precede independent walking, categorize the movements of infants into four different forms of prewalking locomotor strategies plus an "other" category. Infants in all categories were found to go on to show normal motor development. They concluded that normal motor development does not follow a single pathway and that many factors are probably involved in the genesis of locomotor strategies. They suggest that lax ligaments, hypotonia, size of child, asymmetry, and genetic heredity all play a part in the quality of movement the infant shows. Bottos et al[28] also monitored linguistic development. They found no difference in development of this domain among the babies that were in a category that just got up and walked and those that crawled and then walked. They made the point that the locomotor strategies in themselves did not significantly influence neurologic development, in particular linguistic development, of the children. Thus, according to Bottos et al,[28] treatment approaches such as those advocated by Delacato[29] that require children, even those who are already independently able to walk, to go through specific types of locomotor programs (eg, symmetrical crawl, reciprocal crawl, symmetrical creep) are inappropriate.

All of the above mentioned ideas regarding development blend very well with the new systems theory of motor control. With the systems theory, there are many circular loops and levels of control that cannot only work independently but can also work interactively with each other.[30] This theory suggests an interaction in the progression of all systems and subsystems that determines when a motor skill appears and what the quality is of that skill. Als,[31] in her work with preterm infants, postulates a similar theory, the synactive organization of behavioral development. This theory involves four different systems of the organism. The systems, from most biological to most interactional, are the autonomic system, the motor system, the state regulation system, and last, the attentional-interactive system. All the systems interact and may affect the outcome and organization of any motor behavior; likewise, the motor system can influence the other systems. Ultimately, the motor system's organization affects the ability of the infant to interact with the environment and learn.

Interaction of the Domains of Development

Coordination and interaction occurs not only in the systems described by Als[31] but also in a broader sense among different domains of development. Normal development in all domains is intercorrelated, and development in one domain may slow down and stop while the infant concentrates on activities in another domain.[24] The specific developmental relationship of motor and cognitive skills has been examined by Bertenthal and Campos.[32] Their research suggests that some motor experience is necessary for development of certain types of basic cognitive skills. Specifically, Bertenthal and Campos[32] have studied self-produced locomotion and found that it seems to be a necessary factor for infants to learn avoidance of heights, memory of locations, and spatial cognition skills. Based on their findings, they believe, as do many neurobiologists, that there is a primacy of action over reaction in the course of normal development. Thus there are many environmental motor experiences such as self-produced locomotion that facilitate overall developmental changes.

Age, Severity of Disability, and Development

In addition to emphasizing the intercorrelation between domains, the Bobaths[24] also state that,

Treatment should not attempt to follow the sequence of development described, regardless of the age and physical condition of the individual child. Rather, it should be decided what each child needs most urgently at any one stage or age, and what is absolutely necessary for him to participate for future functional skills, or for improving the skills he has but performs abnormally.[24(p11)]

Thus they advocate that the overall aim of the treatment is to make the infant or child as functional as possible with specific goals that vary depending on the individual. To become as functional as possible, the infant or child with a significant amount of motor involvement may need alternative routes rather than following a normal developmental sequence. Likewise, the child with less motor involvement may need rigorous sensory cues and practice to learn more normal and thus more adaptive motor skills.

Molnar[33] advocates some general guidelines relative to the focus of therapeutic treatment at different chronological ages. The younger infant and child, thought to have more plasticity in their neuromuscular systems, may benefit from facilitation of as normal movement as possible. But if movement ability has not progressed in the older child, he or she would require alternative ways to accomplish movement so that environmental retardation would not minimize whatever genetic capability the child might possess. Determining when to make this change of focus of treatment would again be dependent on the individual child. If one believes Bertenthal and Campos'[32] findings that suggest that some motor skills facilitate some very early basic cognitive func-

tions, perhaps therapists should consider alternative means of movement earlier.

To examine the link between independent mobility and self-initiated behaviors, Butler[34] studied the use of early powered wheelchair mobility for children with major motor disabilities. She found that the frequency of self-initiated behaviors in the children examined improved after achievement of independent mobility. With this in mind, therapists should not discourage children from using whatever means they have to maneuver in the environment even if the therapeutic focus is for normal muscle tone and movement patterns.

If a normal developmental sequence is demanded of a child who has extreme difficulty with movement, regardless of age, and alternative means of interacting with the environment are not facilitated, the child may learn that his or her actions have no effect on the environment and a phenomenon of learned helplessness may develop.[35] Campbell,[36] in describing older children, advocates that the motor system does not function in isolation, but rather it provides each of us with a means of interacting withour environment. Campbell[35,36] espouses that therapists using neurodevelopmental approaches need to combine developmental treatment ideas with behavioral analysis techniques and child-directed motivating outcomes. In this way, children may learn to perform independently in areas critical for independence as adult members of society. Especially with children who are severely involved, therapists must consider why we move and thus teach critical movements to improve not only safe and productive interaction with the environment but also functional ability, rather than to provide therapy based on a normal developmental motor sequence. Using techniques from a motor learning perspective could enhance this endeavor.[37]

CONCLUSION

Many issues must be considered when determining whether to follow a normal motor developmental sequence for treatment planning and implementation. First, there are new ideas of the progression of normal development that we can incorporate into earlier theories about motor development. For example, children do not require complete proximal control before beginning to work on distal control. The child would benefit from working on activities in both realms simultaneously. Further, evidence of preprogrammed motor strategies for gait, standing balance, and reaching suggests that therapists should directly facilitate specific motor patterns to achieve these functional goals.

Second, all the motor milestones and their components normally develop in overlapping sequences, with spurts of development and some plateaus or even regressions, while development occurs in other body areas and aspects. Therapists need to consider these overlaps of development and provide motor activities at various intensities and developmental levels.

Third, many variations can occur in the development of motor milestones in terms of quality of movement and onset of the movement, but these variations can lead to motor abilities that are within normal limits. Therapists should continue to consider other factors involved in the quality and onset of movement, such as body size and type or muscle tone and strength. Nonetheless, therapists could allow children more latitude to be unique in their own movement patterns.

Fourth, therapists also need to consider the needs of the child in all the domains of development rather than just the motor area. Sometimes either the frequency of motor therapy should be decreased or the focus of treatment altered to allow extra work in another domain for a period of time. Our ultimate goal for therapy is improvement of functional abilities. With this in mind, therapists need to consider specific motivators for any given child and respond to the child's lead in order to maximize the benefits of therapy and ultimately, function.

Fifth, the age and extent of disability should be considered heavily when determining a therapy plan. Sometimes adherence to a normal motor development sequence per se should be abandoned in order to encourage functional ability. Older children's therapy programs should include very functional age-appropriate activities of interest to the child and family in lieu of emphasis on the components of normal motor development. In the case of a child with severe motoric involvement, it may be more meaningful from the very beginning to emphasize movements for communication and interaction within the environment versus working for normal development of equilibrium reactions and other motor components. In the more cognitively intact child, we should encourage motor behaviors such as alternative forms of independent mobility so that development in the other domains can proceed in as normal fashion as possible.

Having an updated understanding of normal development from all perspectives will help therapists make decisions about children's therapy programs. As our body of knowledge grows, therapists will be challenged to incorporate both the basics of development and many of the subtle complexities into their work with children and families. All aspects of development and its complexities should be reviewed when formulating a therapy program for a child with motor delay or disability. However, each child and family should be considered individually in terms of their current needs and desires. Only then can the best activities and methods be determined to facilitate development of the most functional motor behaviors.

References

1. Bobath B. Facilitation of normal postural reactions and movement in the treatment of cerebral palsy. *Physiotherapy.* 1964;50:246-262.
2. Stockmeyer SA. An interpretation of the approach of Rood to the treatment of neuromuscular dysfunction. *Am J Phys Med.* 1967;46:900-956.
3. Voss DE. Proprioceptive neuromuscular facilitation: the PNF method. In: Pearson PH, Williams CE, eds. *Physical Therapy Services in the Developmental Disabilities.* Springfield, Ill: Charles C Thomas, Publisher; 1972:223-282.
4. Ayres AJ. *Sensory Integration and Learning Disorders.* Los Angeles, Calif: Western Psychological Services; 1972.
5. Domain RJ, Spitz EB, Zucman E, et al. Children with severe brain injuries: neurological organization in terms of mobility. *JAMA.* 1960;17:257-262.
6. Harris SR, Atwater SW, Crowe TK. Accepted and controver-

7. Gordon J. Assumptions underlying physical therapy intervention: theoretical and historical perspectives. In: Carr JH, Shepherd RB, Gordon J, et al, eds. *Movement Science: Foundations for Physical Therapy in Rehabilitation.* Rockville, Md: Aspen Publishers Inc; 1987:1-30.
8. Jacobs MJ. Development of normal motor behavior. *Am J Phys Med.* 1967;46:41-51.
9. Lawlor MC, Henderson A. A descriptive study of the clinical practice patterns of occupational therapists working with infants and young children. *Am J Occup Ther.* 1989;43:755-764.
10. Campbell SK. Editorial. *Physical & Occupational Therapy in Pediatrics.* Spring 1989;9:1-4.
11. Ottenbacher KJ, Biocca Z, DeCremer G, et al. Quantitative analysis of the effectiveness of pediatric therapy: emphasis on neurodevelopmental treatment approach. *Phys Ther.* 1986;66:1095-1101.
12. Ottenbacher KJ. Sensory integration therapy: affect or effect. *Am J Occup Ther.* 1982;36:571-578.
13. Ottenbacher KJ, Peterson P. The efficacy of vestibular stimulation as a form of specific sensory enrichment. *Clin Pediatr (Phila).* 1983;23:428-433.
14. Palmer FB, Shapiro BK, Wachtel RC, et al. The effects of physical therapy on cerebral palsy: a controlled trial in infants with spastic diplegia. *N Engl J Med.* 1988;318:803-808.
15. Parette HP, Hourcade JJ. A review of therapeutic intervention research on gross and fine motor progress in young children with cerebral palsy. *Am J Occup Ther.* 1984;38:462-468.
16. Case-Smith J, Fisher AG, Bauer D. An analysis of the relationship between proximal and distal motor control. *Am J Occup Ther.* 1989;43:657-662.
17. Lawrence DG, Kuypers HGJM. Pyramidal and non-pyramidal pathways in monkeys: anatomical and functional correlations. *Science.* 1965;148:912-975.
18. Shumway-Cook A, Woollacott MH. The growth of stability: postural control from a developmental perspective. *Journal of Motor Behavior.* 1985;17:131-147.
19. Thelan E. Developmental origins of motor coordination: leg movements in human infants. *Developmental Psychobiology.* 1985;18:1-22.
20. Heriza CB. Organization of leg movements in preterm infants. *Phys Ther.* 1988;68:1340-1346.
21. Fetters L. Developmental concepts for therapeutic intervention. In: *In Touch Self-Study Courses: Topics in Pediatrics, Lesson 7.* Alexandria, Va: American Physical Therapy Association; 1990:1-8.
22. Bly L. *The Components of Normal Movement During the First Year of Life and Abnormal Motor Development.* Birmingham, Ala: Pittenger and Associates Pathway Press; 1983.
23. Gilfoyle EM, Grady AP, Moore JC. The spiraling continuum of spatiotemporal adaptation. In: Gilfoyle EM, Grady AP, Moore JC, eds. *Children Adapt.* Thorofare, NJ: Slack Inc; 1981.
24. Bobath B, Bobath K. The neuro-developmental treatment. In: Scrutton D, ed. *Management of the Motor Disorders of Children with Cerebral Palsy.* London, England: Spastics International Medical Publication; 1984:6-18.
25. Bayley N. *Bayley Scales of Infant Development.* New York, NY: The Psychological Corp; 1969.
26. Gesell A. *Developmental Diagnosis.* 2nd ed. New York, NY: Harper & Row, Publishers Inc; 1947.
27. Illingworth RS. *The Development of the Infant and Young*

Child: Normal and Abnormal. New York, NY: Churchill Livingstone Inc; 1960.

28. Bottos M, Barba BD, Stefani D, et al. Locomotor strategies preceding independent walking: prospective study of neurological and language development in 424 cases. *Dev Med Child Neurol*. 1989;31:25-34.

29. Delacato CH. *Neurological Organization and Reading*. Springfield, Ill: Charles C Thomas, Publisher; 1966.

30. Schoner G, Kelso JAS. Dynamic pattern generation in behavioral and neural systems. *Science*. 1988;239:1513-1520.

31. Als H. A synactive model of neonatal behavioral organization: framework for the assessment of neurobehavioral development in the premature infant and support of infants and parents in the neonatal intensive care environment. *Physical & Occupational Therapy in Pediatrics*. Summer-Fall 1986;6:3-51.

32. Bertenthal BI, Campos JJ. New directions in the study of early experience. *Child Dev*. 1987;58:560-567.

33. Molnar GE. A developmental perspective for the rehabilitation of children with physical disability. *Pediatr Ann*. 1988;17:766-776.

34. Butler C. Effects of powered mobility on self-initiated behaviors of very young children with locomotor disability. *Dev Med Child Neurol*. 1986;28:325-332.

35. Campbell PH. Programming for students with dysfunction in posture and movement. In: Snell ME, ed. *Systematic Instruction of Persons with Severe Handicaps*. Columbus, Ohio: Merrill Press; 1987;1:88-210.

36. Campbell PH, McInerney WF, Cooper MA. Therapeutic programming for students with severe handicaps. *Am J Occup Ther*. 1984;38:594-602.

37. Croce R, DePaepe J. A critique of therapeutic programming with reference to an alternative approach based on motor learning theory. *Physical & Occupational Therapy in Pediatrics*. Summer 1989;9:5-33.

Chapter 12

Should the Normal Motor Developmental Sequence Be Used As a Theoretical Model to Progress Adult Patients?

Ann F. VanSant, PhD, PT
Associate Professor
Department of Physical Therapy
College of Allied Health Professions
Temple University
Philadelphia, PA 19140

Studies of motor development were quite common early in this century. Nancy Bayley,[1] Arnold Gesell,[2] Mary Shirley,[3] and Myrtle McGraw[4] were among the most well-known motor development researchers and motor development sequence builders during that early period. The importance of their descriptive surveys of the abilities of infants and children cannot be underestimated. Their work provided the foundation on which further study of the correlates and determinants of age-related change was and continues to be based. Further, their work provided the developmental foundations for our traditional neurophysiologic approaches to physical therapy.[5-7]

Early motor development researchers such as Bayley,[1] Shirley,[3] and Gesell[2] reported an order of appearance of motor skills during infancy and early childhood. Their methods involved repeated observations of numbers of babies at set intervals. They documented the age of accomplishment of skills they were studying and calculated average age of attainment as a method of condensing their data. Figure 12-1 illustrates Shirley's[3] normal developmental sequence leading to bipedal locomotion. It is these average ages that prescribe what we have commonly referred to as the *normal developmental sequence*.

Maybe because developmental sequences traditionally lead to maturity and are therefore directed to an end, the steps have assumed an importance that is inappropriate. Unfortunately, if the mature end-state is predetermined, then the steps leading to that end take on undue significance: somehow the developmental steps become the route to maturity. It is important to remember that the steps to maturity are just the motor behaviors that were the focus of the developmentalists who described the sequence. They are not a magical route to maturity.

Unfortunately, until relatively recently[8,9] little attention has been paid to the variability in the order of accomplishment of infant skills. Touwen[10] found a great deal of variability across infants in the sequence of motor development. This recent finding supports similar conclusions by Shirley[3] more than 50 years ago. The implication of variable

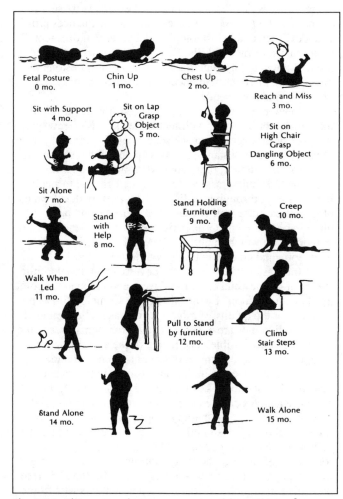

Fig. 12-1. *This series of pictures, reprinted from Shirley,[3] illustrates a normal developmental sequence leading to bipedal locomotion. The sequence is composed of a set of distinctly different tasks and is therefore an intertask developmental sequence. The age of accomplishment has been used to order the tasks into a sequence of development. The sequence is commonly termed the normal developmental sequence.*

orders of accomplishment of motor milestones is great for physical therapy. Variability of motor sequences also requires that we re-examine common hypotheses regarding developmental skills. For example, Is it necessary to creep before one walks? If just one child walks without first creeping, then it is immediately apparent that creeping is not a necessary prerequisite skill for walking.

We have too strictly interpreted motor developmental sequences as a series of prerequisite skills leading to walking. When disabled adults are asked to participate in activities that represent developmental tasks of infancy and early childhood because the activities are considered necessary steps for later function, one may rightfully raise the question, Have we taken this too far?

Does this suggest that developmental sequences have no meaning for us as therapists? I would suggest that developmental sequences are very meaningful. But we should remember that there are different types of developmental sequences, and each can be used in different ways.

The kinds of motor developmental sequences that hold value for us as physical therapists include *intertask* sequences and *intratask* sequences. Intertask sequences provide developmental chronologies of a variety of different motor tasks, or motor skills. Developmental sequences commonly known to physical therapists as motor milestone sequences are intertask sequences. Figure 12-1 portrays Shirley's[3] intertask sequence.

In contrast, intratask sequences outline the development of motor behavior within a single skill. McGraw[4] provided us with several intratask sequences. Figure 12-2, from McGraw,[4] illustrates an intratask sequence for assuming an erect posture. In fact, there are two intratask sequences illustrated. The first task could be termed pulling to standing. Phases A through E of Figure 12-2 portray development of the infant in the pull-to-stand task. The second task, pictured in phases F and G, is performed without benefit of an individual on which to pull up. Phases F and G illustrate developmental change in rising without assistance.

Intertask sequences, or the developmental motor milestones of infancy and childhood, were aptly named "appointments with function" by the late Milani-Comparetti. Despite concern for the quality of motor performance, he reminded us that individuals are expected to care for themselves to the greatest extent possible. The listing of the average age for developmental accomplishments serves as a check on the motor independence of infants and as cues to physical therapists for the functional skills expected of infants. Developmental schedules can be used to determine age appropriate objectives for physical therapy programs for infants who are not yet walking. We should not forget that developmental accomplishments continue after infancy. The ability to perform tasks of running, hopping, jumping, skipping, and galloping are accomplishments of very early childhood. These tasks also should be considered as appointments with function for children. When young children are prohibited these activities because the quality of their locomotor patterns is judged to be inadequate, the young child's opportunity to gain additional functional competence may be thwarted.

We cannot forget that a step of an intertask developmental sequence can be considered prerequisite for

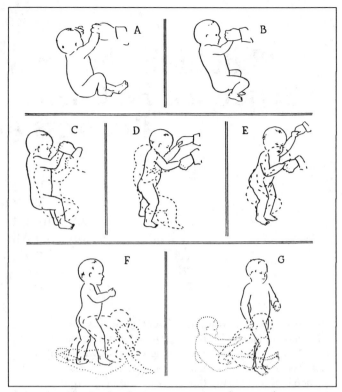

Fig. 12-2. *This illustration, reprinted from McGraw,[4] demonstrates the sequence of development within the task of assuming an erect posture. Technically, two different tasks are illustrated. One task is pulling to erect stance; the other involves rising without pulling up. Phases A through E portray developmental change in the motor behaviour of the infant in the pull-to-stand task. Phases F and G illustrate developmental change in movement patterns used to rise without pulling up.*

later functional accomplishments only if the later appearing task is composed of postural or movement patterns of the early appearing task. For example, keeping the head aligned with respect to the vertical is normally accomplished before the task of standing erect. Vertical head alignment can be considered prerequisite to standing erect because it is a component of the latter task.

Within the intertask sequences of infancy are natural orders of progression of body control against the force of gravity. The center of gravity of the body is progressively elevated above the support surface as the postures of sitting, being on hands and knees, kneeling, and standing are accomplished and as an increasing number of degrees of freedom must be controlled. This natural order also presents a diminishing base of support for the body, requiring a concomitant increase in balance abilities. Although the tasks are scaled in difficulty, they are not necessarily prerequisites for standing.

Intertask sequences should serve as a guide to infants' and children's functional competence and should be a reminder for physical therapists of those tasks that provide physical independence. Intertask sequences do not outline the only route one may take to motor maturity. Adults do not need to practice all the tasks of infancy in preparation for relearning to walk.

We are just now beginning to focus attention on and appreciate intratask sequences. McGraw's[4] sequences can serve as guides for age-related expectations for body movements used by infants to perform tasks such as rolling, getting to sitting, rising to standing, and walking. Age differences in movements used to perform other tasks of daily living are beginning to be described for older children, adolescents, and adults of various ages (see VanSant, life-span motor development chapter in this volume). These intratask sequences can be used as guides when selecting movement patterns to teach patients for the performance of fundamental righting tasks such as rolling and rising from the bed, the chair, or the floor.

It appears that the change in movement patterns used to perform these fundamental skills may be related to gender, changing body dimensions, and activity level. At present, selecting age appropriate movement patterns to teach patients would seem most appropriate until the determinants of these movement patterns are better understood.

From my perspective as a life-span developmentalist, I would suggest that it would be useful to further define age-related tasks of latter childhood; adolescence; and young, middle, and older adulthood. By doing this, we may systematically identify the most common functional tasks of these periods of the life span, and we may create life-span intertask sequences. Compared with the developmental sequences of infancy and early childhood, the latter-life periods are relatively unstudied.

This lack of study may be because we believe we already know the tasks that youth and adults perform. All that may very well be true, but when are the tasks of infancy and childhood commonly given up? How important is a task such as creeping to a teenager or to a middle-aged adult? When do adults commonly give up running? These abilities, although seemingly so variable, are likely to change systematically with age. And for those abilities that are relatively constant across the life span, additional study of age-related change in movement patterns used to perform common tasks would be useful for therapists who are designing rehabilitation programs.

So, would I use the *developmental sequence* as a pattern of progression for adults? No, I would not. The developmental sequence, as an intertask developmental sequence, is simply an outline of the average ages at which infants ac-

quire skills of physical independence. Many of the tasks while appropriate for infants seem inappropriate for adults. Although I see natural orders of progression within intertask sequences, I know that early appearing tasks are not necessary steps to later appearing skills unless, in fact, the early task is a part of the later task. On the other hand, intratask sequences are helpful when selecting which movement patterns one might teach a patient. Intratask sequences provide guides for age appropriate movement patterns.

References

1. Bayley N. The development of motor abilities during the first three years. *Monograph of the Society for Research in Child Development* . 1935;1:1-26.
2. Gesell A. Maturation and the patterning of behavior. In: Murchison C, ed. *A Handbook of Child Psychology*. 2nd ed. Worcester, Mass: Clark University Press; 1933.
3. Shirley MM. *The First Two Years: Postural and Locomotor Development*. Minneapolis, Minn: University of Minnesota Press; 1931.
4. McGraw MB. *Neuromuscular Maturation of the Human Infant*. New York, NY: Hafner Publishing Co; 1945.
5. Knott M, Voss DE. *Proprioceptive Neuromuscular Facilitation: Patterns and Techniques*. New York, NY: Harper & Row, Publishers Inc; 1956.
6. Rood MS. Neurophysiological reactions as a basis for physical therapy. *Phys Ther Rev*. 1954;34:444-449.
7. Bobath K, Bobath B. Treatment of cerebral palsy by the inhibition of abnormal reflex action. *British Journal of Orthopedics*. 1954;11:88- 89.
8. Touwen BCL. Variability and stereotypy in normal and deviant development. In: Apley J, ed. *Care of the Handicapped Child. Clinics in Developmental Medicine, No. 67*. Philadelphia, Pa: J B Lippincott Co; 1978:99-110.
9. Wolff PH. Normal variation in human maturation. In: Conolly KJ, Prechtl HFR, eds. *Maturation and Development: Biological and Psychological Perspectives. Clinics in Developmental Medicine, No. 77/78*. Philadelphia, Pa: J B Lippincott Co; 1981:1-18.
10. Touwen BCL. *Neurological Development in Infancy. Clinics in Developmental Medicine, No. 58*. Philadelphia, Pa: J B Lippincott Co; 1976.

Chapter 13

Motor Development: Traditional and Contemporary Theories

Carolyn Heriza, EdD, PT
Vice-Chair and Associate Professor
Department of Physical Therapy
School of Allied Health Sciences
St. Louis University Medical Center
St. Louis, MO 63104

The field of motor development has been an area under study for the past 50 years. Over four decades ago, Halverson,[1] Shirley,[2] McGraw,[3,4] Gesell,[5] and Bayley[6] made observations of the motor behavior of infants and children that became the basis for a set of influential assumptions about motor development.

The traditional study of motor behavior was characterized by careful and detailed observations of progressive changes in the form of different kinds of motor sequences. These included actions like grasping, rolling, crawling, climbing, and walking. Such patient and exacting observation is the mainstay of good science and is an important component of the current study of motor development.

These observations were made within the zeitgeist of both developing technology and new knowledge about the anatomical structure of the infant's central nervous system (CNS). Coghill,[7] an embryologist, greatly influenced the study of motor development in the thirties and forties. He devoted attention to both the neural and the behavioral development of lower vertebrates, specifically the salamander, and sought to correlate observable changes in the nervous system with overt changes in behavior. From these studies, he formulated fundamental and important generalizations concerning the process of growth, namely that specific behavioral functions are associated with definite anatomical structures of the nervous system. One of the more important influences in the neural control area was the work on reflexes at about the turn of the century by Sherrington.[8] He studied pathological lesions of the human nervous system and classified the major responses to stimuli present in the extremities. He believed that most of our voluntary movements resulted from these fundamental reflexes and proposed that reflexes may be the cornerstone of voluntary movement.

Overall interest in motor development diminished in the 1950s and early 1960s.[9] In the late sixties, there was an exciting rebirth of interest in the topic of motor development with emphasis on feedback and knowledge of results.[10] This perspective was compatible with the information processing approach that was gaining popularity. Another important impetus was an interest in the ecological approach to understanding perception presented by James Gibson.[11]

Today, after a long dormant period, there is again a renewed interest in motor development. Several converging factors have contributed to this revitalization. Techniques for recording movements and muscle activities are becoming precise and sophisticated. Advancements in neurobiology and neuroscience are at a stage where they are starting to help us understand the emergence of motor function. Finally and probably the most important, there is a deepening interest in theoretical issues sparked by the thinking of J. Gibson[11] and the ideas about the physiology of action of the Soviet physiologist, Nicolai Bernstein.[12,13] The theoretical concepts of J. Gibson have been expanded by Eleanor Gibson[14,15] and Reed,[16,17] and those of Bernstein by Kelso and his colleagues in the United States.[18-20] With respect to motor development, Thelen[21,22] and Thelen and his colleagues[23-25] have used these constructs to address how new forms of movement evolve in real and developmental time.

Many of the theoretical concepts that we currently use in physical therapy evaluation and therapeutic intervention have been based on the theoretical constructs developed in the 1930s and 1940s. Specifically, we have adopted a neuro-maturational theory of development purported by McGraw[3] and Gesell.[5] In this theoretical construct, structure precedes function, and changes in motor development are thought to be the results of maturation of the CNS. The nervous system prescribes changes in movement. With development, higher centers of the CNS inhibit lower centers and elicit voluntary movements. Reflexes are the building blocks of voluntary movement. From this perspective, the maturational theory reflects the nature portion of the nature-nurture controversy. Although we have focused on the maturational view point of development, we also have encompassed some of the concepts of the nurture portion of development, or the behaviorist's concepts, in that the development of the infant or child results from learning with the environment being the driving force in development. No contemporary physical therapist would advocate either pole in the nature-nurture or maturation-learning dichotomy. Recently, we have been introduced to the concepts of the interactionist, transactionist, and systems theories of development discussed by Sameroff[26,27] in which both the biological makeup and the environment are important to the developing organism. An example of an interactionist theory is the Piagetian stage theory.[28] However, despite Piaget's focus on the interaction of the organism and the environment as necessary for development, the theory still emphasizes the importance of structure in development and thus is more on the maturational side of the nature-nurture controversy. Additionally, although Piaget emphasized the importance of active movement during the sensorimotor period, his theory does not devote much attention to movement and is primarily a theory of cognition versus motor development. Much of the current research on the sensorimotor stage of development suggests that this stage of development will have to be substantially modified or perhaps even abandoned.[29] Contemporary theories that reflect a systems perspective on development are the synactive theory of development for the preterm infant by Als,[30] the dynamical systems theory,[22] the perception-action theory,[16,17] the structural-behavior theory,[31,32] and the general systems theory proposed by Sameroff.[27,33] Of these, the dynamical systems and the perception-action theories specifically address motor development.

In this chapter, I begin with a discussion of the theoretical concepts of McGraw and Gesell as they pertain to the development of motor behavior. Following this, I introduce the theoretical concepts of the dynamical systems theory espoused by Thelen, providing examples from her research. I then discuss the implications of this theory to the development of the atypical infant. Finally, I discuss the implications of the theory for physical therapy evaluation and treatment. Definitions of important works are found in the Glossary.

THEORETICAL OUTLOOK: TRADITIONAL THEORY

McGraw's Theory of Development

McGraw believed that human behavior emerged in a lawful manner from the structural growth and maturation of the CNS. To discover the relationship between structure and function, she believed that one must observe the onset and form of the overt behavior and correlate this behavior with its anatomical and physiological substrate.[3,4]

McGraw longitudinally described in infants the motor behaviors of swimming, rolling, prone progression, sitting, and erect progression; the postural adjustments to inversion; and grasping. She then correlated these motor changes with her understanding of human neurogenesis and described four periods of neural maturation:

1. A period of reflexive behavior representing the function of lower centers of the CNS.
2. A period of decline in overt expression of reflexes reflecting cortical inhibition of the functioning of lower centers.
3. A period of cortical control over function as indicated by the deliberate or voluntary quality of overt activity.
4. A period of integration of the various neural centers involved in function as evidenced by smooth movements.

Figure 13-1 shows the seven phases of erect locomotion as depicted by McGraw.[3] Reflex stepping is demonstrated in Phase A and the loss of it in Phase B. Phase C, a transition phase, shows the bouncing and stomping activities of a child supported in standing. In Phase D, the infant takes deliberate

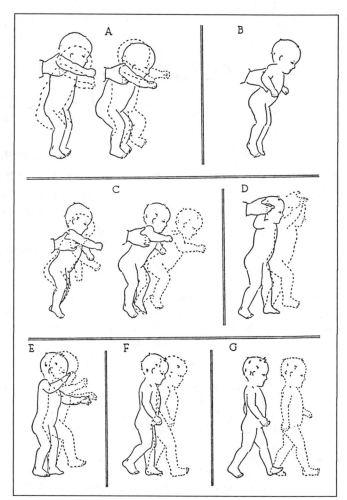

Fig. 13-1. *Seven phases of erect locomotion in human infants. From McGraw.[3]*

steps while supported by the hands. Phases E, F, and G show the refinement of independent walking characterized by increasing postural and balance control and more mature coordination of the legs. With respect to this example, Phase A demonstrates the first phase of the development of walking, the reflexive period; Phase B and C are examples of the decline of early reflexive walking: Phase B shows inhibition of the reflex, whereas Phase C is a transitional period where it is difficult to tell whether the stepping movements are reflexive or deliberate; Phase D represents cortical control as is demonstrated by the deliberateness of walking; and Phases E, F, G, show periods of refinement of the movement representing integration of the various centers of the nervous system.

From her descriptions of changes in motor patterns and her hypothesized correlations with the developing structure of the CNS, McGraw[3] proposed the following principles for the development of motor behavior:

1. There are two major divisions of the CNS controlling neuromuscular functions: the cerebral cortex and the lower levels of the CNS.
2. At birth, the cerebral cortex is not functioning, and movement, mediated by lower centers of the CNS, is reflexive in nature.

3. Some functions remain under the control of lower centers throughout life, such as coughing, sneezing, yawning.
4. Some movements are residuals of phylogenetic functions that have lost their usefulness in the human, such as swimming, the Moro reflex, grasping.
5. As the cerebral cortex develops, it exercises a controlling influence over neuromuscular functions and inhibits lower centers of the CNS.
6. Developmental changes in overt behavior are associated with maturation of the CNS.
7. Development proceeds in a cephalocaudal direction.
8. Growth of the cerebral cortex does not progress uniformly.

McGraw[3] attributed the driving force for developmental change to maturation of the CNS, specifically the increasing role of the cerebral cortex. As the brain matures, function improves. Function emerges from structure and not the reverse. Thus the theoretical framework for McGraw is a prescriptive neuromaturational model of motor development.

McGraw[3] recognized the importance of the longitudinal study of movement in comparison with cross-sectional methods of collecting data. Such longitudinal study focuses on the process of change of motor behavior in comparison with the product outcome of the behavior. Although she stressed the relationship between structure and function with primary emphasis on structure, she also alluded to the possibility that function may change structure. "There is every reason to believe that when conditions are favorable, function may contribute to further advances in structural development of the nervous system. An influential factor in determining the structural development of one component may be the functioning of other structures which are interrelated."[4(p363)] In addition, although McGraw's writings emphasize the importance of the CNS in development, she recently stated that her interest during her studies focused on the multisystems of developmental processes, their emerging and advancing at different times and different rates yet finally interacting, integrating, and synthesizing for the creation of new performances or traits.[34]

Gesell's Theory of Development

Gesell,[5] like McGraw, believed that development was a reflection of the maturational process, placing heavy emphasis on biological variables as providing the impetus to and the guidance for development. Maturation produced progressive changes in structure that closely correlated with changes in function. He considered the human organism to be a complicated action system and described the maturation of the infant as encompassing four areas of development: 1) adaptive behavior, 2) motor behavior, 3) language behavior, and 4) personal-social behavior.

Gesell[5] maintained that development must progress through a particular sequence, that the sequence was invariant from individual to individual, and that the sequence was determined by the biological and evolutionary history of the species. He maintained that the rate of development may vary from child to child but is individually determined by the child's own hereditary background. Although environment may temporarily affect the rate of development, the child's biological factors ultimately control the rate of development.

Based on normative data from observations on developing infants, using cinematography, he identified five basic principles of development: The Principle of Developmental Direction, The Principle of Individuating Maturation, The Principle of Reciprocal Interweaving, The Principle of Self-Regulating Fluctuation, and The Principle of Functional Asymmetry.

The principle of developmental direction. According to this principle, motor development has direction: cephalocaudal (head to tail) and proximal-distal (center to peripheral). Gesell believed that this direction was a function of preprogrammed genetic mechanisms.

The principle of individuating maturation. According to this principle, the process of development is controlled by endogenous (or internal) factors and cannot be influenced by exogenous (or external) factors. Like McGraw, Gesell[5] believed that the development of motor skills was under the control of the CNS. Also, like McGraw, he believed that structure must be present before function could occur. According to Gesell, environment is not the primary stimulus for growth and development; the stimulus resides in the maturational sequences of the organism's development. Learning can occur only when the physical structures have come into being, permitting behavioral adaptation. No amount of specific training before the development of the structure will be effective.

His data for the principle of individuating maturation are found in the frequently cited identical twin training studies where, controlling for genetic differences, one twin was trained and the development of the two twins compared. The stair-climbing study serves as a useful illustration (Fig. 13-2). Twin T received 6 weeks of daily training in stair climbing before the structures necessary to perform the behavior were thought to have developed. Twin C did not receive early training, but when the structures were thought to be mature, he received daily training for 2 weeks. At the end of the experiment, when both twins were the same age, no dif-

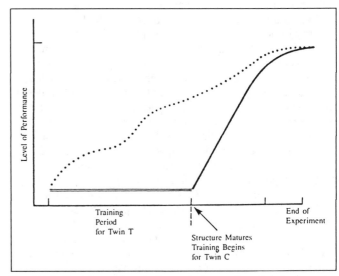

Fig. 13-2. *Prototype of co-twin control experimental studies. From Horowitz,[31] reprinted with permission.*

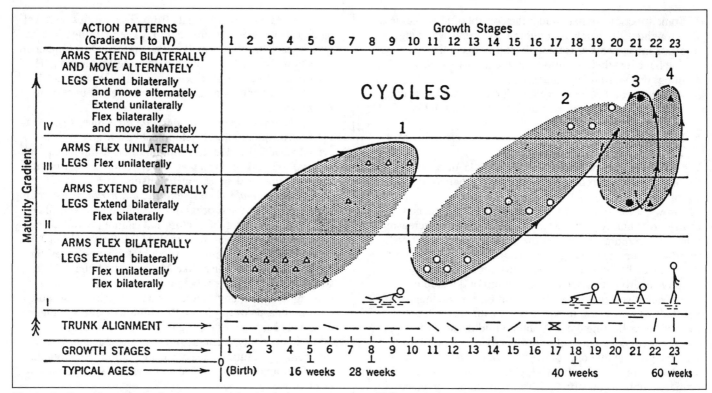

Fig. 13-3. *Growth cycles in the patterning of prone behavior. From Gesell,[5] reprinted with permission.*

ference in stair climbing was noticed. These results were proof for Gesell that maturation alone was the most important variable in development and that early experience and special environmental manipulation could not affect the eventual competence of the behavior.

The principle of reciprocal interweaving. Gesell[5(p349)] defined this principle in the form of a law as follows: "The organization of reciprocal relationships between two counteracting functions or neuromotor systems is ontogenetically manifested by somewhat periodic shifting of ascendance of the component functions or systems, with progressive modulations and integration of resultant behavior patterns." In other words, Gesell saw the development of motor control as the waxing and waning of components combining in multiple ways in a spiral course. At each stage, components regress, emerge, merge, and are replaced, creating new maturational transformation. This spiral pattern of development is apparent when the movement of the arms and legs in the progression of prone development are charted on a maturity grid (Fig. 13-3). This principle reflects the law of reciprocal innervation proposed by Sherrington[8] in which there is action and counteraction that each time takes the organism to a slightly higher level of organized activity.

The principle of self-regulating fluctuation. Self-regulating fluctuation is also a form of reciprocal interweaving that describes development as a see-saw, fluctuating between periods of instability and stability, culminating in more stable responses. The principle reflects the supposedly inherent spiral nature of development with advances, regressions, consolidation, and new advances.

The principle of functional asymmetry. Functional asymmetry is a special case of the principle of reciprocal interweaving. Gesell[5] defined this principle as behavior going through a period of asymmetric development to enable the organism to achieve a measure of symmetry at a later stage. The example used by Gesell to illustrate this principle is the asymmetric tonic neck reflex (ATNR). According to Gesell, the ATNR promotes and channels visual fixation leading to hand inspection, eye-hand coordination, and prehensory approach, eventually leading to unidexterity. The ATNR was thought to be a precursor to later development of symmetrical reaching behavior.

Although Gesell, like McGraw, attributed developmental change to maturation of the CNS, his principle of reciprocal interweaving (which encompasses self-regulating fluctuation and functional asymmetry) reflects a systems view of development.[35] Growth was seen not as a linear process but a spiral one where structure and function jointly mature leading to regression, asymmetries, and reorganization. Although Gesell is best known for his principles of direction of development and individuating maturation, his principle of reciprocal interweaving, which is less known, should be reconsidered; it indeed foreshadows contemporary systems view of motor development.

In summary, McGraw's theory of development proposes that change is dependent on the maturation of the CNS and therefore reflects a prescriptive, hierarchy, linear neuromaturational model of development. In contrast, Gesell's theoretical construct, although it also emphasizes that maturation drives development, reflects principles of systems theory of development. Both of these theories were influenced by the time in which they evolved when considerable emphasis was placed on the structure of the organism as being prepotent to function.

Proof for the Neuromaturational Theory

The principles and theoretical model, or neuromaturational model, proposed by McGraw and Gesell have come into question over the years. First, the proof that changes in motor development are a singular result of the development of the CNS remains indirect. Support for this construct is drawn usually from the literature on animal behavior, from individuals with neurological deficits, or from normative CNS development juxtaposed with normative age-of-appearance data for the selected behaviors. Direct human evidence of the link between CNS maturation and behavior is as yet unavailable and may remain so for many years. Even with the explosion of knowledge about the CNS and its development, the relationships between structure and function are poorly understood.

The direction of development (cephalocaudal, proximal-distal) has been questioned. Thelen's[36] research on stereotypes shows that rhythmical movement is present in the lower extremities before the upper extremities and even before the head and trunk. Fetters[37] has shown that no dichotomy exists between the proximal and distal components in reaching; control develops concurrently. Forssberg and Nashner[38] have demonstrated that postural reactions develop from the base of support; in the standing position, this is distal to proximal. Recent evidence shows that in a stand-to-squat movement to pick up an object, infants first use a knee-ankle strategy and then a hip-knee synergy.[39] Clark,[40] however, has shown that in the control of intralimb coordinated movement in beginning walking, the coordination of thigh reversal with the lower leg's trajectory became more adult-like sooner than the coordination of the lower leg reversal with respect to the thigh's trajectory.

Second, neural maturation alone is not a satisfactory explanation for "causing" developmental change. What is missing is the process of change. If instructions prescribe change, how do these instructions change? How does the nervous system compile, store, and continuously update these neural commands? This degree-of-freedom problem has long been recognized by Bernstein.[12]

Third, instructions, or prescriptions, for movement imply a "top-down" hierarchy executive and ignore the systems nature of movement in which action reflects the interaction of many subsystems organized by the task in a given context.

In sum, the descriptions of movement provided by McGraw and Gesell have identified motor skills and the normative times of appearance and have provided a basis for many standardized assessments of motor abilities.[41-43] They have fallen short, however, in their ability to explain the development of these skills. Although we need to know the natural history of development and be familiar with observed variability at a descriptive level, we also need to have an understanding of the process of developmental change. As indicated by Wolf,[44(p240)] "the induction of novel behavior forms may be the single most important unresolved problem for all the developmental and cognitive sciences."

THEORETICAL OUTLOOK: CONTEMPORARY THEORY

Dynamical Systems Perspective: Contemporary Model

Contemporary models of motor control and development see the CNS as one subsystem of many that dynamically interacts to produce movement. The framework for the dynamical systems theory was inspired from the work of Bernstein[12,13] and guided by the principle of nonequilibrium phenomenon in physics.[45] These concepts have been elaborated on by Kelso et al,[18] Kelso and Tuller,[19] and Kugler et al[20] and expanded more recently to the dynamic pattern theory.[46,47] Thelen and his colleagues[22,23,25,48,49] have extended these concepts to the development of movement.

The dynamical systems perspective provides a new way of conceptualizing motor development. This approach replaces the static language of codes, schemas, and programs with the dynamic concepts of self-organization, stability and change, phase shifts, and attractors. Rather than viewing motor behavior or developing behaviors as the unfolding of predetermined or prescribed patterns in the CNS, this perspective sees motor behavior as emerging from the dynamic cooperation of the many subsystems in a task-specific context. The dynamical systems theory offers a conceptual framework that is free of maturational determinism and primacy as the executor of all movement. Instead, the CNS is seen as a necessary but not sufficient component to explain movement changes. Other elements implicated are the infant's biomechanical, psychological, and social environments.

I would like to elaborate further on the central propositions of the dynamical systems theory with respect to the development of movement.[50] These are as follows: 1) moving and developing organisms are high-dimensional systems, and behavior represents a compression of the degrees of freedom; 2) behavior emerges in a self-organizing fashion as a function of the cooperation of the many subsystems in a task context; 3) moving and developing organisms occupy preferred but not obligatory regions of their state space; 4) new behavioral forms emerge in movement and development as a series of phase shifts; 5) developmental change can be envisioned as a series of stabilizing and destabilizing attractors; and 6) the "control parameters" of the system change over time.

Proposition 1. Moving and developing organisms are high-dimensional systems, and behavior represents a compression of the degrees of freedom.

For humans, particularly new walkers, upright walking is an extremely complex behavior. How does the new walker compress the enormous degrees of freedom from the muscles, bones, joints, neurons, and motor units to the relatively few degrees of freedom observed in walking? Although there are many possible combinations of muscular, skeletal, and neural elements, walking is characterized by a specific movement pattern. In dynamical terms, how can we describe a high-dimensional system composed of many elements, such as neurons, muscles, bones, and joints, by a low-dimensional description of walking?

A dynamical system is any system that changes over time.[51] A high-dimensional system is any system that has many degrees of freedom, that is, many elements that com-

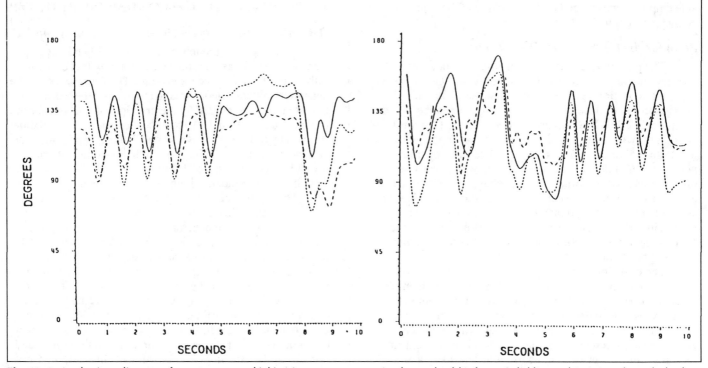

Fig. 13-4. *Angle-time diagrams for spontaneous kicking in two representative I-month-old infants. Solid line = hip joint; short-dashed line = knee joint; long-dashed line = ankle joint. Decreasing joint angles indicate flexion movements; increasing angles indicate extension movements. From Thelen and Fogel,[24] reprinted with permission.*

prise the system. How do you go from the many degrees of freedom inherent in a system to only a few degrees of freedom or from a high-dimensional behavior to a low-dimensional description of this behavior?

Bernstein[12,13] suggested that the many degrees of freedom inherent in the multiple muscles and joints of the body could be organized into larger functional groups, or synergies, that constrain the muscles and joints to act as a unit. These basic units of motor behavior came to be known either as functional synergies[19] or coordinative structures.[19,52-54] But movement is more than muscles and motoneurons. Other elements that participate in movement include sensory, perceptual, and integrative neural components; the respiratory and cardiac subsystems; and many levels of the autonomic subsystem. Thus, in more general terms, units of behavior may be described as coordinated patterns.[46] In dynamical terms, the high-dimensional behavior of any system can be characterized by a low-dimensional description of that behavior. This low-dimensional description has been called an "order parameter," or a collective variable.[22,47] Order parameters characterize movement patterns and they capture, in more simple terms, all the systems that cooperate to produce the movement. This allows us to quantify the coordination of a single limb or the coordination between two limbs. As such, order parameters may be used to describe quantitatively developmental changes in movement behavior.

As defined earlier, a synergy (coordinative structure) is a group of muscles, often spanning several joints, that is constrained to act as a single functional unit.[55] Thus kicking, stepping, and throwing a ball are examples of coordinative

structures, or in more general terms coordinated patterns. Collective variables (order parameters) describe these coordinated patterns. In intralimb coordination, such as the coordination of a single limb seen in kicking or stepping, identified collective variables that characterize the coordinated pattern are as follows: the timing of individual movement phases such as flexion and extension; the phase lags, which are defined as the time between the onset of movement of one joint with respect to another joint; and the relationships of individual joints to each other.[56-58] At the interlimb level of analysis, such as the coordination between limbs as seen in kicking and in supported or unsupported walking, the collective variables (order parameters) have been shown to be the relative temporal and spatial (ie, distance) phasing between the two limbs.[22,40,58-61] Phasing is the proportion of the ipsilateral limb cycle when foot strike occurs in the contralateral limb.

For example, Figure 13-4 shows the time-dependent (angle-time) diagrams of intralimb kicking behavior in two infants at one month of age.[24] Each kick is characterized by four phases: 1) the flexion phase, the time interval in which the infant's foot moves continuously toward the body in a horizontal plane until movement stops or changes horizontal direction; 2) the intrakick pause, the time interval between the cessation of the flexion phase and the initiation of the extension phase; 3) the extension plane, the time interval in which the infant's foot moves continuously away from the body in a horizontal plane until movement ceases or changes direction; and 4) the interkick pause, the time interval be-

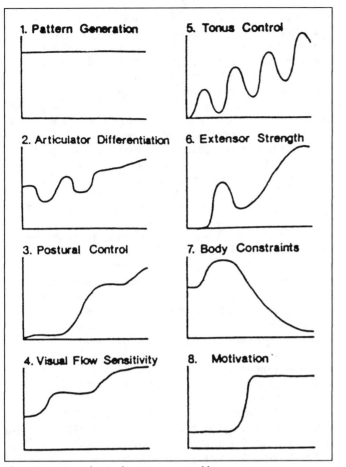

Fig. 13-5. *Hypothetical components of locomotor development, plotted as a function of age. From Thelen,[21] reprinted with permission.*

tween the end of extension and the initiation of the next flexion phase.

Visual analysis indicates that the movement trajectories of the joints are similar between these infants. The quality of the visual analysis of the intralimb coordination can quantitatively be indexed by the order parameters of the relationships of individual joints to each other and the timing of the movement phases. The strength of the relationships between the joints (three pairs for each infant: hip and knee, hip and ankle, and knee and ankle) were strong. In both infants, the timing of the movement phases were constrained, and the flexion phase was shorter than the extension phase.

The spatial and temporal patterning of supine kicks is similar to that of newborn stepping. From kinematic analyses of stepping and kicking in 2-week-old infants, Thelen and Fisher[62] concluded that these are identical movement patterns differentiated only by the posture in which they are produced. Both coordinated patterns demonstrated four distinct phases and both displayed tight temporal and spatial synchrony among the hip, knee, and ankle joints. Thus infants at an early age demonstrated a coordinative pattern of movement, indexed by order parameters, that compressed the multiple degrees of freedom of the kicking or stepping leg to only a few degrees of freedom that represented kicking or early stepping.

When multiple neurons, muscles, joints, and bones of the body are constrained to act together, a self-regulatory system is created in which movement patterns self-organize (ie, spontaneously arise from the interaction of the components). Movement need not be prescribed a priori by the CNS; rather, movement emerges from the dynamic interaction of the contributing components. Coordinated patterns have the characteristics of spatial and temporal order and of stability and flexibility. The stability of the coordinative pattern, indexed by the collective variables (order parameters), captures the spatial and temporal order of the movement we recognize as kicking, walking, or throwing a ball. Flexibility allows the coordinative pattern to adjust to a variety of environmental demands.

Proposition 2. Behavior emerges in a self-organizing fashion as a function of the cooperation of the many subsystems in a task context.

Behavior is multiply determined and task assembled. Humans are complex biological systems in which movement outcome is an interplay of all components of the system in real and developmental time, assembled by the task and context. Real time refers to the self-organization of a movement pattern that is currently ongoing (ie, what the organism does second-by-second, minute-by-minute). Developmental time is the self-organization of movement patterns that change over days, month, or years. No prescription, or code, for the particular movement pattern exists beforehand in the CNS. Rather, the outcome of the movement pattern is the result of the dynamic interaction of the contributing subsystems that organize with respect to the demands of the task and the environmental context of the system. No one subsystem is the executive of the system. Rather, it is function (task and context) that assembles behavior rather than pre-existing instructions.

With respect to developing systems, Thelen[21] has hypothesized eight subsystems involved in the production of the development of walking in the infant (Fig. 13-5).

1. Pattern generation. Pattern generation is synonymous with coordinative structure (ie, a group of muscles spanning many joints that work together as a basic unit of behavior), or in more general terms a coordinated pattern. As indicated previously, intralimb kicking demonstrates a coordinated pattern that is described by the order parameters of joint correlations and constrained movement time of the flexion and extension phases of the kickcycle. The coordinated pattern of kicking has been identified as early as 28 weeks gestational age,[63] and it is probably present even earlier as seen in the fetus with ultrasound. Other forms of coordinated patterns seen in the infant are rooting, sucking, hand-to-mouth, and grasping. Therefore, infants demonstrate organized movement early, and it is this early movement pattern, available from birth, that underlies subsequent motor development.

2. Articular differentiation. Early movement patterns in the legs (intralimb kicking and stepping) are characterized by movement of all joints in tight synchrony. With age, this joint movement becomes disassociated or uncoupled. In early kicking, all three joints move into flexion or extension together. In later kicking and in functional walking, the hip and ankle move together while the knee is out of phase with

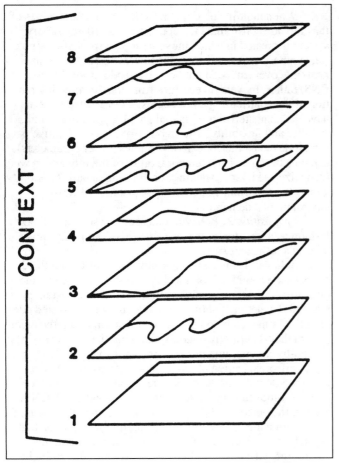

Fig. 13-6. *Hypothetical components of locomotor development shown as a layered system, with parallel but interacting developmental profiles. Outcome at any point in time is context dependent, indicated by the whole system bracket. From Thelen,[21] reprinted with permission.*

the other two joints. Thus early movement patterns of kicking and stepping become uncoupled for functional gait to occur.

3. Postural control. At birth, infants have minimal ability to support their body against gravity. Antigravity responses develop over the first year, beginning with head control, so that by the end of the first year the upright or erect position needed for ambulation is present.

4. Visual flow sensitivity. Visual, proprioceptive, and vestibular input are necessary to maintain posture and to move through the environment. Research has shown that infants are sensitive to visual flow with respect to postural corrections as early as 7 months of age. After the infant begins to walk, this visual flow information is refined as a result of perceptual learning.[15]

5. Tonus control. Tonus control in this hypothetical theory of the development of gait refers to the alternation of flexor and extensor dominance during the first year of life. This reciprocal interweaving of dominance, first described by Gesell,[5] has been demonstrated by studies from Thelen's research.[61,64] Electromyopgraphic studies showed that although both flexors and extensors are activated during the

flexion phase of kicking in infants, flexion predominates. The extension phase is a passive recoil from the initial burst of flexor muscles. At 5 months of age, the character of kicking changes from a strong flexor thrust to both active flexor and active extensor thrusts. At this time, elements of extensor posture are present. However, it is not until about 7 months of age that reciprocal activation of flexor and extensor muscles is seen; even at 1 year of age it is not uncommon to see coactivation of flexor and extensors.[58,65]

6. Extensor strength. Muscle strength is an important component for the development of walking and probably for the acquisition of other developmental motor skills. Thelen[66] has hypothesized that the lack of extensor posture and strength act as rate-limiting factors for independent locomotion.

7. Body constraints. The body grows during the first 18 years of life, particularly during the first 3 years of life. Changes in body size and body composition over the first year influence the development of upright posture and locomotion. Although we have considered the disappearance of early stepping to be the result of maturation of the CNS in which cortical control inhibits the lower level responses, Thelen and Fisher[62] have shown that the disappearance of this "reflex" is related to the increased size of the infant without a concomitant increase in muscle strength. Therefore, infants do not take steps because they cannot lift their heavy legs.

8. "Motivation." By motivation, Thelen[21] means the infant's ability to recognize a task and want to move toward a goal. Even before independent locomotion children will move toward a desired toy or person by rolling, crawling, creeping, or hitching when sitting. If given postural support in the standing position by an adult or by a walker, children will move toward the desired end. Even handicapped infants in motorized wheel chairs will move outward toward desired objects even if they cannot independently walk.[67]

Although these elements have been hypothesized for the development of walking, many of them may also be involved with the development of other postural and movement patterns during the first year such as rolling, sitting, crawling, and creeping. Additionally, there may be other components that are important in the development of upright locomotion and other developmental milestones that as yet have not been identified.

Figure 13-6 shows these eight subsystems as a layered ensemble of subsystems, each with its own developmental timetable and progressing at its own rate. The entire system is enclosed in a bracket in which the movement takes place, including the physical constraints and support of the environment.

By manipulating the environmental context of the system, Zelazo,[68] Thelen and colleagues,[49,60,62,69,70] and Clark and associates[59] have elicited more mature leg coordinations in infants. Some of these behaviors were believed to have disappeared while others were months from when they were normally seen. A summary of the studies on the manipulation of the environmental context as they relate to McGraw's stages of the development of walking is seen in Figure 13-7.

First there is the disappearance of stepping at about 2 months of age. McGraw[3] assigned this disappearance to cor-

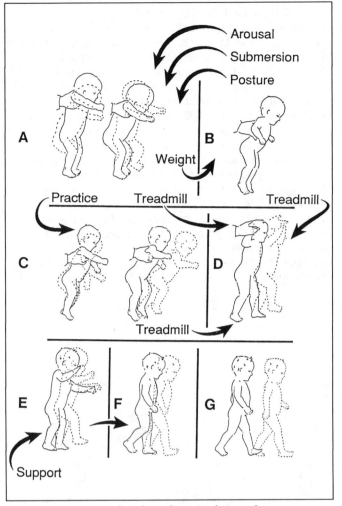

Fig. 13-7. *Summary of studies of manipulation of environmental context related to McGraw's seven phases of erect locomotion. From Thelen,[50] reprinted with permission.*

porting the hands also accelerates the coordination of walking.[59]

These studies call into question the assumption that maturation of the CNS is responsible for changes seen in the development of locomotion. They emphasize the importance of a multisystem perspective for understanding developmental milestones and emphasize the importance of the context in the assembly of task-specific actions. Context may include the social and the physical constraints.

Interlimb coordination between the legs can also be manipulated by changing the context. In supine kicking, for example, small weights placed on one leg of 6-week-old infants systematically affected the amplitude and frequency of kicks in both legs.[71] Weighting caused infants to decrease the rate of kicking in the weighted leg and increase the rate in the unweighted leg. Movement amplitude and velocity were maintained in the weighted leg but dramatically increased in the unweighted leg. A similar phenomenon is seen in treadmill stepping. When 7-month-old infants are placed on a split-belt treadmill where one leg can be driven twice as fast as the other, infants continue to make alternating step. These infants decreased the rate of stepping on the fast belt and increased the rate of stepping on the slower belt to produce an overall rate that was intermediate between the step rate on either the fast or slow belt alone.[72] Further studies in the newborn period confirmed that infants will adjust to changes in treadmill speed and to different belt-speed ratios at earlier ages.[49]

In these examples, infants made involuntary corrections to perturbation in a two-legged system. Alternation of the two legs appears to be preferred movement pattern, and infants will return to it when perturbed. This research provides additional support to the proposition that movement self-organizes with respect to the task and context. These experiments also demonstrate that context is more important than age or phase of locomotor development.

Thus coordinated movement patterns are preferred but are not obligatory, because they are adaptable to the task within environmental demands. These coordinated patterns are not hard-wired but are softly assembled. These coordinated patterns self-organize, exhibiting stability of form but retaining flexibility to adjust to changing conditions within the infant and with respect to the task and the environment.

Because function (task and context) rather than instruction drives behavior, a variety of maturationally available coordinated patterns may be recruited for the same functional end, and conversely, the same coordinated pattern may be recruited for different tasks. The final outcome of the movement is dependent on the task or goal within given contextual conditions (ie, the internal and external environments).

Proposition 3. Moving and developing organisms occupy preferred but not obligatory regions of their state space.

A general characteristic of complex dynamical systems is to settle into preferred but not obligatory coordinated movement patterns. These coordinated movement patterns act as a kind of dynamic magnet, or dynamic attractor, such that when the system is perturbed it tends to return to the preferred movement pattern. Thus coordinated movement patterns can be referred to as dynamic attractors. Dynamic attractors live in state space. *State space* is a hypothetical

tical inhibition. Zelazo[68] however, demonstrated in a classic experiment that simple practice of stepping maintained it in the repertoire of the infant. The stepping response never disappeared. Thelen and colleagues,[62,69,70] in a series of experiments, also showed that the disappearance of stepping is deceptive. If placed in the supine position, infants continued to kick throughout the first year.[62] As discussed previously, supine kicks are kinematically identical to upright steps. Infants who no longer stepped while upright also showed stepping movements when placed in water, and conversely, stepping could easily be inhibited in young infants by placing small weights on their legs.[69] Some infants who would not step when they were calm, stepped when excited.[70] In infants who were in Stages A, B, or C and who performed little or no stepping movements, supporting them over a motorized treadmill elicited steps.[49,60] That is, infants who stepped not at all or in a poorly coordinated manner when the treadmill was turned off, immediately produced movements that approximated much more mature behavior and were more similar to adult-like steps than newborn steps. During the refinement of independent walking, the simple action of sup-

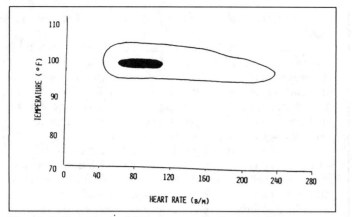

Fig. 13-8. *Hypothetical "fitness space" of a normal human individual showing dynamic range of heart rate and temperature. Individual "prefers" to spend time in the dark center portion, but she is not limited to it. When perturbed, the system normally returns to the center oval. From Thelen,[22] reprinted with permission.*

space that can be defined by any number of variables. For example, Figure 13-8 is a diagram of a system in state space.[22] The *x* and *y* axes may be any dimension that you believe defines the behavioral system you are studying. Here, the hypothetical fitness state space of an individual is depicted by plotting body temperature and heart rate. Normal adults will occupy a preferred region of the space. Illness or excessive exercise may shift you to another portion of the space, but your system will want to return to the dark center spot after perturbation by illness or exercise.

In mechanical systems, such as kicking or stepping, the axes may be composed of the joint angle of a moving limb against another joint angle of the same limb (angle-angle plot) (Fig. 13-9A) or the joint velocity of a limb against the joint angle of the same limb (phase plane plot)[73] (Fig. 13-9B). Each point on the plot represents the state of the system at some time. If the movement pattern is stable, it occupies a preferred space within the plot. In dynamical terms, the preferred space occupied by the behavior is called

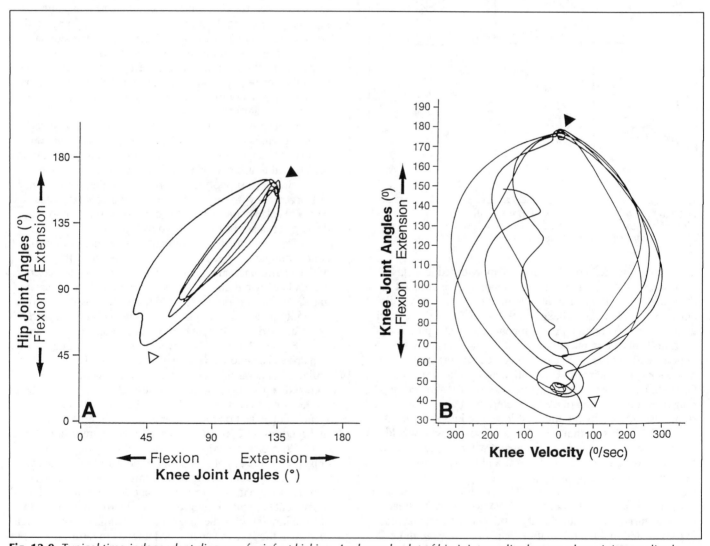

Fig. 13-9. *Typical time-independent diagrams for infant kicking. Angle-angle plot of hip joint amplitude versus knee joint amplitude (A), and phase plane trajectory (phase portrait) of knee joint amplitude and peak velocity (degrees per second) (B). Filled arrows indicate beginning of kick flexion movement; open arrows indicate peak flexion. From Harris and Heriza,[73] reprinted with permission.*

Contemporary Management of Motor Problems

a preferred attractor state space,[22,72] and the plot is called the phase portrait of the system.[39]

The phase portrait in Figure 13-9B is a description of a dynamical system (eg, a behavior or, as in this example, a coordinative pattern) as it evolves over time. Phase plane diagrams progress clockwise. The path the system takes as it changes over time is called the path trajectory. In this example, the path of the knee joint changing over a kick cycle is described by its displacement and velocity. There are five kick cycles in this figure. For all cycles, the trajectories appear to stay in the same region of the state space. In other words, the kick cycles find a region of the state space to which they all settle. This is the preferred region, the "attractive" region, of the state space. This phase portrait, then, is an attractor, a coordinative behavioral pattern of kicking, mapped in state space, as defined by the knee joint's displacement and velocity during kick cycles.

Despite all the degrees of freedom that comprise this biological system, we have a behavior that is described by a two-dimensional geometric model. We have a high-dimensional system characterized by a low-dimensional description.

Three types of attractors have been defined:[22] a point (equilibrium) attractor, a periodic (limit cycle) attractor, and a chaotic (mixing) attractor (Fig. 13-10). A *point attractor* is an attractor in which the trajectory converges onto a single state, or a point. A *periodic attractor*, or limit cycle attractor, is one in which the trajectory forms a closed ring. And the third, the *chaotic attractor* is an attractor in which trajectories are mixed in state space (ie, they are noisy). The example of kicking is considered to be a limit cycle attractor. In fact, lower extremity motions found not only in kicking but also in walking, running, hopping, galloping, and skipping might well be described as limit cycle attractors.[50]

Proposition 4. New behavioral forms emerge in development as a series of phase shifts.

As indicated in the beginning of this discussion, a major question in the development of coordinated behavior is from where do new movement patterns come. The dynamical systems theory proposes that new forms of movement are the result of scalar changes in one or more of the subsystems components including the subsystems of the organism, the environment (physical and social), and the task. Shifts from one qualitative coordinated pattern to another are often nonlinear, or discontinuous.

An often cited example is quadruped gait.[55] A shift from one stable movement form to another, such as from walking to trotting in the horse, occurs without stable intermediate movement states. New forms of movement emerge as a result of changes in critical values of one variable. In the horse example, the variable change is an increase in speed and, therefore, muscle power, which shifts the horse from walking to trotting to galloping. With respect to infant kicking, behavioral state drives the system.[61,70] When the infant is in a sleep or drowsy state, little kicking is noted; as the infant becomes more aroused, the spatial and temporal pattern of kicking is observed; in the crying state, a new pattern emerges, which is a rigid coactivation of all the muscles into stiff immobility.

In dynamical terms, a variable that shifts the move-

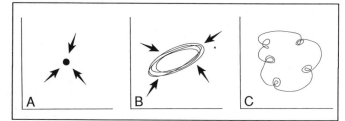

Fig. 13-10. *Three hypothetical attractors plotted in two-dimensional state space: point attractor (A), limit cycle attractor (B), chaotic attractor (C). Arrows indicate that movement trajectories tend to converge on these behavior patterns. Adapted from Thelen,[22] reprinted with permission.*

ment from one form to another is called a control parameter. The word control does not mean that the control parameter contains a prescription for movement change but rather that it acts as an agent for reorganization of the movement.[22] Control parameters may be essential components but nonspecific to the behavior of interest. Control parameters may reside in the infant, for example behavioral state; in the environment, for example gravity; in the social environment, for example the caretaker; or in the goal or task.[22] New coordinated patterns arise because the old patterns become unstable and the system is pushed to a new stable state. Changes in the scalar properties of control parameters are responsible for pushing the system into a new stable state. During phase shifts or transitions, the coordinative movement pattern (dynamic attractor) becomes less stable and more easily perturbed by control parameters.

As discussed earlier, McGraw[3] considered that the shift from one phase to another was the result of the maturation of the CNS. As you know, the change in weight of the infant has been shown to be the control parameter for the disappearance of stepping.[62] Infants gain weight rapidly in the first few months of life, but this weight gain is primarily fat versus muscle. Therefore, infants are unable to lift their heavy legs and cannot produce steps. When these same infants are placed in a supine position, in water, or on a treadmill, stepping and kicking movements are present. Gaining fat is nonspecific and nonobvious to the coordinative pattern of stepping. Yet, scalar changes in the body build of these infants shifted the infant into a new motor milestone.

Control parameters external to the infant, such as the environment or the social context, also shift the infant into new avenues of development. The practice of stepping prevented the infant from going through the phase of nonstepping and facilitated the earlier development of independent walking.[68] The social partner or caretaker may provide elements seemingly "missing" for the performance of a behavior; for example, support at the hand provides postural control, eliciting more mature walking. Experience with the nonsocial environment also is important in organizing the system for coordinated patterns. For example, developmentalists have shown that the onset of self-propelled locomotion (crawling, motorized wheelchairs) provides increased opportunities to explore the environment and to develop more adaptive levels of spatial cognition and social relations.[67,74]

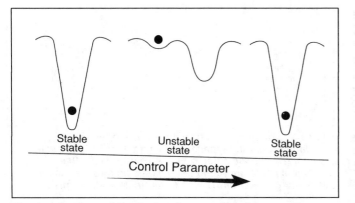

Fig. 13-11. *Phase shifts depicted as a series of deep and shallow wells. Stable states have steep wells; unstable states have shallow wells. At critical scalor changes of the control parameter, phase shifts (transitions) occur from one stable coordination pattern to another. Adapted from Thelen,[22] reprinted with permission.*

Proposition 5. Developmental change can be envisioned as a series of stabilizing and destabilizing attractors.

Dynamical systems theory provides an alternative explanation for the waxing and waning of behavioral forms (reciprocal interweaving) and for the progressive stage-like images of traditional theory. Instead of being the result of maturation of the organism, new forms arise because of the dissolution of stable forms with the subsequent formation of new coordinative patterns. The stability of attractors (coordinative patterns) changes as control parameters are scaled. Attractors lose stability at points of transition, and new preferred coordinated patterns evolve. Because dynamical systems prefer certain configurations, development takes on a stage-like quality.

Previously, we graphically represented a coordinated pattern (attractor) living in state space. We were interested in visually depicting a high-dimensional system in a two-dimensional system to determine whether the behavior was stable or unstable. We indicated that we could use this procedure for any behavior that we wished to observe. Another way to represent graphically a universal picture of an attractor is seen in Figure 13-11. What we see are deep or shallow wells, or attractor basins. It would be extremely difficult for the attractor (depicted as a ball) to climb out of the basin. A shallow basin depicts an attractor that is less stable. Attractors in shallow basins are more easily perturbed and therefore suited for adaptive behavior.[51]

During phase shifts, attractors move from stable states (deep wells) to unstable states (shallow wells) and then to stable states (deep wells). As stated earlier, these changes occur as a result of critical scalar changes in a control parameter. There are two characteristics of a transition stage, or unstable state.[22] First, there is more variability within the coordinated pattern, or attractor, and therefore it can more easily be perturbed. Second, it takes the coordinative pattern longer to return to a stable state if perturbed (relaxation time).

An example of phase shifts is seen in intralimb kicking of infants. Supine kicking was traced from the newborn period until about 10 months of age (Fig. 13-12).[58] During the newborn period, all joints moved in unison. The hip-ankle joints began to uncouple at 2 months of age, and between 4 and 6 months there was further disassociation of the joints. However, this joint individuation was transient because between 5 and 8 months of age the correlation between all pairs of joints again became tighter. At 10 months, the hip and knee became negatively correlated in supine kicking. By this age, the infant showed little of the staccato kick of the earlier period but used the legs in a variety of complex and apparently voluntary patterns.

In summary, the coordinated pattern (attractor) becomes less stable and more easily perturbed by control parameters during periods of transitions. New movement patterns emerge when there is a critical scalar change in a control parameter that results in the attractor moving out of the attractor basin. During this period, the attractor is going through a transition period. Infants may exhibit discrete stages that are stable, but once critical values of control parameters are exceeded, a new stable state or stage may emerge. One or more control parameters may trigger the transition from one stable state (stage) to another and may reside within the infant, such as anatomical growth or neural differentiation, or be outside the infant, such as the social system, the task, or other environmental opportunities and constraints.

Proposition 6. The control parameters of the system change over time.

Remember that we characterized developing systems as composed of many participating, equally important sub-

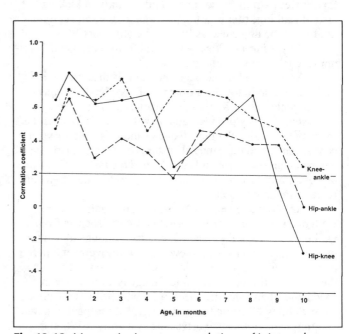

Fig. 13-12. *Mean pairwise cross-correlations of joint angles during a 10-second segment of spontaneous supine kicking of four infants at 11 ages from 2 weeks to 10 months. Values above and below the solid horizontal line are statistically significant. From Thelen,[58] reprinted with permission.*

systems. Over time, each of the interacting subsystems has its own dynamic and nonlinear course of development, and each proceeds at its own developmental rate. Because the contributing components of the system may not mature in a synchronous fashion, and because these components dynamically assemble, one component may compete with, inhibit, or facilitate another component.

Each of the eight elements hypothesized to be necessary for the development of independent walking has its own development profile (Fig. 13-13). At any point in time (ie, Time 1 or Time 2), the resulting behavior is the cooperative interaction of these elements specific to and organized by the context (the task and environment at hand).

For any given task and any developmental status of the components, a preferred coordinated pattern will emerge. Under other conditions (developmental level of the components, the task, or the environment), different movements may emerge. Some elements such as the pattern generation are ready far in advance of the ability to ambulate while others such as postural control and strength mature only after locomotion has been achieved. Each element demonstrates regressions along the developmental trajectory. The maturity of the components is not continuous but demonstrates a nonlinear course of development. Thus no one element alone controls the development of locomotion, but it is the dynamic interaction of all elements in real and developmental time that interrelate to promote the acquisition of gait. There is no "locomotor" switch that turns on at 12 months of age to cause walking.

Although no one element is necessary and sufficient to cause locomotion, Thelen[66] has hypothesized that three elements—postural control, balance, and extensor strength—may constrain the development of walking. It is not until the maturation of these three elements that infants walk. Although other elements in the system are mature before the time of walking, it is not until these components mature that the system shifts into the mode of walking. All components continue to mature and interact with other elements in the system to refine ambulation.

Because changes in the components are nonlinear, a control parameter that shifts the system into new forms of movement at one time may not be the control parameter that is critical at a later time.[22] This point may again be illustrated with the transitions in infant stepping. The control parameter for the first transition, from stepping to no stepping, was the rapid deposition of body fat.[62] The control parameters for the second major transition, from no stepping to stepping again, appears to be related to the ability to stabilize the base of support and shift the weight from leg to leg. Thus muscle strength and balance may be the control parameters.[66] The control parameters for independent walking, the third transition, may be dynamic postural control, balance, and strength.[66]

A dynamical systems view of development, therefore, no longer allows us to give the CNS the preeminent role of change in behavior. There is no single cause or predetermined model, be it genetic, neurological, cognitive, or environmental, for behavioral change. No longer can we consider the infant and young child as passive recipients of information from the environment. We should view them as

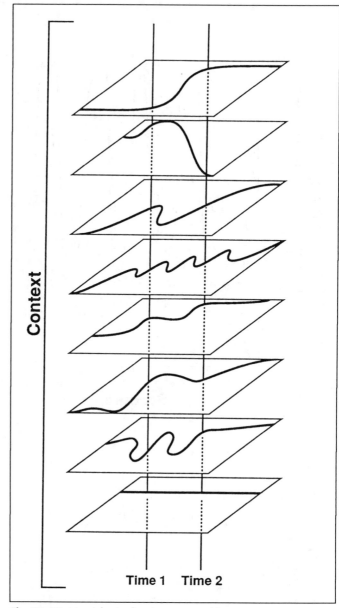

Fig. 13-13. *Hypothetical components of locomotor development as a layered system. Outcome at Time 1 or Time 2 is the result of the self-organization of the components at that point in time within the physical constraints and support of the environment. Adapted from Thelen,[21] reprinted with permission.*

active participants in which movement self-assembles from the many subsystems within the environmental context. Instead of reflexes and reactions demonstrating hierarchial organization and comprising the substrata of movement, we need to consider the concept of groups of muscles and joints, coordinative structures (attractors, coordinated patterns) organized in a heterarchial arrangement, in which all elements participate in the decision for movement.[54]

Dynamical systems perspective for atypical movement and development.

As physical therapists, we have based our evaluation

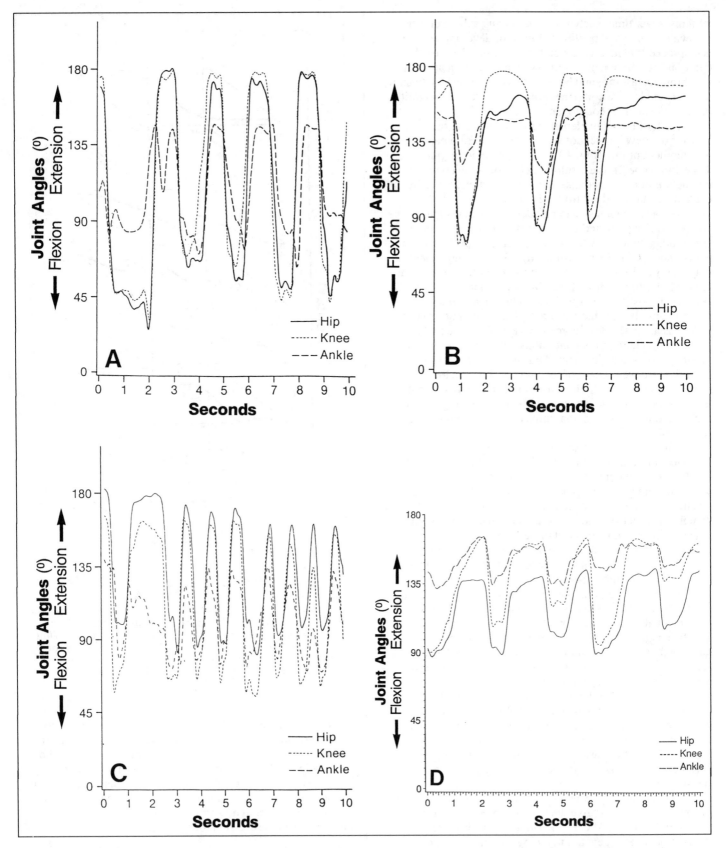

Fig. 13-14. *Angle-time diagrams of joint angles of typical leg movements of four infants: low-risk infant at 34 weeks gestational age (A), same low-risk infant at 40 weeks postgestational age (B), fullterm infant at 40 weeks gestational age (C), and a high-risk infant at 40 weeks gestational age (D). From Heriza,[75] reprinted with permission.*

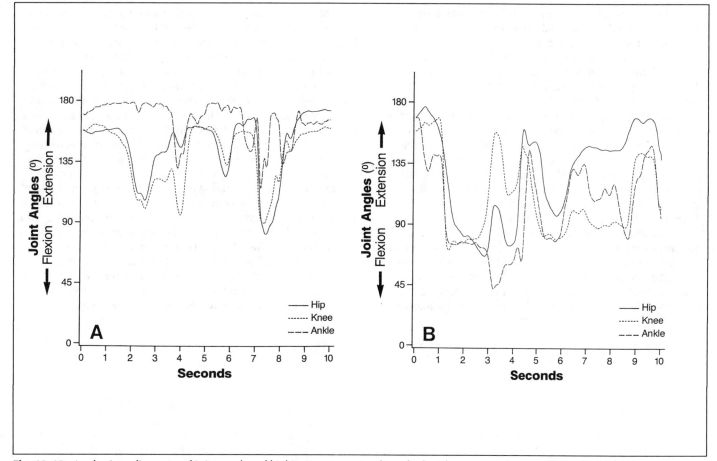

Fig. 13-15. *Angle-time diagrams of joint angles of kicking movements of two high-risk preterm infants at 40 weeks PGA: high-risk infant with Grade IV IVH (A), high-risk infant with Grade IV IVH and hip dysplasia (B). From Heriza,[75] reprinted with permission.*

and treatment of atypical infants and children on developmental theory as it pertains to the development of normal children. To date, this has been the neuromaturational theory of McGraw[3] and Gesell.[5] This theory has formed the basis for the evaluation of reflexes and reactions and of motor milestones, two components of the evaluation process. This theory has also been used in the development of our facilitation treatment programs for individuals with neurological dysfunction. Recent research of the effectiveness of these treatment approaches has not been promising. Many have indicated that perhaps one of the reasons that success was not seen relates to the evaluation tools used to determine effectiveness, specifically motor milestones. This is a quantitative approach addressing a qualitative issue. Another concern is the lack of a well-documented theoretical model to provide guidance to the what, when, where, and how of intervention. Traditional models of motor development have described changes in movement with age but have not adequately explained how movement changes.

The dynamical systems theory may not only be useful as a theoretical theory on which to base the efficacy of physical therapy treatment but also be useful in providing different evaluation tools that may more effectively identify changes in movement. But first, we need to see if the theory can be "transferred," or generalized, to the atypical infant.

Fundamental questions addressed by professionals who care for atypical or handicapped infants and children are as follows:
1. Is the movement of handicapped infants different from that of normal infants?
   If so, in what ways?
   If not, what are the commonalities?
2. Is the development of movement of handicapped infants different from that of normal infants?
   If so, in what ways?
   If not, what are the commonalities?
3. What treatments can be used in the remediation of motor dysfunction for atypical infants?

In discussing these issues, I will use the results of studies of atypical infants that address the dynamical systems perspective. There have been few studies, but they are growing in numbers. I specifically will use results of my studies on preterm infants,[56,57,75] treadmill stepping of infants with Down syndrome by Ulrich and associates,[76] stepping of infants with Down syndrome by Clark,[51] and treadmill stepping of preterm infants by Davis (D. Davis, MS; personal communication; June 1990). As with the discussion of the theoretical model of the dynamical systems theory, I will organize the discussion of the movement of atypical infants according to the six propositions.

Proposition 1. Moving and developing organisms are high-dimensional systems and behavior represents a compression of the degrees of freedom.

Are the movement patterns of kicking and stepping of atypical infants different from those of normal infants? Are the collective variables (order parameters) for these movements the same or different?

Kicking behavior of low-risk and high-risk preterm infants with documented intraventricular hemorrhages (IVH) are similar to that of fullterm infants at 40 weeks corrected age.[56,57,75] The vast degrees of freedom are reduced to that of a few representing the observable movement of intralimb kicking, a coordinated pattern. Figure 13-14 shows the angle-time diagrams of kicking behavior of four infants at different gestational and postgestational ages (GA, PGA).

Although visual analysis indicates some differences in the movement trajectories among the infants, the pattern of intralimb kicking is similar. The quality of the visual analysis on the intralimb coordination can be indexed quantitatively by the following collective variables (order parameters): the relationships of individual joints to each other, the

phase lags between joints during kicking, and the timing of the movement phases. The strength of the relationship between the joints (three pairs for each infant: hip and knee, hip and ankle, and knee and ankle) were strong. This was particularly true of the hip and knee; that is, when the hip flexed the knee flexed, and when the hip extended the knee extended. All possible pairwise correlations of the joints were significant. Thus the movement of the joints of one leg are constrained to act as a unit of movement. A high-dimensional system is explained by a low-dimensional behavior. No significant differences existed among the groups of infants. This close synchrony of movement denoted by the high interjoint correlations were confirmed by small phase lags between the movement of the joints. A phase lag is the elapsed time between either the onset of flexion or the point of peak flexion of the movement of one joint with respect to another joint, divided by the duration of the kick period. These small phase lags demonstrated that the joints started moving or reached peak excursion in perfect unison. Timing of the flexion and extension phases of the kick cycle is another order parameter for the movement pattern of intralimb

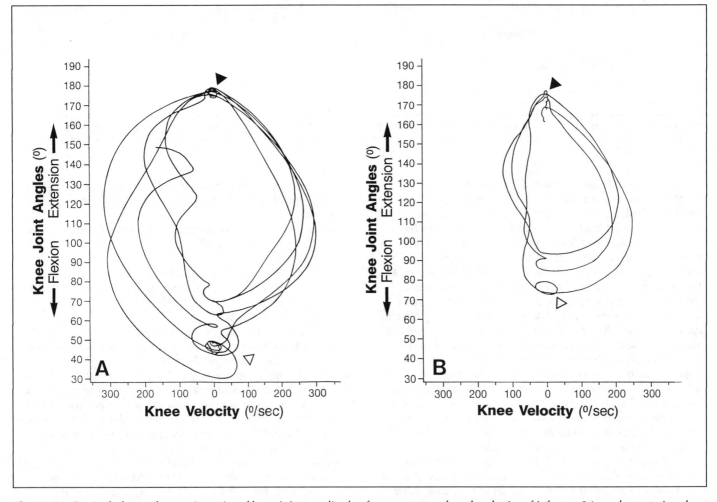

Fig. 13-16. *Typical phase-plane trajectories of knee joint amplitude of movement and peak velocity of infant at 34 weeks gestational age (A) and at 40 weeks postgestational age (B). The filled arrows indicate the beginning of kick flexion movement; open arrows indicate peak flexion. From Heriza,[57] reprinted with permission.*

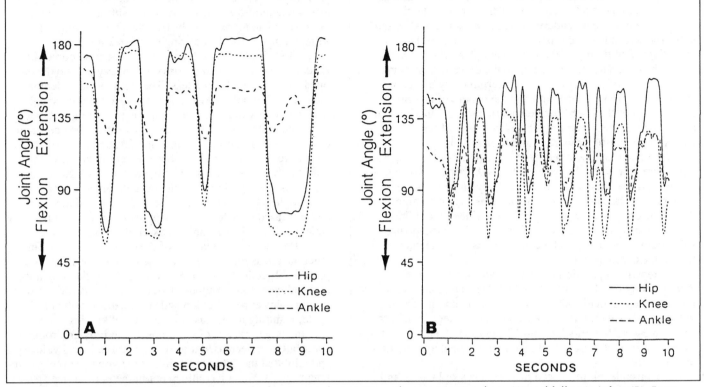

Fig. 13-17. *Joint angles of typical leg movements of preterm infant at 40 weeks postgestational age (A) and full-term infant (B). From Heriza,[56] reprinted with permission.*

kicking. In all infants, the timing of the movement phases were similar. Although there was a trend for the younger or sicker infants to have longer flexion and extension phases, there were no significant differences among the groups. Thus, for intralimb kicking, the collective variables that described the movement pattern were strength of the joint correlations, phase lags between joints, and movement time of flexion and extension. All infants, regardless of age, environment, or risk factors, demonstrated a coordinative pattern of kicking, indexed by collective variables (order parameters) that compressed the multiple degrees of freedom to a few, representing kicking. Thus, when grouped, the kicking behaviors of preterm infants (low- and high- risk) are similar to that of normal infants and can be described by the same collective variables: joint correlations, phase lags, and timing of the movement phases.

Although, as a group, high-risk preterm infants demonstrated coordinative movement patterns of kicking at 40 weeks PGA, some infants showed individual profiles in which kicking appeared disorganized.[75] In Figure 13- 15, the time dependent diagrams show that the ankle is out of phase with the knee and hip in infant A, a preterm infant with a grade IV IVH; the knee is out of phase with the hip and ankle in infant B, a preterm infant with a grade IV IVH and hip dysplasia. Although the timing of the movement phases of flexion and extension were similar to that of other infants, the strength of the correlations between the joints were weak, and the phase lags were long. This was especially true for the hip and ankle and the knee and ankle for in-

fant A, and for the hip and knee and the knee and ankle for infant B. Therefore, two order parameters that describe the coordinative pattern of early kicking movements and that differentiate between organized and disorganized movement could be used as evaluative tools for kicking: joint correlations and phase lags between joints.

Proposition 2. Behavior emerges in a self-organizing fashion as a function of the cooperation of the many subsystems in a task context.

Preterm infants. Although the pattern of kicking was stable among low- risk preterm infants, differences were found in the amplitude and velocity of movement, the pauses during the kick cycle, and the joint angles at the initiation of kick flexion and at peak flexion.[57] With age, low-risk preterm infants demonstrated a trend to kick more in 3 minutes than younger preterm infants, reflective of shorter pauses. Figure 13-16 shows typical phase-plane plots of the knee of a low-risk preterm infant at 34 to 36 weeks GA (A) and this same infant at 40 weeks PGA (B). As a group, older low- risk preterm infants showed significantly decreased movement amplitude and peak velocity in comparison with the younger age.

At 40 weeks PGA, all low-risk preterm infants were more extended at all joints, especially the ankle, in comparison with fullterm infants.[56] Figure 13-17 shows the typical angle-time displacement of the joint angles of the hip, knee, and ankle of a low-risk preterm infant at 40 weeks PGA and a fullterm infant. These same infants also paused more during kicking in 3 minutes in comparison with fullterm infants, resulting in longer kick periods and a trend to kick less.

If the movement pattern is the same, as indexed by the collective variables (order parameters) of joint correlations, phase lags, and timing of the movement phases, what explains the differences? According to the dynamical systems theory, movement outcome is not determined by a pattern of strict muscle firings alone but from the pattern of neuromuscular firings of the coordinative pattern and from mechanical and dynamic considerations such as measures of body build, passive viscoelastic properties of muscles, and muscle strength. The movement outcome is the result of the cooperative interaction of all the participating subsystems in developmental and real time and is not coded anywhere in the nervous system. Because there is no pre-existing instructions to define the coordinative pattern of kicking, the order of kicking is the result of the self-organization of the participating subsystems. Kicking spontaneously arises from the interaction of the components.

Stepwise regression analysis of arousal level; measures of body build; passive muscle "tone"; and joint extensibility on the kinematic variables of duration, amplitude, and velocity did explain differences in movement seen in infants between 34 to 36 weeks GA and 40 weeks PGA and between low-risk preterm infant at term equivalent age and fullterm infants.

Arousal level influenced the frequency of kicking and

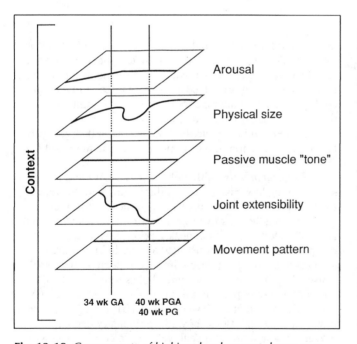

Fig. 13-18. *Components of kicking development shown as a layered ensemble of subsystems, each with its own developmental timetable and progressing at its own rate. Entire system is enclosed in a bracket representing the context in which the movement takes place including physical constraints and supports of the environment. (Components for preterm infants at 34 to 36 weeks GA and at 40 weeks PGA and for fullterm infants at 40 weeks GA.) Adapted from Thelen,[21] reprinted with permission.*

joint angles at peak flexion. Infants who were highly aroused demonstrated short pauses, resulting in short kick periods and an increase in the frequency of kicking. These same infants showed small angles at peak flexion.

Body build also influenced movement outcome. Infants who rapidly became stocky and heavy or who developed chubby legs, kicked less. These infants also demonstrated small amplitude excursions associated with small peak velocities and large angles at the beginning of flexion and at peak flexion. These results may reflect asynchronous development of muscle strength and fat such that infants who were fat or who quickly became fat did not have the muscle strength to kick their heavier, stockier legs.

Passive muscle tone influenced the interkick pause and joint angles at the beginning of kick flexion. Infants who had increased muscle tension demonstrated short pauses and small angles at the beginning of kick flexion.

Possible interpretations of the differences in kicking outcome are as follows: 1) Increased arousal level, which is presumably reflected in more energy delivered to the muscles and more motor output, including kicks, contributed to small angles at peak flexion and short pauses in the kick cycle, resulting in increased frequency of kicking; 2) with age, the larger masses of the limbs in a gravity environment contributed to decreased movement amplitude and velocity and inhibited the extreme flexion of the youngest preterm infants; and 3) the long confinement in the intrauterine space for fullterm infants may bias muscles and joints toward flexion, contributing to the flexor dominance of the fullterm infants. Therefore, the movement changes in low-risk preterm infants with age and the differences in kicking between low-risk preterm infants at 40 weeks PGA and fullterm infants may largely be of nonneural origin and not solely be caused by maturational changes in the CNS.

The differences in kicking reflect the assumption of the dynamical systems perspective that the outcome of the movement is the result of the dynamical interaction of the subsystems in real and developmental time. As adapted from Thelen,[21] Figure 13-18 depicts a developing system as a layered ensemble of subsystems, each having its own developmental timetable and progressing at its own rate. The entire system is enclosed in a bracket representing the context in which the movement takes place, including the physical constraints and supports of the environment. At 34 to 36 weeks GA, 3 days postintrauterine environment, the various subsystems dynamically organize in real time to produce infant kicking; at 40 weeks PGA, these same subsystems, which have matured and experienced 6 weeks of extrauterine environment, self-organize to produce kicking; and at term, 40 weeks GA, these same subsystems, which have experienced the intrauterine environment for an additional 6 weeks, self-organize for kicking. Thus, although the pattern of coordination of kicking of preterm infants at different ages and fullterm infants is identical, the context varied between time spent in the intrauterine or extrauterine environment and the components of the system (ie, body build, arousal level, passive muscle tone, and joint extensibility) varied with age. These variations can explain differences seen among the infants.

Down syndrome infants. Six infants with Down syn-

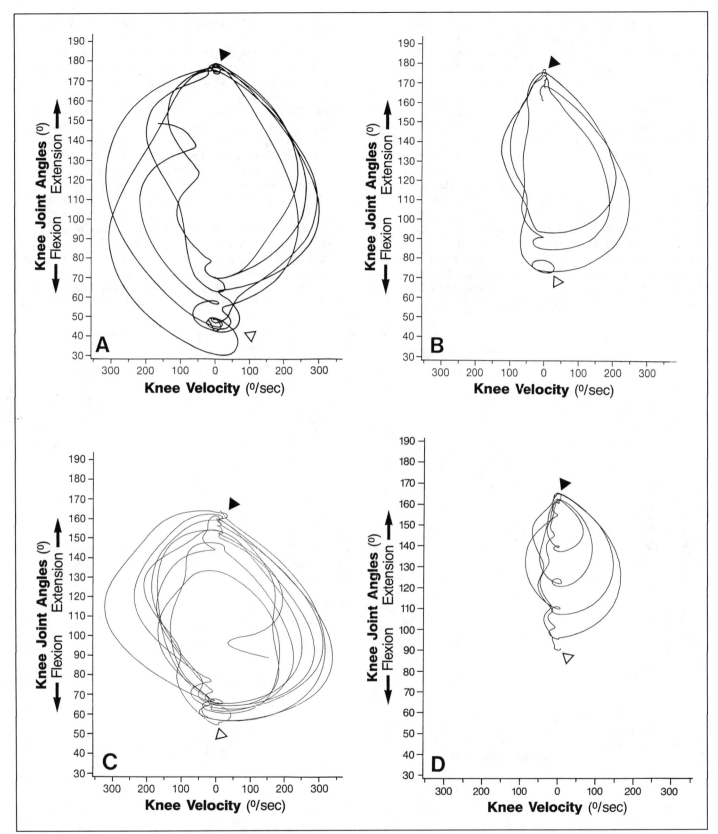

Fig. 13-19. *Phase-plane trajectories of knee of four representative infants: low-risk infant at 34 weeks gestational age (A), same low-risk infant at 40 weeks postgestational age (B), fullterm infant at 40 weeks gestational age (C), and high-risk infant at 40 weeks postgestational age (D). The filled arrows indicate the beginning of kick flexion movement; the open arrows represent peak flexion. From Heriza,[75] reprinted with permission.*

drome, aged 8 to 11 months, were placed on a motorized treadmill to produce stepping patterns in advance of voluntary stepping.[76] Like normal infants, these infants produced alternating step-like patterns well in advance of independent walking. The context (ie, the treadmill) organized their systems to produce stepping in contrast to preexisting instructions. Infants did not voluntarily control this stepping because virtually no steps would be taken as a baseline before the belts were moving, and they stopped "walking" when the belt was turned off. Not only did these infants produce alternating steps, but the collective variable (order parameter) that represent stepping on the treadmill was similar to that of normal infants (ie, the time phasing between the two limbs). The alternating leg pattern occurred when one limb began its cycle while the other limb was in the middle of its cycle. The infants with Down syndrome were also sensitive to speed changes of the treadmill and were able to adapt their stepping pattern to the change. As the belt speed increased, these infants, as do normal infants, stepped more frequently, resulting in shorter cycles. There was, however, greater vari-

ability in the number of steps and the duration of the step cycle in the infants with Down syndrome.

Preterm infants. Treadmill stepping can also be elicited in preterm infants as young as 1 month corrected age (D. Davis, personal communication). Again, the treadmill organized the components of the system to produce stepping. There were no preexisting instructions for treadmill stepping versus stepping without the treadmill, as indicated by the nonsteps during the prebaseline and postbaseline phases when the treadmill was not moving. The pattern of stepping was more mature than that seen in fullterm infants of comparable age. The steps looked more like those seen with 7-month-old infants. Perhaps a reason that preterm infants can take more mature-like steps earlier than term infants is that they have more extensor posturing in the legs than fullterm infants. Thelen[66] has hypothesized that lack of extensor posturing and strength of the legs may be a control parameter that rate-limits independent walking.

Proposition 3. Moving and developing organisms occupy preferred but not obligatory regions of their state space.

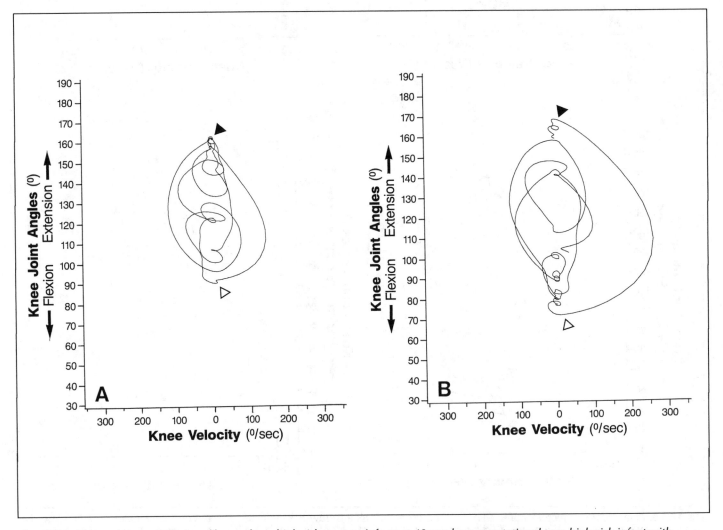

Fig. 13-20. *Phase plane trajectories of knee of two high-risk preterm infants at 40 weeks postgestational age: high-risk infant with Grade IV IVH (A), high-risk infant with Grade IV IVH and hip dysplasia (B). The filled arrows indicate the beginning of flexion movement; the open arrows represent peak flexion. From Heriza,[75] reprinted with permission.*

Contemporary Management of Motor Problems

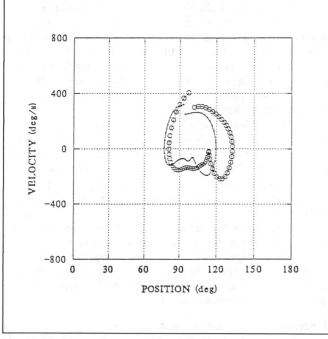

Fig. 13-21. *Phase plane portraits of the thigh of two 3-month-old walkers. Trajectory marked o-o is a normal infant; other trajectory is an infant with Down syndrome. From Clark,[51] reprinted with permission.*

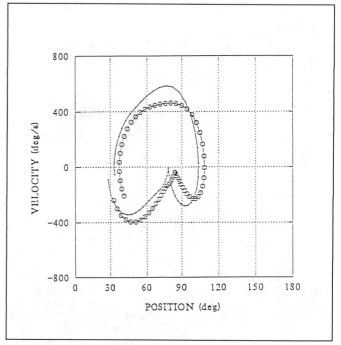

Fig. 13-22. *Phase plane portrait of the lower leg of two 3-month-old walkers. Trajectory marked o-o is a normal infant; other trajectory is an infant with Down syndrome. From Clark,[51] reprinted with permission.*

Preterm infants. The intralimb coordinated behavior of kicking can be described in terms of phase plane trajectories, or phase portraits, of the motion by plotting kicking as a function of the position and velocity of a joint. Figure 13-19 shows the corresponding phase plane trajectories of the knee of the previous representative infants at different GA and PGA.

Visual analysis indicates that the movement trajectory of the knee is confined to a particular region of the plot and shows that a particular ordered pattern exists in all infants, having the form of simple closed curves with oscillations or loops at the beginning and end of the movement phases. The amplitudes and peak velocities of the kick movements for each infant are similar with the exception of the high-risk infant movements that show variability of amplitude and peak velocity for the four kicks. There are no self-intersections (ie, no self-crossings or reversals of movement at zero velocity) during the flexion and extension movements. In other words, intralimb kicking occupies a preferred but not obligatory region of the abstract state space. This preferred repetitive cyclic behavior of kicking is considered a stable attractor state and can be classified as a limit cycle attractor.

Although as a group the 40-week-PGA high-risk preterm infants demonstrated preferred behavioral patterns that acted as stable attractors, some infants showed individual profiles.[75] Phase plane diagrams of these infants demonstrate differences in the abstract state space. In Figure 13-20, A is an infant with a grade IV IVH; B is an infant with a grade IV IVH and hip dysplasia. In general, the kicks show simple closed curves with oscillations at the extremes of the movement. There is variability in the amplitude and the velocity of the kick movements in these infants. And in contrast to

the phase plane plots of other infants, self-intersecting loops are present, (ie. self-crossings or reversals of movement at zero velocity). These loops vary in size and are proportional to the amplitude or pace of the retrograde motion. These reversals tend to occur during the extension phase of the movement, especially in infant A. Thus these plots appear to occupy various portions of the state space rather than the preferred regions of the space, and perhaps the movement pattern could be said to be a chaotic attractor.

Down syndrome infants. Figure 13-21 is a phase portrait of the thigh of two infants who have been walking for 3 months.[51] Although both infants have the same amount of experience walking (ie, 3 months), they are about 1 year apart chronologically. Both of these plots represent limit cycle attractors (ie, they both represent a geometrically shaped closed ring in state space). Because both plots do not lie atop one another, there are some small differences. The swing phase of the gait cycle (the large circular portion on the top of the plot) is similar for both infants. There are some differences in the stance phase of the gait cycle (bottom of the plot). These differences, however, are primarily related to the displacement of the movement rather than to the shape of the plot. The phase portrait of the lower leg segment of the same step-cycle of these two infants shows more similarity (Fig. 13-22). The attractor for walking demonstrates that it is stable and occupies a preferred region within the state space. Therefore, although the infant with Down syndrome did not walk for almost 1 year after the normal infant, walking behavior seems to be similar for an infant who has had 3 months' experience walking.

Thus phase plane portraits can be used as evaluation tools and do differentiate between nonhandicapped infants

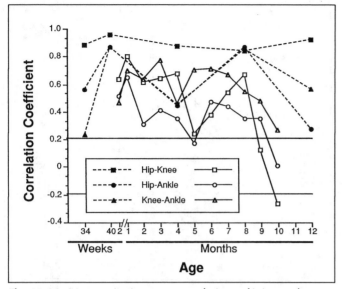

Fig. 13-23. *Mean pairwise cross correlations of joint angles during a 10-second segment of spontaneous supine kicking of four infants (solid line, open symbols) at 11 ages from 2 weeks to 10 months and one infant with a Grade IV IVH (dashed line, solid symbols) at five ages from 34 weeks postgestational age to 12 months adjusted age. Values above and below the solid horizontal lines are statistically significant. Adapted from Thelen,[58] reprinted with permission.*

and those with possible neurological dysfunction. The portraits were similar between nonhandicapped infants and infants with Down syndrome who have been walking the same amount of time.

Proposition 4. New behavioral forms emerge in movement and development as a series of phase shifts.

Preterm infants. One high-risk infant was followed during the first year. This infant, who was born at 26 weeks GA and had a documented grade IV IVH, showed organized movement at 40 weeks PGA as demonstrated by the collective variables (order parameters) of high joint correlation, small phase lags between the movement of the joints, and constrained movement times. Figure 13-23 shows mean pairwise cross correlations of joint angles during spontaneous supine kicking of four normal infants and the one infant with a grade IV IVH. Although this movement pattern began to disassociate at 4 months corrected age for the infant with IVH, just as seen with fullterm infants, the joint correlation of the infant with IVH became stronger at 8 months, with the hip-knee correlation remaining strong at 12 months corrected age. The kicking pattern stayed close to the preferred pattern at 40 weeks PGA.

In this case, the pathology may be defined as maintenance of an early preferred attractor state with the inability to uncouple the early coordinated movement pattern. Because the infant did not show the expected pattern change with development, a critical question is why not? What control parameters, be they intrinsic or extrinsic, prevented this transition, or what control parameters were missing? Possible intrinsic control parameters may be body build, passive muscle tone, muscle strength, muscle stiffness, cognitive level, and motivation. Possible extrinsic control parameters may be lack of experience in the upright position and de-

creased practice in walking. As kicking and walking have been shown to be the same movement pattern,[62] lack of experience in the upright position with the promotion of stepping may be an extrinsic control parameter that shifts the infant from a tight reciprocal kick pattern in early infancy to an uncoupled kicking pattern that evolves during the second half of the first year in conjunction with the development of independent walking.

Proposition 5. Developmental change can be envisioned as a series of stabilizing and destabilizing attractors.

Preterm infants. Data on only one infant have been analyzed over the first year of life. This infant demonstrated a stable attractor state over the first year.

Proposition 6. The control parameters of the system change over time.

Preterm infants. Again, data from only one infant have been analyzed over the first year. Because this infant showed no changes in the pattern of kicking, this proposition cannot be addressed at this time. However, a plausible question is whether the control parameters are different or the same as those for normal infants.

Summary of Data on Atypical Infants

These data suggest that the dynamical systems approach to understanding movement can be applied to atypical populations. The patterns of coordination seen in intralimb kicking and stepping and in interlimb stepping on a treadmill demonstrate that high-dimensional systems with many degrees of freedom can be reduced to low-dimensional behavior with few degrees of freedom. All components of the system (ie, musculoskeletal, neurological, arousal level, body build, passive elastic properties of muscles, and muscle strength) self-organize to produce preferred movement patterns in real and developmental time. These preferred movement patterns are assembled by the function of the task within the constraints of the immediate environment; this thought is in contrast to the traditional view that preexisting instructions assemble the movement pattern. These preferred movement patterns occupy preferred regions of the state space and, as such, can be considered stable dynamic attractors.

For intralimb kicking, movement dysfunction may have resulted from 1) the muscles and joints of one leg not being organized as a preferred movement pattern because additional variables interfered with the natural timing of a movement such as seen in kicking or 2) one or more control parameters may have caused rate-limiting or masking of another component in real or developmental time such that, in at least one infant, transitions to more functional movement patterns were prevented. Although the components of the system dynamically self-organized, the resultant movement pattern may have been too rigid in some infants and too random and disorganized in others.

Although these data support tenets of the dynamical systems theory, questions remain with respect to atypical movement. Are there different types of abnormal movement patterns (eg, obligatory preferred attractor states, disorganized or chaotic attractor states)? If so, are there different control parameters involved in the different types of movement dysfunction with respect to constraining developmental progression? Are the transition periods and control parameters hypothesized by Thelen[66] for normal infants the same for atypical infants? Which control parameters are the most powerful at specific transition periods, and if identified, can we use these parameters for intervention with infants with atypical movement?

IMPLICATIONS OF THE DYNAMICAL SYSTEMS THEORY FOR CLINICAL PRACTICE

The implications of the dynamical systems theory for the atypical or handicapped infant and child are just now being explored. The understanding of how this theory influences the evaluation and treatment of these infants is in its infancy. Because the dynamical systems theory is interested in the process of how new movement is generated, this theory has implications for the infant, child, or adult with movement dysfunction. A goal in therapeutic intervention is to maximize function. The atypical infant or child may be learning new ways to move or may be "relearning" movement if dysfunction occurred after the acquisition of a movement skill. Whether an action pattern is a new movement skill (ie, never having been learned) or a relearning of a previousmovement skill, the infant or child is still learning a new form of movement behavior. The theoretical model of conceptualizing development proposed by Thelen[21] can provide a framework for the evaluation and treatment of infants and children with movement dysfunction (Fig. 13-6). The subsystems can be any subsystems that we evaluate. The context can be any environment, and the task any task. Although no specific treatment techniques are inherent in this theoretical model, this theory can guide us in clinical practice. It is the role of the physical therapist to generate therapeutic intervention techniques.

Evaluation

According to the dynamical systems perspective, movement outcome is the result of the dynamic interaction of the components of the system within the current context of action. Therefore, there are three areas that should be addressed when evaluating the movement of patients: the various subsystems, the environment (physical and social), and the task. At this point you and I are probably saying we already do this, and indeed, we do. However, our assumptions as to why we do this evaluation may vary slightly or perhaps take on new meaning. Although we evaluate many subsystems, we emphasize the importance of the CNS in directing movement outcome. Although we know that the environment is important, we conduct our evaluations, perhaps out of necessity, in a clinical setting versus the home or school setting. We tend to emphasize the physical environment versus the social environment. We do look at function, but we look from the perspective of motor milestones as they unfold in developmental time. In contrast to working with adults, many motor milestones are functional for children, but perhaps we can expand our repertoire of tasks.

Subsystems. As therapists, we evaluate many subsystems: the musculoskeletal system (including joint mobility, muscle strength, and static postural alignment), movement patterns (including motor milestones, reflexes and reactions, coordination between posture and movement, balance, endurance, functional performance in ADL), sensation (visual, vestibular, proprioceptive, auditory, tactile), and perception. Our assumption for evaluating these subsystems is to identify which subsystem(s) is constraining functional movement. For example, if the patient is a neurologically impaired patient, we emphasize the CNS; if an orthopedically involved patient, we emphasize the musculoskeletal system. In the dynamical systems model, the assumption underlying the various component evaluations is that the outcome of the movement is the result of the dynamic interactions of all components. No one system causes movement or movement dysfunction. All systems are important in movement outcome.

Task context. We often do not test the various subsystems within a task context. For example, muscle strength and joint range are frequently tested in nonfunctional positions. We may consider identifying age appropriate tasks for the infant and young child that we are evaluating and then determining whether the infant or child has the muscle strength and joint range to accomplish the task.

Environment. We use the same environment to test movement patterns. By changing the environment during testing, we will be able to ascertain whetherthe infant or child can adapt to the changing context or whether the same movement pattern is used in all instances. We are interested in not only whether the child can perform the behavior in a coordinated manner but also whether she can demonstrate flexibility in movement patterns to changing environmental conditions. Changing environments will allow us to look at the stability and flexibility of movement patterns. It also will provide important information into the types of environment or environmental support that produce the movement patterns in which we are interested. For example, we need to know if the infant can adapt her locomotion pattern from walking on a solid support to moving on foam or grass.

New evaluation concepts. The dynamical systems theory offers us additional evaluation strategies such as identifying the collective variables, transition periods, and control parameters. We need to be able to do the following:

1. Identify the collective variables (order parameters). With respect to intralimb coordination, these have been shown to be joint correlations, phase lags, and movement times in the lower extremities. The number of decelerations and accelerations in reaching, called movement units, has also been useful in children with cerebral palsy.[77] With respect to interlimb coordination in the legs, the phasing of the limb with respect to time and distance have been shown to be helpful in the analysis of movement. There are probably other order parameters that are yet unidentified.

2. Identify transition periods. This can be addressed by the variability of the movement pattern and the amount of time that it takes for the pattern to return to a stable pattern after perturbation. At transition periods, you should see more variability in movement patterns, and these patterns should more easily be perturbed.

3. Identify control parameters. Control parameters are those variables that may constrain (limit) a movement pattern. Because weight has been demonstrated as a control parameter in infant kicking and stepping, this variable and other anthropometric measures such as height (sitting and

standing), head circumference, and circumference and length of limbs should be assessed.

Assessment tools. Assessment tools that may add to the evaluation of infants and young children are the use of videography, kinematics, electromyography, and kinetics. Because we are interested in movement patterns, using videography will be an important part of our evaluations. In contrast to developmental tests that address motor milestones, videotape analysis holds the potential for analyzing movement in its component parts with respect to the context in which the movement occurs. Kinematic analysis is used often in conjunction with videography. It is a sensitive measurement system that quantifies the quality of movement by capturing the dynamic quality of the movement; describing the movement according to the objective kinematic variables of time, velocity, amplitude, and acceleration; and providing a permanent record of the movement. Kinematic data can be displayed graphically either as time-dependent (angle-time) representations in which the patterns of joint displacement are plotted as a function of time or as time-independent representations such as angle-angle diagrams and amplitude velocity phase plane trajectories. We have also called these diagrams phase portraits and have used them to display attractors in state space. These plots result in a visual permanent record of the movement that can be reviewed for evaluation purposes, compared with other movement sequences of the same infant, or compared with movement patterns of other infants. These plots not only provide useful interpretative data about the movement path of a body segment with respect to time or the movement path of one body segment versus another but also provide the movement path's velocity, direction, and magnitude.

Kinematic analysis is necessary to evaluate the kinetics of movement, or the distribution of forces, that provide information on the underlying cause of movement disorders. In addition, kinematic analysis can be coupled with electromyography for insights into the neural control of movement.

From a dynamical systems perspective, our evaluation should identify the following: 1) age appropriate tasks that are performed well and those that cannot be performed; 2) transition periods; 3) control variables that are constraining movement (either endogenous factors that reside within the infant or child or exogenous factors that reside in the environment or social context); and 4) contextual variations, that is, stability of movement patterns across varying contexts.

Treatment

Based on the dynamical systems perspective, the following principles may be useful in physical therapy intervention:

1. Promote function.

According to the dynamical systems theory, function (task and context) assembles behavior. These tasks or goals must be age appropriate. This concept demands that we perceive the infant and child as active participants in the therapy sessions versus their being passive recipients of our therapy.

Age appropriate tasks or goals do not dictate that we follow the developmental sequence in our promotion of func-

tion. For example, creeping is not necessarily a prerequisite for standing and walking. Although the majority of children in our culture transverse the stage of creeping on their way to the attainment of independent walking, this is not true for other cultures.[78,79]

2. Identify the transitional phases.

The transitional phases are the optimal times to effect changes in movement. It may be the time that you have the best opportunity to change the movement pattern. Before the transitional phase, the movement is very stable and resistant to perturbation. You may think of physical therapy as perturbing the system. If the movement pattern is very stable (ie, if there is a strong attractor and the behavior pattern lies in the bottom of the well), it is going to be very difficult to shift the movement pattern to a more mature pattern. The shift is more easily accomplished, however, if the infant or child is in a transitional state, which is characterized by variability of the movement pattern and by an increased time delay in returning to the stable movement pattern. During these states, behavior is in a shallow well and the movement pattern is more flexible and more adaptable. It is at these times that the infant or child should be given the opportunity to explore options for movement and to find stable solutions. Infants must be able to explore movement actively to arrive at the best possible movement strategies for that functional goal or task. Function is paramount.

The role of the physical therapist is to assist the infant or child to find a stable movement solution, but the infant must find the solution. The stable solution can only be found in function. The physical therapist can assist by 1) providing a variety of experiences directed toward functional goals or tasks, 2) selecting age appropriate tasks, 3) structuring the environment, and 4) manipulating control parameters that constrain the movement.

3. Manipulate control parameters that constrain the desired functional task or goal.

Control parameters 1) reside within the infant or within the environment, including the physical and social environment; 2) have their own developmental course; 3) may constrain movement at one time period and support it at another time; and 4) may have a big influence on movement outcome during transition periods or a little influence during nontransitional periods.

Control parameters may be arousal level, body build, postural control, or muscle strength. They must have a scalar property, that is, they must have a continuum of possible ranges such that they can be scaled up or down. Some of these control parameters may be manipulated to enhance the functional motor task or goal; others may be managed by providing the missing component during the execution of the task.

Although infants possess the neuromuscular pattern to walk earlier than 12 months, they do not walk because of the lack of adequate strength or postural control to accomplish this activity. If they are supported under the axilla, which helps support their weight and provides postural control, these infants take coordinated steps. As they grow and become larger, body weight and lack of muscle strength constrain the infant from taking steps. When placed in water, which provides support to the weighted limbs, and if supported under the axilla, these infants also take steps. If placed on a treadmill, these infants take steps. Thus, in therapy, if the control parameters that are constraining the movement pattern from being exhibited are manipulated, or if the control parameters can artificially be provided, more mature forms of movement can be produced.

A control parameter may be missing from the environmental repertoire of an infant. For example, in the high-risk preterm infant who did not uncouple the tight synchrony of early kicking, a discussion with mother indicated that this infant was rarely placed in the upright standing position. If the practice of movement in the upright position shifts the pattern of ambulation from an immature to a mature pattern, and if kicking and stepping are the same movement pattern, then this experience should also shift the uncoupling of the joints in kicking.

4. Change the context, or environment, in which the movement pattern exists.

This may include the social environment as well as the physical environment.

a. Physical context. Tasks should be practiced in a number of different environments to promote the flexibility of movement patterns while maintaining stability. The environment may need to be modified to support posture and movement. Other architectural engineering may include the use of adaptive equipment including orthotics. These could also be considered as managing control parameters that are missing.

b. Social context. The social context is extremely important for infants and young children. Parents and caretakers should be trained to promote functional movement patterns. Activities incorporated into the daily routine of care giving of the infant or young child provide increased opportunity to explore various movement patterns and find solutions for particular functional tasks or goals.

5. Practice, practice, practice: experience, experience, experience.

Think how frequently infants and young children practice a newly found movement pattern. When infants first learn to pull to stand, they constantly pull up, fall, pull up, fall, and pull up. During practice, the infant experiences and learns two types of information: the relationship of the infant to the environment, and the interrelationship of body segments within a gravitational field. Practice of movements can be goal directed, as in pull to stand, and can be nongoal directed, as in spontaneous kicking. Spontaneous kicking in the early months of life is nongoal directed, being endogenously driven by arousal level. With age, kicking comes under intentional control, being exogenously driven to explore objects, make noise, or signal caretaker.[80] Although experience strengthens movement patterns, it only does so in a context in which the movement strategy is functional.

In a classical study of the effect of practice of early stepping movements on the onset of ambulation, researchers demonstrated facilitation of the walking response through brief daily exercise of the stepping reflex.[68] Infants who received formal handling in cultures that promote development of motor tasks accomplished these activities earlier than infants who did not receive this handling.[78]

6. Focus on the process of change in movement patterns versus outcome measures.

Generally, the efficacy studies on the effectiveness of physical therapy interventions have used change in gross motor milestone attainments as the outcome variable. This measure is a product measure and does not address how the infant or young child is progressing toward accomplishing a motor activity. We have discussed factors that may address how movements evolve based on the dynamical action system such as 1) the identification of collective variables (order parameters) that might be expected to change during an intervention program of physical therapy and 2) the use of phase planes plots to address the state space in which the movement pattern occurs.

With respect to treatment, the use of these factors, over time, may demonstrate those changes that physical therapy can effect. Thus a way to look at the process of change is to do serial evaluations. Case studies and the single subject design can be used to determine the efficacy of physical therapy treatment. These formats also provide a way to document progress that can be used for accountability for the government and third party payers. They also provide a database on the movements of infant and young children that will aid research efforts for the clinical scientist.

CONCLUSIONS

This is an exciting time for physical therapists. The field of motor development has lain dormant for 50 or more years. The lack of knowledge on how movement develops has led us to continue using theoretical concepts that in their time were appropriate. But it is time to relook at our assumptions for the evaluation and treatment of infants and young children, modify them as indicated, and perhaps consider contemporary models of motor development as an alternative theoretical framework for the evaluation and treatment of infants.

Acknowledgment

My work reported on in this chapter was supported in part by a grant from the Foundation for Physical Therapy.

GLOSSARY

Action. Movement with a goal.

Angle-angle plots. Joint angle of one joint plotted against the simultaneous joint angle of another joint of the same limb.

Attractor. Geometric form that describes behavior in state space; what the behavior of the system settles down to or is attracted to.

Attractor state space. Hypothetical space defined by any number of variables of a preferred coordinated pattern.

Chaotic attractor. Attractor, or coordinated pattern, in which the trajectory of the behavior forms a complicated structure in state space; referred to as a noisy attractor.

Constrain. Confine, limit, restrain, restrict.

Context. Constraints and supports of the environment in which a task is completed.

Control parameter. Variable that shifts the behavior from one form to another; has to have a scalar quantity; does not control the change but acts as an agent for reorganization of the behavior.

Coordinated pattern. Unit of behavior composed of many elements (variables) organized into larger functional groups that constrain the multiple elements to act as a unit.

Coordinative structure (synergy). Organization of multiple muscles and joints of the body into larger functional groups or synergies that constrain the muscles and joints to act as a unit.

Degrees of freedom. Many elements (variables), each of which is free to vary; in this context, does not refer to spatial degrees of freedom.

Developmental time. Self-organization of movement patterns that change with time, with respect to days, months, or years, versus movement patterns that change over seconds or minutes.

Dynamic. Spontaneous self-organization of elements (variables) into observed units of behavior.

Dynamic attractors. Preferred coordinated patterns determined by the morphology of the system, the energy flow through the system, and the task and environmental constraints.

Dynamical system. Any system that changes over time.

Function. Task and context.

High-dimensional system. A system composed of many elements (variables, dimensions, degrees of freedom).

Limit cycle (periodic) attractor. Attractor, or coordinated pattern, in which the trajectory of the behavior forms a closed ring (curve) in state space.

Low-dimensional system. A system described by the fewest number of elements (variables, dimensions, degrees of freedom) possible.

Order parameter (collective variable). Low-dimensional description of a unit of behavior that describes quantitatively the behavior.

Path trajectory. Path the movement takes as it changes over time.

Phase plane plots. Joint angle of one joint plotted against the simultaneous velocity of the same joint.

Phase portrait (state-space picture, phase-space portrait). State space filled with trajectories converging onto attractors; geometric representation of the behavior of the system in state space; an attractor, that is, a preferred coordinated pattern, mapped in state space.

Phase shift. Transitions, often nonlinear, from one preferred qualitative coordinated pattern to another preferred qualitative coordinated pattern; for example, from walking to trotting in the horse.

Point (equilibrium) attractor. Attractor, or coordinated pattern, in which the trajectory of the behavior forms a single fixed point in state space.

Real time. Self-organization of a movement pattern that is currently ongoing (ie, what the organism is doing second by second, minute by minute).

Self-organization. The system, composed of a number of elements, organizes spontaneously from the dynamic interaction of the elements; no representation, prescription, or motor program need exist.

State. A point in state space representing the state of the system at a given time.

State space (phase space). Hypothetical space defined by any number of elements (variables); abstract space whose coordinates are the degrees of freedom of the system.

System. Network composed of a number of interacting elements (variables) that contribute to the unit of behavior.

Time-dependent graphics. Angle-time plots, or time series plots; amplitude, or displacement, of a joint plotted as a function of time.

Time-independent graphics. Angle-angle plots; phase plane plots.

References

1. Halverson HM. An experimental study of prehension in infants by means of systematic cinema records. *Genetic Psychological Monographs*. 1931;10:107-286.
2. Shirley MM. *The First Two Years: A Study of Twenty-Five Babies: Postural and Locomotor Development*. Minneapolis, Minn: University of Minnesota Press; 1931;1.
3. McGraw MB. *The Neuromuscular Maturation of the Human Infant*. New York, NY: Hafner Press; 1945.
4. McGraw MB. Maturation of behavior. In: Carmichael L, ed. *Manual of Child Psychology*. lst ed. New York, NY: John Wiley & Sons Inc; 1946:332-369.
5. Gesell A. The ontogenesis of infant behavior. In: Carmichael L, ed. *Manual of Child Psychology*. 2nd ed. New York, NY; John Wiley & Son Inc; 1954:335-373.
6. Bayley N. The development of motor abilities during the first three years. *Monographs of the Society for Research in Child Development*. 1935;1:1-26.
7. Coghill GE. *Anatomy and the Problem of Behavior*. New York, NY: Cambridge University Press; 1929.
8. Sherrington CS. *The Integrative Action of the Nervous System*. New York, NY: Scribner Book Co; 1906.
9. Pick HL. Motor development: the control of action. *Developmental Psychology*. 1990;25:867-870.
10. Adams JA. Response feedback and learning. *Psychol Bull*. 1968;70:486-504.
11. Gibson JJ. *An Ecological Approach to Visual Perception*. Boston, Mass: Houghton-Mifflin Co; 1979.
12. Bernstein N. *Coordination and Regulation of Movements*. New York, NY: Pergamon Press Inc; 1967.
13. Whiting HTA, ed. *Human Motor Action: Bernstein Reassessed*. New York, NY: Elsevier Science Publishing Co Inc; 1984.
14. Gibson EJ. Exploratory behavior in the development of perceiving, acting, and the acquiring of knowledge. *Ann Rev Psychol*. 1988;39:1-41.
15. Gibson E, Schmuckler MA. Going somewhere: an ecological and experimental approach to development of mobility. *Ecological Psychology*. 1989;1:3-25.
16. Reed ES. An outline of a theory of action systems. *Journal of Motor Behavior*. 1982;14:98-134.
17. Reed ES. Changing theories of postural development. In: Woollacott MH, Shumway-Cook A, eds. *Development of Posture and Gait Across the Lifespan*. Columbia, SC: University of South Carolina Press; 1989:4-24.
18. Kelso JAS, Holt KG, Kugler PN, et al. On the concept of coordinative structures as dissipative structures: II. Empirical lines of convergence. In: Stelmach GE, Requin J, eds. *Tutorials in Motor Behavior*. New York, NY: Elsevier Science Publishing Co Inc; 1980:49-70.
19. Kelso JAS, Tuller B. A dynamical basis for action systems. In: Gassaniga M, ed. *Handbook of Cognitive Neuroscience*. New York, NY: Plenum Publishing Corp; 1984:321-356.

20. Kugler PN, Kelso JAS, Turvey MT. On the concept of coordinative structures as dissipative structures: I. Theoretical lines of convergence. In: Stelmach GE, Requin J, eds. *Tutorials in Motor Behavior*. New York, NY: Elsevier Science Publishing Co Inc; 1980:3-47.

21. Thelen E. Development of coordinated movement: implications for early human development. In: Wage MG, Whiting HTA, eds. *Motor Development in Children: Aspects of Coordination and Control*. Boston, Mass: Martinus Nijhoff Publisher; 1986:107-120.

22. Thelen E. Self-organization in developmental processes: can systems approaches work? In: Gunnar M, Thelen E, eds. *Systems and Development: The Minnesota Symposium on Child Psychology*. Hillsdale, NJ: Lawrence Erlbaum Associates Inc; 1989;22:7-11.

23. Fogel A, Thelen E. Development of early expressive and communicative action: reinterpreting the evidence from a dynamic systems perspective. *Developmental Psychology*. 1987;23:747-761.

24. Thelen E, Fogel A. Toward an action-based theory of infant development. In: Lockman J, Hazen N, eds. *Action in Social Context*. New York, NY: Plenum Publishing Corp; 1989:23-63.

25. Thelen E, Kelso JS, Fogel A. Self-organizing systems and infant motor development. *Developmental Review*. 1987;7:39-65.

26. Sameroff AJ. Early influences on development: fact or fancy? *Merrill-Palmer Quarterly*. 1975;21:267-294.

27. Sameroff AJ. Developmental systems: contexts and evolution. In: Mussen PH, ed. *Handbook of Child Psychology*. 4th ed. (Formerly *Carmichael's Manual of Child Psychology*.) New York, NY: John Wiley & Sons Inc; 1983;1:237-294.

28. Piaget J. *The Origins of Intelligence in Children*. New York, NY: International Universities Press Inc; 1952.

29. Mandler JM. A new perspective on cognitive development in infancy. *American Scientist*. 1990;78:236-243.

30. Als H. Toward a synactive theory of development: promise for the assessment and support of infant individuality. *Infant Mental Health Journal*. 1982;3:229-243.

31. Horowitz FD. *Exploring Developmental Theories: Toward a Structural/Behavioral Model of Development*. Hillsdale, NJ: Lawrence Erlbaum Associates Inc; 1987.

32. Horowitz FD. Commentary: process and systems. In: Gunnar MR, Thelen E, eds. *Systems and Development: The Minnesota Symposia on Child Psychology*. Hillsdale, NJ: Lawrence Erlbaum Associates Inc; 1989;22:211-218.

33. Sameroff AJ. Commentary: general systems and the regulation of development. In: Gunnar MR, Thelen E, eds. *Systems and Development. The Minnesota Symposia on Child Psychology*. Hillsdale, NJ: Lawrence Erlbaum Associates Inc; 1989;22:219-235.

34. McGraw M. Professional and personal blunder in child development research. *Newsletter for Society for Research in Child Development*. Winter 1985 (suppl).

35. Thelen E. The role of motor development in developmental psychology: a view of the past and an agenda for the future. In: Eisenberg N, ed. *Contemporary Topics in Developmental Psychology*. New York, NY: John Wiley & Sons Inc; 1989:3-33.

36. Thelen E. Rhythmical stereotypies in normal human infants. *Animal Behavior*. 1979;27:699-715.

37. Fetters L, Fernandez B, Cermak S. The relationship of proximal and distal components in the development of reaching. *Journal of Human Movement Studies*. In press.

38. Forssberg H, Nashner LM. Ontogenetic development of postural control in man: adaptation to altered support and visual conditions during stance. *J Neurosci*. 1982;2:545-552.

39. Ashmead DH. Infant posture and prehension during deep knee bends. Presented at the International Society for Infant Studies; April 22, 1990; Montreal, Canada.

40. Clark JE, Truly TL, Phillips SJ. A dynamical systems approach to understanding the development of lower limb coordination in locomotion. In: Block H, Bertenthal B, eds. *Sensory-Motor Organization and Development in Infancy and Early Childhood*. Hingham, Mass: Kluwer Academic Publishers. In press.

41. Knoblock H. *Manual of Developmental Diagnosis: The Administration and Interpretation of the Revised Gesell and Amatruda Developmental and Neurologic Examination*. Hagerstown, Md; Harper & Row, Publishers Inc; 1980.

42. Bayley N. *Manual for the Bayley Scales of Infant Development*. New York, NY: Psychological Corp; 1969.

43. Frankenberg WK, Dodds JB. The Denver Developmental Screening Test. *J Pediatr*. 1967;71:181-185.

44. Wolf PH. *The Development of Behavioral States and the Expression of Emotions in Early Infancy*. Chicago, Ill: University of Chicago Press; 1987.

45. Haken H. *Synergetics, an Introduction: Non-equilibrium Phase Transitions and Self-organization in Physics, Chemistry and Biology*. 3rd ed. New York, NY: Springer-Verlag New York Inc; 1983.

46. Kelso JAS, Schoner G. Self-organization of coordinative movement patterns. *Human Movement Science*. 1988;7:27-46.

47. Schoner G, Kelso JAS. Dynamic pattern generation in behavioral and neural systems. *Science*. 1988;239:1513-1520.

48. Thelen E. Coupling perception and action in the development of skill: a dynamic approach. In: Block H, Bertenthal B, eds. *Sensory-Motor Organization and Development in Infancy and Childhood*. Hingham, Mass; Kluwer Academic Publishers. In press.

49. Thelen E, Ulrich BD. Hidden precursors to skill: a dynamical systems analysis of treadmill-elicited stepping during the first year. *Monographs of the Society for Research in Child Development*. In press.

50. Thelen E. Conceptualizing development from a dynamical systems perspective. Presented at Dynamics in Development Workshop: Society for Research and Child Development; April 26-27, 1989; Kansas City, Kan.

51. Clark JE. On viewing atypical and normal development as dynamical systems. Presented at the International Conference on Infant Studies; April 21, 1990; Montreal, Canada.

52. Easton TA. On the normal use of reflexes. *American Scientist*. 1972;60:591-599.

53. Kelso JAS, Southards DL, Goodman D. On the nature of human interlimb coordination. *Science*. 1979;203:1029-1031.

54. Turvey MT. Preliminaries to a theory of action with reference to vision. In: Shaw R, Biansford J, eds. *Perceiving, Acting, and Knowing: Toward an Ecological Psychology*. New York, NY: John Wiley & Sons Inc; 1977;211-265.

55. Tuller B, Turvey MT, Fitch HL. The Bernstein perspective: II. The concept of muscle linkage or coordinative structure. In: Kelso JAS, ed. *Human Motor Behavior: An Introduction*. Hillsdale, NJ: Lawrence Erlbaum Associates Inc; 1982.

56. Heriza CB. Comparison of leg movements in preterm infants at term with healthy full-term infants. *Phys Ther*. 1988;68:1687-1693.

57. Heriza CB. Organization of leg movements in preterm infants. *Phys Ther*. 1988;68:1340-1346.

58. Thelen E. Developmental origins of motor coordination: leg movements in human infants. *Dev Psychobiol.* 1985;18:1-22.

59. Clark JE, Whitall J, Phillips SJ. Human interlimb coordination: the first 6 months of independent walking. *Dev Psychobiol.* 1988;21:445-456.

60. Thelen E. Treadmill-elicited stepping in seven-month-old infants. *Child Dev.* 1986;57:1498-1506.

61. Thelen E, Ridley-Johnson R, Fisher DM. Shifting patterns of bilateral coordination and lateral dominance in the leg movements of young infants. *Dev Psychobiol.* 1983;16:29-46.

62. Thelen E, Fisher DM. Newborn stepping: an explanation for a "disappearing" reflex. *Dev Psychol.* 1982;18:760-775.

63. Heriza CB. *A Kinematic Analysis of Leg Movements in Premature and Full-Term Infants.* Edwardsville, Ill: Southern Illinois University at Edwardsville; 1986. Dissertation.

64. Thelen E, Fisher DM. The organization of spontaneous leg movements in newborn infants. *Journal of Motor Behavior.* 1983;15:353-377.

65. Thelen E. Learning to walk: ecological demands and phylogenetic constraints. In: Lipsitt LP, Rovee-Collier C, eds. *Advances in Infancy Research.* Norwood, NJ: Ablex Publishing Corp; 1984:213-249.

66. Thelen E. Evolving and dissolving synergies in the development of leg coordination. In: Wallace SA, ed. *Perspectives on the Coordination of Movement.* New York, NY: Elsevier Science Publishing Co Inc. In press.

67. Butler C. High tech tots: technology for mobility, manipulation, communication, and learning in early childhood. *Infants and Young Children.* 1988;1(2):66-73.

68. Zelazo PR, Zelazo NA, Kolb S. "Walking" in the newborn. *Science.* 1972;176:314-315.

69. Thelen E, Fisher DM, Ridley-Johnson R. The relationship between physical growth and a newborn reflex. *Infant Behavior and Development.* 1984;7:479-493.

70. Thelen E, Fisher DM, Ridley-Johnson R, et al. Effects of body build and arousal on newborn infant stepping. *Dev Psychobiol.* 1982;15:447-453.

71. Thelen E, Skala KD, Kelso JAS. The dynamic nature of early coordination: evidence from bilateral leg movements in young infants. *Dev Psychol.* 1987;23:179-186.

72. Thelen E, Ulrich BD, Niles D. Bilateral coordination in human infants: stepping on a split-belt treadmill. *J Exp Psychol [Hum Percep].* 1987;13:405-410.

73. Harris SR, Heriza CB. Measuring infant movement: clinical and technological assessment techniques. *Phys Ther.* 1987;67:1877-1880.

74. Kermoian R, Campos JJ. Locomotor experience: a facilitator of spatial cognitive development. *Child Dev.* 1988;59:908-917.

75. Heriza CB. Implications of the dynamical systems approach to understanding infant kicking behavior. *Phys Ther.* In press.

76. Ulrich BD, Ulrich DA, Collier JH. Motor development in Down Syndrome infants: a new approach to understanding. Presented at the International Society for Infant Studies; April 21, 1990; Montreal, Canada.

77. Kluzik J, Fetters L, Coryell J. Quantification of control: a preliminary study of effects of neurodevelopmental treatment on reaching in children with spastic cerebral palsy. *Phys Ther.* 1990;70:65-78.

78. Hopkins B, Westra T. Motor development, maternal expectations, and the role of handling. *Infant Behavior and Development.* 1990;13:117-122.

79. Super CM. Environmental effects on motor development. *Dev Med Child Neurol.* 1976;18:561-567.

80. Schneider K, Zernicke RF, Ulrich BD, et al. Understanding movement control in infants through the analysis of limb intersegmental dynamics. *Journal of Motor Behavior.* In press.

81. Ulrich BD, Jensen JL, Thelen E. Stability and variation in the development of infant stepping: implications for control. In: Patla AE, ed. *Adaptibility of Human Gait: Implications for the Control of Locomotion.* New York, NY: Elsevier Science Publishing Co Inc. In press.

Chapter 14

Merging Neurophysiologic Approaches with Contemporary Theories

I. Setting the Stage for Discussion

Darcy Umphred, PhD, PT
Associate Professor
Graduate Program in Physical Therapy
University of the Pacific
Stockton, CA 95211

The following presentations are the result of three representative panelists from this portion of the program being asked to prepare papers reflecting their views and integrating their concepts with the contemporary theories of motor control and motor learning as discussed at this conference and as found in the literature.

The first presentation, submitted by Dr. Jackson, represents a more traditional method of discussing a treatment philosophy and therefore does not directly integrate in writing the threads between her specific philosophy and the motor control-learning research findings. Dr. Jackson's success as a clinician, however, reflects the obvious use of appropriate reinforcement scheduling, learner participation, and open-loop systems that actually link her philosophy with the contemporary theories. Although the following presentation of Dr. Jackson may not identify specifically how the theories are integrated, readers can gain an advantage in meeting the challenge to integrate those thought processes themselves.

The second presentation reflects the ideas of a colleague who is in close contact both clinically and theoretically with professionals who are researching motor control and motor learning. Dr. Montgomery's unique clinical skills and expertise have given her a perspective that allows traditional philosophies to be threaded with contemporary theory. She has chosen to accept both traditional and contemporary theories and study the relationships. She has seen successes in the clinic where variables are difficult to control, while also studying specifics in the research laboratory. Realizing there are numerous clinical interactions for which a valid and clear rationale has not been identified, Dr. Montgomery is constantly pursuing new knowledge.

The third presentation reflects a colleague's attempt not only to integrate traditional approaches with contemporary theories but also to integrate those materials with the specifics presented at the II STEP conference. Mrs. Minor came to the conference with a preconceived paper that merged two traditional approaches with her interpretation of motor control theory. While at the conference, she integrated her original paper with materials presented during the

3 days before her presentation. Her presentation in this volume, therefore, represents not only the integration that was occurring in her mind during the conference but also the continuation of that process while she was preparing her final copy.

SETTING THE STAGE

As today's moderator I not only have the privilege to introduce our distinguished speakers but also have the responsibility of making sure the objectives for the day's presentation have been met. Our primary objective is to integrate contemporary theories of motor control, motor learning, and motor development with traditional neurophysiologic approaches and current theories of practice. The objective is quite simple. The task is very awesome. There is no way within the limited time frame of today that we can present even an overview of all approaches and theories, either traditional or current. Thus the panel and I will try to identify a process that colleagues use when trying to link their early learning and clinical practice experiences with current research findings and theories of motor control, motor learning, and motor development.

Colleagues such as Signe Brunnstrom, Berta Bobath, Mary Fiorentino, Margaret Knott, Dorothy Voss, Margaret Rood, Moshe Feldenkrais, Jean Ayers, Temple Fay, Sally Semans, and many others have laid the foundation for what might be referred to as traditional neurologic rehabilitation over the last 20 to 30 years. This foundation has lead to current clinical practice in the area of central nervous system (CNS) function, whether the focus be on neonates, children, adolescents, adults, or elderly persons. These clinicians' contributions to our professional growth over the last few decades should never be overshadowed by new knowledge. What these people have given to us not only encompasses their words regarding treatment but also their cumulative philosophies that people have the potential to learn and change irrespective of damage or alteration in CNS function. Each one of these very talented colleagues tried to share with the profession what he or she was seeing and doing when evalu-

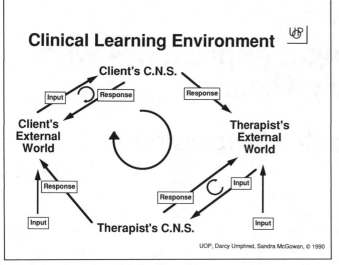

Clinical Learning Environment

Client's C.N.S.

Input — Response — Response

Client's External World — Therapist's External World

Response — Input

Response — Input

Input — Therapist's C.N.S. — Input

UOP, Darcy Umphred, Sandra McGowan, © 1990

Fig. 14-1. *Depiction of early clinical learning environment.*

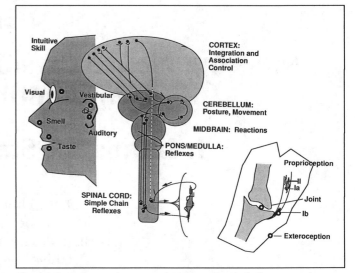

Intuitive Skill

CORTEX: Integration and Association Control

Visual

Vestibular

CEREBELLUM: Posture, Movement

Smell

Auditory

MIDBRAIN: Reactions

Taste

PONS/MEDULLA: Reflexes

Proprioception

II Ia

Joint

SPINAL CORD: Simple Chain Reflexes

Ib

Exteroception

Fig. 14-2. *Relevant aspects of a client through the eyes of a founder of an early therapeutic approach.*

ating and treating patients. Their students interpreted and verbally communicated those thoughts and tried to explain why the procedures were working better than those traditional procedures taught in school. In reality, only a very small amount of what any one of those people was actually doing or processing at any one moment in time was probably communicated. Thus much of the mystique or gift held by each of these people still remains a mystery.

In trying to meet our objective of integrating current and traditional theory, we must understand how early theory developed and has changed. Initially, our early colleagues, or founders, were confronted with a clinical environment (Fig. 14-1). This environment consisted of the client, the clinician, and all the external factors that affect both the therapist and the recipient of health care. Each clinician used her or his own education, prior experiences, learning styles, affective uniqueness, observational strategies, kinesthetic skill, and genuine love for learning in order to develop a framework to understand, interpret, evaluate, and treat their clients. Even though the founders had teachers or guides that directed their early paths, they were confronted with problems their teachers had not addressed. They also had a belief that more could be done than was being done to help clients gain function. All these founders were keen visual observers with highly developed kinesthetic ability. They saw a client with many sensory modalities, a motor response system, and a mysterious internal processing system yet to be understood and researched (Fig. 14-2). Each founder discovered methods and sequential treatment procedures that were more effective than approaches taught to them. Each looked at behavioral responses and tried to figure out ways to alter behavior through input. The input techniques that each one of these clinicians found helpful and successful when treating clients became incorporated into his or her approach. Some techniques focused more on one modality than another. Some founders were more successful in one position of treatment than another; therefore, that position became the one of choice for that particular approach.

Some founders felt strongly about having a valid neu-

rophysiologic basis for their approaches and tried to explain why techniques worked based on the understanding of the CNS at that moment in time. Others did not delve into the basic sciences to find a rationale; instead, they used behavioral and observable responses of the clients as the rationale for acceptable treatment. Initial positions for treatment, specific methods, and sequential treatment procedures have changed within each approach over the last few decades. New generations of people have added to the depth and breadth of each approach. Some knowledge, however, was not available, such as that of internal processing, procedural and declarative learning, and motor control function as we know it today. Therefore, the rationale for the success of each clinician was often based, in today's framework, on inaccurate or invalid content. Yet no one who had the privilege of observing the "magic" hands of these clinicians would deny their ability to alter motor control, to help the client regain motor skill, and to increase the quality of life for the individual they treated.

When relating these founding methodologies to CNS organization, our founders were aware of sensory input as a method of altering CNS processing and thus motor output (Fig. 14-3). In those earlier years, motor output was categorized into two systems. First was the pyramidal system that was thought to control intentional movement, especially fine motor skills. The second was referred to as the extrapyramidal system. This system was conceptualized as a hierarchical system. Many sequential treatment procedures were based on this hierarchy, and sequences were selected to integrate each step or level in the hierarchy. As the second, third, and fourth generation therapists removed from these founders, we need to be careful not to place concrete structures around fluid treatment sequences. The founders would certainly adapt any treatment procedure if the technique did not lead to the goal that was set. These gifted clinicians were creative in how they approached clients. Although they identified sequences and treatment procedures, they always let the client's CNS guide them in the specifics on a moment-to-moment interaction.

In the last 10 to 15 years, the ideas of motor control, motor learning, or procedural learning have evolved. Many involved in this evolution began to question the ideas and treatment sequences taught in school. As procedural learning and the feedforward-feedback interaction within the motor system was studied, the emphasis on the motor system became paramount. The focus on input systems as the primary guide to treatment began to split philosophical camps between traditional and contemporary theories of treating neurologically involved patients (Fig. 14-4).

Motor control and motor learning theorists began to study the motor system and its complexity. The importance of the basal ganglia and cerebellum, with their influence over nuclei within the brain stem and their ultimate influence over the spinal motor generators, took precedence over input systems. The study of the motor system initially focused on the normal intact CNS throughout life. As study of normal motor control branched into areas of motor impairment, the questions of appropriate evaluation and treatment procedures were presented and debated. These questions and research findings at times split further the camps between contemporary and traditional treatment procedures. Some colleagues are still arguing. Yet, from my perception, we are still in an early evolutionary process. These two philosophies of CNS organization come together clearly when the remaining components of the CNS are placed in the model (Fig. 14-5). There is an emotional-cognitive system that screens the input and directs the motor output. Such colleagues as Vernon Brooks and Josephine Moore and I are looking into the integration of procedural and declarative learning and the complex interaction of all systems when we each analyze behavioral responses. The limbic and the cognitive systems' influences over motor control can never be ignored, nor was it ever ignored by the founders of the various approaches. They may not have known cognitively or been able to discuss these issues verbally, but they certainly took them into account when interacting in a flowing sequence with their clients. If we look at a slide sequence of a child jumping off a park bench, the child will demonstrate for us the interaction

of all his systems and will nonverbally tell us that we must never lose sight of the whole picture, no matter what our specific focus or philosophy might be.

First, we might perceive this child in a feedforward mode that clearly identified with motor theory today. At first glimpse, he climbs onto the bench, walks along, jumps off, lands, and is off to do it again. If we look more clearly at the moment he starts to walk off, it becomes obvious he is about to experience something new. He is about 15 ms before heel strike in a feedforward mode. Yet the plan is walking, not jumping. As he continues to walk, he is now falling. Feedback becomes critical. Understanding which systems he will use will help us analyze how he interprets the environment. Obviously, olfaction and gustatory input are not the critical systems for task-specific success. Auditory input would influence the system if someone yelled or warned the child of the impending danger. This massive alerting might have altered his responses in less desirable ways. The cutaneous system is both cold and wrapped in maintained pressure through clothing, thus its influence over learning would also be minimal. The visual system is intent on looking at the ocean. It will quickly be directed to look at the ground once the vestibular system is activated. Thus this system will play a significant role in cognitive analysis and recall. The proprioceptive and the vestibular systems are two systems that will play a critical role in feedback and learning. What the CNS expects and what it is receiving is a mismatch. This child must scan his memory of past motor experiences to find something similar. What he will find is something labelled "falling." This plan will prepare him for impact with earth. The selected plan will not necessarily lead to smooth coordinated movement because there is not time. It will lead to the necessary force, speed, direction, range, balance, and synergies necessary to prevent injury upon impact. When looking at the facial expression on the child, which reflects attention and cognitive-emotional focus on the task, it becomes obvious that the limbic and cortical structures were involved actively throughout the entire process. Once the child understands what happened, his facial intensity relaxes. He

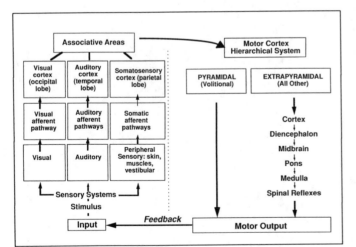

Fig. 14-3. *Using sensory input as a method of altering motor output.*

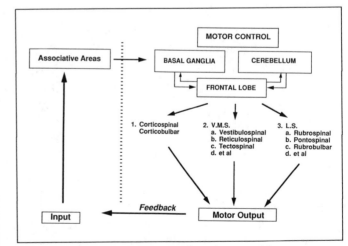

Fig. 14-4. *Using input systems as the primary guide to treatment of neurologically involved patients.*

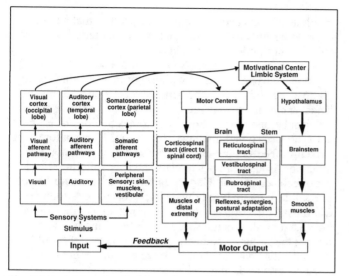

Fig. 14-5. *Adding the limbic and cognitive systems to screen input and direct motor output.*

nonverbally says, "I know what just happened. I am going to go try that again and again and again." Why does he do this? He likes the challenge and the success and is motivated to repeat the activity. All three of these components are limbic and cognitive and would reflect declarative learning. Yet it will lead to procedural learning or semiautomatic motor plans.

The one consistent characteristic of all the founders of the various approaches was their fabulous ability to motivate their clients. Irrespective of the techniques, those people seemed to know when to demand more, when to stop and let clients rest, when to give guidance, and when to withdraw their assistance. This integration of treatment skills is beyond our understanding today, and as our knowledge develops, will necessitate the III STEP conference. Today, we are here to listen to colleagues discuss a process of integration and to let each of you participate in the procedure. I apologize if your specific frame of reference or treatment philosophy is not mentioned this morning. In the afternoon session, each of you will have time to link your experiences with contemporary theories. I hope we will all grow and learn from each other and feel at ease about our differences.

II. The Feldenkrais Method: A Personalized Learning Model

Osa L. Jackson, PhD, PT
Associate Professor
Physical Therapy Program
School of Health Sciences
Oakland University
Rochester, MI 48309-4401

Can you imagine enjoying learning?
Can you agree that your comfort is your responsibility?

The purpose of this chapter is to introduce the Feldenkrais Method as a personalized learning model for individuals in a rehabilitation-physical therapy process. The Feldenkrais Method is for all who work with their bodies, such as performing artists and athletes, and for those who work to enhance the abilities of others, such as teachers, physical therapists, and other health care professionals.

The Feldenkrais Method is a unique way to approach learning. The perspective of interest is not as much what you do as a teacher-therapist but how the learner-patient can use the awareness-information. The questions posed are whether the learning is useful to the patient and whether the individual can replicate the function. The beginning of a learning process is choosing the attitude of positive expectancy, that there is indeed a possibility that the learning will be useful and enjoyable. A critical component is that in everything that is done, the individual feels their participation is important. Another dimension of learning is the perception by the learner that it feels safe and at a pace that is manageable for them. The last major ingredient is the choice of taking personal responsibility (also called internal authority) for the sense of ease or adaptation in the learning process. The overall goal of a lesson (a learning session) is to create an enhancement of the sensorimotor communication so the learner will spontaneously adopt another pattern or strategy because of its obviously increased utility as defined by the learners' use of improved stability, lightness, or control.

HISTORY

Moshe Feldenkrais, DSc, (1904-1984) was a physicist and engineer. He was the first European to receive a black belt in the Japanese martial art of judo, writing five definitive books on its technique and theory. As an athlete, when he became incapacitated by a severe knee injury he chose to apply all his experience gained in working with people like Frederick Joliet-Curie to develop a strategy to gain functional use of his knee again. The work to explore ways of activating the nervous system to improve his overall movement ability began in 1942, and he published his first book in 1949, describing his theories about the relationship between human movement and the nervous system.[1] By 1954, his work was so popular in Israel that he left his post as professor of physics at Weismann Institute and devoted himself to helping others to learn to improve their health. In 1972, Feldenkrais was invited to the United States; today there are over 1000 trained practitioners worldwide. The training involves 32 weeks of daily classes spread over a 3- to 4-year period and presented in a standardized format as specified by the accrediting agency (The Feldenkrais Guild).

Basic Concepts

The essence of learning is to expect refinement or improvement over time. It is therefore expected that the learning model will evolve and become able to describe the human process more clearly as the next generation of teachers-therapists emerges.[2]

1. The learning process involves a conversation between you and me. The term *teacher* will be used to describe the role of the therapist. The term *learner-student* will be used to describe the role of the patient.
2. The learning process is expected to be an enjoyable experience. As the teacher interacts with the learner-student, the experience needs to be perceived as respectful, warm, and friendly.
3. The activity of the teacher is to develop the process (organize the process) so that the learner-student cannot help but have the integrative experience. Another way to state this is that the learner-student literally trips over the process and learns spontaneously, with no willpower effort except the choice of being aware of the process.
4. To facilitate learning, the learner-student needs to have enough time. Time involves giving the person the opportunity to get used to the novelty of every aspect of the interaction, including adapting to the presence of the teacher.
5. Learning is like a dance between two individuals who each have a unique life history. Both the teacher and the learner-student have an entire emotional, cognitive, environmental, and social individuality; these factors all influence the motor functions that the person can perform. Just as when two persons begin to dance, learning is an interaction with an agreement that one person leads and one follows. As the therapist learns to function in one role (as a teacher), it is important to be open and able to shift to functioning in the other role (as a listener/learner). Learning is an ongoing exploratory conversation involving both

of the individuals and their abilities to function comfortably in either role.

6. The teacher needs to begin with the attitude of a listener who desires to learn about the current liabilities and perceptions of the learner-student.

7. "Thinking means finding new ways of doing. In order to receive an insight of learning, your system needs a confrontation with a challenge it has not yet had."[3] Awareness Through Movement (ATM) and Functional Integration (FI) both meet this requirement.

Awareness Through Movement is a strategy for learning that can be done as a person lies down, sits, kneels, or stands. The teacher verbally guides the learner-student to explore how to carry out a sequence of movement activities. The person is requested to make the movements gentle, usually small, and usually slow to allow exploration of options other than the habitual strategies used for moving. Each movement sequence is designed to 1) enhance the ability of the learner-student to find his own most functional pace, 2) increase his sensorimotor awareness, and 3) discover the easiest ways to execute the challenge (the instructions) presented. The increased awareness and relaxation help the learner-student discover the movement patterns that make each effort easier, lighter, or more useful. The ATM can be done alone (using an audiotape), with a teacher, or in a group. The overall goal of the ATM is to help the learner-student move efficiently for the intended function.

Functional Integration is a learning process where the fully clothed individual learns primarily by the guided touch (kinesthetic) and movement provided by the teacher. The learning can be carried out lying down, sitting, kneeling, or standing. The intent and process of the FI is identical to that of an ATM except the teacher provides kinesthetic-visual-verbal information as it is needed to assist the learner-student develop a more efficient way to do the desired function. The FI is done usually in private and adapted to the special learning goals of the individual patient. The FI and ATM combined allow an individual to learn in the two key settings in life: independently with some interaction with another person and in a group. The aim is to help the learner-student organize to move with minimum effort and maximum efficiency, not through muscular strength but through an increased consciousness of how it feels and through an ability to use himself to carry out the desired function.

Special Teacher-Learner Relationship

The initial conversation (verbal or nonverbal) is about how the teacher can "assist" the learner-student in the internal process of changing to enhance function.[4] Function is defined as the ability to carry out the intention of the desired action. Action alone without awareness or intent is not considered functional.

The I-Thou relationship described by Schacht[4] summarizes the communication process of learning. Schacht[4] notes that the focus of responsibility for action is on the learner-student. The entire interaction for learning is to support the learner-student in the initiating mode. A component of this is to talk about "me and you." The discussion is not opened to objectify the leg, the pain, or the disease. All conversation (verbal or nonverbal) is between and about me (the teacher) and you (the learner). Using the current sensorimotor abilities of the learner, the teacher points out and clarifies or cues things that are usable for the learner. The outcome is that the teacher and the learner come to sense that the interaction is creating change.

Pain is viewed as a signal that a less than optional organization is occurring, and it is a natural signal that calls for a refinement or modification of the current process. The Feldenkrais Method does not elicit pain as a part of the teacher/learner interaction. A sensorimotor exploration is carried out to inventory the learner's-student's awareness of preliminary warning signs of overexertion or dysfunction. It is viewed as desirable for the learner-student to be able to notice tiredness, heaviness, or mild incoordination as preliminary warning signs before pain.

To begin the learning process, the following are critical concepts to examine.

1. What corrections or refinements will the learner's-student's nervous system make spontaneously given new or additional sensory or motor information? An example of sensory information is light contact, done slowly and perceived as pleasant by the learner-student, to outline the contours of the scapula, ribs, and clavicle. The intent is to enhance the learner's-student's kinesthetic image of that body segment. An example of motor information is to provide small, gentle (pleasant as perceived by the learner), rapid, passive range of motion to the ankle (in the supine position) to observe how the motion travels up the body to the cervical spine. The motor information of gentle passive motion to the ankle allows an exploration of the learners-student's pattern of neuromuscular organization without great effort on the part of the learner-student. The skill of the teacher is to select the appropriate sensorimotor cues and use them in the best pace and sequence.

2. The only procedures that are instructive and relevant are what the learner-student takes in and can use. The art of teaching is to provide information that is at a pace and in a format perceived as pleasant and that is able to be carried out by the learner. All motions are a possible source of information. It is critical to note that information is mediated through the emotional-cognitive integrative mechanisms of the learner. The teacher who wants to create spontaneous learning therefore needs to begin with what the learner can receive and can feel at ease. As the learner-student feels safe and his confidence builds, the teacher can invite the learner-student to experiment with new movements and ideas.

3. The primary postural activity of the trunk is influenced most easily by spontaneous learning. The ability to refine the ease of motion in the trunk is critical to the ease of total motion of the person. The neuromuscular organization of the head, neck, and trunk is the foundation for all functional refinement in the use of the extremities.

4. The teacher's learning occurs from noting exceptions to preset notions of what "should" happen according to the textbook. The human exceptions mean that the informa-

tion in the textbook is not quite accurate. If the learner-student does it, it is real.

LEARNING PROCESS

The learner's-student's perception and awareness is the primary focus, providing the critical cues to the teacher. The learner-student guides the interaction by noting the expressions of ease or lack of ease. The person has a unique personal history (including body-movement memories), which also is true of the teacher. The key is to use the learner's-student's perception for deciding where to start. The initial position chosen is usually the one that is most familiar or easiest for the person. The rationale is that this provides the least distraction resulting from pain. The goal is to start so the learner-student can focus on the teacher's verbal and nonverbal cues.

How can I do this as a teacher? By answering the next questions. What are the missing pieces in the patient's self-awareness? How do I help the individual to fill in that missing sensorimotor information?

As an example, as I observe an individual it appears that when his heel strikes the ground there is not a natural participation of the movement up the body to create a smooth walking pattern. To help the individual refine the sensorimotor process, the first step is to determine how he constructs his reality. What strategies are easy for this individual to take in and make use of in applying new information? What are all the components of the preferred learning strategies?

The second aspect in beginning to interact is to take into account what perceptions the individual has about his walking pattern. If the learner- student is very sad about the loss of the functional motor pattern, then my interaction will begin and proceed differently than if the patient is very angry about the functional motor loss. Another critical factor to take into account is which perception of his reality he chooses to act on. For example, if an individual is experiencing a lot of secondary gain from a loss of motor function, and if this is the perception of reality he is acting on (his anger still present), then my process of teaching refinement in the motor skill also needs to address this choice on the part of the learner-student. Neurolinguistic Programming is a formalized strategy for examining how to replicate desired behavior. The work of Carl Pribram, Milton Erickson, and Richard Bandler was studied intensely by Feldenkrais and there are recognizable components of their work in the Feldenkrais Method.

The teacher works with the learner-student to increase his awareness of the number of useful options to carry out the desired function. The teacher guides the trials with kinesthetic, visual, and auditory cues that create the awareness of other options beside the habitual, or usual, way for the learner- student to carry out the function. In addition, the teacher provides ongoing cues to help eliminate things that separate the learner-student from his desired experience.

The Feldenkrais Method is a sensorimotor strategy to improve desired function(s). The focus is on the entire phenomena, including the function (eg, walking) and the interacting components with their special relationship to each other at every movement and moment of the function. The interaction of learning is between teacher and learner-student. The sense of improvement or learning is measured by the self-estimation of the learner as far as possible. Note: Formal documentation is still developed for assessment, progress, and reassessment, but it is a separate process from the student-teacher interaction. The learner-student would only be involved in documentation as he or she values the involvement.

Motor behavior-adaptation is a function of complex sensorimotor processes that are primarily unconscious. It is presumed that once a function can be reproduced by the learner, spaced repetition (a home program) will be provided because it can be useful to "anchor" the feel for the new function and the desire to use the new function. The overall goal is to create an enhancement of the sensorimotor communication so the learner will spontaneously adopt another pattern (not continue to use the habitual) because of the obviously increased utility of the process as defined by the improved sense of stability, lightness, or control. The skill of the therapist relates to the choices of modifying the myriad of variables that can create the learning experience. For example, if the valued function of the learner-student is the ability to look up with ease and without pain, all the aspects discussed previously come into play. The teacher then develops an exploratory learning process that will help the learner-student refine the valued function.

For example, Alon[3] uses the sequence below as one of many hundreds of approaches to exploring and refining the function of looking up. The 2-minute experiment is as follows:

In a sitting position, raise your head upward and try to see the ceiling. Make a note how this movement works for you. At what point in your reach do you have a feeling of difficulty? What happens to your breathing?

Now, shift your attention to the feet. Take off one shoe and extend that foot forward, as far as your sole stays flat on the floor. Begin to slowly flex your toes downward, dragging them along the floor closer to your heel. In this position, lift the ball of the foot from the floor and decrease the angle of bending in the ankle. All this time, the heel is still anchored to the floor. This is an unusual combination of movements involving the foot. Allow the foot to return to its comfortable place on the floor and repeat the whole sequence several times.

In the next step, place your foot in full contact with the floor again, but this time bend the toes upward, raising them in the air while the ball of the foot stays on the ground. Alternate several times between the two movements, from bent ankle to outstretched ankle, with the heel planted all the time on the floor. The toes point to the floor when the foot comes up, and they are turned to the ceiling when the ball of the foot rests on the floor. See if you can reduce the amount of effort which you invest in bending the ankle and the toes. Notice that in order to design a strange arrangement which perhaps is totally new to you, you have to use a device other than direct physical power. Identify within yourself this quality of listening and clarification—it is this quality which makes the difference between exercise and learning.

Now bring the foot back to its usual place, and again lift your head so as to look at the ceiling. Has your scan of the ceiling now been made a bit easier than it was earlier?[3]

The outcome of the above experiment for yourself will guide you to refinement in your understanding of the interrelationship of motor function. The motor learning is not about a leg, a pain, or a stroke. Using the personalized learning model, the motor learning process becomes an interaction between me and you. As compared with the motor learning model and the traditional learning model (as noted in this volume), the personalized learning model provides the following conceptual differences:

1. Functional outcomes result in the urge to use the valued functions spontaneously (as identified or agreed on by the learner-student, whichever is possible).
2. Open-loop tasks emphasize providing new sensory awareness that the learner will choose to use.
3. Tasks are oriented first to encourage spontaneous learning of function and then to use the function in carrying out another familiar function, which assures ease of use.
4. Function is carried out in various positions in environment to assure ease of use and ability to adapt (explore strategies), and the environment is organized for comfort and ease and sense of safety for the learner.
5. Exploration is repeated, with the goal of finding the easiest, softest, and most efficient way to execute function.
6. Awareness of the response and adaptation to the response enhance utility of the next trial effort.[5] The feedback model is not used because the mechanical model of thinking is not desired. The cybernetic model of learning is more applicable to human learning because it is presumed that this model will also be refined over the years to improve the accuracy of describing the human learning process. Note: There is not a definition of correct performance except as it is defined by the learners' sense that a

particular strategy for executing the functional movement feels easier, lighter, or more efficient to use.

This paper on the Feldenkrais Method is but a general summary. I hope that this initial discussion will provide a springboard for research and lead to many future refinements in the personalized learning model. Like a child of 4-years of age who is given a large rubber band for the first time, you are encouraged to experiment with the many sequences that are available and to study the literature. It is usually easier to learn to shoot the rubber band for the first time if you have a teacher, although it is possible to experiment and learn the function if you are on your own.

The Feldenkrais Guild can provide you with the names of trained ATM Feldenkrais teachers (persons with a minimum of 2 years of instructions), trained Feldenkrais Practitioners (persons with a minimum of 4 years of instruction), and the names of certified Assistant Trainers (a minimum of 7 years' activity in the work) and Trainers (a minimum of 11 years in the work) who are available to assist you with your exploration of motor learning.

Acknowledgment

A special thank you goes to Mark Reese, Feldenkrais Trainer, for his editorial assistance with the manuscript.

References

1. Feldenkrais M. *Body and Mature Behavior*. New York, NY: International Universities Press Inc; 1949:2.
2. Zemach-Bersin D, Zemach-Bersin K, Reese M. *Relaxercise: The Easy New Way to Health and Fitness*. New York, NY: Harper & Row, Publishers Inc; 1990:3.
3. Alon R. *Mindful Spontaneity: Moving In Tune With Nature: Lessons in the Feldendrais Method*. New York, NY: Prism Press-Avery Publishers; 1990:5.
4. Schacht WD. The special patient-therapist relationship created by "hands on" practitioners," *Physical Therapy Forum*. July 2, 1990;6.
5. Feldenkrais M. *The Potent Self: A Guide to Spontaneity*. New York, NY: Harper & Row, Publishers Inc; 1985.

III. Neurodevelopmental Treatment and Sensory Integrative Theory

Patricia C. Montgomery, PhD, PT
Therapeutic Intervention Programs, Inc.
2217 Glenhurst Road
St. Louis Park, MN 55416

My task today is to provide an example of how a clinician who uses assessment and treatment principles from both a neurodevelopment treatment (NDT) and sensory integrative (SI) perspective has altered my overall theoretical framework to incorporate contemporary models of motor control and motor learning.

THEORETICAL FRAMEWORK

First, I will review my interpretation of the major tenets of NDT and SI. These may be different than yours, and if Berta Bobath or Jean Ayres were presenting this material their descriptions and emphasis would certainly be different. Theoretical frameworks are a little like the party game of whispering messages from one individual to another: components get altered and reinterpreted based on a number of factors along the way.

I will ask you first to read the following quotes and be able to tell me if you think they were written by Bobath or Ayres.

The CNS acts as a coordinating organ for the multitude of incoming sensory stimuli, producing integrated motor responses adequate to the requirements of the environment.[1(p1)]

Postural responses have their major integrating mechanisms in that part of the brain that lies below the cortex . . . , the very automaticity of postural reactions leads to their being taken for granted, even in the remedial situation.[2(p77)]

In workshops where I have listed several similar quotes, most therapists attributed "sensory-related" statements to Ayres and "motor-reflex-tone-related" statements to Bobath. In fact, the first quote is from Bobath and the second quote is from Ayres. Both theorists emphasized sensory and motor elements of behavior, and I have found no difficulty in my clinical pediatric practice combining these theories into an assessment and treatment model.

I illustrate the major principles of NDT and SI as outlined below:

NDT identifies the problem as release of abnormal and widespread reflex patterns of posture and movement from inhibition, specifically brain stem, cerebellum, midbrain, basal ganglia, and cortex.

SI identifies the problem as inadequate integration or interpretation of sensory feedback and the inability to use sensory input well as feedback or to use sensory systems to anticipate and plan ahead for motor acts.

NDT bases approach on normal development, compensations of movement, and habitual motor patterns that may lead to muscle imbalance-contractures.

SI bases approach on normal development, neurophysiology of sensory systems, and assessment through standardized battery of tests and clinical observations.

NDT emphasizes the following concepts: automatic postural adjustments, sensory structures for eliciting postural responses; muscle tone; "fixes" to compensate for low muscle tone; development of mobility, awareness of movement potential, active muscle development, and graded muscle control.

SI emphasizes the following concepts: subcortical or brain stem mechanisms, importance of postural mechanisms, multisensory neuronal integration, the "adaptive" response, and sensory processing leading to "end products" of function.

General goal of theory in NDT: to establish a treatment program that uses repeated active movements (isolated or in patterns), resisted by gravity, body weight, or manual pressure, to achieve a balance between muscle groups and to decrease the effects of abnormal tonal influence on automatic responses and movement patterns.

General goal of therapy in SI: to provide and control sensory input, especially vestibular and somatosensory, in such a way that the individual spontaneously forms the adaptive responses that integrate those sensations.

In this 20 minute presentation, I have chosen to emphasize an assessment model and have based the overall framework on information from motor control theorists, especially Brooks.[3] Information from motor control research[4] is especially applicable to treatment principles. However, I will not have time to cover that material today.

I illustrate the major components of my assessment model as outlined below:

ASSESSMENT: INTEGRATED MODEL

I. Cognitive-motivational elements
   A. Arousal level
   B. Selective attention to environment-task(s)
   C. Desire to move
   D. Understands task(s)
   E. Rules formed
   F. Praxis (motor planning)
II. Motor programming elements
   A. Initiation of movement

B. Varies speed of movement
C. Synergies-movement patterns
   1. Number (limited-variety)
   2. Functional versus nonfunctional (normal versus abnormal)
   3. Spontaneous versus evoked
   4. Postural synergies (stability)
   5. Volitional synergies (mobility)
D. Cessation of movement
III. Sensory feedforward and feedback
   A. Sensory systems
      1. Visual
      2. Auditory
      3. Somatosensory (proprioceptive-tactile)
      4. Vestibular
      5. Olfactory
      6. Gustatory
   B. Feedforward (active-volitional movement)
   C. Feedback (active or passive or both through handling and environment)
IV. Biomechanical constraints
   A. Muscle elongation
   B. Joint range of motion
   C. Alignment during task(s)
V. Developmental milestones-skills
   A. Reflex patterns-postural responses
   B. Gross motor skills
   C. Fine motor skills
   D. Behavioral (social-emotional)
   E. Cognitive-language development
   F. Self-care (feeding-dressing-toileting)
VI. Goals
   A. Patient
   B. Family
   C. Therapist
   D. Other (ie, physician-educator-occupational therapist)

You will note that I have incorporated many NDT and SI principles in the assessment model with varying degrees of emphasis. The NDT theory has especially been helpful in my observation of movement in determining the "motor programming" elements and in describing postural responses.[1,5] The SI theory has particularly been useful in assessing cognitive-motivational elements, sensory systems, and praxis.[2,6]

When assessment is completed, the task is to determine goals for intervention. One method is deciding what behavior is being "interfered with" and then planning treatment around this concept.[7] For example, if the child in a supine position turns his head, assumes an asymmetrical posture, and cannot bring his hands to his mouth or hands together at midline, the asymmetry can be considered to interfere with certain motor behaviors. It is not as critical that we "know" that this is an asymmetrical tonic neck reflex, or a lack of symmetry, or a sensory disregard of one side of the body, but that we all observe and describe the motor behavior. We may then have a therapeutic goal of decreasing asymmetry, and we can measure it with behavioral objectives if the child has changed or met a specified goal after a period of intervention. For example, after 2 months of therapy, the child will volitionally be able to bring either hand to his mouth and will be able to bring his hands together at midline for hand-to-hand contact and manipulation of objects.

Although it is helpful if our theoretical frameworks contain similar elements based on current research and knowledge in motor control, motor learning, and motor development, it is essential that we carefully observe behaviors, accurately describe these behaviors, and always use functional measurable objectives to determine change.

References

1. Bobath B. *Abnormal Postural Reflex Activity Caused by Brain Lesions*. 3rd ed. Rockville, Md: Aspen Publishers Inc; 1985.
2. Ayres AJ. *Sensory Integration and the Child*. Los Angeles, Calif: Western Psychological Services; 1979.
3. Brooks VB. *The Neural Basis of Motor Control*. New York, NY: Oxford University Press Inc.; 1986.
4. Schmidt RA. *Motor Control and Learning*. Champaign, Ill: Human Kinetics Publishers Inc; 1982.
5. Bly L. *The Components of Normal Movement During the First Year of Life and Abnormal Motor Development*. Chicago, Ill: Neurodevelopmental Treatment Association; 1983.
6. Ayres AJ. *Developmental Dyspraxia and Adult Onset Apraxia*. Torrance, Calif: Sensory Integration International; 1985.
7. Connolly B, Montgomery P, eds. *Therapeutic Exercise in Developmental Disabilities*. Chattanooga, Tenn: Chattanooga Publishing Co; 1987.

IV. Proprioceptive Neuromuscular Facilitation and the Approach of Rood

Mary Alice Duesterhaus Minor, MS, PT
Assistant Professor
Physical Therapy Program
Maryville College-St. Louis
St. Louis, MO 63141

This paper has been prepared as a commentary on points raised previously during this conference and how these points relate to the approaches of Rood and of proprioceptive neuromuscular facilitation (PNF) in managing a patient with disability. To understand the specific issues and points referenced, the reader is referred to the proceedings papers from this conference. Reference to all speakers and significant points is not possible. I have selected those points I believe are most appropriate to be addressed in this forum

Friday morning, Kay Shepard (see Shepard, this volume) told us that theory encompasses contemplation and observation. According to Shepard, a theory is an abstract idea, or collection of ideas, used to explain physical or social phenomena. Margaret Rood, the originator of the Rood approach, and the originators of the PNF approach contemplated the then-current literature and observed patients in clinical settings. Based on this contemplation and observation, they began to formulate a theory, or a philosophy, or an approach to the management of individuals with physical disabilities. A common premise of both approaches, indeed of physical therapy in general, is that patients possess the potential for improvement.

Dr. Herman Kabat,[1] a neurophysiologist before he was a physician, tried to apply in the clinic what Sherrington had demonstrated in the laboratory. Reading Kabat's articles, particularly those in the *Permanente Foundation Medical Bulletin*,[2,3] the reader can gain a sense of the excitement and learning that occurred during this period of experimentation. Working with Kabat were physical therapists such as Margaret Knott.

Rood was a contemplative person. I have an image of her sitting on a rock in a desert with at least two trains of thought running through her mind. One train of thought is the literature she read extensively. The second train of thought is of patients she had observed. Occasionally, these two trains of thought were coupled as one, providing her with an insight to a phenomenon of patient motor performance or a method to enhance patient performance. Rood would take a fragment from the literature, embroider it in a way that made sense to her, and use the resulting tapestry to explain a model of patient deficits, a rationale for treatment interventions, and an explanation of patient responses to her interventions.

Rood and the originators of PNF believed that their therapeutic interventions worked, but their justifications or rationales would need to be re-examined in light of new information. I believe these theories were meant to be evolving and changing, rather than static, theories of patient management.

Rood's therapeutic interventions demonstrated that a response was possible. And PNF was to be used to build in and upon the desired response. As part of patient evaluation, we want to know about the integrity of the neuromuscular system. As part of patient treatment, we want to modify or shape motor response. Rood is associated with the phrase "sensory input gives motor output that gives more sensory input." Initially, Rood[4] used exteroceptive inputs, and later she relied more on proprioceptive inputs. Rood used sensory input for two basic reasons:

1. To test the system: Was the patient's neuromuscular system intact enough to produce any motor response?
2. To modify or shape motor response: a therapeutic intervention.

The sensory inputs of Rood and PNF are similar, although PNF emphasizes their use for therapeutic intervention. In their teachings, Dorothy Voss and Rood commented that they considered Rood's therapeutic interventions to be preliminary to those used in PNF. The catchword used was "Rood is crude PNF."

The hierarchical model of the nervous system together with the structure-before-function theory were used as rationale for both approaches. Certainly, the hierarchical model has been questioned at this conference this past weekend (see Horak and Guiliani, this volume). The theory that newer, higher centers of the nervous system have the most control of function is not consistent with the currently developing theory of how the nervous system functions. New research findings seem to imply that central nervous system function is explained better by the new theory than the old. The hierarchical system, as usually described to explain Rood and PNF, may be too simplistic. A theory based on the hierarchical system does not seem to stand up well under the light of new research findings.

The complete relationship of neural structure to function is not clear. Functions of most structures are known, but I do not believe anyone has deciphered what are all the interconnections between structures, which structures can act as control centers, or when a center is a control center. I believe, for example, that until a certain amount of myelinization (structure) has been achieved, certain motor responses

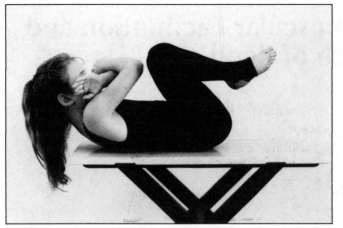

Fig. 14-6. *Skeletal functions sequence: flexor withdrawal supine.*

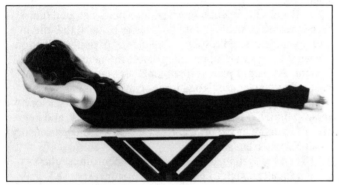

Fig. 14-7. *Skeletal functions sequence: pivot prone.*

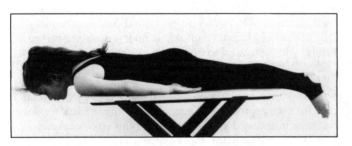

Fig. 14-8. *Skeletal functions sequence: neck cocontraction.*

are not possible. It is not always obvious from observation of function that a person has a structural deficit. Despite such a deficit, function may be within normal limits. At other times, functional deficits resulting from structural deficits are obvious. Research literature and clinical experience both seem to indicate that the degree of functional deficit observed in acquired loss of structure (such as from a CVA) varies with the extent of structural loss, age, and type of onset.

The function of a missing structure cannot just be replaced. Often, we do not know enough about the interactive functions of the missing structure. An example is parkinsonism. If we think of molecules as structures, we know that

"drugs" can be used to replace missing molecules. Yet an individual's motor behavior is not usually totally "normal," even with the replacement. Each event of sensory input is much more transient than a drug whose effects may last several hours or days. Such transient events cannot replace a missing structure. Sensory input is used for several reasons, such as giving patients a new point of reference or a different method for controlling performance. It has never been a tenet of the approaches of either Rood or PNF that sensory input is to be used as a permanent replacement for a lost structure.

The idea of task, or goal, oriented movement versus "exercise" has also been discussed. Carry over of movement to functional ability from exercise has been questioned. Rood emphasized two functional sequences: the vital functions sequence and the skeletal functions sequence. The vital functions sequence includes the following: 1) inspiration; 2) expiration: crying, sneezing, coughing; 3) sucking and swallowing fluids; 4) phonation; 5) chewing and swallowing solids; and 6) speech articulation.

The skeletal functions sequence includes the following: 1) flexor withdrawal supine, 2) roll over, 3) pivot prone, 4) neck cocontraction, 5) prone on elbows, 6) quadruped, 7) standing, and 8) walking. (Figures 14-6, 14-7, and 14-8 illustrate flexor withdrawal supine, pivot prone, and neck cocontraction.) Most of these tasks are functional goal-oriented tasks.

Two types of movement patterns are associated with PNF: one type is represented by the spiral diagonal patterns of the extremities and trunk and the other type by the total patterns of a developmental sequence of motor skills. The diagonal patterns were determined by kinesiological study to be optimal combining components of motion for each joint of a segment and for the segment as a whole. Muscles thought to be prime movers were identified. Patterns of movement were emphasized because they more closely resembled normal movements than did the isolated joint movements of the earlier "traditional" approaches.

Total patterns used in PNF are the major motor milestones of the normal developmental sequence of motor skills (see VanSant and Heriza, this volume). The theory of sequential mastery of tasks in the developmental sequence has been a guiding principle of PNF. At the same time, however, proponents of PNF recognize that not all individuals follow the same sequence of developmental activities. An individual task has its own developmental sequence. The critical factors necessary for achieving functional skills gained by following the developmental sequence are still not understood. Perhaps now emphasis must be shifted to examining activities of the developmental sequence for critical biomechanical and other factors. Activities of the developmental sequence progress from stable postures requiring little motor function to unstable postures requiring the use of multiple systems, not just the motor system, to be functional.

The PNF approach emphasizes total patterns as having both clinical and functional significance. For example, if I determine a patient is unable to switch smoothly between contractions of trunk flexors and trunk extensors, I might choose to have the patient perform the activity of rolling.

While the desired (clinically significant) muscle activity is being performed, the patient is learning the functional task of turning in bed. Not all tasks used are functional in all situations. For example, creeping may be a functional means of locomotion at home even for an adult, but it is not an acceptable means of locomotion in the community.

The goal of PNF treatment is to "engram" movement patterns as close to normal as possible into the central nervous system. This is achieved by providing enough initial assistance to the patient to allow the patient to produce desired responses. The assistance (proprioceptive, exteroceptive, teloreceptive cues) is then withdrawn until the patient is independent in the task. Independence means the patient has learned the task and retained the task for future use.

Long-term goals (LTGs) are stated to the greatest extent possible in terms of measurable, observable, and functional behaviors. The LTGs should answer the question, "What will the patient look like when he completes physical therapy?" Both the approach of Rood and of PNF assume that the goal of treatment is the improvement of a patient's functional abilities. Short-term goals (STGs) are also measurable, observable patient behaviors. The STGs are aimed at correcting deficits that prevent a patient from achieving a LTG. The LTGs and STGs are organized sequentially. The time to reach goals varies with each patient.

In both approaches (Rood and PNF), there are times when a patient is a passive recipient of input. Even under these conditions, a patient-produced response is expected. Particularly when using PNF, a patient's cognitive processes are engaged in performing an exercise. A patient's attention is focused on the task at hand. Different strategies are used with children and with patients who have attention deficits or are in a coma, but the goal is always to develop or maintain active patient participation.

Rood made us very aware of the importance of the patient's emotional state. She described patients as being on an emotional continuum. Therapists are responsible for continually reassessing where on the continuum the patient is and for selecting treatment interventions based on the patient's present ability to participate. Motor learning requires the learner to be a doer and a processor. The patient can only do and process if intervention is specifically tailored to the current status of the patient. Therapists must assess (see Keshner, this volume) the total patient: the affective state, the cognitive state, and the neuromusculoskeletal system. Based on results of these evaluations, therapists can then construct the treatment environment to enhance motor learning and retention of desired skills.

To many patients, particularly those with acquired disability, their world is in chaos. This chaos includes many areas of function: psychological, social, and neuromusculoskeletal performance. As therapists, we try to control the level of chaos confronting the patient. It is understandable and impossible to take away entirely all degrees of chaos. We try to control the chaos so patients can demonstrate increased functional ability. As patients begin to deal with chaos by producing some stability or order, the therapist should decrease control so the context of environment represents a more realistic environment. This should be continued until each patient is satisfied that he is the best that he can be at this time.

Rood and Signe Brunnstrom were especially sensitive to a patient's ability to cope in a way that preserved his dignity. I have observed two negative responses to overwhelming chaos. One response is to shut down, or withdraw. The other response is to become agitated. Neither state promotes learning and retention or allows the patient to maintain his dignity. A therapist controls the environment, allowing the patient to be a successful problem solver, thereby maintaining or enhancing his motor control and dignity. A therapist can exert control in many ways, such as by giving guidance in the form of sensory inputs, verbal cues, or demonstrations; limiting environmental complexities; or selecting appropriate tasks.

The PNF approach emphasizes that motor learning must take place for the patient to improve and that treatments can be designed to promote motor learning. New research offers more precise information about methods to promote motor learning (see Schmidt and Winstein, this volume). The type and timing of feedback to be given and the practice schedules have been described. Many PNF treatment interventions incorporate these methods to promote motor learning. Typically, patients practice using block style practice; feedback is provided as a summary at the end of one or more blocks of practice. Because PNF treatments emphasize practicing whole tasks, transitions between segments of a task are included. When a patient reaches a segment of a task he cannot perform adequately, that segment is practiced within the whole task, maintaining task context. Practice promotes retention of a skill. Practice also produces fatigue, changing the task context. Using the PNF approach, the patient works to promote improved motor performance in several appropriate tasks while alternating among these tasks during one treatment session, minimizing the negative aspects of practice that change task context.

Acknowledgments

I extend thanks to Dr. Scott D. Minor for editorial and photographic assistance and to Sarah R. Minor for photographic assistance.

References

1. Voss DE, Ionta MK, Myers BJ. *Proprioceptive Neuromuscular Facilitation Patterns and Techniques*. 3rd ed. Philadelphia, Pa: Harper & Row, Publishers, Inc; 1985.
2. Kabat H. Studies on neuromuscular dysfunction: XI. New principles of neuromuscular reeducation. *Permanente Foundation Medical Bulletin*. November 1947;5.
3. Kabat H. Studies on neuromuscular dysfunction: XII. Rhythmic stabilization, a new and more effective technique for treatment of paralysis through a cerebellar mechanism. *Permanente Foundation Medical Bulletin*. January 1950;8.
4. Stockmeyer SA. An interpretation of the approach of Rood to the treatment of neuromuscular dysfunction. *Am J Phys Med*. 1967;46:900-961.

V. Concluding Remarks on Merging Concepts

Darcy Umphred, PhD, PT
Associate Professor
Graduate Program in Physical Therapy
University of the Pacific
Stockton, CA 95211

Today began with an objective: to merge concepts of current theories of practice in neurological treatment with contemporary theories of motor control, motor learning, and motor development. How this merger will affect practice with respect to patient evaluation and treatment and how it will affect teaching is yet to be discovered. The future began with a birth and a growth process. It seemed fitting to wrap up this session with an overview of the evolution of our profession. We might go back to the early decades of this century (Fig. 14-9). At that time many individuals searched beyond their learning to create new and progressive approaches to patient care. Individuals such as Delorme with progressive resistive exercise (PREs), Hettinger and Müller with brief maximal exercise (BME) and later with brief resisted isometric maximal exercise (BRIME), Zinovieff with the Oxford approach, Phillips with bracing, and many others laid the foundation for traditional therapeutic exercise. These ideas were the corner stones for early treatment procedures incorporating manual resistance, sling suspension and wall pulleys, and use of machines such as the Delorme table and boot or the N-K table. The use of modalities began at the same time, and although not discussed today, the topic needs to be included. As the clinical knowledge bank grew, a fork in our path was made that separated the focus of client care into orthopedic and neurologic areas. On the orthopedic path between the years of 1940 and 1960, two very powerful camps developed: osteopathic theory and therapeutic exercise. As physi-

cal therapists, we encapsulated our focus of cardiopulmonary and peripheral-spinal orthopedics under therapeutic exercise and did not identify ourselves with osteopathic procedures. As the orthopedic area evolved during the last 30 years, many more approaches developed that integrated therapeutic exercise and manipulation with the unique strategies identified by the founders of the various treatment methodologies (Fig. 14-10). The area of orthopedics encompasses acute to long-term care and includes individuals at both ends of the normative scale with regard to function. The future focus, problems, and questions presented to an orthopedic therapist are very similar to those presented to any other specialist within the field of physical therapy. Therefore, going back and looking at how the neurologic path developed seems appropriate (Fig. 14-11).

The same early approaches were the founding influence for all those people developing their methodologies between 1940 and 1960. Obviously, traditional therapeutic exercise was still the primary focus of education. Yet colleagues such as Rood, Brunnstrom, Knott, Voss, Fiorentino, Ayers, Feldenkrais, Bobath, Fay, and others were making their powerful individual impact on the growth of our profession. As the next generation of colleagues observed, learned, and began to help teach the various approaches, another fork in the developmental path could be seen in the late 1960s (Fig. 14-12). The majority of the profession veered toward specific treatment based on an identi-

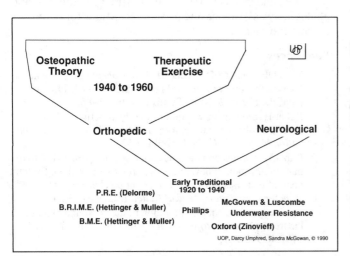

Fig. 14-9. *Overview of early therapeutic approaches.*

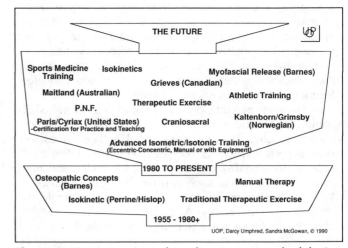

Fig. 14-10. *Representative orthopedic treatment methodologies over the past 30 years.*

fied approach. In school, most students were introduced to one or more of these approaches depending on the experience and knowledge of the faculty members. A small group of colleagues veered away from this specific-approach philosophy toward an integrated-approach model. These models tried to incorporate all approaches into an integrated whole. Evaluation and treatment was not based on a specific philosophy but rather on a problem-solving approach. Each model included behavioral development and movement analysis, the basic science of brain function, and the unknown variable of the learning environment. The specific words and focus varied within each model, as they did in the specific-treatment-based approaches, yet each individual who tried to teach using this integrated philosophy believed each colleague would, in reality, develop his own unique approach. The best way to develop this unique approach would be to have all options available.

Before we look at the future of the neurological approaches we need to look at one additional area of education that lays the foundation for the development of motor control, motor learning, and motor development (Fig. 14-13). Basic science began initially with four major areas: anatomy, physiology, psychology, and pathology of man. The basic sciences still remain as intact, intricate parts of our educational schema today. Out of these basic areas have evolved the applied sciences. The specific numbers of unique subdivisions within any category are large. When many of our colleagues returned for advanced study following their basic physical therapy education, they began to integrate basic and applied science with their therapeutic background. That evolution naturally lead to the study of motor development, motor learning, and motor control.

This II STEP conference was initially conceptualized by a few colleagues who saw a critical need to tie together the current state of the art of physical therapy. All areas of our profession could not be included in this short time frame, thus the focus was placed on neurology and pediatrics. If time had permitted, we would have included such current practice areas as orthopedics and cardiopulmonary

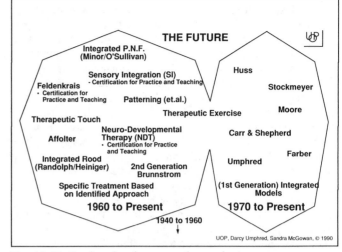

Fig. 14-12. *Further development of neurologic treatment methodologies by identified approaches.*

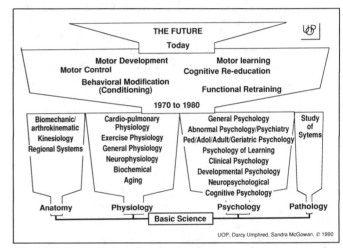

Fig. 14-13. *Foundations for the development of motor control, motor learning, and motor development.*

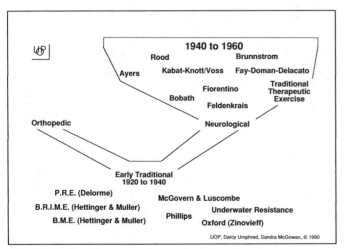

Fig. 14-11. *Development of neurologic treatment methodologies over time.*

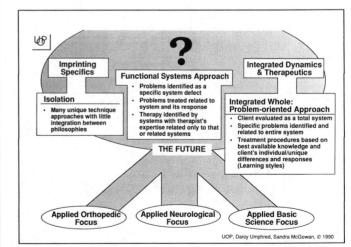

Fig. 14-14. *Examples of possible therapeutic approaches of the future.*

and such specialty areas as electrodiagnosis, biofeedback, electromography, research, and administration. Presenting today's ideas and practices leads to the future. Where that future will lead might be anywhere (Fig. 14-14). It might lead to an approach such as Imprinting Specifics where many unique techniques within any specific specialty area, such as neurology, need not be integrated. Each approach identifies its boundaries. A Functional Systems approach may be another path of choice. With this focus, problem areas would be identified as a specific system defect and therapy would be identified by systems with therapist's expertise relating only to that or related systems. That is, the orthopedic therapist need not concern themselves with the central nervous system or vice versa. We may select an approach called Integrated Dynamics and Therapeutics. In this model, a problem-oriented approach becomes the primary emphasis with a client always being viewed as a total system. The specific problems identified would always relate back to all systems within the human body. Treatment procedures would be based on the best available knowledge and the client's individual-unique differences and responses. Our future may to some extent incorporate all three categories and some not mentioned. Our development began with a breath or an idea. That development has evolved through many stages and has crossed many bridges. Some of the paths followed have re-quired risks and were thought to be dangerous. Yet once we reached the other side we saw the learning. I hope the many paths walked and bridges crossed will lead to a greater understanding of the whole.

In the last 20 years we have gained tremendous breadth in all areas of knowledge as it relates to the brain and all systems controlled by the brain. That knowledge has stimulated development of new philosophies, integration of old ones, and change. Change will lead to future knowledge and cognitive growth. We have come together to share that knowledge and growth. Yet the critical question still remains, Have we also grown in wisdom?

We need the wisdom to remove ourselves from our egos, to divorce ourselves from preconceived "truths," and to acknowledge ideas and philosophies of others even if they differ dramatically or are in conflict with our own. Have we grown to accept differences as potential avenues for future growth versus battles to be won?

Our future is ours. The knowledge will come. The wisdom will not develop unless we choose to open our minds and hearts to those universal threads that will lead us to that understanding.

This day was a day of integration. It will be exciting to be part of the future. It is yours and mine.

Chapter 15

Framework for the Measurement of Neurologic Impairment and Disability

Suzann K. Campbell, PhD, PT, FAPTA
Professor of Physical Therapy
University of Illinois at Chicago
Chicago, IL 60612

Increased attention to the art and science of measurement is necessary for improving physical therapy (PT) for clients and accountability to the public. The art entails deciding what to measure and when in the course of a condition that is changing on the basis of both natural history and therapeutic intervention. The science entails knowing how to assess important areas of function and dysfunction with reliability, validity, and efficiency for the client and therapist. Both the art and the science aspects of measurement are problematic because the constructs we need to assess regarding the movement dysfunction of patients with central nervous system (CNS) disorders have not adequately been defined.

My assumptions regarding measurement in PT are the following:

1. Measurement in PT is not conducted in a systematic, theoretically based manner. In other words, a conceptual framework is needed for measuring the impairments and disabilities associated with CNS dysfunction affecting movement.

2. One reason for the lack of a conceptual framework for measurement is that the constructs of importance, especially so-called quality of movement, have not been defined operationally.

3. Clinical measurement and decision making are hindered by lack of diagnosis-specific data on abnormal motor control processes, motor learning with an abnormal CNS, and characteristics of the therapeutic process. Improvements in assessment and treatment efficacy depend on increased understanding of these processes and mechanisms.

In this chapter, I will 1) provide an overview of the problems of measurement in PT, 2) discuss the lack of a conceptual basis for assessing movement dysfunction, 3) offer a broad conceptual framework both for describing disability and for measuring dysfunction, and 4) provide examples for applying such a conceptual framework.

MEASUREMENT PROBLEM IN PHYSICAL THERAPY

A significant body of research literature describes the lack of reliability of clinicians' judgments.[1] In fact, most published studies on the topic of clinical decision making in medicine report that using an equation to make diagnostic decisions is more accurate than even the most experienced physicians' judgments.[2] Yet the rules for developing a mathematical equation for predicting a diagnosis always come from clinicians. This means, of course, that clinicians do not reliably follow their own rules. Failure to do so does not reflect arbitrary decision making; rather, each patient presents the health professional with a complex problem, and none seems more complex than the patient with neurologic impairment. Identifying the often multiple problems of each patient is a challenging cognitive task in which the clinician must manipulate hypotheses, observations, and facts. The task can easily exceed the capacity of the ordinary human mind, with negative effects on the reliability of decisions.

Besides the fact that complex mental operations are involved, judgments made by clinicians vary for a variety of reasons: 1) biologic variations in sensory acuity from assessment to assessment, 2) nonsystematic application of diagnostic criteria to clinical evidence, 3) errors of omission or commission in gathering evidence, 4) tendency to record inference rather than evidence, and 5) bias in judgment caused by what the clinician expects to find.[1-3] When observing patients, clinicians immediately begin to generate hypotheses regarding what is wrong and then proceed by looking for data ruling *in* favored hypotheses rather than ruling *out* alternatives.[4]

Introduction of a systematic protocol involving standardized assessments guards against each source of unreliability in judgment except the first. For example, the directions for administering and scoring standardized tests provide specific criteria for judging the quality of observed behaviors. Testing each client according to a set protocol guards against errors of omission. Scoring rules for objective quantification of tested behaviors leads to the recording of factual observations rather than inferences. Finally, use of a standard protocol guards against the application of biased expectations in interpreting the meaning of observations and should lead to high interrater reliability.

Corroboration of key clinical findings by repetition of tests, blind assessment of clients by colleagues, and use of decision analysis algorithms to standardize and simplify the cognitive process of interpreting complex sets of data are other means for improving the reliability of clinical judgments.[1,2,5] Decision analysis algorithms are based on published data on clinical outcomes of large populations of patients so that probabilities of various outcomes can be calculated for a patient with a specific combination of characteristics. For example, it would be possible to develop a decision algorithm for predicting outcome of PT for a patient after a cerebrovascular accident (CVA), based on the type of lesion, rate of recovery in the first two months, and other pertinent factors.

If recommendations such as these improve the accuracy of patient assessment, why do few physical therapists use standardized protocols for assessing clients with CNS dysfunction, or alternatively, why are they dissatisfied with the protocols they do use? The reasons that a measurement problem continues to exist despite recently increased attention to it are multiple. They include 1) education, 2) lack of tests and perceived nonapplicability of the tests in existence, 3) the time involved in completing a thorough assessment of the multiple problems of neurologically impaired patients, 5) an antiquantitative bias on the part of practitioners, 6) lack of a data base on the natural history and underlying pathologic processes involved in the control of movement by an abnormal CNS, 7) lack of a conceptual framework for structuring measurement, and 8) failure to define the constructs of interest. Each of these cannot be described here in depth, but the more theoretically interesting aspects related to construction of a theoretical framework for measuring movement dysfunction will be discussed.

Physical therapists do not receive much instruction in measurement nor much training in use of formal tests during their educational experiences. Educational program faculty usually do not teach tests used only by specialists, and clinical instructors are unlikely to provide formal training in measurement if clinicians make little use of tests. Therapists, then, tend to rely on anecdotal records to capture problems and change in their clients.[3] These tend to be nonsystematic in regularity of recording and content; they focus on deficits being treated rather than on the competencies and functional performance of the client. Consequently, only clinics that have a data base approach to record keeping, along with a quality assurance program to insure timely recording of the same types of data on all patients of a specific type, are likely to have records that are useful for any program evaluation purpose.

The reasons therapists typically give for not using formal testing usually include the time involved and the lack of useful data resulting from the tests available. Clinicians want tests that 1) assess quality of movement, including postural alignment and control, balance, and coordination, 2) capture improvement in clients who change slowly, and 3) measure functional skills.[6] If such tests were available, benefits relative to cost might allay concerns regarding the time involved.

Despite the fact that therapists have articulated what they want in a measurement tool, a fundamental problem is failure of the profession to define adequately the constructs of importance within some logical conceptual framework for viewing neurologically based movement dysfunction. Currently available measures have been incongruent with therapeutic exercise models (which are totally lacking in objective assessment strategies), but new tests are only slowly becoming available because we have not clearly defined the essentials to assess; they have not been articulated in a measurable way. The classical conceptual framework for mea-

surement suggests that therapists should assess, with separate tests, performance components like strength, endurance, and flexibility, but results from available tests have not lead to helpful solutions to the movement problems of clients even though deficits in these dimensions may be important. The result is that the validity of these tests in assessment of neurologically impaired patients has been questioned rather than the concepts redefined for application to those clients.

The concepts that have previously seemed important in patients with neurologic dysfunction included abnormal movement synergies, righting and equilibrium reactions, postural tone, and movement transitions from one position to another. Surely it is understandable if clinicians fail to make the connection between the tests they have learned and their daily concerns regarding patient treatment and outcome.

Although a new model for neurologic rehabilitation put forward by Carr and colleagues[7] is based on contemporary concepts of motor programs and on research and theory in motor learning, this approach also lacks an integrated measurement model for comprehensive assessment. Additional new models for patient treatment based on dynamical systems theory or distributed control system concepts undoubtedly will arise as a result of the II STEP conference. II STEP papers may culminate in a metabasis for patients with neurologic dysfunction and a renewed challenge in the art and science of measurement for PT. As new models are articulated, assessment strategies that fit the model and provide a means for measuring their efficacy are essential. Although these assessment strategies may incorporate already existing tests, such as the Barthel Index,[8] it is likely that some of the traditional measures for assessing strength and endurance will warrant a fresh look. They may need to be reincorporated into thinking about neurologic impairment or revised to meet the needs of the new conceptual models. Certainly, assessments of functional tasks within defined environmental contexts must be incorporated.

DEFINING IMPAIRMENT AND RECOVERY

Three basic and interrelated problems hinder the development of a conceptual framework for measurement of movement dysfunction in clients with neurologic disorders. These are 1) lack of a natural history data base to define the positive symptoms of CNS dysfunction that typically develop and that must be prevented to limit disability while we strive to improve the performance deficits of clients in the realms of strength, endurance, and coordination; 2) failure to define the constructs of interest in developing new tests; and 3) lack of understanding of motor control processes in each type of CNS disorder that are basic to establishing diagnostic categories and improving treatment. In short, our science lags behind our therapeutic art, and both lack a unifying theory.

Natural History

Lack of a data base on the natural history of neurologic disorders is a major problem. Here is one question that will illustrate my point. How, when, and under what conditions does equinus contracture develop in children with cerebral palsy (CP)? They are not born with contractures, although presumably they are born with (or sustain shortly after birth) the brain damage resulting in CP. In a study of range of motion in children under 2 years of age with CP, we found significant hamstring muscle contractures in many children, but limitations in ankle dorsiflexion were rare (S.K. Campbell, I.J. Wilhelm, D.S. Slaton; unpublished data; 1987). Yet later, inhibitive casting, toe walking, and tendon of Achilles lengthening are major issues in PT for children with CP. Olney and colleagues[9-11] have shown that the single major problem in the gait of children with hemiplegic and diplegic CP is in control and power at the ankle. We do not know how or whether the problem of poor force output relates to plantar flexor hypoextensibility. Tardieu and colleagues[12,13] have suggested that there are at least two reasons for development of hypoextensibility of the gastrocnemius-soleus muscle group: failure of muscle plasticity to accommodate increasing skeletal growth or overuse of the muscles during daily activities. Yet not all children with spastic CP develop hypoextensibility in this muscle group. Who does? Why? When? Can it be prevented? Can the need for orthopedic surgery be reduced? These are important questions that can be answered with a large clinical data base.

On the other hand, information on natural history can refute long-held assumptions and force a fresh look at old problems. Wing and colleagues,[14] for example, recently reported that contrary to expectation, recovery of flexor movements at the elbow in five patients after a CVA was not necessarily faster or more complete than recovery of extension. Furthermore, recovery of movement velocity reached an asymptote in about 20 weeks although rate and degree of recovery varied. The movements studied were performed so that the force of gravity was eliminated. The coordinative structure of elbow and shoulder differed from normal; however, isolated movements at the elbow were no more impaired than two-joint movements. Is the ability to perform selective control at the elbow in these patients possible because the force of gravity is eliminated? If impaired force control is a major problem as Sahrmann and Norton[15] have suggested, would gravity-eliminated exercise be useful in treatment? Can rate or degree of recovery in the first 20 weeks be improved by PT? If so, will improvement in selective control of movement be correlated with improved functional recovery? These and other important questions are generated by case studies such as this.

Construct Validity of Measures

The second problem that hinders the establishment of efficacious testing protocols is failure to define the measurement constructs of major interest. A construct is an idea resulting from the logical arrangement of facts. In measurement theory, it means the concept a test purports to measure. Measurement texts list various types of validity; these include content, construct, and criterion-related validities.[16-18] Construct validity relates to the theoretical basis of the test and whether, through research, the test has been demonstrated to behave the way it should in practical application. For example, if a motor test behaved differently in samples with different levels of cognitive ability, one might suspect that intelligence was contaminating the results and invalidating the intended assessment of motor performance. Or, for

many years physical therapists may have thought they were assessing muscle tone during passive movement when biomechanical hypoextensibility of muscle structures also was involved. A test can typically measure only one construct well unless it consists of a number of subscales, each reflecting independent constructs. Unfortunately, many of the tests in use in PT appear to be made up of items measuring multiple underlying factors.

Many years ago, important clinicians working in the area of CNS-based movement dysfunction recognized that performance categories such as strength did not fit neurologic disorders very well. They began to speak of assessing the quality of movement, and we have been mired down in it ever since. Quality is not a single construct. Rather, it is a metaconcept that may not easily be measured objectively in the clinical setting.

Each of the classical approaches to therapeutic exercise emphasizes different aspects of quality, all of which are probably important. Some of the variables it seems to encompass include postural set for movement, including weight shifting and postural alignment, stability or balance, postural tone, coordination of joints involving ability to use selective controls, and smoothness of movement. Recently, an occupational therapist designed the Miller Infant and Toddler Test as an assessment of quality of movement in children; Miller[19] defined quality as being variety and frequency of movement, especially movements that change the position of the body. A further complication is the recent recognition that poor quality of movement results not only from aberrant motor control processes but also from the biomechanics inherent in muscle extensibility and other nonneural components.[20,21] This view fits well with a dynamical systems approach to understanding motor control but only makes the measurement problem more complex.

Quality of movement, then, does not appear to represent a single or simple construct. We must define it in order to measure it. Alternatively, we might decide to measure its components (after defining them) or to choose some variable that results from the components that comprise quality, such as smoothness of movement, speed, or efficiency. To complicate matters further, it may be true that the problems contributing to poor quality of movement in each type of neurologic condition are fundamentally different. If so, it might be impossible to develop a single test that captures the unique characteristics of reduced quality in all neurologic patients unless the underlying muscle activation patterns and resulting forces are measured.

In attempts to develop solutions to this difficult problem, my concern is that we may discard prematurely the valuable clinical observations from the past in favor of new efforts to simplify the problem. An example is the current discussion of the importance of muscle tone. Most people have believed for a long time that tone is a component contributing to the quality of movement; however, we now appear to be switching from a focus on postural tone and abnormal reflexes as the most important underlying mechanisms creating movement dysfunction to discarding these concepts entirely. I would suggest that we have not adequately defined the construct for clinical purposes and have not yet done enough research. Current knowledge regarding the role of muscle tone in movement dysfunction is based on studies involving only a small number of subjects of various types, studied under different protocols with a narrow definition of spasticity.[15,20-22] Furthermore, findings from one diagnostic entity may be applied to other diagnostic entities without ever questioning whether that is appropriate.

Sahrmann and Norton[15] have suggested that abnormal muscle tone is not as important as the lack of normal force production and the prolonged activation of agonists in distorting the movement of patients with spastic hemiplegia; they support their point of view by referring to work that has shown that tone reduction in spastic patients is not correlated with improved function. Similar ideas are reported in the literature on spastic CP, along with the suggestion that mechanical restraint of movement that therapists perceive to be "increased tone" may be more related to altered mechanical properties of muscle, not to neurologically based reflexes.[20] These papers and work by Olney and colleagues[9-11] demonstrating poor force output by ankle plantar flexors during the push-off phase of gait in children with CP clearly show that force production is a major and important problem in clients with spasticity caused by CP and CVA. The corollary that abnormal tone does not hinder movement is not as convincing. Despits obvious evidence that the short latency stretch reflex does not by itself create restraint of movement in at least some patients with CP and CVA, more severely impaired patients have been studied inadequately, as have faster movements and movements involving eccentric contractions. For example, Milner-Brown and Penn[21] reported that in patients with CP and severely impaired ability to reciprocally activate muscles to keep an alternating movement going, hyperactive stretch reflexes further degraded movement.

Finally, the questions of how, why, and when a muscle becomes hypoextensible and whether the stretch reflex or other abnormal reflexes are important in that phenomenon have not yet been answered. If prevention of disability is as important as promoting functional improvement, these questions need more study before abnormal tone is dismissed as insignificant.

Furthermore, the research on the role of abnormal tone in impaired movement is based on a definition of spasticity as being an increase in the velocity-dependent stretch reflex.[22] This is not what a physical therapist means by abnormal tone. The construct must be defined in clinically meaningful terms and then measured to determine its role in aberrant movement. Semantics is obviously important here— if the term spasticity is left to those who have redefined it as a short latency velocity-dependent reflex, then what to call the clinical problem must be decided.

The dynamical systems model provides one way to hypothesize a basis for abnormal postural tone as the complex process that it is. The distributed control model can also be used because it suggests that different components of the motor control system contribute to different aspects of movement regulation. In any case, the outcome of movement in the presence of an abnormal CNS is a result of what the remaining functional parts of the system can do to best accomplish the goals of movement that remain. Over time, that "best it can do" performance may change the very compo-

nents of the system as compensatory mechanisms operate in a dynamically functioning system.

The model presented by Horak at the II STEP conference (see Horak, this volume) for understanding postural tone includes the biomechanics of muscle structures, selective voluntary control of muscle activation, responses to stretch, and patterns of muscle activation. This model allows us to hypothesize about the factors contributing to abnormal tone and how it might develop and whether it is a separate problem from that of decreased force production and other aspects of aberrant coordination. One possibility for how the components produce the "spasticity syndrome of CP," as Craik (R.L. Craik, PhD; personal communication; July 1990) has suggested we might call it, is as follows. Key roles of the motor-sensory cortex include contributions to regulation of force production and selective activation of muscles.[23] In the case of some functions, like individual fine control of the fingers, no other area of the CNS can compensate if the area of the motor-sensory cortex that relates to hand control is destroyed irrevocably. Thus some areas of the brain have more uniquely developed control functions— a concept that is important in understanding the "encephalization" of function in higher primates. The pathology of spastic CP is thought to involve damage to gray or white matter in the motor-sensory cortex or its descending corticospinal and other tracts, which include both sensory and motor pathways.[24] When a lesion involves motor-sensory cortex, it makes sense that one result would be decreased ability to develop force in agonist muscles. Yet individuals experiencing such lesions are motivated to move by the goal of accomplishing tasks. They not only have to function with a system that has impaired ability to produce force in selected muscles, but have probably been confined to bed with resultant disuse atrophy of muscles, impairing the ability to produce tension, especially rapid production. In a system that attempts to accomplish a goal through interaction of a set of dynamic components, the system might magnify, or increase the gain of, sensory input to improve task accomplishment—exactly what a dynamical control system model would predict. We would note the presence of increased gain by observation of an increase in the short latency stretch reflex, but incoming sensory afferents also project widely in multisynaptic spinal circuits and to high levels of the CNS. The result might involve prolonging the activity of the agonist muscle in order to create enough force to reach the goal, as Sahrmann and Norton[15] have found, or activating accessory muscles to create more force or stability, as seems to be especially common in CP.[15,21,25] The result might begin to look like spasticity.

We might also predict that the individual would constrain the degrees of freedom of the motor system in order to decrease the need to contend with reactive forces, especially if postural set preceding movement inadequately prepares the body for accepting such forces. Over time, the system would be expected to respond by changing the nature of the muscles, the processing of sensory information, or any other parts of the dynamic system that have the plasticity to respond interactively to promote improved goal attainment. In the developing nervous system, effects might be different than in a previously well-established motor control system.

For example, Myklebust[26] has shown that reflex organization in children with spastic CP differs from that in adult-onset brain damage, and Leonard[27] has shown a failure to transform an immature gait pattern into one in which phasic alternating muscle contractions occur. These effects might be viewed as compensatory strategies in terms of motor learning, adjustments in operation of neural circuitry, and possibly actual changes in physical structure. By-products might be contractures or limited freedom of movement.

My theory regarding mechanisms underlying the clinical observation of abnormal postural tone in spastic syndromes caused by CP and CVA includes the following: 1) the presence of coactivation of muscles in situations where this is not a pattern typically chosen by a normal control system, 2) the lack of selective activation of appropriate agonists, and 3) the poor timing of the muscles in a coordinative structure (both prime movers and postural muscles making up a synergy). Over time, changes in muscle fibers and elasticity of muscle structures take place. Evidence exists in the literature that changes in these features improve movement and can lead to functional gains as well.[28,29] The reader should note that my theory suggests that abnormal tone is a separate problem from decreased force production and, at least in part, is a compensatory strategy that creates biomechanical complications over time. Tests of this hypothesis should then include separate measures of force and tone and attempt to demonstrate that they involve separable processes. The implication is also clear that ways to prevent abnormal tone development should be sought in addition to ways to increase force production. Alternative theories should obviously be tested that might imply that force and tone are part of the same process and are inseparable; therefore, they are not cause and compensation, respectively.

The most important message, however, is that research is needed to test alternative hypotheses in well-defined populations and that the answers have clear and important implications for future practice. Critical questions are as follows:

1. Can force production be improved in patients with spasticity?
2. Can selective control of muscle activation and postural set for movement be improved?
3. Can spasticity be prevented, and if so, does it matter?
4. Can the course of natural recovery be altered by intervention?

If the answers to each of these questions is *No,* then the goals of PT must lie in ways to compensate for functional deficits with assistive technology and teaching alternative strategies for accomplishing functional tasks.

Why is there such a problem in defining what we should measure, when, and how? One reason is that we do not yet know enough about the underlying processes that create aberrant movement in patients with different types of neurologic impairments. In particular, we have not identified the components that are *primary*. Lack of selective control and poor force production now appear to be key issues in spastic conditions, but we have almost no data on these variables and no specific tests, although a few items have been used in research that represent an initial intent to measure selective control. Confusion also exists regarding what any

one test can do; tests in use are expected to measure multiple constructs and perform multiple tasks. This is unrealistic.

TYPES AND USE OF TESTS

Before returning to the problem of defining a conceptual framework for measuring neurologic dysfunction and capturing the essence of quality of movement, a description of the purposes that tests must fulfill is appropriate. From the physical therapist's point of view, tests are required to do three things: discriminate (identify normal as normal and abnormal as abnormal), predict, and evaluate (document that change has occurred).[30] A *discriminative index* distinguishes between individuals with and without a specific problem. For example, developmental scales like the Bayley Scales of Infant Development,[31] Gesell Revised Developmental Schedules,[32] and Peabody Developmental Motor Scales[33] are intended to discriminate children who are developmentally normal from those who are below average or definitely abnormal in achieving motor milestones. Scales like these, age-normed on large populations and standardized to insure reliability and validity, are used in developmental diagnostic clinics where identification of children who need therapy is an important goal. Therapists often expect tools like these to be useful in planning and assessing treatment; however, that is only likely if PT increases the rate of motor milestone development. Furthermore, there is a tendency to use these test scores as if they were error-free. Although a single score is obtained from testing, the child's so-called "true" score actually lies somewhere within a range of scores surrounding the obtained score that is defined by the test's standard error of measurement (SEM).[17] The SEM is related to the test's reliability. Thus no single test score provides perfect discrimination between normal and abnormal.

A second purpose of tests is prediction. A *predictive index* classifies people into categories based on a predicted later outcome.[30] The SEM is once again highly useful for analyzing the degree of confidence that can be placed in an individual's score on such a test. Other calculations are necessary, however, to express the degree to which a test can be expected to predict successfully a future outcome or discrimination among a population of individuals with and without a specific problem. The statistics that are important to know to assess the overall validity of a test are the sensitivity (ability to identify abnormal as abnormal) and the specificity (ability to identify normal as normal).[34-37] These calculations are made based on data placed in a fourfold table summarizing the performance of individuals on two measures: the test of interest and a gold standard diagnostic measure obtained at the same time (for a discriminative index or screening test) or at some later point (for a predictive index).

Prediction is a major purpose of the Movement Assessment of Infants (MAI) which was designed originally to assess 4-month-old infants to predict their risk for CP.[38] The sensitivity of the MAI at 4 months of age when compared with a physician's diagnosis of CP at age 3 to 8 years in 152 high risk infants was reported to be 73.5%.[39] The specificity was 62.7%. In this study, the MAI was better than the Bayley motor scale for predicting abnormality (73.5% vs 35.3%), but much worse at identifying those children who would be normal (62.7% vs 94.9%). The two tests appear to assess somewhat different but equally important characteristics; perhaps use of both scores in a decision analysis algorithm would improve prediction. It is important for the clinician to understand, however, that the actual predictive accuracy of a positive or negative result on an individual client who is assessed varies with the prevalence of the condition of interest in the population.[35] The reader should refer to Feinstein for more explanation of this phenomenon.[35]

An *evaluative index* is used to measure change in function over time or with intervention.[30] For example, the newly available Gross Motor Function Measure is intended for use in measuring change in children with CP and was designed specifically for use in measuring the out-come of PT for such children.[30,40] A companion measure, the Gross Motor Performance Measure, is under development for the purpose of assessing the more qualitative aspects of motor performance, such as postural alignment, weight shift, and selective control of movement in individual joints.

It is usually impossible to use a single test for the purposes of both discrimination and evaluation or of prediction; therefore, in selecting tests for use in clinical practice, the therapist must carefully identify the major purpose for using a specific test and review information on tests under consideration to judge whether they are suitable.

Clearly, tests available for use by physical therapists vary in purpose and have different underlying theoretical constructs. To use them more effectively, they should be judged relative to the needs of a general framework for assessing patients in which a combination of tests is selected on the basis of their unique specific purposes and the overall goals of a comprehensive assessment. Certainly, room remains for development of new tests, and the availability of a general conceptual framework for measurement would help to identify what they are.

CONCEPTUAL FRAMEWORK FOR DESCRIBING AND ASSESSING NEUROLOGIC DISABILITY

Although any number of conceptual frameworks could be generated, one possible approach for organizing the measurement of neurologic dysfunction will be presented. The framework has two parts. One part is related to defining and categorizing patient problems with dichotomous variables for the purpose of describing patient populations and making gross assessments of problems and outcomes. A second part is related to measuring specific aspects of problems in more detail for treatment planning, out-come assessment, and prevention.

The World Health Organization's (WHO) international classification of impairment, disability, and handicap (ICIDH) model is a hierarchical system for categorizing patient problems that simultaneously documents areas in which there are no problems, thus providing a comprehensive description of the client in a variety of skill areas.[41] The system in brief is as follows: various levels of problems are encountered when analyzing any disabling condition, and measurement of such a condition can take place on each of these levels: pathology, impairment, disability, and handicap. The lowest level is that of *pathology*—the target disorder. Pathology refers to the underlying disease or injury process at the

organ level and is the usual focus of physicians and laboratory personnel.

The patient usually presents to physical therapists with concerns described by the second level: *impairment*. Impairments consist of the signs and symptoms of the condition at the level of the total organism, the human body. Problems at this level are measured when strength, range of motion, or spasticity are assessed or when a client is described as having spastic hemiplegia or diplegia. This level has been the main focus of PT assessment in the past.

Disabilities comprise the third level and consist of the behaviors of the person within his or her immediate environment. Skills in this category include behavior, communication, personal care, locomotion, body disposition, dexterity, and other skills specific to the individual. Categorized under locomotion and body disposition are tasks such as walking, traversing, climbing, transferring, lifting, reaching, kneeling, and maintaining posture. For the individual involved, problems at this level result in disturbance of goal-directed behaviors. Recent emphasis in PT has been focused on task-oriented behaviors of this type and on the need for better tools to measure dysfunction and improvements with intervention. The Pediatric Evaluation of Disability Inventory (PEDI) under development by Haley and colleagues[42] is designed with the WHO ICIDH system as its basis.

The ultimate level of dysfunction is *handicap*. Herein lies the very personal meaning of the disabling condition for the individual as he or she functions in society fulfilling life roles. Within this level are included any limitations in the areas of employment, fulfilling family roles, educational attainment, travel, and leisure activities. Handicap is defined primarily from the perspective of the individual involved and the significant persons in the individual's social and family network. The ICIDH categories are orientation, physical dependence, mobility, occupation, social integration, and economic self-sufficiency.

The ICIDH system uses a digit-coding system to classify each problem as present or absent. Additional digits can be added to designate the severity of the problem and the potential for improvement. It is possible also to add individualized categories, if needed. Therapists will find that some essential categories, such as developmental activities appropriate for children, are missing.

One value of this classification system is that both problem areas and nonproblem areas are defined so that a complete picture of competencies and disabilities is obtained. Furthermore, it is easily comprehended by professionals of all disciplines and by clients and family members. Tests used in conjunction with the ICIDH system to provide for more in-depth assessment should focus on *one* level and not combine items assessing both disability and impairment. This model is useful in defining constructs to measure across the various levels in order to structure a battery of tests for the assessment of patients with neurologic dysfunction. Unique test batteries might be needed for each specific condition for describing impairment if the underlying mechanisms producing aberrant movement differ from condition to condition. At the level of impairment, tests are needed for categorizing patients within and across types of disorders in order to establish diagnostic categories of movement dysfunction specific to PT. At the level of disability, however, tests should not need to be diagnostic-specific.

To accompany the ICIDH system, I would like to suggest a conceptual framework for measurement of impairment and disability by physical therapists. It is certainly only one of many possible models, but it incorporates major areas of importance in capturing the essence of disability for planning treatment, assessing outcome, and preventing complications. The model has four elements described by the acronym SAFE. After describing the model, I will attempt to give examples of how we might organize and summarize assessment results for a child with hemiplegic CP using this model. Other brief examples of how the model highlights important aspects of patient performance will also be given.

These are the components of a SAFE model of assessment:

S in the model stands for Safe. It suggests that in our planning for and intervention with patients, we should aim to do no harm, to prevent potential harm, and to reduce disability and handicap resulting from neurologic impairments. Planning the prevention of secondary problems, such as contractures, need for surgical intervention, or orthopedic complications because of overuse or strain of joints and ligaments, requires specific documentation of dysfunction predisposing to such complications. It is listed as a special category of assessment in order to 1) highlight the importance of always considering the potential future consequences of what we do and what we fail to do, based on the natural history of the individual condition and 2) emphasize that few assessments we use on a routine basis have a prognostic component to them. That is, we frequently fail to anticipate and measure unwanted complications prospectively. This is the level at which we must attend to abnormal postural tone and reflexes if for no other reason than they predispose to complications. Assessments in this area would involve primarily tests for impairment, such as range of motion, postural abnormalities, and skin breakdown.

In the area of secondary impairment, adhering only to a model of normal performance will fail. The physical therapist's model for measurement and treatment of neurologic conditions must take into account the potential for complications because, first, treatment seldom produces a normally functioning system and, second, PT, in some cases, will reach its potential for improving deficits in performance. The only remaining goal may be prevention of secondary impairment and disability. Furthermore, providing a unique component for this area in a measurement system may be helpful in documentation for reimbursement for preventative and maintenance services.

A search of classical clinical literature, current case histories, and old patient files may be useful in developing a list of impairments that have a high probability of occurring under specific predisposing conditions. Consistent recording of these problems in patient records should be useful in future program-evaluation research, especially when new treatments are incorporated into patient management and results compared with historical records on clients treated under different regimens.

A in the SAFE model stands for measurement of Adaptive behavior. I postulate that the two most important adaptive behaviors needed by ourpatients are *locomotion* and *manipulation,* or eye-hand function.[7] When impairments result in disability in these two behaviors, it is likely that there will be functional difficulties in a variety of areas and potential handicap in functioning in society if not reduced by therapeutic exercise or compensated for by use of assistive devices, orthoses, and so on. Tests selected for assessing adaptive behaviors would include measure of gait and hand function at the observational level in the clinical setting and assessment of body stability during translation and posture stability during seated functional activities. Such tests might also include developmental milestone tests for children. Problems identified in performing adaptive behaviors would lead the therapist to search for underlying causes, such as weakness or balance disorders, as the problem-solving process continues. When identified sources of dysfunction have been corrected or compensated for with assistive devices, attention would again focus on other areas in the conceptual model. For example, in a patient management problem presented recently at a professional meeting, gait assessment of a child with myelomeningocele identified difficulty with stability at the knee and ankle during weight acceptance and single limb support, inadequate hip extension during midstance and terminal stance, foot drag during swing, and lateral lean of the trunk. The child had weak hip extensors and Zero strength in ankle muscles, hip abductors, and hip adductors. Use of locked ankle-foot orthoses and Lofstrand® crutches improved the appearance of his gait and significantly increased its velocity. The new gait pattern, however, appeared to submit the knee to high rotatory forces, raising questions regarding the long-term potential for damage to the knee and concerns about the safety (Safe component of the model) of this intervention.

F in the model stands for Functional assessment and includes assessment of the use of adaptive behaviors in functional contexts. Such activities include locomotion in the community, transfers, and eye-hand coordination in functional activities such as dressing and eating. Here the primary focus of assessment is whether the individual can accomplish tasks such as these in daily life so as to be functional for the person, regardless of quality or efficiency. Separate tests should not be needed for different disabilities, although norms for different diagnostic groups would be useful. Assessment of adaptive behaviors in the clinic and functional behaviors in specific contexts both address the ICIDH disability category, but at different levels.

Ultimately, the results of functional assessment will be correlated with the degree of handicap experienced by the individual in society; however, this is not the primary focus of PT assessment. Degree of handicap is the outcome of all assessments by the rehabilitation team when viewed in relation to the individual's stated goals, ambitions, and typical life roles. Thus assessment at the level of handicap is a team function, and the team includes the client. Handicap also refers to society's response to disability and its willingness to accommodate and integrate individuals with special needs. These concerns, of course, should be addressed by the therapist during interviews of the patient throughout rehabilitation to gather his or her concerns regarding limitations on the quality of life and the client's ideas regarding the value and goals of therapy.

E stands for Efficiency, and I wish to postulate that this assessment is the unique province of physical therapy, specifically because I believe it to be our primary focus at many different levels of the impact of the disability on the individual client. Unlike assessment of Adaptive behavior and Function, which represent two levels of assessment of disability, efficiency crosses levels in the ICIDH model. At the level of functional ability, efficiency would include assessment of how much time it takes the person to perform activities like dressing and crossing the street. At the level of impairment, it might be appropriate to assess endurance, fatigue or pain with exercise, or mechanical efficiency of gait (from cinematography). Efficiency might be an appropriate variable to represent quality of movement as a primary focus of physical therapy assessment and intervention, across levels of movement dysfunction.

A quick method to summarize efficiency in many activities might be to assess speed or ability to accomplish continuous activity either for a stated period of time or for a number of repetitions per unit of time. Measurement of effects of intervention can be done easily with tools such as a stopwatch or a videocorder. Although assessments would need to be individualized for each client, they could be summarized across clients for program evaluation purposes, with statistics such as percentages or rates of improvement.

As VanSant (in this volume) has suggested, there are undoubtedly age-related and disability-related norms for how fast movement is likely to be for best efficiency. Olney,[11] however, has suggested that there are two other ways that physical therapists might document that intervention has improved mechanical efficiency. One is to use a measure of heart rate to show either that the activity previously tested and found wanting is now performed at the same speed with a lower heart rate or that the same activity can be performed faster with the same heart rate. This will be a good approximation of increased efficiency because heart rate has been found to correlate quite well with energy cost, but only if testing conditions are carefully controlled, the number of samples of behavior required to minimize variability is determined, and no fitness effect is likely to have occurred.

A second method that might prove acceptable is use of the Physiological Cost Index, or PCI.[11,43] The PCI uses two primary variables: heart rate and walking velocity. The equation is as follows: heart rate while walking minus heart rate (bpm) divided by average speed of walking (meters/min). This index has two advantages: 1) an adjustment is built in for fitness and 2) speed of movement is included in the equation. Finding a lower PCI after intervention could be accepted as evidence of improved efficiency if the reliability of the measure is demonstrated to be satisfactory.[11]

From a research point of view, we need to learn more about the kinematics and the muscle activation patterns that characterize the various types of neurologic disabilities common in PT practice. This is absolutely critical to learning why the motor control system has selected the coordinative structures used by the patient and what therapy must accomplish to improve the efficiency of a patient's movement.

Study of patients is critical because either patterns that are efficient for normal individuals may never be possible for clients or patterns that are not a close approximation to normal may be more efficient for them.

As a first approximation, Olney[11] suggests that clients with spasticity will have more efficient movement if it becomes less jerky, contains less coactivation of antagonists or of multiple muscles in synergic patterns, and contains less static work (ie, fewer periods when isometric contraction is occurring); also, there will be less overlap of energy generation and absorption. The final proof would be an overall reduction in metabolic cost.

The experienced pediatric therapist will immediately say, "What about the child who bunny-hops to crawl about?" There is no doubt that it provides a fast, efficient movement pattern allowing functional mobility for the child with CP. The SAFE model, however, would lead one to consider the preventive aspects of assessment of movement patterns, considering the future consequences of current functionally useful movement in abnormal patterns. Most pediatric physical therapists believe that use of such a habitual movement pattern leads to tightening hamstring muscles, is correlated with "W-sitting" that has other characteristics conducive to production of deformities, and inhibits practice of reciprocal creeping patterns that provide more practice in interlimb and intralimb coordination that is similar to patterns used in walking. Here we need to consider models of abnormal development, motor control, and motor learning and cannot just consider what is functional for the child. This combination of attention to improved function through promoting improved efficiency of basic gross motor activities along with prevention of future complications is what makes PT truly unique in rehabilitation.

Although not all of the measures needed to structure assessment within a SAFE conceptual framework are currently available, the following case example may help to show how it could work.

Case Report

History. Jimmy was born weighing 7 lb 13 oz after a full-term pregnancy with no problems.[6] At 3 months of age, Jimmy had a high fever with seizures and an apparent left cerebral infarct. After abnormal electroencephalogram results, he was placed on phenobarbital. At 4 months of age, he was observed to ignore his right side and did not use his right hand at all. He was referred to PT for treatment of right hemiplegia at the age of 5 months.

Six-month assessment. Jimmy was assessed with the Peabody Developmental Motor Scales at 6 months of age. On the Gross Motor Subscale, he received a raw score of 85 for a developmental quotient of 95, indicating that his gross motor abilities were well within the average range for his chronologic age. He was able to sit independently, achieve hands-and-knees position and rock back and forth, pivot a little in the prone position, and stand with support. He had excellent head control and was able to balance when sitting and playing with toys. In sitting, however, his trunk slumped slightly toward the right, and the right leg tended to maintain a stiff extended posture. When balance was perturbed in sitting, he reacted with protective extension reactions on both sides; however, the right arm was ineffective in preventing a fall. In supported standing, most of the weight was born on the left leg, and the right knee tended to remain locked in extension, apparently for stability.

Because of Jimmy's neglect of the right arm, the Fine Motor Subscale of the Peabody was scored separately for the right and left arms, with items requiring use of both arms added into the score for each side. Jimmy obtained a raw score of 70 for a developmental quotient of 104 for use of the left hand, again well within the average range. The right arm, however, performed at a level more appropriate to a 2-month-old child, and his score for the right arm was 51, outside the range of normal for his chronologic age. The percentile rank score for the left arm was 61, for the right less than 2, meaning that he scored less well than 98% of children his age on the right side. Jimmy was able to use the left hand to pick up small objects with an inferior-pincer grasp and used it to bang, shake, and manipulate objects. The right hand had a crude grasp, but it was used mostly in concert with the left hand and with poor aim when reaching for objects. The shoulder muscles on the right were tight, interfering with reaching, and the arm tended to be used only in synergic patterns. The right hand appeared to have either a strength deficit or, more likely, a sensory deficit. For example, when a cotton ball was placed in the right hand out of his sight, the hand grasped reflexively, but he seemed unaware of it.

The PT diagnosis was a right hemiplegia with more involvement in the arm than the leg. Jimmy's ICIDH description is as follows:

IMPAIRMENT
71.06 Mechanical impairment of right shoulder
72.20 Spastic hemiparesis of right side
97.10 Sensory impairment of right side
DISABILITIES
53.0 Reaching up
58.0 Postural disability
61.3 Moving objects
61.4 Handling objects
62.0 Fingering disability
63.0 Gripping disability
64.0 Holding disability
80.03 Play, exploration disability
HANDICAP
None

Treatment goals included improvement of hand and arm function on the right side; lengthening of the tight muscles of the right shoulder and the trunk; achievement of erect posture and stability in sitting; and more equal distribution of weight in sitting, standing, and four-point postures.

Nine-month assessment. Jimmy was reassessed with the Peabody Scales at age 9 months. On the Gross Motor Subscales, he received a raw score of 118 for a developmental quotient of 108, just above average for chronologic age. Considering the SEM of the test, the increase of 13 points from 6 to 9 months shows a significant increase in gross motor development. He was cruising around furniture, creeping, pulling to stand, and taking several steps with just one hand held. During these activities, Jimmy used the right leg quite well, although it occasionally stiffened, and he tended to put more weight on the left leg. He pulled to standing by

stepping forward on the left foot almost exclusively, although he was able to do it with the right if encouraged.

Because Jimmy's movement patterns were functionally appropriate for his daily play activities, he could be considered to perform adequately in Adaptive behavior and Function. A videotape of his creeping performance, however, revealed that he was unable to creep rapidly, probably because of inability to have both extremities on the same side moving at the same time (presumably a result of inadequate postural stability). Furthermore, large vertical excursions of the trunk occurred during creeping, demonstrating poor conservation of energy. Thus movement efficiency would be considered to be compromised. These problems could be documented quantitatively by measures of inter-limb and intralimb coordination taken from frame-by-frame analysis of the videotape or by calculations of speed of creeping.

On the Fine Motor Subscale of the Peabody, Jimmy received a raw score of 61 for the right hand for a developmental quotient of 74, or almost 2 SDs below the mean for age (a functional age equivalent of 6 months at 9 months chronologic age). The change from the 6-month assessment represents significant improvement in Adaptive behavior but is still below the average range for age. He was able to grasp large objects with the right hand but held them only briefly. He used the right hand to bang objects and tried, without success, to rake in small objects. He continued to have a tendency to tighten up in the flexors of the right hand and continued to give the appearance of lacking sensation on the right. Thus the *S* area in the SAFE model continues to raise concerns and the need for preventative action in treatment planning (and for a reliable means for documenting range of motion in CP[44]). The right hand was used actively as a helping hand with the left to hold large or heavy objects and to clap. On the left side, Jimmy received a raw score on the Peabody of 80 for a developmental quotient of 95, about average for age. He lacked a fine-pincer grasp for tiny objects on the left and usually held large objects using the whole hand on the radial side rather than using just the fingers. Overall functional performance in eye-hand coordination had not changed significantly relative to age peers because the change from a score of 104 to 95 is within the range of chance expectation.

Overall, Jimmy's updated ICIDH description would reflect the following changes: Mechanical impairment of the right shoulder (71.06, tight muscles) no longer exists so impairment has decreased. In the area of disabilities, 53.0 (reaching up) and 58.0 (postural problems in sitting) have resolved. Handling, gripping, and other hand functions continue to be disabled but can be scored with the extra digit codes to reflect severity and potential for improvement. The fourth digit code would be at level 1 for difficulty in performance and the fifth digit code at level 2 for improvement (but not full recovery) potential without the need for aids or assistance. As Jimmy learns to walk, new concerns regarding posture, balance, potential to develop contractures, and movement efficiency will arise that can be documented with the ICIDH system. Ultimately, these designations would provide a complete summary record of the waxing and waning of Jimmy's motor control, musculoskeletal, and functional performance problems and of the therapist's assessment of the severity of Jimmy's problems and potential for improvement.

Acknowledgment

I gratefully acknowledge the American Physical Therapy Association for permitting me to adapt and reprint material from my lesson entitled "Using Standardized Tests in Clinical Practice," from *In Touch Home Study Course: Topics in Pediatrics, Lesson 11*.

References

1. Sackett DL, Haynes RB, Tugwell P. *Clinical Epidemiology: A Basic Science for Clinical Medicine*. Boston, Mass: Little, Brown & Company Inc; 1985.
2. Dawes RM, Faust D, Meehl PE. Clinical versus actuarial judgment. *Science*. 1989;243:1668-1674.
3. Campbell SK. Measurement in developmental therapy: past, present, and future. In: Miller LJ, ed. *Developing Norm-Referenced Standardized Tests*. New York, NY: The Haworth Press Inc; 1989:1-13.
4. Elstein AS, Bordage G. Psychology of clinical reasoning. In: Dowie J, Elstein A, ed. *Professional Judgment*. New York, NY: Cambridge University Press; 1988:109-129.
5. Shewchuk RM, Francis KT. Principles of clinical decision making: an introduction to decision analysis. *Phys Ther*. 1988;68:357-359.
6. Campbell SK. Using standardized tests in clinical practice. In: *In Touch Home Study Course: Topics in Pediatrics, Lesson 11*. Alexandria, Va: American Physical Therapy Association. In press.
7. Carr JH, Shepherd RB, Gordon J, et al. *Movement Science: Foundations for Physical Therapy in Rehabilitation*. Rockville, Md: Aspen Publishers Inc; 1987.
8. Mahoney FI, Barthel DW. Functional evaluation: The Barthel Index. *Maryland State Medical Journal*. 1965;14:61-65.
9. Olney SJ. New developments in the biomechanics of gait in children with cerebral palsy. In: *In Touch Home Study Course: Topics in Pediatrics, Lesson 1*. Alexandria, Va: American Physical Therapy Association; 1989:1-13.
10. Olney SJ, Costigan PA, Hedden DM. Mechanical energy patterns in gait of cerebral palsied children with hemiplegia. *Phys Ther*. 1987;67:1348-1354.
11. Olney SJ. Efficacy of physical therapy in improving mechanical and metabolic efficiency of movement in cerabral palsy. *Pediatric Physical Therapy*. In press.
12. Tardieu C, Huet de la tour E, Bret MD, et al. Muscle hypoextensibility in children with cerebral palsy: I. Clinical and experimental observations. *Arch Phys Med Rehabil*. 1982;63:97-102.
13. Tardieu G, Tardieu C, Colbeau-Justin P, et al. Muscle hypoextensibility in children with cerebral palsy: II. Therapeutic implications. *Arch Phys Med Rehabil*. 1982;63:103-107.
14. Wing AM, Lough S. Turton A, et al. Recovery of elbow function in voluntary positioning of the hand following hemiplegia due to stroke. *J Neurol Neurosurg Psychiatry*. 1990;53:126-134.
15. Sahrmann SA, Norton BJ. The relationship of voluntary movement to spasticity in the upper motor neuron syndrome. *Ann Neurol*. 1977;2:460-465.
16. Sattler JM. *Assessment of Children*. 3rd ed. San Diego, Calif: J M Sattler Publisher; 1988;8:28-29, 168.
17. Anastasi A. *Psychological Testing*. 6th ed. New York, NY: Collier Macmillan Publishers; 1988:133-138.
18. American Psychological Association. *Standards for Education and Psychological Testing*. Washington, DC: American Psychological Association, 1985.
19. Bonder BR. Planning the initial version. In: Miller LJ, ed. *Developing Norm-Reference Standardized Tests*. New York, NY: The Haworth Press Inc; 1989:15-42.
20. Berger W, Quintern J, Dietz V. Pathophysiology of gait in children with cerebral palsy. *Electroencephalog Clin Neurophysiol*. 1982;53:538-548.
21. Milner-Brown HS, Penn RD. Pathophysiological mechanisms in cerebral palsy. *J Neurol Neurosurg Psychiatry*. 1979;42:606-618.
22. Young RR, Koella WO, eds. *Spasticity: Disordered Motor Control*. Chicago, Ill: Year Book Medical Publishers Inc; 1980.
23. Evarts EV. Role of motor cortex in voluntary movements in primates. In: Brookhart JM, Mountcastle VB, eds. *Handbook of Physiology. The Nervous System—Motor Control*. Bethesda, Md: American Physiological Society; 1981;2(pt 2):1083-1120.
24. Hill A, Volpe JJ. Seizures, hypoxic-ischemic brain injury, and intraventricular hemorrhage in the newborn. *Ann Neurol*. 1981;10:109-121.
25. Barolat-Romana G, David R. Neurophysiological mechanisms in abnormal reflex activities in cerebral palsy and spinal spasticity. *J Neurol Neurosurg Psychiatry*. 1980;42:333-342.
26. Myklebust BM, Gottlieb GL, Penn RD, et al. Reciprocal excitation of antagonistic muscles as a differentiating feature in spasticity. *Ann Neurol*. 1982;12:367-374.
27. Leonard CT, Hirschfeld H, Forssberg H. Gait acquisition and reflex abnormalities in normal children and children with cerebral palsy. In: Amblard B, Berthoz A, Clarac F, eds. *Posture and Gait: Development, Adaptation and Modulation*. New York, NY: Elsevier Science Publishing Co Inc; 1988:33-45.
28. Parke B, Penn RD, Savoy SM, et al. Functional outcome after delivery of intrathecal baclofen. *Arch Phys Med Rehabil*. 1989;70:30-32.
29. Latash ML. Penn RD, Corcos DM, et al; Short-term effects of intrathecal baclofen in spasticity. *Exper Neurol*. 1989;103:165-172.
30. Rosenbaum PL, Russell DJ, Cadman DT, et al. Issues in measuring change in motor function in children with cerebral palsy: a special communication. *Phys Ther*. 1990;70:125-131.
31. Bayley N. *Bayley Scales of Infant Development*. New York, NY: The Psychological Corp; 1969.
32. Knobloch H, Stevens F, Malone A. *A Manual of Developmental Diagnosis: The Administration and Interpretation of the Revised Gesell and Amatruda Developmental and Neurological Examination*. New York, NY: Harper & Row, Publishers Inc; 1980.
33. Folio MR, Fewell RR. *Peabody Developmental Motor Scales and Activity Cards: Manual*. Hingham, Mass: DLM Teaching Resources; 1983.
34. Stangler SR, Huber CJ, Routh DK. *Screening Growth and Developmnt of Preschool Children: A Guide for Test Selection*. New York, NY: McGraw-Hill Inc; 1980:51-55.
35. Feinstein AR. *Clinical Epidemiology: The Architecture of Clinical Research*. Philadelphia, Pa: W B Saunders Co; 1985:434-439.

36. Sackett DL. Clinical diagnosis and the clinical laboratory. *Clin Invest Med.* 1978;1:37-43.

37. Sox HC. Probability theory in the use of diagnostic tests. *Ann Intern Med.* 1986;104:60-66.

38. Chandler L, Andrews M, Swanson M. *Movement Assessment of Infants.* Rolling Bay, Wash: Infant Movement Research; 1980.

39. Harris SR. Early detection of cerebral palsy: sensitivity and specificity of two motor assessment tools. *Journal of Perinatology.* 1987;7:11-15.

40. Russell D, Rosenbaum P, Cadman D, et al. The Gross Motor Function measure: a means to evaluate the effects of physical therapy. *Dev Med Child Neurol.* 1989;31:341-352.

41. *World Health Organization. International Classification of Impairments, Disabilities, and Handicaps.* Geneva, Switzerland: World Health Organization; 1980.

42. Haley SM, Faas RM, Coster W, et al. *Pediatric Evaluation of Disability Inventory.* Boston, Mass: New England Medical Center; 1989.

43. Butler P. Engelbrecht M, Major RE, et al. Physiological cost index of walking for normal children and its use as an indicator of physical handicap. *Dev Med Child Neurol.* 1984;26:607-612.

44. Harris SR, Smith LH, Krukowski L. Goniometric reliability for a child with spastic quadriplegia. *J Pediatr Orthop.* 1985;5:348-351.

Chapter 16

Abnormalities of Motor Behavior

Rebecca L. Craik, PhD, PT
Associate Professor
Department of Physical Therapy
Beaver College
Glenside, PA 19038
Adjunct Assistant Professor
School of Veterinary Medicine
University of Pennsylvania

Abnormalities of motor behavior is such an all encompassing topic that I was tempted initially to cite numerous references that detail the sequelae commonly seen in a person following injury. Greenspan,[1] for example, described deficits associated with 28 persons who had multiple sclerosis from ages 5 months to 34 years. Problems cited by Greenspan[1] included cerebellar ataxia, intention tremor, paralysis or paresis in one to four extremities, sensory loss or paresthesia, visual field deficit, proprioceptive loss, tic douloureux, dysphasia, dysarthria, euphoria, depression, dementia, fatigue, constipation, and bladder dysfunction. Nine percent could climb stairs and 18% could ambulate independently. Although useful for general descriptive purposes, the list of symptoms does not describe the relationship between symptomatology and functional ability. Instead of listing symptoms, I will discuss some of the factors that contribute to abnormal motor behavior and relate them to the discussions of motor control theory and measurement. My most common example of abnormal motor behavio.. will be problems in the adult with hemiplegia secondary to a stroke.

PURPOSE

What are the topics in a discussion of abnormal motor behavior that cross all disabilities resulting form central nervous system (CNS) injury? Knowledge of the neural mechanisms responsible for the production of abnormal behavior may help in understanding the origin of some of the motor behavior. Know the relationship between the variables examined in a classic neurological assessment and the abnormal motor behavior may allow the clinician to evaluate the efficacy of the traditional assessment. Certainly a discussion of abnormal motor behavior should include the integrity of individual muscles, the ability of the muscles to produce a coordinated movement, and, finally, the ability to accomplish a functional activity. There is also the more global issue of the "gold standard" that should be used to define abnormal motor behavior. Each of the above topics will be addressed in this chapter.

DEFINITION OF MOTOR BEHAVIOR

A definition of abnormal assumes a definition for normal motor behavior. Variables that have been measured to describe motor behavior include muscleactivity; joint motion, joint velocity, or joint acceleration; limb trajectories; joint or limb torque; and metabolic cost.[2] An operational definition of coordinated behavior should include the variable(s) controlled by the nervous system. At this time, there is not consensus about what variables the system is trying to control, so it is necessary to describe behavior using a variety of variables.

A very simplistic definition is offered by DeLong[3] who defines coordinated movement solely from the aspect of the muscle. DeLong states that three conditions must be met in order to achieve a coordinated movement: 1) the proper muscles must be selected, 2) the selected muscles must be activated and inactivated in the proper sequence and at the correct time, and 3) the muscles must be activated with the correct amount of tension. It is appealing to develop an operational definition for coordinated behavior based on the muscles' ability to meet the above criteria successfully. The relationships between patterns of muscle activation and limb behavior, or final functional outcome, must clearly be demonstrated, however, before such a definition is acceptable. Such relationships have not been demonstrated definitively in the research literature.

My definition of normal coordinated behavior will therefore be based on the assumption that appropriate muscle activations will result in appropriate intralimb coordination of the joints. Using the lower extremity as an example, appropriate intralimb coordination helps to ensure that the necessary torque is developed at the correct time to propel the body smoothly through space during the stance phase or to clear the swinging limb during swing. The appropriate timing of movements among limbs, or interlimb coordination, will effect an efficient movement of the body and the limb through space.

Final outcome of movement may be the controlled variable rather than the appropriate timing of individual muscle, joint, or limb movement. A final outcome of a swinging limb during walking is the accurate placement of the foot at ground contact. If final outcome is the controlled variable, then muscle, joint, limb, and interlimb components would be viewed as subsystems of the final goal.

My definition of normal motor behavior therefore includes the proper sequencing and tension development by the muscles, the necessary intralimb and interlimb joint excursion and sequencing, and adequate torque development. These subsystems work together to produce an efficient and accurate motion of the body to complete a task successfully. Such a model assumes intact sensation and unimpaired cognitive ability.

CLASSIC NEUROLOGICAL ASSESSMENT

A traditional way to describe performance following injury is to detail the results of a classic neurological assessment. There is an implicit assumption that we are assessing the integrity of pathways when such an assessment is performed. Many clinicians assess the integrity of a variety of reflexes, evaluate tone, and test for sensory integrity. This testing is usually performed with the patient in a recumbent or semirecumbent posture. What is the origin of this testing and how do the outcomes of these tests relate to voluntary motor behavior?

The classic neurological assessment is based on a hierarchical motor control theory (see Horak, this volume). The hierarchical model assumes that deficits observed following a CNS lesion are the direct result of a release of more primitive or automatic behaviors from higher control. Jackson [4(p218)] described the presence of positive and negative symptoms following CNS injury. *Positive symptoms* were described as exaggerated or distorted performances of surviving neurons released from their normal integrative relationship with structures that are damaged. *Negative symptoms* were described as deficits in normal behavior resulting from destruction of pertinent tissues. So the classical assessment is designed to examine the presence of the positive and negative symptoms.

If stroke, head injury, or cerebral palsy are examples of upper motor neuron syndromes, the positive symptoms include abnormal postures; exaggerated proprioceptive reflexes producing spasticity; and exaggerated cutaneous reflexes of the limbs producing flexion withdrawal spasms, extensor spasms, and the Babinski response.[5,6] The negative features are shock, weakness, loss of coordination, and, particularly, loss of manual dexterity. Although evaluations may include assessment of all of these features, the focus in the research literature and in treatment has been on spasticity.

The presentations that have preceded this one have suggested that we should consider factors in addition to the nervous system when trying to detail the mechanisms responsible for movement dysfunction. What factors account for what is measured as "spasticity" in a traditional neurological assessment? I will address three: neural mechanisms, viscoelastic properties, and weakness. The neural mechanisms that may account for hyperreflexia will be addressed first.

NEURAL MECHANISMS

For historical purposes, it may be valuable to look at the mechanisms responsible for spasticity by comparing the

knowledge at the time of the original NUSTEP conference[7] with the knowledge of today.

A myriad of classic definitions for spasticity exist and most of them include the concept that spasticity is a disorder of spinal proprioceptive reflexes, manifested clinically as tendon jerk hyperreflexia and as hypertonia, increased muscle tone that becomes more apparent the more rapid the stretching movement.[5]

Twenty years ago hyperreflexia was proposed to occur because of aberrant activity in the simple monosynaptic reflex pathway, which consisted of the afferents from muscle receptors, the receptors' central connections to agonist motor neurons, and the efferents to the agonist muscles (Fig. 16-1).[5] The tendon jerk was used to assess this monosynaptic segmental reflex arc. The percussion applied to the tendon induced action potentials in group Ia afferents from the primary muscle spindle endings. The aberrant continuous activity of the gamma efferent (fusimotor) system was proposed to account for continuous firing of the Ia afferent by maintaining the spindle's sensitivity to stretch.

Muscle tone is clinically assessed as the resistance felt in a muscle to passive elongation.[5] Rapid passive elongation leads to more resistance. Excessive afferent input to the simple segmental pathway from the muscle spindle was also proposed to account for the presence of hypertonia. The melting away of resistance that occurs in the clasp-knife phenomenon was explained by the presence of Golgi tendon organ (GTO) activity that disynaptically inhibited the agonist's motoneuron (Fig. 16-1). The theory was that the GTOs were excited when the spastic muscle tension exceeded a certain level.[5] Activation of the GTOs was proposed to inhibit the

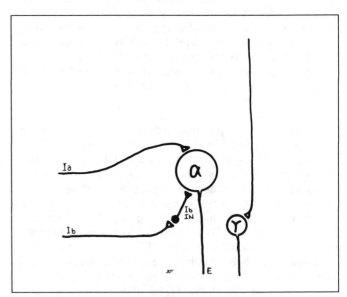

Fig. 16-1. *Simplistic view of the connectivity associated tapping a tendon. The agonist motor neuron (E for physiological extensor) is receiving input from the monosynaptic Ia input from the muscle spindle and the Ib input from the Golgi tendon organs. Note the presence of supraspinal input on the gamma motor neuron.*

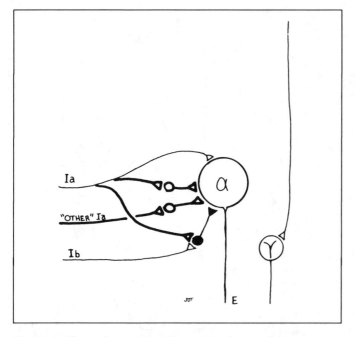

Fig. 16-2. *Illustration revising Figure 16-1 by proposing activation of additional afferent input.[5] Note the presence of polysynaptic and monosynaptic Ia input.*

motor neurons responsible for the initial muscle contraction and result in relaxation, or a melting away of tension.

Recent evidence raises questions about each aspect of these assumptions. Three recent reviews provide an excellent summary of current research and theories about the neural mechanisms that may be responsible for hypertonia.[5,8,9] The reviews are detailed so I will only superficially address the neural mechanisms by summarizing some of the information in the three reviews. The following discussion will focus on the response of the gastrocnemius-soleus muscle, collectively called the triceps surae, to a tendon tap. Burke describes the percussion input as taking 10 ms to reach its peak and lasting as long as 40 ms.[5]

First, percussion of the Achilles tendon can repeatedly excite Ia afferents from the triceps surae. The stimulus to the Achilles tendon can also activate Ia afferents in the intrinsic muscles of the foot and in the antagonist muscles of the anterolateral compartment.[5] Mechanoreceptor and other cutaneous afferents in the skin of the foot and leg may also be excited by the percussion stimulus (Fig.16-2). With all of the receptor types than can be stimulated, it is not surprising that the tendon jerk can produce much more than monosynaptic input to the motoneuron pool within the time of the initial percussion until the first motor response.

Second, the afferent circuitry is now viewed as more than a monosynaptic pathway to the stretched muscle's motoneuron pools.[5,8,9] The Ia afferents from he stretched muscle have been proposed to be carried by the agonist and synergists motoneuron through oligosynaptic pathways as well as monosynaptic pathways (Fig 16-2). There is adequate time for the motor neurons recruited first in the reflex discharge to affect recruitment of higher- threshold motor neurons through recruitment of the Renshaw inhibitory pathway.

There is also adequate time for the antagonist muscles afferents to influence the agonist motor neuron pool.

Third, there is not significant background fusimotor drive directed to spindle endings in relaxed human subjects.[10] The hypothesis is being rejected that tone in the healthy subject is the result of tonic muscle contractiondriven by gamma (fusimotor) input. Spindle endings have been shown to be sensitive in the absence of gamma input for tendon percussion to produce a tendon jerk.

Fourth, the GTO afferents are no longer the explanation for the melting away produced during the clasp-knife phenomenon.[5] Other receptors proposed include secondary spindle afferents, nonencapsulated mechanoreceptor that use group II, III, and IV afferents; and joint mechanoreceptor. These afferents, along with cutaneous afferents,are collectively called flexor reflex afferents (Fig.16-3).

In summary, current research on neural mechanisms requires that the tendon tap or a quick manual stretch be viewed as adequate stimuli to much more than the Ia monosynaptic afferents from homonymous muscles. If the discussion of the neural mechanisms associated with hyperreflexia is limited to the segmental mechanisms that result in involuntary muscle activation following a tendon tap, one must recognize that output to the muscle following a percussion input may result from the summation of a host of different inputs including excitatory inputs from Groups Ia and II muscle spindle afferents, inhibitory inputs from interneuronal connections from antagonistic muscle, and presynaptic inhibition initiated by descending fibers. In addition, there

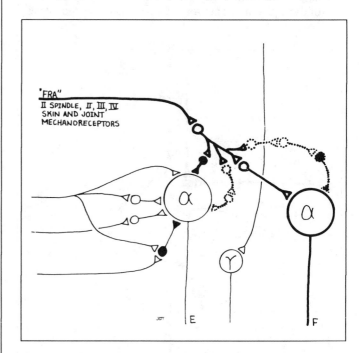

Fig. 16-3. *Illustration including the presence of the flexor reflex afferents (FRA) that have been proposed to account for the clasp-knife phenomenon.[5] The bold lines highlight the principal FRA input to the physiologic extensor that is also the agonist (E) in this case and to the physiologic flexor that is the antagonist (F). Evidence suggests that the pathways indicated by dotted lines may also be present.*

may also be time for the cutaneous afferent input to influence the muscle's response to a tendon tap.[5]

Recognizing that the spinal cord circuitry is more complicated, what model can be used to describe hyperreflexia? Again, 20 years ago, investigators were trying to distinguish between spasticity produced because of an overactive gamma system (gamma spasticity) and that produced because of an overactive alpha motor neuron (alpha spasticity).[11] In today's view of neuronal circuitry the question is if the hyperreflexia results from an abnormal afferent input or from abnormal processing of the afferent input after it reaches the spinal cord.[5]

Although all of the neuronal circuitry has not been examined, what is known provide new insight. For example, there is no evidence in the animal models used to simulate the human upper motor neuron syndrome that demonstrates overactivity of the fusimotor or gamma system.[5,8] Nor is there evidence, at this time, that humans with spasticity are demonstrating hyperreflexia because of excessive spindle activity as measured from Ia afferents.[5] Of course, the assumption is that the absence of excessive spindle activity is indirect proof of overactive fusimotor drive. At this point, most research supports the hypothesis that problems in the spinal cord circuitry (alpha spasticity) rather than problems with the gamma system result in excessive spindle activity. Although it is possible that the alpha motor neurons are altered directly as a result of injury, there is no substantial evidence to support a change in intrinsic membrane properties at this time.[8] It appears that the synaptic input to the motor neurons is changed following injury rather than the intrinsic properties of the alpha motor neurons. Two connections that have

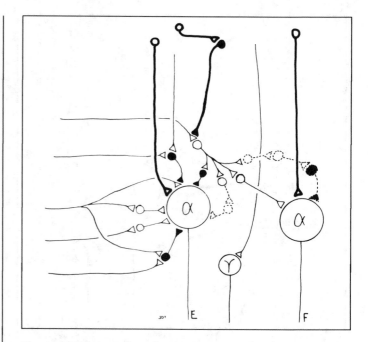

Fig. 16-5. *The neural mechanisms associated with spasticity have become very complex. Compare this illustration to Figure 16-1 to recognize the level of complexity associated with spinal cord circuitry. Additional circuitry not included in the figure are the Renshaw cell and the Ia inhibitory neuron. See text for details.*

been investigated that may alter the monosynaptic reflex pathways are the presynaptic inhibition and the Ia inhibitory neuron.[5]

Presynaptic inhibition to the Ia afferents can be provided by several systems including descending tracts (Fig. 16-4).[5] In the normal nervous system, the CNS can modulate the monosynaptic Ia pathway by the presence of this presynaptic inhibitory connection. Loss of descending input may, therefore, reduce the supraspinal modulation of the monosynaptic pathway and contribute to hyperreflexia.

The Ia inhibitory neuron is the other site with wide ranging influence that may be affected by CNS disease. The Ia inhibitory neuron can be excited by the supraspinal pathways, propriospinal pathways, homonymous groups Ia afferents, and flexion reflex afferents.[5,7,8] It inhibits the antagonistic motoneuron pool. The Ia inhibitory neuron is inhibited by the Renshaw cell. There is evidence in some persons with spasticity that reciprocal inhibition is impaired.[12] For example, the triceps surae has been shown to inhibit reciprocally the tibialis anterior, but the tibialis anterior does not reciprocally inhibit the triceps surae in some of the persons with spasticity. An alcohol injection into the triceps surae motor point, which presumably compromises Ia afferents, produced increased voluntary tension in the tibialis anterior without compromising volitional activity in the triceps surae. Tanaka[12] views this as evidence for disturbed reciprocal innervation.

In summary, during the past 20 years the neural mechanisms associated with spasticity have gone from a neural control model that proposed that spasticity was the result of fusimotor hyperactivity to a recent model where there ap-

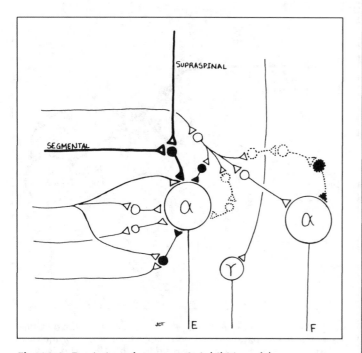

Fig. 16-4. *Depiction of presynaptic inhibition of the monosynaptic Ia muscle spindle input. The bold lines indicate that the presynaptic input can be modulated by supraspinal and peripheral afferent (segmental) input.*

pears to be a disorder in supraspinal and spinal interneuron inhibitory modulation of various pathways (Fig.16-5). Despite the extensive research that remains to be done, the recent model is consistent with a system model for motor control where the spinal cord is viewed as a control site rather than part of the final common pathway controlled by supraspinal input. Many other circuitry connections must be examined before the neural mechanisms and their relationship to spasticity are understood. For example, we must examine the role of the Ib input, the Renshaw cell, and the role of plasticity in contributing to hyperreflexia and hypertonus.

I was compelled for three reasons to address some of the neural mechanisms associated with spasticity despite the conclusion that much more work must be done: 1) any treatment will be some way alter the nervous system and, therefore, we should have an hypothesis or a theoretical framework for the way in which we affect the nervous system; 2) as clinicians who are assuming more responsibility for our patients we must understand the rationale for physician's giving particular drugs or offering particular surgeries; and 3) there is recent evidence to suggest that spasticity may be an indirect rather than a direct effect of injury. If spasticity is the organism's attempt to reorganize, then we need to know if we can maximize it.

VISCOELASTIC PROPERTIES

Mechanisms

Recent investigators have stressed the role that nonneural elements play in the production of muscle tone.[5,8] The viscoelastic changes that occur following CNS injury include changes in the compliance of the muscle andassociated connective tissue in the muscle, tendons, ligaments, and joint structures; changes in muscle fiber properties; and changes in joint alignment. For example, changes in the mechanical-elastic characteristics of muscular and connective tissues are certainly important. Tardieu et al[13] demonstrated that muscle loses sarcomeres rapidly when immobilized in a shortened position, making the muscle less compliant, or stiffer, when tested through its normal range. In this example, an increased resistance to passive movement may be produced by passive elements rather than active elements. What effect do the viscoelastic properties have on functional behavior?

Viscoelastic Properties and Function

Tardieu et al[14] and Dietz and Berger[15] developed models for quantitative analysis of toe-walking, based on the contribution of both the active and passive components of muscle and connective tissue. Tardieu et al[14] examined toe walking in children with cerebral palsy. The total moment developed about the ankle joint during locomotion and the passive moment developed by the ankle in supine posture were assessed. A ratio (R) was used to describe the relationship between the passive moment and the total internal moment. The R gives an indirect measure of the role of muscle activation, which is defined as the active moment. For example, the smaller the R the greater the role played by the neural circuitry and the smaller the role played by the mechanical-elastic components of muscle and connective tissue. The

R value was used to categorize the patients. The healthy subjects who walked on their toes had a lower R value than the same healthy subjects who walked using a heel-toe gait. The model predicts this outcome: more muscle activity is required for toe walking in individuals with intact nervous systems than is required to perform heel-toe walking, hence a lower R value for the healthy toe walkers. The children with cerebral palsy who demonstrated toe walking gait were also divided into two groups: one group demonstrated toe walking primarily because of muscle activity and the other group demonstrated toe walking primarily because of contractures (ie, changes in the passive component of the muscle). Similar findings were reported by Dietz and Berger[15] who studied 54 adults with hemiplegia or incomplete paraplegia and 10 children with cerebral palsy.

Three important points can be made from the results of the studies just cited: 1) the passive component of the muscles can contribute to the resistance the clinician feels when passively stretching a muscle; 2) excessive muscle activity may not produce "classic" postures such as toe walking in cerebral palsy, excessive plantar flexion during stance in head injury, or flexed arm in stroke; and 3) testing of the ankle function in the supine posture may not predict performance of the ankle during the stance phase of gait.

WEAKNESS

Muscle weakness has recently been rediscovered as a factor that may influence the rehabilitation of patients following a CNS injury.[16] The concept of weakness following CNS injury has been reported in the literature, but it has not been a focus of treatment for patients with neurological disorders, during the past 20 years. This is surprising because we have directed so much attention to the positive symptoms proposed by Jackson. Jackson[5(p402)] also listed weakness as one of the direct negative symptoms resulting from CNS injury. Perhaps the ability of the muscle to generate tension was neglected because of the view that hyperreflexia, hypertonia, and abnormal synergy patterns interfered with testing. Has the integrity of the muscle itself changed following injury and does this change affect the person's ability to generate torque in order to move from one position to another?

Neural mechanisms

In persons with intact nervous systems, muscle tension is increased by recruiting additional motor units; increasing the number of large, high threshold motor units; and increasing the firing rate in the already firing units. Weakness may be defined as the inability of the patient to generate normal levels of tension, force, or torque. Reported changes in the muscle tissue suggests that it may not be as "strong" as it was before injury. Individuals with injury secondary to stroke demonstrate atrophy in the remaining muscle units on the paretic side, fast fatigable motor units with increased contraction times, and motor units that are more easily fatigued.[17,18] The loss of motor units and the presence of what appears to be denervated muscle fibers have both been reported in humans.[19] Hypotheses of altered recruitment order and of decreased motor unit firing rates are proposed to account for weakness, but the evidence is still conflicting.[8] Bourbonnais and Vanden Noven[20] recently reviewed the literature that further discusses the mechanisms that may result in the muscle weakness reported following stroke.

Clinical findings

Is weakness present following CNS injury and is there a pattern of weakness? In the late 1890s, Wernicke and Mann[21] reported that the weakest muscles following a stroke were extensors of the upper extremity and flexors in the lower extremity. Muscle testing was qualitative. Several authors have recently quantified the presence of weakness in the upper extremity of patients with stroke.[21,22] The recent findings do not support the earlier work, which had suggested that the extensors were the more severely affected. In recent reports, the most severely affected muscles were hand grip and finger and wrist flexors. Least affected muscles included elbow extensors and shoulder adductors and abductors. It is also important to note that muscles ipsilateral to the lesion also demonstrated weakness compared with control subjects; shoulder adduction and wrist extension were the most involved.

Additional study needs to be completed before a complete picture of weakness following CNS injury is obtained. At this time, however, note that the traditional patterns of weakness immediately following injury are in question and that the uninvolved extremity can also be involved. The relationship between weakness noted during muscle testing and the muscle's ability to generate tension during a functional task needs to be examined. The presence of weakness in an individual muscle is not important by itself; what is important is how or if the weakness affects behavior. Muscle weakness may reduce the capacity of a muscle to generate the torque necessary to maintain posture, to initiate movement at the correct time, or to control movement.

SPASTICITY AND MOVEMENT

What is the relationship between the spasticity identified in the classic neurological test and the behavior seen during functional activity? What roles are changes in the viscoelastic properties and weakness playing during the production of volitional movement? I recognize that many clinicians treat patients who demonstrate hyperreflexia and hypertonia that interfere with such simple tasks as positioning the patient in bed. I do not mean to belittle the relationship between the positive symptoms and function in these cases. I am concerned, however, about the predictive validity of a supine test of hyperreflexia and hypertonus for the behavior demonstrated during the completion of a volitional, functional motor activity.

Giuliani[23] recently reported that a clinician called to ask advice about a motor control problem with the patient. When asked to describe the problem, the clinician reported that the patient had "very severe spasticity in his left leg, moderate spasticity in his right leg, and a lot of hypertonus in his trunk." How does this description assist us in understanding the person's movement behavior? Why did the clinician assume that the problems presented were resulting in abnormal movement? Is there a linear relationship between the Jacksonian positive symptoms and function?

Sahrmann and Norton[24] were among the first investigators to compare the muscle's response to a stretch reflex during passive limb movement with the muscle's response during volitional movement. There was a positive correlation between the severity of biceps hyperreflexia and the speed of rapid, repetitive movements. If analysis stops there, one might assume that the hyperreflexia was responsible for the behavior. But a correlation does not imply cause and effect. Sahrmann and Norton went on to report that the temporal patterns and distribution of electromyographic (EMG) activity during active movement were not produced by antagonistic stretch reflexes. The results of this study suggested, instead, that the slowness of movement was produced by insufficient activation of the agonist. This finding may be an indication that weakness plays a role in generating abnormal motor behavior.

Knutsson and Martensson[25] reported on EMG patterns in 24 patients with spastic paraparesis. The first finding was the marked interindividual difference in motor disability among the patients. Some patients were able to walk several kilometers but others were wheelchair bound. Patient variability was also noted in their inability to develop torque in voluntary isokinetic knee joint extension and flexion. Some patients were unable to perform the movements at one or several of the preselected speeds, and others developed torques within normal limits. A general trend noted, however, was that the majority of patients had more difficulty producing fast rather than slow voluntary movements. Three EMG findings were proposed to account for this response. Some patients did not demonstrate adequate activation of the prime movers. Other patients demonstrated coactivation of agonists and antagonists. A third group of patients demonstrated antagonistic restraint, suggesting facilitation of stretch reflexes.

Watkins et al[26] also used isokinetic testing to assess torque production in the quadriceps and hamstring muscles and found significantly less peak torque in patients with hemiplegia than in healthy subjects. Watkins et al[26] also reported additional motor control problems such as a longer time for the involved muscles to produce tension and a longer interval between reciprocal contractions.

A study recently completed by Bourbonnais et al[27] suggests that there is also spatial selection problem with muscle following CNS injury. Spatial selection is defined as the selection of a muscle to be activated over a broad angular range in a symmetric pattern. Normally, muscle activity increases with increasing force, and the peak of muscle activity is located at the angle of calculated maximum mechanical advantage. For example, normal elbow flexor muscles are activated maximally in the direction of flexion. In the study, persons with spastic paretic limbs did not exhibit the same spatial patterns of muscle activation.[27] The relationship between and the angular range and spatial orientation was disturbed. In the persons with hemiparesis, the biceps brachii showed a substantial shift in the angle of peak EMG, and the muscles were maximally activated 90 degrees or even 135 degrees away from the normal angle.

A criticism of the studies just cited is that the investigators were examining muscle activity in an "artificial," or laboratory, context. Bourbonnais et al,[27] for example, required an abnormal posture of the upper extremity and an isometric contraction to examine the spatial activation of the biceps brachii. Several authors have noted the absence of hyperreflexia during the execution of a functional task despite the presence of hyperreflexia in classic supine testing. Disturbance during quiet standing and ambulation are commonly cited examples.

Dietz and Berger,[28] for example, reported a delayed and reduced agonist EMG response rather than an early unwanted antagonistic response to an unexpected unilateral perturbation during quiet standing in 12 patients with paraparesis and 12 patients with hemiparesis. Badke and Duncan[29] reported several aberrant patterns of muscle activation in adults with hemiplegia including synchronous contraction of several or all lower extremity muscles tested, inconsistent patterns of muscle activation throughout each trial, and distorted sequences of muscle activation.

Knuttson and Richards[30] noted that although some of their patents with spastic hemiparesis showed signs of exaggerated stretch reflexes during ambulation, others demonstrated a muscle pattern dominated by either a paresis of agonists or an abnormal, widespread muscle coactivation.

Summary

Although the variability among patients is high in the studies just cited, a general concept emerges. A lower threshold to stretch (hyperreflexia) was commonly demonstrated during a passive test; the same velocity of stretch imposed on the ankle unexpectedly during quiet standing or voluntarily duringthe stance phase of gait did not evoke the same muscle activity seen during supine testing. The results of the studies just reviewed suggest that there may not be a relationship between hyperreflexia or hypertonia measured during classic static testing and the behavior obtained during a test of functional performance. The results of these studies also suggest the need to consider other factors in producing abnormal motor behavior, such as the two factors discussed above: viscoelastic changes and weakness.

I am not suggesting that the examination of spasticity should be abandoned. At this point, however, it seems necessary, at the very least, to consider the role of spasticity while the patient is attempting to produce a volitional movement of the extremity. For example, the studies just cited suggest that there is an alteration in the time course and spatial selection of EMG activation in agonist and antagonist muscles during volitional activity. The literature suggests that in persons with a stroke the control problems of an individual joint include impaired agonist control and antagonist relaxation. Poorly timed and ineffective simultaneous cocontraction of agonists and antagonists may also occur. Individual muscle factors that impair behavior include the muscle's ability to initiate and terminate activity at the correct time and to develop peak activity at the correct time.

Perhaps it is more useful to describe spasticity as the incorrect timing or spatial activation of the antagonist during a volitional movement. In this contest, spasticity is one of several abnormalities patients may have in selecting the correct muscles and in activating and inactivating them at the correct time. Each of the abnormal activation patterns reviewed above may produce "uncoordinated" motor behavior.

MECHANISM SUMMARY

The factors just examined as contributors to abnormal motor behavior are hyperreflexia, hypertonia, weakness, abnormal spatial and temporal activation and inactivation of muscle activity, and viscoelastic properties. The list is not meant to be comprehensive. There is an obvious lack, for example, of discussion related to sensation, perception, and cognitive ability. What I tried to do is put spasticity in perspective. During the past 20 years, much new knowledge has been gained about the neural mechanisms associated with spasticity. Concomitantly, investigators have come to recognize that other nonneural factors may be just as important in producing abnormal motor behavior.

OUTCOME MEASURES

In going back to the definition of coordinated behavior offered by Delong,[3] it is apparent that persons with CNS injury demonstrate uncoordinated motor behavior. Is this important? The relevant clinical questions are, What is the task, what strategy is the patient using to solve the task, and is the strategy selected the most efficient one? If the strategy is not efficient, what factors should be considered to help the patient solve the problem? Rather than looking for such factors as hyperreflexia andweakness, let us look at the person's ability to perform functional tasks. What is the relationship between abnormal patterns of EMG activation and the ability to perform functional tasks?

In preparing for this presentation, I went back 10 years into some of our often used clinical journals to look for articles that described outcome following injury. The purpose of the search was to discover detailed descriptions of abnormal motor behavior. Instead, I came out of the stacks in the library with articles describing outcomes using classic neurological assessments, biomechanical analysis, or a variety of standardized assessment tools. The problems with such lists of symptoms has already been discussed, so I would like to focus on other outcome measures.

Biomechanical studies

I cannot adequately review the biomechanical literature in this chapter, but I would like to cite several examples to highlight the usefulness and limitations of biomechanical studies. Wall and Turnbull[31] described the walking performance of 25 adults with residual hemiplegia ranging in duration from 18 months to 2 years. The functional ambulators were described as slow and asymmetrical in their performance. The subjects spent a longer time in support on the nonaffected extremity and rushed through support on the affected limb.

Burdett et al[32] quantified the kinematics of lower extremity performance in persons with hemiplegia. The speed of walking was 15% of normal, and step lengths were 37% shorter than normal. The subjects demonstrated a wide base of support and an increased toe-out angle. Footstrike was characterized by decreased hip flexion and excessive knee flexion and ankle plantar flexion. Toe-off was characterized by increased hip flexion and decreased ankle plantar flexion. The hip and knee demonstrated limited flexion and excessive ankle plantar flexion during midswing. There are many other studies that look at other biomechanical variables.[2]

For the most part, the biomechanical studies have been descriptive and, therefore, are useful in characterizing some of the abnormalities in coordination. Such studies, however, are costly and time-consuming; therefore, sample size is often small, and selection criteria are often equipment- specific, limiting the generalizability of the results. Many biomechanical studies focus on outcome and neglect to categorize the patients carefully, using a clinical assessment tool. Readers are therefore not aware of individual variability in performance or the relationship between severity of involvement and biomechanical performance. Another limitation of biomechanical studies is that they are often limited to the laboratory setting rather than being representative of the person's natural environment. Laboratory conditions may produce better than usual behavior or different behavioral strategies that are not seen under more natural conditions. Despite the limitations, developing a careful quantitative description of a person's motor control problems is an exciting avenue that requires further exploration.

Standardized Assessment Tools

The categories of standardized assessment tools include activities of daily living (ADL), instrumental activities of daily living (IADL), assessment of motor function, and multidimensional functional assessment.[33] The difference between ADL and IADL is that ADL activities are involved with self- centered activities, such as hygiene, dressing, and feeding, whereas IADL activities are those in which the person interacts with the environment, such as when performing domestic functions and enjoying leisure time activities.

Many of the examples cited are assessment tools used with persons who sustained strokes, but the list is neither comprehensive for stroke assessment tools nor comprehensive for other neurologic disabilities. The major categories, however, are relevant for outcome studies regardless of disease. Each of the motor assessment tests examines motor function limited to the involved side and balance. Some of the tests, like the Sensorimotor Assessment of Stroke Patients, developed by Fugl-Meyer et al,[34] also assess sensation, joint motion, and pain. Multidimensional tests go beyond the description of physical abilities to include examination of psychosocial sequelae such as social interaction and personal adjustment.

Do any of these tools assist in providing a description of the relationship between abnormal motor behavior and functional ability? Granger et al,[35] for example, described the functional status of patients before the onset of stroke, at rehabilitation admission, at discharge, and at 6 months after discharge. The Barthel Index (BI) was used to evaluate the physical ability of 539 patients; they had an average admission BI score of 37 and a mean discharge BI score of 66. Seventy percent of the patients were discharged to the community, and 68% were still in the community 6 months after discharge. Of the 206 patients discharged with BI scores of 60 or lower, 41% were living in the community 6 months after discharge. Of the 333 patients discharged with BI scores of 61 or higher, 85% were living in the community. The authors also evaluated the impact of the stroke on psychosocial behavior; therefore we can use this study as an example of outcome studies that are multidimensional assess-

ments and not just assessments that look at ADL or IADL. Although this type of study provides much useful information, such as mortality predictions, average length of hospital stay, and final disposition, no insight is gained about the types of motor behavior that were used by patients to achieve their living status. One can speculate that there are both physical and psychosocial reasons why the patients not achieve a perfect BI score of 100. Although the behaviors measured in these types of outcome studies are ultimate goals of treatment, the studies do not provide any insight into the motor strategies that are common, necessary, or successful in performing ADL tasks.

Fugl-Meyer et al [34] and Carr and Shepherd[36] are among the clinicians who have developed motor assessment tests that examine the integrity of motor behavior. The Fugl-Meyer assessment (FMA) used Twitchell's and Brunnstrom's descriptions of sequential stages of motor recovery, following injury, based on a hierarchical model. Carr and Shepherd[36] assumed a systems motor control theory in developing the Motor Assessment Scale (MAS) to measure such functional capabilities as moving from a supine to a sidelying position or from sitting to standing. Both of these assessments assume that there is a specific way to accomplish a task. The FMA is based on sequential recovery and the MAS is based on the theory that there is a stereotyped "normal" approach to solving a motor problem. Although these tests have been shown to be valid and reliable and provide us with a score of a patient's abilities, they do not describe abnormal motor behavior. If the purpose of the assessment is to understand abnormal motor behavior, then the tests just cited do not give the clinician insight into that behavior. Either the FMA or the MAS may be useful in categorizing patients and then determining if patterns of abnormal behavior are associated with different categories. Such research must be done if we are going to understand the abnormalities of motor behavior.

THE GOLD STANDARD

The issue of what is normal or abnormal motor behavior is the final issue to address. What should we use as the "gold standard" by which to evaluate patient's performance? What is normal? This is a very difficult question to pose, and Suzann Campbell addressed some of these issues in her presentation at this conference (see Campbell, this volume). What is our standard? Is normal function our standard? If normal behavior is the standard, when what aspect of normal is of interest? Should tone be normal? Should motor coordination be normal? Should final outcome be normal?

Let us use lower extremity function as example. Should the force generating capability of the muscle be assessed along with passive and active range of motion? If the standard is the normal muscle, then who's normal muscle? Should the normal be standardized for age, height, weight, gender, and activity level? In going form the activity of an individual muscle to the whole limb, the questions are equally confusing and unanswered. What movement patterns should be observed to determine whether a person is demonstrating normal movement? Should the task be functional? Is the speed of movement important? How many trials should be initiated? Should the learning that might take place during the test be considered? How should function be assessed? Is functional assessment measuring the ability to complete a task or the quality of task success?

Clearly, the most common clinical approach to evaluation is to compare the patient's performance to some normal standard. The normal standard is commonly defined as the manner in which an individual with an intact nervous system performs the activity. If the purpose of the assessment is to describe how a patient's performance differs from the normal standard, than an accurate assessment requires that all the differences between the patient's performance and the standard should result from the patient's disability. Factors such as height, weight, age, gender, practice, and speed of movement have to be considered in developing the standard.[2] Ann VanSant suggested that an indication of normal may be the presence of variability in performance or the ability to complete the task using a variety of strategies (see VanSant, this volume). This factor should also be incorporated into the development of the standard.

An investigator who is interested in describing the effect of CNS pathology on the control of movement may legitimately select a normal group for comparison. The use of a normal standard for clinical evaluation of gait, however, may not describe functional deficits. If normal performance is the standard, the scale may not be sensitive enough to detect changes in abnormal function that occur as a result of treatment.

Use of a normal standard may be inappropriate if the goal of treatment is functional ability.[37] For example, gait deviations are often adaptive if the treatment goal is the ability to move from the chair to the sink. The cosmetic appearance of the gait may be irrelevant, and the selection of a normal standard may not help in planning a treatment program. In fact, the patient's progress in achieving a functional gait may be hindered if the treatment is directed at making the patient walk normally rather than at helping the patient solve a problem in the most efficient manner.

Testing conditions are also important, regardless of the standard. If the purpose of the gait evaluation, for example, is to assess the functional limitations in ambulatory ability, gait should be assessed on a variety of surfaces. The conditions under which an assessment is performed will determine whether the assessment describes the person's functional ability.

A major limitation in the current evaluation tools of motor behavior is the lack of appropriate test schemes and reference data. There are a lack of standards that can be used to develop realistic treatment goals.

GENERAL SUMMARY

In moving our thinking from neural mechanisms associated with the production of abnormal movement to muscle strategies used to produce movement and from movement concerns to functional abilities, we still find a lot of unanswered questions about abnormal motor behavior. What is the relationship among all of these areas? If we define coordinated motor behavior as being related to muscle activation, joint sequencing, and torque production, which muscles and joints should be examined? Is it appropriate to discuss a muscle pattern when only a few muscles about the joint are as-

sessed? If an experiment requires a certain level of performance, can we generalize the findings to include the responses of patients who must be excluded from the test? If experiments are time consuming and costly and therefore are done with a small sample, how "generalizable" is the outcome? Does the knowledge of abnormal patterns of muscle activation and inactivation serve as a good tool or treatment planning? It appears that we still have many more questions than we have answers. I do not think that we have enough evidence to discard one theory and embrace another, nor do I think that we have enough evidence to suggest that there is an optimal way to define or, let alone, assess abnormal motor behavior. However, the work during the past 20 years has increased the number of theories and the number of tools available to test the propositions associated with the theories of motor control. So now our challenge is to get on with it.

References

1. Greenspan B, Stineman M. Multiple sclerosis and rehabilitation outcome. *Arch Phys Med Rehabil.* 1987;68:434-437.
2. Craik RL, Oatis CA. Gait assessment in the clinic: issues and approaches. In: Rothstein JM, ed. *Clinics in Physical Therapy: Measurement in Physical Therapy.* New York, NY: Churchill Livingstone Inc; 1985;47:169- 206.
3. DeLong M. Central patterning of movement. *Neurosciences Research Program Bulletin.* 1972;9:10-30.
4. Landau WM. Spasticity: the fable of a neurological demon and the emperor's new therapy. *Arch Neurol.* 1974;31:218-219.
5. Burke D. Spasticity as an adaptation to pyramidal tract injury. In Waxman SG, ed. *Advances in Neurology: Functional Recovery in Neurological Disease.* New York, NY: Raven Press; 1988; 47:401-423.
6. Siegler EL, Beck LH. Stiffness: a pathophysiologic approach to diagnosis and treatment. *J Gen Intern Med.* 1989;4:533-540.
7. An exploratory and analytical survey of therapeutic exercises: proceedings of Northwestern University Special Therapeutic Exercise Project. *Am J Phys Med. 1967;46:9-1135.*
8. Katz RT, Rymer WZ. Spastic hypertonia: mechanisms and measurement. *Arch Phys Med Rehabil.* 1989;70:144-155.
9. Schomburg ED. Spinal sensorimotor systems and their supraspinal control. *Neurosci Res.* 1990;7:265-340.
10. Burke D, McKeon B, Skuse NF. The irrelevance of fusimotor activity to Achilles tendon of relaxed humans. *Ann Neurol.* 1981;10:547- 550.
11. Drachman DA. Disorders of tone. *Am J Phys Med.* 1967;46:525- 535.
12. Tanaka R. Reciprocal Ia inhibitory pathway in normal man and in patients with motor disorders. In: Desmedt JE, ed. *Motor Control Mechanisms in Health and Disease.* New York, NY: Raven Press; 1984:433-441.
13. Tardieu C, Lespargot A, Tarbary C, et al. For how long must the soleus muscle be stretched each day to prevent contracture? *Dev Med Child Neurol.* 1988;30:3-10.
14. Tardieu C, Lespargot A, Bret MD. Toe-walking in children with cerebral palsy: contributions of contracture and excessive contraction of triceps surae muscle. *Phys Ther.* 1989;69:556-662.
15. Dietz V, Berger W. Normal and impaired regulation of muscle stiffness in gait: a new hypothesis about muscle hypertonia. *Exp Neurol.* 1983;79:680-687.

16. Duncan PW, Badke MB, *Stroke rehabilitation: the recovery of motor control*. Chicago, Ill: Year Book Medical Publishers Inc; 1987.

17. Edstrom L, Grimby L, Hannerz J. Correlation between recruitment order of motor units and muscle atrophy pattern in upper motoneurone lesion: significance of spasticity. *Experimentia*. 1973;29:560-561.

18. Dietz V, Ketelsen UP, Berger W, Quintern E. Motor unit involvement in spastic paresis: relationship between leg muscle activation and histochemistry. *J Neurol Sci*. l986;75:89-103.

19. Spaans F, Wilts G. Denervation due to lesions of the central nervous system. *J Neurol Sci*. 1982;57:291-305.

20. Bourbonnais D, Vanden Noven S. Weakness in patients with hemiparesis. *Am J Occup Ther*. 1989;43:313-319.

21. Colebatch JG, Gandevia SC. The distribution of muscular weakness in uppermotor neuron lesions affecting the arm. *Brain*. 1989;112:749-763.

22. Bohannon RW, Smith MB. Assessment of strength deficits in eight paretic upper extremity muscle groups of stroke patients with hemiplegia. *Phys Ther*. 1987;67:522-525.

23. Giuliani CA. Should we measure spasticity, tone and other ugly terms? In: *Proceedings of the Forum on Neurological Physical Therapy Assessment*. Alexandria, Va: Neurology Section, American Physical Therapy Association; 1990.

24. Sahrmann SA, Norton BJ. The relationship of voluntary movement to spasticity in the upper motor neuron syndrome. *Ann Neurol*. 1977;2:460-465.

25. Knutsson E, Martensson A. Dynamic motor capacity in spastic paresis and its relationship to prime motor disfunction, spastic reflexes and antagonistic coactivation. *Scand J Rehab Med*. 1980;12:93-106.

26. Watkins MP, Harris BA, Kozlowski BA. Isokinetic testing in patients with hemiparesis: a pilot study. *Phys Ther*. 1984;64:184-189.

27. Bourbonnais D. Vanden Noven S, Carey KM, Rymer WZ. Abnormal spatial patterns of elbow activation in hemiparetic human subjects. *Brain*. 1989;112:85-102.

28. Dietz V, Berger W. Interlimb coordination of posture in patients with spastic paresis: imperial functions of spinal reflexes. *Brain*. 1984;107:965-978.

29. Badke MB, Duncan PW. Patterns of rapid motor response during postural adjustment when sitting in healthy subjects and hemiplegic patients. *Phys Ther*. 1983;63:13-20.

30. Knutsson E, Richards C. Different types of disturbed motor control in gait of the hemiparetic patients. *Brain*. 1979;102:405-430.

31. Wall JC, Turbull GI. Gait asymmetries in residual hemiplegia. *Arch Phys Med Rehabil*. 1986;67:550-553.

32. Burdett RG, Borello-France D, Blatchly C, Potter C. Gait comparison of subjects with hemiplegic walking unbraced, with ankle-foot orthosis, and with air-stirrup brace. *Phys Ther*. 1988;68:1197-1203.

33. Lindmark B. *Evaluation of Functional Capacity after Stroke with Special Emphasis on Motor Function and Activities of Daily Living*. Uppsula, Sweden: University of Uppsula; 1988. Dissertation in ACTA Universitatis Uppsaliensis, vol 174: Comprehensive Summaries of Uppsula Dissertations from the Faculty of Medicine. Uppsala, Sweden: University of Uppssula; 1988.

34. Fugl-Meyer AR, Jaasko L, Leymen I, et al. The post-stroke hemiplegic patient. *Scand J Rehabil Med*. 1975;7:13-31.

35. Granger CV, Hamilton BB, Gresham GE. The stroke rehabilitation outcome study: I. General Description. *Arch Phys Med Rehabil*. l988;69:506-509.

36. Carr JH, Shepherd RB. A motor learning model for rehabilitation. In: Carr JH, Shepherd RB, Gordon J, et al, eds. *Movement Science: Foundations for Physical Therapy Rehabilitation*. Rockville, Md: Aspen Publishers Inc; 1987:31-92.

37. Holden MK, Gill KM, Magliozzi MR. Gait assessment for neurologically impaired patients: standards for outcome assessment. *Phys Ther*. 1986;66:1530-1539.

Chapter 17

Recovery Processes: Maximizing Function

Rebecca L. Craik, PhD, PT
Associate Professor
Department of Physical Therapy
Beaver College
Glennside, PA 19038
Adjunct Assistant Professor
School of Veterinary Medicine
University Of Pennsylvania

Research efforts have increased to identify both central nervous system (CNS) and behavioral changes following CNS injury. The findings suggest that classical theories of CNS function may no longer be appropriate. Although there are still very few clinical studies documenting change in behavior following injury, the basic science research proposes that the mammalian nervous system is capable of reorganization following injury. The purpose of this presentation is to review some of the evidence for plasticity following injury and to discuss some of the factors that may influence recovery.

Plasticity is an abused term. The dictionary defines plasticity as the capacity to change.[1] Neuroanatomists define plasticity as the presence of morphological evidence of an altered state of organization. Electrophysiologists define plasticity as a change in the efficiency of a synapse. Biologists use the word mutability to describe change in a muscle fiber or some component of the fiber. Psychologists define plasticity as the ability of the animal to respond in a new way. Clinicians use the term behavioral plasticity when the patient demonstrates acquisition of performance following injury. The most appropriate definitions of plasticity relate to the anatomical and electrophysiological changes in the CNS following injury.[2] Clinicians cannot see plasticity, but they can observe the effect of plasticity or changes in function.

This presentation will be divided into two parts. In the first half, some of the literature that describes plastic changes within the CNS following injury will be reviewed. In the latter part of the presentation, other factors that may influence recovery of function will be discussed.

NEURAL CONTROL MODEL

Most of the knowledge about the nervous system has been derived from experiments in animals. The classic way in which experiments were done was to produce an experimental lesion and to examine the result. Neuroanatomists followed anterograde and retrograde degeneration to formulate tracts. Physiologists recorded electrical activity from immobilized, lesioned, and anesthetized animals. Behaviorists looked at the residual behavior following injury and ascribed a function to the tissue that had been lesioned. The experiments led to the development of a hierarchical model for nervous system function. The hierarchical model was often coupled with the concept of localization of function.[3] The theory associated with localization of function is that the brain can be viewed as a collection of organs, each with its own functional assignment. This model provides a nervous system that is very rigid after maturation. In 1928, Cajal[4] (p49) went on to impose further constraint on the nervous system's flexibility by concluding that nerve pathways are fixed and immutable following maturation. He stated that everything can die within the CNS and that nothing can regenerate. A model of the nervous system that includes hierarchical control, localization of function, and lack of regeneration does not provide a dynamic framework to explore mechanisms that could account for recovery of function.

The distributive control model (system model) provides a view of a nervous system that offers 1) numerous reciprocal connections both between and within levels of the nervous system, 2) information and motor commands that flow in all directions not just from the top down, 3) function that is not assigned to a single area but is viewed as a cooperative effort among regions of the nervous system, and 4) a site of control that differs depending on the task to be executed.[5] Some of the most dramatic suggestions of the nervous system's ability to reorganize have been demonstrated in the somatosensory cortex.[6] In studies using neonatal and adult mammalian models, such as primate, cat, raccoon, and rat, it has been shown by different laboratories that the cortical somatosensory map organization can be modified at all times between conception and death. For example, following amputation of a digit in adult monkey or raccoon, the deafferented portion of the cortical map is "filled in" by adjacent digit representations. Surrounding digit representations become larger. This electrophysiological evidence suggests that more neurons over a larger cortical area are processing sensory information from the remaining digits, which results in improved tactile acuity. If we adopt a dynamic model of CNS activity, then rather than assigning function to the lesioned part and talking about symptoms produced by the lesion we should be concerned with what the rest of the nervous system does following injury.[7] The focus is, therefore,

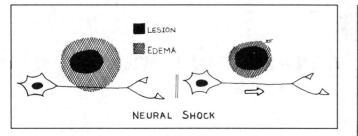

Fig. 17-1. *Depiction of recovery of synaptic effectiveness. On the left, edema blocks conduction through the axon. The right figure depicts resolution of the edema that should allow nerve conduction to resume. (Modified from FitzGerald.)*

away from the lesion site and onto the capabilities of intact structures.

PLASTICITY

A distributive neural control model provides a more optimistic view of the nervous system's capacity to reorganize following injury. Research in a number of different laboratories suggest that there are, in fact, a variety of events occurring within the mammalian nervous system following injury. This review will address some of the mechanisms. Recognize, however, that no single mechanism has been proposed to account for return of all function following injury. Laboratories have to focus attention on one mechanism. If these single mechanisms are occurring in the human nervous system following injury, they may be occurring collectively to account for recovery.

Neural Shock Resolution

Von Monakow[8] defined *diaschisis* as the temporary disruption of function affecting neuronal processes far from the site of the lesion. Damage to the nervous system deprives other intact regions of normal afferent inflow that had previously come from the injured area. The result is that symptoms are produced from the intact as well as the injured areas. The resolution of diaschisis may therefore be used to account for some of the return of function following injury. If the intact areas recover from loss of some afferent input, symptoms produced because of disruption in the intact areas will dissipate. The resolution of diaschisis does not account for losses that result from destroying neurons or for compensatory responses for such losses. *Neural shock* is a term that includes diaschisis and synaptic effectiveness.[9]

Recovery of Synaptic Effectiveness

This concept is very similar to the concept of diaschisis except that the neurons that are compromised are directly affected at the site of the lesion rather than indirectly affected by loss of some afferent input.[9] Edema at the injury site, for example, may compress axons and produce a physiological block in conduction (Fig. 17-1). Blood supply to neurons may be disrupted temporarily and result in loss of function. Timely reduction of the edema or restoration of blood supply will restore some lost function.

The term *neural shock* is more commonly used today to include the concept of temporary injury to intact areas in the CNS. Resolution of neural shock is often used to explain

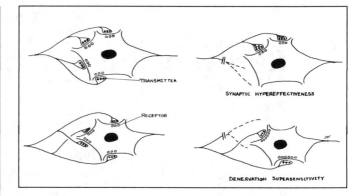

Fig. 17-2. *Synaptic hypereffectiveness: the two figures at the top. Upper left figure depicts the intact state in which neurotransmitter is released from axon terminals (terminal boutons). Upper right figure depicts an increase in neurotransmitter in the remaining boutons. Denervation sensitivity: the two figures at the bottom. Lower left figure depicts the target cell receiving four terminal boutons. The lower right figure depicts the postsynaptic membrane becoming more sensitive to the reduced supply of neurotransmitter. (Modified from FitzGerald.)*

the return of tone in an initially flaccid paralysis. Very little research has been done to confirm the relationship between neural shock and functional behavior. Glassman[10] demonstrated that gradual recovery from punctate lesions in the primary sensory-motor cortex that abolished a conditioned response in cat correlated with the return of normal sensory evoked potentials. Additional work must be done to confirm or reject the concept.

Synaptic Hypereffectiveness

The theory about recovery resulting from synaptic hypereffectiveness grew out of work in the peripheral nervous system.[11] Partial denervation was originally proposed to produce an increased release of acetylcholine from remaining efferent fibers in skeletal muscle fiber. It was subsequently discovered that changes in the postsynaptic membrane accounted for the heightened sensitivity to acetylcholine. Evidence for presynaptic hypereffectiveness in the CNS also is lacking at this time.

Denervation Supersensitivy

Although the theory of synaptic hypereffectiveness suggested change in remaining presynaptic fibers, denervation supersensitivity is viewed as a postsynaptic phenomenon.[11,12] Again, this theory derives from research done in the peripheral nervous system. Additional specific receptors in the postsynaptic membrane are proposed to appear to respond to the neurotransmitter that is released (Fig. 17-2). The postsynaptic membrane will increase its reactivity to a released neurotransmitter. This phenomenon has been observed in the mammalian nervous system. One of the problems in Parkinson's disease is that neurons producing dopamine are lost in the substantia nigra. The neurons within the striatum that are deprived of input become "more sensitive" to the dopamine released from the remaining fibers. The enhanced sensitivity that may be produced through the denervation supersensitivity may therefore account for some of the recovery. Immediately following the injury function is lost because the system is unable to generate action potentials in its partially denervated state. Increasing the number of receptors or increasing of the responsiveness of the remaining receptors may then allow the limited input to drive the postsynaptic cell and produce a function.

Persistence of Hyperinnervation

During maturation, the brain overproduces neurons, possibly twice as many as needed.[13] If one subscribes to the theory that the elements in the nervous system are committed to specific functions early in life and that synaptic connections are genetically programmed, then the presence of hyperinnervation would imply that the extra neurons would die. If, on the other hand, one subscribes to a more dynamic view of synaptic organization, then the presence of hyperinnervation may assist in the recovery of injury for the younger mammal. There is evidence using young animal models that two recovery mechanisms may occur because of the hyperinnervation: 1) axons may not follow the maturational "order" to retract in the presence of injury and 2) growing axons may reroute to a different location in the presence of injury.[13,14] I will give a specific example of this later. There is no indication at this time whether this phenomenon is limited to maturing nervous systems.

Recruitment of Silent Synapses

The concept of either silent synapses or latent pathways is becoming more than a theory (Fig. 17-3). The best known work is by Berman and Sterling[15] and Kratz et al.[16] Kittens had one eye sutured shut for 4 months. The sutures were removed and recordings from the occipital cortex indicated that only 10% of the neurons responded to light. Normally, 80% of the neurons respond to a light stimulus. The

good eye was surgically removed, which resulted in an immediate increase (40% of the neurons responded) in the occipital cortex cells associated with the previously sutured eye. This type of research suggests that functional connections were present but were masked under normal conditions.

Sprouting

Although there is evidence for axonal regeneration in mammalian nervous system, the amount of regeneration is limited. Most research in the area of sprouting cites growth of axonal branches following injury.[12] *Regenerative sprouting* occurs when the cut axon responds by issuing side-branches (Figs. 17-4A and B). *Collateral sprouting*, or reactive synaptogenesis, occurs when side branches from nearby uninjured axons are produced and have synapses at sites vacated by injured axons. Liu and Chambers[17] reported collateral sprouting in 1958, and a myriad of researchers have confirmed this earlier finding. The sprouting has been reported to begin between 4 days and 2 weeks following injury.

Vicarious Function

Vicarious function does not relate to actual neuronal changes but to behavioral outcomes following injury. Vicarious function theory assumes that functions attributed to the damaged portion of the nervous system can be taken over by areas not previously concerned with that function.[18] Function lost to unilateral cortical damage, for example, would be assumed by the undamaged homologous structure on the other side of the brain, by uninjured areas on the same side, or by a brain stem region. Proponents of localization of func-

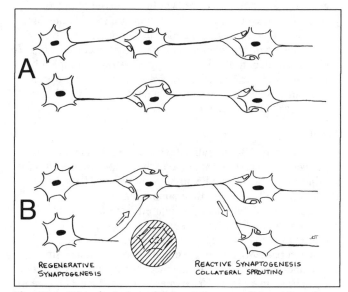

Fig. 17-4. *(A) is depiction of the preinjury condition. Note the two pathways and the presence of three neurons in each pathway. (B) illustrates how regenerative and reactive synaptogenesis may compensate for the injury. Regenerative sprouting is depicted by the extension of the left axon to connect to a new site following degeneration of the original target cell. Reactive synaptogenesis is depicted by the uninjured neuron providing collaterals to supply the neuron deprived of some of its input. (Modified from FitzGerald.)*

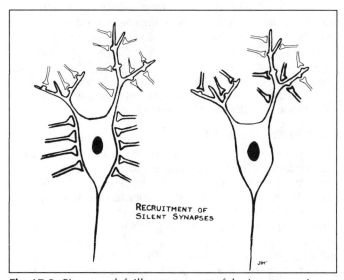

Fig. 17-3. *Figure on left illustrates some of the input to an intact neuron. The terminal boutons located close to the axon hillock have degenerated secondary to injury. The theory of recruiting silent synapses suggests that the terminal boutons may be more functional.*

tion have difficulty with the concept of vicarious function. The original definition of *vicariation* suggests that the recovered behavior should be identical to the behavior lost because of injury.[19] In their discussion of vicarious function, Slavin et al[18] argue that recovery of identical behavior is too strict a criterion and certainly depends on the precision of the assessment. Slavin et al[18] propose that vicariation may be the appropriate "umbrella" term to encompass all of the neural mechanisms that occur following injury. In this context, vicariation assumes that loss of function will occur following brain damage and that the nervous system has the capacity to develop alternative strategies that may lead to recovery. The alternative strategies may occur because of such factors as recruitment of silent synapses and persistence of hyperrinnervation. The original definition of vicarious function assumes recovery of identical behavior; the definition offered by Slavin et al[18] is broader in scope and does not limit improvement to recovery of identical behavior. Because the two definitions of vicarious function lead to different outcome expectations, it is important to know which definition of vicarious function is used by an author when reading the literature.

Compensation

Compensation, or behavioral substitution, is another outcome-based theory that proposes that the person solves the problem in a different way than was done before injury.[12] Alternative behavioral strategies are adopted to complete the task. Compensation may occur because different receptors and muscles and new strategies are adopted by the damaged system to perform the task.

The difference between the original definitions of vicariation and compensation was in the recovery outcome produced following injury. Vicariation assumed that undamaged tissue could produce the identical behavior demonstrated before injury whereas compensation occurred when the task was accomplished successfully using a completely different motor strategy.[19] If the reader adopts the proposal by Slavin et al,[18] compensation would be one of the descriptors under the umbrella term of vicariation.

Summary

As I stated at the outset, each of the mechanisms just reviewed may account for some of the change that occurs following injury. It should be obvious, however, that there is evidence for plasticity in the mammalian nervous system and that Cajal's statement that injured neurons can only die must be modified. Although some of the research has attempted to relate a change in a neural mechanism to a change in behavior, the experiments have not demonstrated cause and effect. Several of the mechanisms just discussed may operate in synergy, for example, to produce a change in behavior.

Although there is no evidence that interrelates the anatomical and physiologic changes that follow injury, it is tempting to speculate how the various mechanisms may relate. For example, initial recovery of function may result from the resolution of neural shock at the injured site; additional recovery of function may occur if denervation supersensitivity enhances the neural environment for recruitment

of silent synapses and reactive or regenerative synaptogenesis at the sites of injury. Change in behavior may also occur secondary to compensation. As suggested by Slavin et al,[18] the processes may be described collectively as vicariation. Much additional work must be done before we have an understanding of the capacity of the mammalian nervous system and particularly the human nervous system.

It is important to recognize that the plastic changes may result in maladaptive behavior as well as adaptive behavior.[12] Perhaps spasticity, for example, is the result of reactive synaptogenesis as peripheral sensory afferents fill the vacant synaptic sites occupied by degenerating supraspinal input. The plasticity literature certainly leads one to question the Jacksonian concept of positive and negative symptoms being direct effects of injury. The positive and negative symptoms may be the result of CNS reorganization that occurs following the injury.[7]

The research to date on plasticity supports the hypothesis that the CNS is an extremely dynamic system. In a theoretical paper, Finger and Almli[20] suggest that such events as sprouting and supersensitivity have nothing to do with the nervous system's attempt to recover or to obtain improved behavior. Finger and Almli[20] suggest that improved behavior may be either a lucky event or an "epiphenomenon." An alternative theory is that neural reorganization is an ongoing process in the normal nervous system and that it is a coincidence when the normal processes assist recovery in the normal brain. This hypothesis gains support in light of the following observations: 1) the variability in the behavior seen following injury and 2) the suggestion that the neural recovery mechanisms may lead to both adaptive and maladaptive behavior. The variability in functional outcome despite similar location and extent of a lesion has been accounted for by such factors as prelesion experience, genetic endowment, and motivation. Some of the variability may also be attributed to the type and level of plasticity.

Although research to date on plasticity raises more questions than provides answers, the research supports the hypothesis that the CNS is dynamic andcapable of restoring and reorganizing. More recent work is focused on identifying CNS processes that retard, prevent, or further injure the neuron's plastic ability. I always leave this literature incredibly excited and optimistic about our future ability to maximize recovery following CNS injury.

RECOVERY OF FUNCTION

Attention has been focused on the neural mechanisms that account for behavioral changes following injury, without a definition for recovery having been provided. Clinicians who have spent time with patients having neurological disorders can readily cite anecdotes about patients who demonstrated improvement following CNS injury. Almli and Finger[12] cite three examples. The first example is the 1-year-old infant who suffers damage to Broca's speech area and goes on to develop normal speech. The second example is the adult who sustains head trauma and demonstrates gross memory deficits for several days but goes on to have apparently normal cognitive processes. The third example is an adult who sustains a massive left cerebrovascular accident but goes on to learn to write with his left hand and become independent in the use of a wheelchair. The three examples provide insight into the complications associated with defining improvement.

Le Vere et al[12] define *recovery* as a complete regaining of identical functions that were lost or impaired after brain damage. Such a precise definition of recovery allows discrimination among the terms recovery, sparing of function, and compensation of function.

Sparing of function occurs when behavioral deficits are not found after brain injury.[12] Sparing differs from recovery because recovery requires the loss of function after injury. Therefore, the child who demonstrated normal language ability following brain damage demonstrated sparing of function.

Compensation of function, or behavioral substitution, also is different from our definition of recovery of function.[12] Compensation occurs when the individual is able to accomplish the goal using a different strategy. The example cited above of the patient with the stroke illustrates compensation. The man was able to write by substituting the use of his left hand for his right hand.

Therefore, to demonstrate recovery of function using the Le Vere et al[12] definition, the following conditions must be met: 1) there has to be an initial deficit and 2) the behavior that is returned must be identical to the one that is lost. The very careful clinical description, by the clinician, of behavior following CNS injury will allow the scientist to gain a better understanding of what the human nervous system is capable of doing following injury. Currently there is sufficient anecdotal evidence to suggest that all three behavioral outcomes occur in the human. It is certainly probable that each of the three phenomenon occur in patients; it would not be surprising if the three phenomenon were present for three different behaviors within the same individual. It is important, however, when reading the literature on plasticity or recovery to understand the author's definition of improvement following injury.

NONPLASTIC FACTORS THAT INFLUENCE RECOVERY

Since recovery of function has been demonstrated in humans and in animal models, a whole myriad of new questions are being addressed. Many factors influencing behavior and recovery of behavior following injury including genetic endowment, past experience, motivation to learn, and health of the body at the time of injury. I would like to focus on additional factors. For example, Will the age of the individual or the animal effect CNS reorganization? Does the entire nervous system respond the same way to injury? Does the extent of the lesion or the rapidity of the insult affect CNS reorganization? And finally, What are the behavioral consequences of these biological phenomena?

Age

A long-established observation is that a CNS injury sustained in infancy often produces fewer and less severe aftereffects than does the same lesion in a mature nervous system. For example, studies on the ability of rats to solve maze problems have shown that 7% cortical ablation in the adult is equivalent to a 50% ablation in a young rat.[21] Kennard[22] focused attention, in the 1930s, to the age factor with her ex-

periments on monkeys. She removed the motor cortex and found that younger animals were able to walk, climb, feed, and demonstrate prehension while older monkeys were unable to perform the tasks.

This sparing of function, which is most often cited in the human, is related to the language example cited above. When the dominant hemisphere sustains damage in persons older than 12 years of age there is usually aphasia in varying degrees of severity.[9] But when injury occurs to the child who is less than 2 years of age, speech and understanding of speech appear untouched.

The Kennard principle has been questioned in light of recent work, which I will briefly review. Schneider's[14] research illustrates some of the observations that have been made about the effect of age on recovery. Schneider selected the golden hamster as the animal model in his study because its nervous system at birth is equivalent to the nervous system of a human fetus at 3 months of age. Use of this animal, therefore, allows one to study early developmental events without having to perform in utero experiments. The animal reaches maturity at 3 months of age. The neonatal animals, with larger lesions than adult animals, demonstrated the presence of visual pattern discrimination in tasks in the presence of bilateral occipital cortex or superior colliculus lesions. Although the neonates demonstrated some impaired function, they were still able to perform the visual tasks while the adults were unable to perform the task. Morphology in the neonates indicated an alternative pathway involving the superior colliculus and pulvinar. The extent of spared behavior in the neonates correlated with the sparing of behavior. These results suggest that both the cortex and subcortical structures are capable of effectively reorganizing following neonatal injury. Two additional findings are worthy of note, however. If one superior colliculus was lesioned instead of both, the neonatal animals demonstrated maladaptive behavior: they reached to the visual cue in the wrong direction. Although the neonates demonstrated a degree of sparing in visual discrimination ability, they demonstrated a retarded ability to perform an instrumental learning task such as opening a door to get water. The adults, on the other hand, demonstrated no difficulty with this task. The results of these and other studies raise questions about the Kennard principle.

The loss of other functions to spare such functions as speech has been demonstrated in children. Woods[23] found that the IQs of children with spared speech following brain damage in the first year of life were well below average and below those of children who suffered brain damage later in life. Milner[24] also suggested depressed or retarded cognitive development in children who had demonstrated spared speech following injury. The preservation of one function and compromise of other functions suggests that a crowding effect may be produced. When a function is spared, careful evaluation of other behaviors must be completed in children when spared function is demonstrated. Research to date has, therefore, qualified the significance of age-related variables; perhaps function is spared in young individuals but function may be spared at the cost of compromising some other behavior.

Another variable that must be considered in relation to the apparent "better" recovery in the young is the postinjury time. Goldman[25] reported that ablation of the dorsolateral frontal cortex spared performance in the young animals on a delayed response task, but the deficit was present when the infants were retested as adults. In this case, the animals grew into the lesion. A possible explanation for this finding is that the insult occurred before that function was served by that cortical region; in infancy some other part of the nervous system may have assumed the control. This has also been demonstrated in human infants who have cortical lesions that produce hemiparesis in adults. Initially, the children show no apparent motor damage for at least 3 months. When the child begins to walk, spasticity, abnormal reflexes, and uncoordinated movements emerge.

The opposite case has also been reported; that is, deficits seen immediately after brain injury recede as the subject grows older. Goldman[25] reported that lesions to the orbital prefrontal cortex initially caused severe impairments on a delayed alternation task, but the impairments disappeared with maturation. This finding suggests that the animals grew out of the lesion.

Therefore, when considering the effect of age on recovery, several variables must be taken into account: 1) the area of the brain where the injury has occurred (eg, sparing is usually less in subcortical regions), 2) the maturity of the brain region rather than the age of the individual, 3) the task that is being assessed, 4) the time following insult, and 5) the loss of other behaviors.

These studies again demonstrate the dynamic capacity of the CNS and stress the need to evaluate more than the behavior you assume is allocated to a specific region and to follow-up the children who have apparently demonstrated spared function.

Nature of the Lesion

The clinical observation has often been made that slow growing lesions such as tumors produce less profound effect than a sudden insult such as a gunshot wound or a stroke.[26] Dax[26(p154)] reported in 1836 that aphasia did not accompany temporal lobe tumors that had reached the size of sudden insults. Jackson[26(p155)] talked about the effect of momentum (mass times velocity) on sparing of function following lesions and used the example of hemorrhage versus a tumor. The other observation is that slow growing lesions produce more permanent, immutable changes than occurs following a sudden insult.

Slow growing lesions have been studied under laboratory conditions by analyzing the effect of serial lesion. A small lesion is made, the animal is allowed to recover, then the lesion is enlarged, and so on. Travis and Woolsey[27] reported that a one stage lesion to Brodman's areas 4 and 6 resulted in animals that were immobilized on the bottom of the cage whereas the same size lesion produced under serial conditions resulted in an animal that had no difficulty righting itself, feeding, and walking; function was spared.

One can speculate on the mechanisms that may produce these outcomes, mechanisms such as axonal sprouting, less transneuronal damage, less scarring, and time for rerouting pathways. There is no single theory to account for this behavior at this time. This uncertainty may explain some of the variability seen in patients who have the same functional

diagnosis but demonstrate a wide variety of behavioral abilities.

Experiential Factors

The experiential factors addressed will be limited to the effects of environment, pharmacological treatment, and treatment on recovery following CNS injury.

Environment. The question of the effect of the person's environment on recovery raises the age-old question of "nature versus nurture." Research in psychology literature suggests that an enriched environment leads to improved performance.[28] Much of this work has been done using rats. A nonspecific enriched environment includes social housing (more than one rat per cage), areas for the animals to climb, and objects for the animals to manipulate. A deprived environment is one in which the animal lives alone in a regular-sized cage that has litter, food, and water. Increased maze performance has been demonstrated by animals living in an enriched environment. Morphological changes are reported to accompany this improved behavior, changes such as an increase in the amount of dendritic spines, larger synaptic boutons, an increased protein synthesis, and an increase in brain weight.

Human infants provided with mobiles over their cribs and brightly colored and patterned sheets were reported to demonstrate visual reaching 45 days before children who were not exposed to similar visual stimuli.[29]

Such studies have raised much controversy that is yet to be resolved. For example, will early development of skills develop a plateau so that the "deprived" subjects will catch up? Will early enrichment lead to "crowding out" of other cognitive functions?

Held et al[30] conducted an experiment that raises additional issues for our consideration. Six groups of rats were used in the experiment: rats that lived in enriched environments before and after surgery, animals that lived in impoverished environments before and after surgery, animals that lived under each of the above conditions but underwent sham surgery, animals that lived in enriched conditions before surgery but in impoverished conditions after surgery, and animals that lived in impoverished conditions before surgery but in enriched conditions after surgery. The surgery involved removal of primary motor cortex. Held et al[30] assessed the time that it took the animals to run on a beam, and they also measured the kinematics of the hind limb. The animals who had lived in enriched environments demonstrated no deficit in running time while the impoverished animals demonstrated a slower running time. The animals that were only enriched preoperatively ran better than the animals who were only enriched postoperatively. Using the presurgical kinematic data as a control, the preoperatively enriched-postoperatively enriched animals and the sham animals demonstrated restitution of function. All other animals demonstrated substitution of function.

Studies such as this raise additional questions. Do particular preinjury experiences protect or in some way enrich the nervous system so that injury is not as profound? Does postlesion nonspecific enrichment enhance recovery? Did the enriched environment encourage active participation that might not otherwise have occurred? The literature on nonspe-

Contemporary Management of Motor Problems

cific enrichment suggest that it might enhance the general adaptive capacity of the individual. Much more work needs to be done in this area.

Pharmacologic intervention. Twenty years ago, it was apparent that the scientists working in drug companies had accepted the doctrine of Cajal and believed that the damaged CNS was incapable of recovery following injury. The drugs available to treat patients were directed at calming the overactive nervous system or resolving some of the positive symptoms such as spasticity. Antispasticity drugs were the primary focus of treatment at that time.

In the past 10 years there has been a dramatic change in this area of research. Research on pharmacologic intervention is directed toward enhancing the environment for possible reorganization or, at least, retarding unnecessary additional destruction.

Fetal tissue transplants have been used to stimulate regeneration in a damaged nervous system or to replace lost cells. Research in fetal tissue transplant has gone beyond the animal model and has been used in humans with Parkinson's disease.[31] The concern about fetal tissue transplants ranges from ethical concerns related to the use of aborted tissue to the long-term viability of the transplanted tissue. For example, very recent data suggest that transplants may never develop a normal blood-brain barrier to circulating blood borne molecules.[31] This means that systemic substances could enter the brain through the grafts and be potentially dangerous. Hormones and steroids could, for example, penetrate the brain more freely and accelerate degenerative processes. Fetal tissue can grow so extensively in the presence of estrogen that the fetal tissue can act as a space occupying tumor.

Spinal transplants of neurons secreting various neurotransmitters have had limited but promising outcomes. Serotonergic implants in spinalized animals can aid in achieving recovery of sexual reflexes.[32] Noradrenergic implants in spinalized animals are capable of inducing a rhythmic activity in the hindlimbs similar to locomotion.[33]

Fetal tissue transplants may prove to be only an intermediate step in pursuit of the final solution.[31] If the neurochemicals responsible for the neurotrophic changes can be isolated from neurons and glial cells that secrete them in the young tissue grafts, then the grafts will be unnecessary.

Neurochemicals secreted by neurons and glial cells have been implicated in producing neurotrophic changes. The neurochemicals consist of various neural and glial proteins, peptides, and lipids. I cannot provide a comprehensive list of neurochemicals, but I will try to cite some of the more common factors.

Lipton and Kater[34] provide a review of the role that neurotransmitters such as acetylcholine, glutamate, and dopamine can play in influencing neuronal cytoarchitecture. It is hoped that it will be possible to use the knowledge of the effects of neurotransmitters to induce regeneration. Most of this research is still in the early investigative stage. Much additional work needs to be completed before there is an adequate understanding of the "dose" of neurotransmitters and their interaction with other neurotransmitters or other agents such as nerve growth factor.

Nerve growth factor was discovered 35 years ago, but its significance in the CNS has only recently been investigated.[35] Nerve growth factor is a biologically potent protein. Small amounts appear to have profound effects in guiding axonal growth and diminishing lesion effects. Microtubule- associated protein 2 is a structural protein concentrated in dendrites. There is evidence that this protein is involved in determining the changing morphology of dendrites during plasticity. Growth-associated protein 43 promotes neural sprouting. Melanocortins are neuropeptides that have been shown to improve the quality of axon repair.[36]

Over 50 different gangliosides, or glycosphingo lipids, have been identified in the brain.[37] Monosialoganglioside is an important one found inneuronal plasma membranes. Systemic administration of this ganglioside immediately following a brain injury appears to assure the best possible recovery in the rat. There is 33% less tissue edema following this administration, and damaged neural membrane function is stabilized. In addition, gangliosides have been reported to protect neurons from neurotoxins and hypoxia and to reduce axon degeneration following injury.

Another area of investigation is involved with the matrix, or the supporting cells (eg, glial cells), and its role in aiding or inhibiting regeneration.[38]

This superficial review of some of the research allows the reader to appreciate the complexity of the processes involved in CNS reorganization. At this time, there is not one single pharmacologic agent that will enhance reorganization following injury regardless of site of injury, type of injury, or age of the individual. The research at this time is still involved in characterizing the processes and the chemicals involved in reorganization. Included in this research is understanding the optimal nonneural environment that will promote reorganization.

Treatment. Can we examine the effect of therapeutic intervention on facilitating recovery? There are studies demonstrating that treatment has no effect on recovery of function. Waylonis et al[39] examined patients with strokes, who were in a nursing home, and concluded that recovery was equivalent between patients who had or had not received treatment. There are those clinicians who believe that patients with strokes are better left alone. This therapeutic nihilism is, in my mind, untenable. The studies that have made such claims are poorly constructed and do not lend support to such a hypothesis.

I am not in a position to evaluate the quality of one treatment approach over another in affecting outcome. And, unfortunately, it is not easy to go to the literature and find studies supporting the contentions either. There is still a paucity of research attempting to document the time, course, or quality of recovery achieved by particular techniques in well-controlled studies of adequate sample size. Some of the newer techniques such as electrical stimulation and biofeedback have been examined. Studies can be found that attempted to control variables and match subjects to evaluate the effectiveness of treatment, but we are still on the tip of the iceberg. Such studies, however, are providing the rationale for the treatments being used in the clinic and are stressing the need for the clinician to document recovery carefully.

Three issues that may affect recovery and that are related to treatment will be addressed: when to treat, how long to treat, and how forcefully to treat.

The results of the environmental enrichment studies suggest that treatment should be early.[30] This finding is further supported in a study by Black et al,[40] who induced motor cortex lesions in rhesus monkeys. One group began postoperative training immediately and continued training for 6months. The other group had no treatment for 4 months and then underwent a similar 6 months of treatment. The early group achieved 82% recovery, and the late group achieved 67% of their preoperative recovery. Additional studies like this support the concept that early intervention is most useful.

When I went to physical therapy school, I was taught that most recovery was achieved in the first 6 months and that treatment after that time was not indicated. Although the majority of recovery occurs in the first 6 months for most adults with hemiplegia (stroke), this rule does not hold true for patients with incomplete spinal cord injury or for persons with head injury. Tueber,[41] for example, demonstrated that Korean war soldiers who sustained head trauma demonstrated improvement 15 years postinjury. Wannstedt and Herman[42] studied a group of 20 patients who had hemiplegia an average of $2^1{}_2$ years duration and found that 16 of the 20 patients were able to learn in an average of seven sessions to stand with symmetrical weight bearing on their lower extremities and to shift weight. Therefore, we cannot assume that recovery is limited to 6 months in all patients with hemiplegia.

Bach-y-Rita[43] suggests that patients reach periods of plateau during which time both the clinician and the patient become frustrated with the rate of recovery. But as with learning, these periods of plateau may not be permanent and therefore a period of no-treatment might be followed by a treatment period in which recovery is again achieved. Such a hypothesis suggests the need to evaluate progress continually and to follow-up consistently.

The other issue is how aggressive our treatment should be. The most dramatic results to date have been achieved in the forced-use paradigms where vigorous training and forced usage are claimed to enhance the rate and extent of recovery following injury. Ostendorf and Wolf[44] presented a case study for an adult with hemiplegia of 18-months duration and reported no apparent change in the efficiency and quality of movement but an increase in the frequency of purposeful behavior by the involved extremity during the restraint period.

The effect that treatment intervention or the factors just cited have on recovery remains elusive. Animal models provide more control of variables and the parallel examination of the behavior and the nervous system. The use of animal models allows for the formulation of theory, and the propositions of the theory can be tested in the clinical setting. Research cannot be limited to animal models because the lesions are usually experimentally induced rather than naturally occurring and the role of motivation and cognition cannot be assessed. The need for clinicians to document carefully their patients' responses following injury is vital not only to third party payers but also to investigators who are trying to understand the mechanisms associated with recovery following injury.

SUMMARY

This presentation has provided an extremely superficial overview of some of the work that is on-going to understand the mechanisms that may lead toimproved recovery. It is obvious that there is much to be learned. I hope, however, you will feel as optimistic as I do about the possibility that the future for the person with CNS injury holds promise for enhanced functional abilities.

Acknowledgments

I thank Dr. Carol Hand, Department of Biological Sciences, Idaho State University, and Dr. Jean Held, Department of Physical Therapy, University of Vermont, for providing materials and ideas to assist with the preparation of this manuscript. I also thank Kimberly Gallo for assisting me with manuscript preparation and Jamie Tomlinson for doing the art work.

References

1. *Webster's New Collegiate Dictionary*. Springfield, Mass: G & C Merriam Co; 1973.
2. Finger S, Stein DG. Physiological plasticity. In: Finger S, Stein DG, eds. *Brain Damage and Recovery: Research and Clinical Perspectives*. New York, NY: Academic Press Inc; 1982:103-134.
3. Finger S, Stein DG. Localization in the central nervous system. In: Finger S, Stein DG, eds. *Brain Damage and Recovery: Research and Clinical Perspectives*. New York, NY: Academic Press Inc; 1982:13-28.
4. Finger S, Stein DG. Regeneration in the central nervous system. In: Finger S, Stein DG, eds. *Brain Damage and Recovery: Research and Clinical Perspectives*. New York, NY: Academic Press Inc; 1982:49-61.
5. Herman RM, Grillner S, Stein PSG, eds. *Neural Control of Locomotion*. New York, NY: Plenum Publishing Corp; 1976.
6. Wall JT. Variable organization in cortical maps of the skin as an indication of the lifelong adaptive capacities of circuits in the mammalian brain. *Trends in Neuroscience*. 1988;11:549-557.
7. Burke D. Spasticity as an adaptation to pyramidal tract injury. In: Waxman SG, ed. *Advances in Neurology: Functional Recovery in Neurological Disease*, New York, NY: Raven Press; 1988;47:401-423.
8. von Monakow C; Harris G, trans-excerpt. Die lokalisation in grosshrirn und der abbau der funktion durch kortikale harde. In: Pribram KH, ed. *Mood, States and Mind*. New York, NY: Penguin Books; 1969:27-37.
9. Glassman RB, Smith A. Neural spare capacity and the concept of diaschisis: functional and evolutionary models. In: Le Vere TE, Almli RB, Stein DG, eds. *Brain Injury and Recovery: Theoretical and Controversial Issues*. New York, NY: Plenum Publishing Corp; 1988:45-69.
10. Glassman RB. Recovery following sensorimotor cortical damage: evoked potentials, brain stimulation and motor control. *Exp Neruol*. 1971;33:16-29.
11. Finger S, Stein DG. Sueprsensitivity as a recovery model. In: Finger S, Stein DG, eds. *Brain Damage and Recovery: Research and Clinical Perspectives*. New York, NY: Academic Press Inc; 1982:271-286.
12. Almli CR, Finger S. Toward a definition of recovery of function. In: Le Vere TE, Almli RB, Stein DG, eds. *Brain Injury*

and Recovery: Theoretical and Controversial Issues. New York, NY: Plenum Publishing Corp; 1988:1-4.

13. Le Vere ND, Gray-Silva S, Le Vere TE. Infant brain injury: the benefit of relocation and the cost of crowding. In: Le Vere TE, Almli RB, Stein DG, eds. Brain Injury and Recovery: Theoretical and Controversial Issues. New York, NY: Plenum Publishing Corp; 1988:133-150.

14. Schneider GE. Is it really better to have your brain lesion early? A revision of the "Kennard Principle." Neuropsychologia. 1979;17:551-583.

15. Berman N, Sterling P. Cortical suppression of the retinocollicular pathway in the monocularly deprived cat. J Physiol (Lond). 1976;255:263-273.

16. Kratz KE, Spear PD, Smith DC. Postcritical period reversals of effects of monocular deprivation on striate cortex cells in the cat. J Neruophysiol. 1976;39:501-511.

17. Liu C-N, Chambers WW. Intraspinal sprouting of dorsal root axons. Archives of Neurology and Psychiatry. 1958;79:46-61.

18. Slavin MD, Laurence S, Stein DG. Another look at vicariation. In: Le Vere TE, Almli RB, Stein DG, eds. Brain Injury and Recovery: Theoretical and Controversial Issues. New York, NY: Plenum Publishing Corp; 1988:165-179.

19. Goldberger ME. Recovery after CNS lesions in monkeys. In: Stein DG, Rosen JJ, Butters N, eds. Plasticity and Recovery of Funciton in the Central Nervous System. New York, NY: Academic Press Inc; 1974:265-337.

20. Finger S, Almli CR. Brain damage and neuroplasticity: mechanisms of recovery or development? Brain Research Review. 1985;10:177-186.

21. Tsang YC. Maze learning in rats hemidecorticated in infancy. J Comp Psychol. 1937;24:221-254.

22. Kennard MA. Cortical reorganization of motor function: studies on a series of monkeys of various ages from infancy to maturity. Archives of Neurology and Psychiatry. 1942;48:27-240.

23. Woods BT. The restricted effects of right hemispheric lesions after age one: Wechsler test data. Neuropsychologia. 1980;18:65-70.

24. Milner B. Sparing of language functions after early unilateral brain damage. Neuroscience Research Bulletin. 1974;12:213-216.

25. Goldman P. An altenative to developmental plasticity: heterology of CNS structures in infants and adults. In: Stein DG, Rosen JJ, Butters N, eds. Plasticity and Recovery of Function in the Central Nervous System. New York, NY: Academic Press Inc; 1974:149-174.

26. Finger S, Stein DG. Fast- versus slow-growing lesions and behavior recovery. In: Finger S, Stein DG, eds. Brain Damage and Recovery: Research and Clinical Perspectives. New York, NY: Academic Press Inc; 1982:153-173.

27. Travis AM, Woolsey CN. Motor performance of monkeys after bilateral partial and total cerebral decortication. Am J Phys Med. 1956;35:273-310.

28. Finger S, Stein DG. Environmental experimental determinants of recovery of function. In: Finger S, Stein DG, eds.

Brain Damage and Recovery: Research and Clinical Perspectives. New York, NY: Academic Press Inc; 1982:175-202.

29. White B, Held R. Plasticity of sensorimotor development in the human infant. In: Rosenbluth J, Allinsmith W, eds. The Causes of Behavior: Reading in Child Development in Educational Psychology. Boston, Mass: Allyn & Bacon Inc; 1966:60-70.

30. Held JM, Gordon J, Gentile AM. Environmental influences on locomotor recovery following cortical lesions in rats. Behav Neurosci. 1985;99:678-690.

31. Stein DG. Practical and theoretical issues in the uses of fetal brain tissue transplants to promote recovery from brain injury. In: Le Vere TE, Almli RB, Stein DG, eds. Brain Injury and Recovery: Theoretical and Controversial Issues. New York, NY: Plenum Publishing Corp; 1988;249-272.

32. Privat A, Mansour H, Rajaofetra N, et al. Intraspinal transplants of serotonergic neurons in the adult rat. Brain Res Bull. 1989;22:123-129.

33. Yakovleff A, Roby-Brami A, Guezard B, et al. Locomotion in rats transplanted with noradrenergic neurons. Brain Res Bull. 1989;22:115-121.

34. Lipton SA, Kater SB. Neurotransmitter regulation of neuronal outgrowth, plasticity and survival. Trends in Neuroscience. 1989;12:265-270.

35. Hart T, Chaimas N, Moore RY, et al. Effects of nerve growth factor on behavioral recovery following caudate nucleus lesions in rats. Brain Res Bull. 1979;3:245-250.

36. Neural regeneration. In: Seil FJ, Herbert SE, Carlson BM, eds. Progress in Brain Research. New York, NY: Elsevier Science Publishing Co Inc; 1987.

37. Karpiak SE, Li YS, Mahadik SP. Ganglioside treatment: reduction of CNS injury and facilitation of functional recovery. Brain Injury. 1987;1:161-170.

38. Collins GH, West NR. Prospects for axonal regrowth in spinal cord injury. Brain Res Bull. 1989;22:89-92.

39. Waylonis GW, Keith MW, Aseff JN. Stroke rehabilitation in a midwestern city. Arch Phys Med Rehabil. 1973;54:151-174.

40. Black P, Markowitz RS, Cianci SN. Recovery of motor function after lesions in motor cortex of monkey. In: Outcome of Severe Damage to the Central Nervous System. New York, NY: Elsevier Science Publishing Co Inc; 1975:65-83.

41. Teuber HL. Recovery of function after brain injury in man. In: Outcome of Severe Damage to the Central Nervous System. New York, NY: Elsevier Science Publishing Co Inc; 1975:159-190.

42. Wannstedt GT, Herman RM. Use of augmented sensory feedback to achieve symmetrical standing. Phys Ther. 1978;58:553-559.

43. Bach-y-Rita P. Brain Plasticity as a basis for therapeutic procedures. In: Bach-y-Rita P, ed. Recovery of Function: Theoretical Considerations for Brain Injury Rehabilitation. Baltimore, Md: University Park Press; 1980:225-263.

44. Ostendorf CG, Wolf SL. Effect of forced use of the upper extremity of a hemiplegic patient on changes in function. Phys Ther. 1981;61:1022-1027.

Chapter 18

Perceptual Issues in Motor Control

Patricia C. Montgomery, PhD, PT
Therapeutic Intervention Programs, Inc
2217 Glenhurst Road
St. Louis Park, MN 55416

In this conference on motor control, we are interested in *how* humans move. In addition to understanding *how* we move, we need to understand *why* we move. We move because we *want* to, we *need* to, or we are *forced* to. In fact, we consider nonpurposeful behavior-movement to be pathological. Individuals with brain injuries or deficits also move because they want, need, or are forced to do so. Physical therapy assessment and intervention, then, must be concerned not only with the mechanisms underlying how we move (eg, selection and sequencing of appropriate synergies, force and timing of muscle contraction) but also with the mechanisms underlying why we move. If an individual with a brain injury or deficit does not perceive there is reason to move, the issue of how he moves does not exist. The purpose of this presentation is to discuss perceptual issues in motor control.

Analyze the various reasons why you move during a single day. For example, as you wake in the morning you may find that your arm is numb because you have been compressing your shoulder and you need to move to restore circulation to your arm. You decide to get up and walk to the kitchen to prepare breakfast because you are hungry. You may not want to eat if you are trying to diet, but the internal message from your stomach is to "feed me." You need to eat for basic physiological survival.

You step outside and discover it is raining. As you slip on the front step, you are forced to respond with a balance reaction to prevent a fall. You then actively use a number of motor strategies, perhaps shortening stride length, grabbing a hand rail, or widening the base of support, to prevent future falls. Later in the day, you go to an indoor driving range and practice your golf swing. You really do not need to do this, nothing in the environment is forcing you to practice these movements, it is simply something you want to do.

These are simple examples of why we move. We have the ability to perceive our internal environment (eg, hunger, thirst) and our external environment. We are motivated to move based on our interpretation and understanding of internal and external events. Different parts of our brain analyze the features of our internal and external environments. It is this analysis of our body and environment that results in perception. The motor systems provide us with the ability to move and act, but we only do so based on our perceptions and motivation.

WHAT IS PERCEPTION?

Definition

Experimental physiologists have proposed the idea of *psychoneural identity*, referring to the total of physiochemical neural events in the brain that are what we call sensation, perception, consciousness, and behavior.[1(p116)]

Sensation Versus Perception

Many meanings have been attached to the term sensation and perception. From a historical perspective, sensations refer to certain immediate, qualitative experiences, such as "warm" produced by a relatively simple and isolated stimulus.[2] The study of sensation has primarily been directed to the structure, physiology, and general activity of specific sensory receptors.

Mountcastle[3,4] explained how a set of sensory maps on the sensory cortices forms our images of the world. The individual performs abstractions and inferences from these maps to form a perception of the environment. "Behavior is based on the perceived environment and not on the real environment."[1(p116)]

Perception, then, has generally referred to psychological processes that encompass meaning by relating past experience, memory, and judgment to the sensations experienced. Although there are distinctions between sensation and perception, these are not clear-cut and are better considered as a chain of interdependent processes.[2] "We can thus identify a train of biological activity: stimulation from the external environment, impinging on sense receptors, which in turn produce neural activity, terminating in the behavioral phenomena of sensation and/or perception."[2(p1)]

Neurophysiologists have proposed that we measure physical and chemical properties of our external environment through sensory organs.[5] Therefore, the brain depends on the properties of these receptors for information. In psychophysical studies of sensory functions, the focus has been on stimulus-response relationships; for example, determining absolute thresholds for detection of stimuli or relating the amplitude of a stimulus to its perceived intensity. Therapists are familiar with senses studied, including vision, hearing, smell, taste, touch (including temperature and pain), balance (vestibular), and proprioception (joint position and muscle length). Despite high sensitivity and resolution, the receptors do *not* convey an exact reproduction of the outside world. Although the brain uses stereotyped electrical signals to process information, information relayed by sensory receptors is subject to processing and inhibition at various levels of the CNS before reaching the cortex. Various sensory systems also have different representations in the brain of various species.[5] In lower vertebrates, the olfactory system dominates so they live in a world of odors. In man, visual sensations dominate so we live in a world of colors and contours.

According to Brooks,[6(p39)] "sensorimotor integration is the key to motor control." Personal sensory perceptions, however, do not always match the intensity or quality of sensory inputs; the sensory inputs are "edited." Brooks refers to the development of motor set prior to movement as a countdown to rocket launch. The individual uses past experience and present mood and attention to the task, then preparations are made "to implement the intention."[6(p111)] Perception, then, is preparatory to movement.

PSYCHOLOGICAL THEORIES OF PERCEPTUAL LEARNING

Various models have been proposed for the processes underlying perceptual learning and can be described as *association, enrichment,* or *response-oriented* theories.[7] In the early 1700s, "associationists" suggested that elementary sense impressions were welded with images of past impressions to form meaningful perceptions. Stated differently, we learn to integrate or associate sensory information to form increasingly more complex perceptions. It has been suggested that the CNS combines and integrates information from various receptors to produce an "ensemble" of information to overcome any ambiguities that may occur with isolated signals.[8] The basic "enrichment" model is that perception begins with elementary sensory processes that are supplemented by other processes.[7] Many of these other processes, such as inferences and hypotheses, are cognitively oriented. Other enrichment models place greater emphasis on the constructive and problem-solving nature of perception. For example, Piaget considers perception as an active, constructive process. Another group of theories may also be classified as enrichment theories, but the other processes are considered responses rather than conceptual or inferential mechanisms. Response-oriented theories can be divided into two groups: one that considers perception to derive from motor activity (motor copy theory) and one that considers perception as an improvement in discrimination (for a detailed review of theories of perceptual learning, see E. Gibson[7]).

J. Gibson[9] outlined a differentiation (discrimination) theory in his book, *The Ecological Approach to Visual Perception.* Current theories suggest that vision depends on the eye, which is connected to the brain. Gibson[9(p1)] suggested that "natural vision depends on the eyes in the head on a body supported by the ground, the brain being only the central organ of a complete visual system." He described *natural vision* as the normal human condition without experimental constraints on the visual system, so that we look around, approach something interesting, move around it to see it from all perspectives, and move from one visual vista to another. Gibson's view of perception rejects the notion that we process sensory inputs and convert them into perceptions by

operations of the mind. He described a radically new way of thinking about perception, emphasizing the extracting of invariants from the stimulus flux. He described objects, places, and events in terms of the *affordances* of the environment, or what these experiences offer us. Gibson's model is "direct" as compared with the "indirect" processes described by other theorists.

The anatomical parts of the visual system in Gibson's view are the body, head, and eyes. All the parts being equipped with muscles, they all move relative to the environment. Gibson[9] suggests that their purpose is perceptual exploration. At all levels, the activities of the systems are adjustments instead of reflex reactions to stimuli or motor or other responses of any kind. The body explores the environment by locomotion and the head explores the ambient array by turning. The eyes explore samples of the array by eye movements (exploratory adjustments). At the level of the eyelid, lens, pupil, and retinal cells, "optimizing adjustments" may be made. "The visual system hunts for comprehension and clarity. It does not rest until the invariants are extracted. Exploring and optimizing seem to be the functions of the system."[9(p219)] This description of perception as an active, internally programmed process fits well with our current emphasis on the aspects of motor control that are internally generated. The process of visual exploration is consistent with Gibson's description of the "ambient optic array," which consists of adjacent visual solid angles that are nested (Figs. 18-1, 18-2). Each solid angle has its base in a feature of the environmental layout. The features themselves are nested in superordinate and subordinate units. The eye-head system can explore hemispheric solid angles of the earth and sky, and we can perceive large murals with sweeps of the eyes. We perceive a printed page with small saccades and use the tiniest saccades of all to thread a needle.

Why do we have perceptual learning? One hypothesis is that there is survival value in the ability to adapt to ever changing environments. Another hypothesis is that higher organisms are more capable of perceptual learning as a result of increasingly greater complexity in brain development.[10]

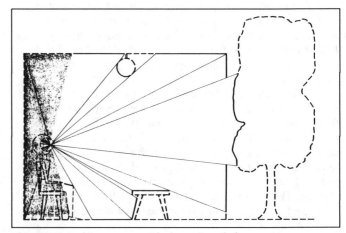

Fig. 18-1. *Ambient array with the point of observation occupied by a person (from Gibson,[9] reprinted with permission).*

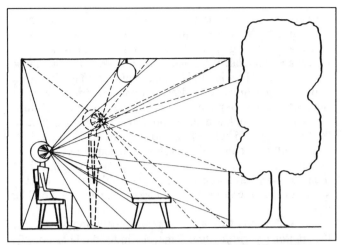

Fig. 18-2. *The change of the optic array brought about by a locomotor movement by the observer. The thin solid lines indicate the ambient optic array for the seated observer, and the thin dashed lines the altered optic array after standing up and moving forward. The difference between the two arrays is specific to the difference between the points of observation, that is, to the path of locomotion. Note that the whole ambient array is changed, including the portion behind the head. Also note that what was previously hidden becomes unhidden (from Gibson,[9] reprinted with permission).*

Perception is the process of obtaining first hand information of the world about us. Gibson[9] suggested the critical element is man's ability to extract information from the stimuli present in the environment rather than to change something in the environment or to do something to it. In Gibson's[7] view, perceptual learning is an increasing ability to extract information from the environment, or *differentiation*. In other words, we learn to make increasingly finer discriminations of the stimulus. This is an active, not passive process involving exploring and searching. As Gibson[7(p4)] stated, "we do not just see, we look; we do not just hear, we listen."

Neurophysiological and psychological studies of perceptual issues are complementary, and these fields of research continue to explore one of the most essential human functions: perception.

PERCEPTUAL ISSUES

Nature Versus Nurture

For many years, a fundamental argument existed regarding whether development and perceptual learning were due solely to innate-genetic factors or to experiential-environmental factors.[11] Most theorists would now agree that learning and development are dependent on interaction between these two influences. We know, for example, that the fundamental structure of the brain is determined genetically, but it is only a starting point.[10] Full configuration of the brain is a protracted process after birth, guided by stimuli, information, and challenges specific to the individual's environment.

In the 1940s, Hebb[12] reviewed cases of individuals, blind since birth, who had some vision restored. He concluded that some visual perception was innate (ie, figure-

ground) and some was learned (ie, form or pattern). These observations helped diffuse the "either-or" controversy. The current view is that some of perception is innate, and some is learned.[11] This is a logical and safe conclusion. But exactly what is innate and what is learned? These questions are important to physical therapists because the answer related to how "normal" and brain-damaged individuals function and are relevant to decisions of whether to intervene and how to intervene. Walk and Pick[11(pxiv)] stated that "in investigating what is learned and what is innate we are also investigating plasticity, the extent to which the organism (human) adapts to the environment, the most appropriate period for plasticity, if there is any, and its permanence."

Critical Periods

What is a critical or sensitive period? It refers to a time in the life of a human or animal when a particular type or types of stimulation are needed.[11] If this stimulation does not occur, behavior appropriate to the species does not develop or occur.

As techniques were developed for recording electrical activity from individual neurons in an intact animal brain, we discovered how the visual system functions in the detection and recognition of shapes. Hubel and Wiesel[13-17] completed a series of studies in cats demonstrating how single cells in the visual system detect specific environmental features such as lines, edges, and angles. These cells were described by the pattern of retinal stimulation to which they were best activated, or the cell's receptive field. It was also determined that the neurons that displayed functional similarities in the visual cortex were arranged in columns, and approximately 80% of the cells could be activated binocularly.

Hubel and Weisel[14] demonstrated in young kittens that receptive field organization, binocularity, and functional architecture were all similar to that of the adult cat. Subsequently, they restricted visual input to one eye while allowing normal visual input in the other in kittens from birth to 3 months of age.[17] After this period of monocular deprivation, most cortical cells in the cortex could only be driven by the experienced eye. Those cells that could be activated by the deprived eye had grossly abnormal receptive fields. Their research suggested that visual experience is necessary to maintain and to further develop the specificity of cells present in the very young animal, and the major effects in the kitten are from 3 weeks to 3 months postnatally (ie, the critical period in the kitten's visual system).

It is interesting to note the effect of limiting early visual experience to lines and edges of a single contour. Spinelli and co-workers[18] raised kittens from birth to 3 months of age, with the kittens wearing specialized goggles so one eye saw only vertical and the other eye only horizontal lines. At 12 weeks of age, electrical recordings indicated that cells of the visual cortex only responded to the particular orientation to which they had been exposed. No oblique fields were found, and all cells were monocular. One hypothesis is that the visual cortex adapts during maturation to the nature of the visual experience.[19] A more acceptable hypothesis is that "exposure to a particular orientation is necessary to maintain and sharpen the innately determined response pattern of a given neuron, while cells which are not properly activated become nonfunctional."[19(p28)] In this same study, modifications of cells in the sensory cortex were found.[18] The kittens were trained to lift a front paw to avoid a mild shock when seeing a danger signal (ie, horizontal line) versus a safe signal (ie, vertical line). The area mapping the trained forearm was several times larger than the area mapping the untrained one. A very high percentage of the cells responded to the danger stimulus; a smaller percentage responded to the safe stimulus; and other cells responded to normal, everyday stimuli. A second study demonstrated that the motor representation of the trained forearm was about four times as large as that of the opposite, untrained forearm.[20] Of polysensory cells, cells responsive to the orientation of the danger stimulus were three times more frequent than other types.

Animal research into critical periods has not been limited to the visual system. The course of vocal development varies in birds, being inflexible in some and plastic in others.[21] The domestic chicken, for example, raised in isolation develops normal species-specific sounds. Most songbirds, in contrast, when raised in isolation or with birds of a different species develop abnormal songs. It is hypothesized that each bird has a blueprint of its species song to help it select the correct song to copy when exposed in a natural setting to the songs of many species. There are varying critical periods in different bird species when auditory exposure has effects on subsequent song development.

It is important to keep in mind, however, that the influence of or interaction between genetic and environmental influences may be different in different parts of the brain. Hubel and Wiesel[22] reviewed research on sensory areas of the immature brain, suggesting susceptibility to a variety of influences that determine anatomical, functional, and biochemical organization. Shwartz and Goldman-Rakic[23] discussed research on the primate prefrontal association cortex (PFC). Damage to the PFC in primates results in cognitive and behavioral defects similar to those found in humans with frontal lobe damage. Studies showed specificity and the presence of an adult-like pattern of organization in these areas of the brain 1 month before birth. One hypothesis is that these areas are less responsive to environmental factors than previously studied sensory areas.

We know that spatial resolution is poor in the 2-month-old human infant. It appears to improve rapidly, however, and approaches adult levels by 6 monthsof age.[24] There is evidence that suggests the human visual system is susceptible to modification by abnormal visual exposure. The ability to perceive forms (visual acuity) and binocular functions (steropsis) have both been shown to be influenced by abnormal early visual input. Examples are amblyopia and early astigmatism that often result in varying degrees of permanently reduced visual acuity. Mitchell[24] suggested that the length of time during which the visual system is modifiable by abnormal vision input varies from the cat (up to 4 months of age) and monkey (up to 6 months of age) to the human visual system (perhaps up to 6 years of age).

Feature Detectors

Evidence exists for feature detectors in human sensory systems. Gibson[9] described *optical flow patterns* that are rays of light striking the eye from every visible part of the environment. We know something is approaching our eyes if the rate of change of angles of light from all edges of an object are identical. We usually respond with a strong avoidance reaction. This is called *looming* and often elicits strong avoidance reactions in children and young animals, suggesting that this type of pattern may be genetically programmed. The human infant has been found to perceive the distinctive features of speech before linguistic experience.[25] It has been suggested that young children should be exposed to the sounds present in a wide variety of languages to enhance their auditory perception and improve production of these same sounds when foreign languages are learned at an older age.

At the end of what information-processing theory calls the *stimulus- identification* stage, the individual has analyzed information in the stimulus array and should know what is happening in the environment.[8] This most "peripheral" level of processing is a memory system for holding information presented for a brief period of time. This process has been proposed for each type of sensation, but most research has been done on visual short-term sensory store. It has been suggested that this short-term sensory store is fairly literal in that the information recorded is the same as it enters the system, with simple transformations done by "analyzers" that interpret information as angled, vertical, rough, colored, and so on. It has been proposed that irrelevant information does not become entangled with relevant information because we have selective attention, allowing us to screen out irrelevant and pass relevant information into short-term memory.

Summary

Researchers have demonstrated that certain experiences are capable of inducing massive changes in the structure and function of visual, somatic, and motor cortex of otherwise normally reared kittens.[10] These plasticity triggering experiences have been shown to "induce adaptive changes in dendritic trees, dendritic bundles, functional properties of single cells in visual and somato-sensory cortex, and even in the shape of the cortical representation of the body surface and motor map.[10(p21)] These changes that occur appear to be permanent and result in modifications of the animal's behavior. The brainresponds to experience with adaptive changes in its structure; a structure that is initially determined by genetic factors. It is proposed that this response of the brain is most powerful during certain critical periods of development.

There are many questions regarding feature detectors and critical periods that are important in rehabilitation. For example, we do not know what happens if a group of "abstracting neurons" responsible for certain perceptions is destroyed.[1] Can other neurons take over their functions? If this occurs, how does it occur? Through what kind of learning? What are the requirements? If a group of neurons takes over these functions, what happens to their original functions?

To what extent do critical periods exist in humans? How do these affect the development of sensory and motor functions in the human infant? Why do critical periods exist? Perhaps they exist to achieve the best possible match for a specific environment. According to Spinelli et al,[10] the higher the animal species the more plasticity and configuring of the brain. The advantage is greater adaptability. The issue for physical therapists is when to deliver the optimal sequence of sensory experience and motor tasks, because timing may be as crucial as the type of information provided.

NEUROLOGIC SUBSTRATE FOR PERCEPTION-MOTIVATION-COGNITION

Brooks[6] described higher, middle, and lower levels of motor control (Figs. 18-3, 18-4). The higher level consists of cognitive and emotional-motivational elements and leads to the motor plan, or decisions regarding "what I want to do." This is in contrast to the middle level that consists of sensory and motor cortex, basal ganglia, brain stem, and cerebellum and is involved in the execution of the motor program, or "how I am going to do it." The lower level consists of the spinal cord, muscles, and joints and is responsible for the execution of movement (includes biomechanical aspects).

A number of central nervous system (CNS) structures are involved in motor planning, including the limbic cortex and association cortex that provide the neural substrate for "recognizing, selecting, attending to, and acting on relevant sensory information in an awake state."[6(p24)]

The limbic system, particularly the hypothalamus, enables us to respond in order to guarantee species survival. When we see a glass of water, if we are thirsty we make a decision to drink. Limbic drives evolve into general ideas and motor goals through subsequent corticocortical processing.[6] The cortico-limbic-thalamic pathway is essential for quick, insightful learning, incorporating the hippocampus

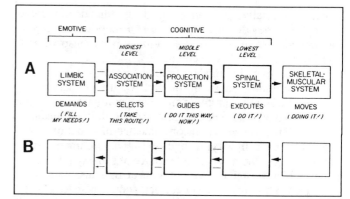

Fig. 18-4. *Cartoon summary highlighting the motivational function of the limbic system in motor control. Direct and indirect connections indicated as heavy and light arrows. Feedforward connections (A) and feedback between equivalent systems in (B). (From Mesnlam MM. The functional anatomy and hemispheric specialization of directed attention. In: Trends in Neuroscience. New York, NY: Elsevier Science Publishing Co Inc; 1983;6:387. Reprinted with permission from Elsevier Publications, Copyright 1983.)*

and amygdala for memory functions. With knowledge of results of movement, we remember what we planned, how it felt, and if we achieved our goal.

Emotions are closely related to sensory processes, state of arousal, and cognitive experiences.[26] These factors enable us to perceive the significance of a particular stimulus. Drive, or motivation, refers to the tendency to "translate into action the plans or reactions elaborated in response to internal and external cues and to their perceived value for the individual."[26(p116)] Behavioral disorders may either be secondary to social factors or the direct consequence of brain dysfunction.

PERCEPTION: ROLE IN MOTOR CONTROL AND LEARNING

Feedback

Physical therapists are familiar with the role of sensory information during movement as a method of feedback. Sensory peripheral feedback from the evolving movement is sent back to CNS centers that compare what was intended with what is actually happening.[6] Knowledge about proficiency of movement appears to be critical to motor learning.[8] Knowledge of how such feedback information works is important, not only theoretically but also practically, because it forms the basis for decisions about intervention in patients with motor control problems. *Intrinsic feedback* is what we receive through the various sensory channels as we move.[8] *Extrinsic feedback* is often in verbal form such as from a coach who tells us how long it took to run a race, from the visual and auditory cues in a video game, or from a physical therapist who tells a patient that movements are correct.

Feedforward

Although many types of sensory input can be used for feedback, the feedback process is too slow in many instances to be effective for planning movement.[6] Rapid move-

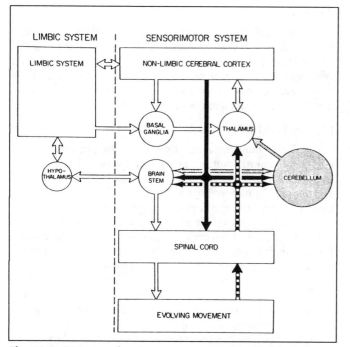

Fig. 18-3. *Diagram of major components of the limbic and sensorimotor systems (separated by broken line) (from Brooks,[6] reprinted from* Physical Therapy *with permission of the American Physical Therapy Association).*

ments, especially, are planned in advance and do not require feedback. They do, however, require perception. In preprogrammed movement, the expectation of what sensory input will result is taken into account.

In an evolving model of motor control, with emphasis on programming that is "inside-out," we need either to assess, accurately, on-going environmentally imposed disturbances to our posture or to predict the possibility of disturbances. Then we need to incorporate that information into the motor plan. In varying multisensory environments, we need to select the most reliable source of sensory information. When we stand in a tilted room at an amusement park we know what we see is *not* correct, and we plan to rely on proprioceptive and vestibular information to program an upright posture. Schmidt[8] suggested that one of the most potent variables for responding in a natural environment is the anticipation of upcoming events.

Motor learning involves both sensory and motor systems. We remember not only how we made the successful movement, but also how it felt.[6] If the motor task is completed successfully, and we recognize that success (throughintrinsic or extrinsic feedback or a combination of both), then we commit the neural and muscular activity to "motor memory," or what Brooks[6] would term a *subprogram*. If he is correct when he suggests that we improve motor skill through programmed movements only after we understand the behavioral goal for which the movements are to be used, then physical therapists need to determine appropriate behavioral goals for patients during rehabilitation and assist in the process of intrinsic and extrinsic feedback. If our treatment is to be effective, the patient must eventually be able to analyze his environment independently, anticipate and plan behavioral goals, and implement these goals through motor programs.

PERCEPTUAL DYSFUNCTION

Perceptual dysfunction is a vast topic. We can consider disorders in perception in two general areas. One is difficulty with receiving and interpreting information from the environment, the other is in receiving and interpreting information from our own bodies. How the environment changes from moment to moment will determine our motor behaviors.[8] We need to extract patterns of movement from the environment. In addition, the patterns of movement of our own bodies (detected through visual, auditory, vestibular, and propricoceptive receptors) determine our motor behavior.

Perception of the Environment: Arousal-Attention

We know that normal human subjects placed in dark, soundproof rooms often have changes in perceptual and cognitive abilities, leading to hallucinations and delusions.[5] These effects can occur after as few as 8 hours of isolation. It has been suggested that reduction or elimination of input through the reticular activating system leads to a decrease in overall activity of the cerebral cortex and upsets the balance necessary for alertness, attention, and control of sleep and wakefulness, which are the factors that account for perceptual and cognitive functions. Emotional reactions to deprivation probably depend, in part, on hypothalamic mechanisms.

The frontal lobe is involved in cognitive selection processes that help us determine how to focus our attention.[26] Physical therapists are familiar with patients who have deficits in their arousal system, such as patients who are either lethargic or over-aroused or patients with problems with selective attention. Perseveration, or the inability to shift attention from one task to another, is common in brain-damaged individuals.

Feature Extractors

If we agree with the premise that behavior depends on certain features in the environment, then we have to consider that particular behaviors may not occur if the neurons that normally extract those features are damaged.[1] In rehabilitation, we hope that the patient can develop alternative strategies, but the total behavior pattern will probably be degraded to some extent if some features of the environment cannot be detected.

Perception of Our Bodies Through Movement

Although Taub's[27] work in monkeys demonstrated that feedback from a deafferented forelimb was not essential for movement, the animals were not normal in their movements, especially when fine finger movements were needed. When sensation is impaired, feedforward processes and feedback from movements may be deficient. Ratcliff[28] categorized spatial disorders of humans into those of sensory analysis and those of more complex disorders affecting personal or extrapersonal space. A classic example of sensory disregard of the body is the patient with right-hemisphere, especially parietal lobe, damage who neglects to use the left side of the body or shaves only the right side of the face.

Summary

Many, if not all, of our brain-damaged patients have sensory deprivation or dysfunction. This may be the result of a combination of normal processes such as those associated with aging, of a disease process such as multiple sclerosis or Parkinson's disease, or of a brain injury such as occurs in a cerebrovascular accident or cerebral palsy.

PERCEPTUAL RECOVERY

The higher mental functions, including perception, cognition, and motivation, are among the most important in motor control. We hope for improvement in these areas through rehabilitation; however, some authors consider these functions the least likely to improve.[1]

Several mechanisms have been proposed that may result in perceptual recovery or an improvement in function.[29] For additional information, refer to Craik's chapter, in this volume, on "Recovery Process: Maximizing Function." Goldman[30,31] described a theory of "differential recovery," after studying brain lesions in infant monkeys. Recovery varied depending on such factors as how "committed" or "plastic" a brain area was and if there were other areas of the brain that could compensate for functions impaired by the brain lesion; the functional sequelae varied depending on whether the brain relied on those areas for performance of specific skills in the immature versus mature animal. Monkeys in Goldman's studies made "progressive" or "regressive" recoveries from brain lesions.

Sensory substitution is another proposed recovery or compensation mechanism and is particularly relevant to a discussion of perception. When a person becomes blind, he does not necessarily lose the capacity to "see," he loses the sensory end organ.[32] However, a substitute end organ, such as a miniature television camera, can be placed under the motor control of the blind person. The optical signals received by the camera can be transducedinto stimuli applied to another sensory system, such as the tactile system, for relay to the brain. Under these conditions, even a congenitally blind person can be trained to use the information as "visual."

An example of a sensory substitution task that physical therapists are familiar with is the use of electromyographic needles or surface electrodes that convert proprioceptive information from muscle contraction into visual or auditory displays. Favorable results of biofeedback in patients with hemiparesis, torticollis, and dystonia have been reported by Brudney and co- workers.[33]

The ability of one sensory system to convey information normally mediated through another requires plastic neural mechanisms. Evidence for neural plasticity comes from studies of recovery of function after brain lesions, neuronal changes associated with learning, alteration in evoked potentials, and sensory deprivation and enrichment studies documenting changes in cortical structure and chemistry. The brain apparently has some plastic mechanisms that allow it to respond to new functional requirements and to training; these mechanisms provide physical therapists with an opportunity to enhance sensory and perceptual rehabilitation.

PERCEPTION, MOTOR CONTROL, AND PHYSICAL THERAPY

Obviously, there is much more we do not know about perception than we know. Although we do not fully understand perceptual mechanisms, it does not mean that we should not attempt to assess and facilitate efficient perception during the rehabilitation process. Ayres made a similar case for the study of sensory integrative functions when she stated the following:

Exactly how sensory integration occurs in the brain remains elusive, but that fact is not an excuse for avoiding an issue basic to all learning. It must be faced and dealt with in as adequate a manner as possible, with full recognition of the limitations involved and with the realization that any conceptual framework is in some respects erroneous. It will require constant revision as new knowledge unfolds.[34(p41)]

Major Questions Relevant to Rehabilitation

Do we consider how perception relates to motor control or motor learning? Do we agree that attention, motivation, and cognition all affectmotor behavior and that the perception of our external and internal environment (ie, how stable is the environment and how stable is our posture in that environment) affects the posture we assume and the movements we make? If we agree that patients as well as

normal individuals select appropriate movement strategies (translated into motor programs) based on varying environmental conditions, then we must conclude that how accurately an individual perceives that environment is crucial to efficient motor behavior. If we are interested in measuring how a patient's motor behavior changes in different contexts, we must know how the patient's perception in these contexts varies. The question is, Does an individual have a motor control problem because he cannot plan or program a movement, or is he unable to plan or program a movement efficiently because he does not accurately perceive the environment or his own movement? If we agree that these are important considerations, then we need to know if the patient understands what is to be done, or what his task is at the moment. And, is he able to determine by himself the most effective way to do a task and to make subtle corrections based on feedback?

Do we consider how a critical period may relate to the objectives of physical therapy intervention? Even if we could assume that critical periods affect primarily the sensory-perceptual systems of the human CNS, the resulting effects would still be related to motor dysfunction. For example, if during a critical period environmental deprivation or injury resulted in decreased ability to process vestibular-visual input, the individual may be limited later in the ability to select appropriate movement programs in situations of vestibular-visual conflict. Are there critical periods of optimal development of some motor functions? An example would be the clinical model that ambulation should be delayed in a child with cerebral palsy until some qualitative "ideal" of control of movement in sitting or standing has been obtained. Does delaying ambulation past a critical period (when the child is motivated to ambulate and the CNS is trying to accomplish the task with a particular body mass and center of gravity relationship) perhaps retard the acquisition of the motor behavior when attempted at a later time?

Do we consider how motor dysfunction may affect perception? It has been argued that we need hard-wired programs to support our movements so higher levels of the CNS can do their functions (ie, perception-cognition, language) efficiently.[35] DeQuiros and Schrager[35] suggested that when the CNS is forced to use cortical processing for balance and posture (functions that should be automatic), cognitive and language development in children are impaired. Does neuromotor dysfunction (ie, a problem at the level of motor programming) interfere with perception, either on a neurophysiological or behavioral level, by diverting perceptual attention from what is happening in the environment or the body to that of producing a motor behavior?

Do we consider that movement may be a "sensory strategy"? We must consider that the way an individual moves might be a strategy to obtain sensory information or enhance perception. One example is the person with a visual defect who turns his head from side to side to obtain as much visual information as possible. Similarly, an individual with a hearing impairment may tilt or turn his head to enhance auditory perception. Do the teeth- grinding and body rocking movements of some developmentally delayed children represent a strategy to obtain vestibular-proprioceptive input? Sensory programs have been demonstrated to decrease self-stimulatory behaviors.[36,37] Perhaps the use of a hip strategy (bending forward and backward at the hips) represents a way to increase or maximize vestibular input in patients with vestibular deficits. Does the hemiplegic patient avoid weight bearing on one lower extremity because he cannot select or elicit the correct motor program, because he is unable to receive proprioceptive information or interpret that information while weight bearing on the limb, or because of both? Movement as a "sensory strategy" is an especially important consideration. If a patient's motor pattern-behavior is not considered optimal, we may try to change it. What if the motor pattern is being used to obtain sensory input or improve perception and we interfere with or prevent that process? Have we helped the patient or only changed the degree or type of his sensorimotor problem?

Do we assess the patient's perceptual abilities? In rehabilitation and in basic and applied research, we should consider sensory-perceptual variables that are specific to the patient and to the rehabilitation process. Perceptual variables specific to the patient include the patient's perceptual appreciation of his own body and of the environment. How accurate is the perception of self-produced movement (ie, vestibular-proprioceptive)? Do we know if the patient is accurately perceiving environmental stimuli? Does the patient know (perceptually) what is happening in the environment? If the patient does not accurately perceive his own body or the environment, how are his intentions and attempts to move affected? Does the patient selectively screen relevant and irrelevant information in the environment and from his own body? Do we assess these processes? Can we train these processes? Can we offer substitutes or alternative strategies?

Analyses of perceptual functions have most often been done by psychologists or occupational therapists, and disorders of the visual-perceptual system have been studied to the greatest extent, including optometric processes, such as accommodation, ocular movement, and convergence, and visual-perceptual functions.[38] Methods that have been proposed for assessment of general sensory-perceptual functions in children and adults are often qualitative.[39-42] There are standardized test batteries that have been designed to assess specific aspects of perception in children[43-48] and in adults.[49-51] Additional tests need to be developed to assess a wider variety of sensory-perceptual functions of various groups of patients with differing motor dysfunction. In particular, tests of sensory organization, such as The Clinical Test for Sensory Interaction in Balance,[52] help us understand the complex interaction of multisensory processing to postural and skilled movement. Unless we do appropriate perceptual assessments of patients, it is difficult to discover the pertinent relationships between perception and motor control.

Do we consider the perceptual environment during rehabilitation? There are sensory and perceptual variables specific to the rehabilitation process. Environmental variables include the size and temperature of the room, auditory (ie, radio, voices) and visual (ie, lighting, color of walls, floor) content of the room, textures and types of equipment and floor surfaces, and room odors (olfactory). Therapist-generated sensory variables also are important, and exam-

ples include visual (physical appearance, body size, color of clothing), auditory (tone, pitch, quality of voice), olfactory (body odor, perfume), proprioceptive and vestibular (handling techniques), and tactile (handling techniques, texture of clothing). Do we know how these variables interact with the rehabilitation process administered to an individual with specific perceptual and motor problems?

Do we alter treatment based on the patient's perception? I admire Ayres for attempting the enormous and brave task of trying to study perceptual processes as she developed the theoretical framework of sensory integration.[53,54] Her approach to the patient and key elements of intervention meld nicely into our current view of perceptual function and motor control. The major characteristics of intervention emphasize individualized treatment with sensory input based on the patient's needs and responses. Activities are rich in proprioceptive, vestibular, and tactile input and require active participation of the patient. Goal directed, purposeful activities determined by the patient are used whenever possible.

SUMMARY

Perception is a key element of motor control. Although physical therapists are experts in movement dysfunction, we must be careful not to focus our attention too narrowly on motor behavior. If we are to improve our assessment and rehabilitation strategies, we must continue to attend to perceptual issues and not leave this area of patient assessment and treatment to other professionals. Sensory information from the environment and the body are important in making decisions involved in many higher-level motor skills.[8] However, this interaction is so complex that researchers often choose to try to minimize these factors by studying movement behavior "focusing on those skills for which the primary determinants of success are the movements themselves."[8(p6)]

Researchers should incorporate perceptual issues into studies of motor control whenever feasible to increase our understanding of basic perceptual mechanisms. Physical therapists in the clinic can contribute to the understanding of perceptual issues by accurately assessing patients; monitoring long-term changes; and documenting the natural history of various brain injuries, perceptual abilities, and effects of intervention.

References

1. Sedgwick EM. Clinical neurophysiology in rehabilitation. In: Illis LS, Sedgwick EM, Glanville HF, eds. *Rehabilitation of the Neurologic Patient*. Boston, Mass: Blackwell Scientific Publications Inc; 1982:115-117.
2. Schiffman HR. *Sensation and Perception: An Integrated Approach*. New York, NY: John Wiley & Sons Inc; 1976:1-15.
3. Mountcastle VB. The view from within: pathways to the study of perception. *Johns Hopkins Medical Journal*. 1975;136:109-131.
4. Mountcastle VB. Brain mechanisms for directed attention. *J R Soc Med*. 1978;71:14-18.
5. Ottoson D. *Physiology of the Nervous System*. New York, NY: Oxford University Press Inc; 1983;chap 24, chap 32.
6. Brooks VB. *The Neural Basis of Motor Control*. New York, NY: Oxford University Press Inc; 1986.

7. Gibson E. *Principles of Perceptual Learning and Development*. Englewood Cliffs, NJ: Prentice Hall Inc; 1969.

8. Schmidt RA. *Motor Control and Learning*. Champaign, Ill; Human Kinetics Publishers Inc; 1982

9. Gibson JJ. *The Ecological Approach to Visual Perception*. Boston, Mass: Houghton Mifflin Co; 1979.

10. Spinelli DN. Plasticity triggering experiences: nature and the dual genesis of brain structure and function. In: Gunzenhauser N, ed. *Infant Stimulation: Pediatric Round Table: 13*. Skillman, NJ: Johnson & Johnson Baby Products Co; 1987.

11. Walk RD, Pick HL, eds. *Perception and Experience*. New York, NY: Plenum Publishing Corp; 1978.

12. Hebb D. *The Organization of Behavior*. New York, NY: Wiley Press; 1949.

13. Hubel DH, Wiesel TN. Receptive field, binocular interaction and functional architecture in the cat's visual cortex. *J Physiol (Lond)*. 1962;160:106-154.

14. Hubel DH, Wiesel TN. Receptive fields of cells in striate cortex of very young, visually inexperienced kittens. *J Neurophysiol*. 1963;26:944-1002.

15. Hubel DH, Wiesel TN. Binocular interaction in striate cortex of kittens reared with artificial squint. *J Neurophysiol*. 1965;28:1041-1059.

16. Hubel DH, Wiesel TN. Cells sensitive to binocular depth in area 28 of the macaque monkey cortex. *Nature*. 1970;225:41-42.

17. Hubel DH, Wiesel TN. The period of susceptibility to the physiological effects of unilateral eye closure in kittens. *J Physiol (Lond)*. 1970b;206:419-436.

18. Spinelli DN, Hirsch VH, Phelps RW, et al. Visual experience as a determinant of the response characteristics of cortical receptive fields in cats. *Exp Brain Res*. 1972;15:289-304.

19. Rothblat LA, Schwartz ML. Altered early environment and effects on the brain and visual behavior. In: Walk RD, Pick HL, eds. *Perception and Experience*. New York, NY: Plenum Publishing Corp; 1978:7-36.

20. Spinelli DN, Jensen FE. Plasticity, experience, and resource allocation in motor cortex and hypothalamus. In: Soody CD, ed. *Conditioning*. New York, NY: Plenum Publishing Corp; 1982.

21. Konishi M. Auditory environment and vocal development in birds. In: Walk RD, Pick HL, eds. *Perception and Experience*. New York, NY: Plenum Publishing Corp; 1978:105-118.

22. Hubel DH, Wiesel TN. Functional architecture of macaque monkey visual cortex. *Proc R Soc Lond [Biol]*. 1977;193:2-59.

23. Schwartz ML, Goldman-Rakic P. Development and plasticity of the association cortex. In: Gunzenhauser N, ed. *Infant Stimulation: Pediatric Round Table: 13*. Skillman, NJ: Johnson & Johnson Bady Products Co; 1987:30-40.

24. Mitchell DE. Effect of early visual experience on the development of certain perceptual abilities in man. In: Walk RD, Pick HL, eds. *Perception and Experience*. New York, NY: Plenum Publishing Corp; 1978:37-75.

25. Eimas PD, Miller JL. Effects of selective adaptation on the perception of speech and visual patterns: evidence for feature detectors. In: Walk RD, Pick HL, eds. *Perception and Experience*. New York, NY: Plenum Publishing Corp; 1978:307-345.

26. Rapin I. Children with brain dysfunction. In: *The International Review of Child Neurology*. New York, NY: Raven Press; 1982:115-117.

27. Taub E. Movements in nonhuman primates deprived of somatosensory feedback. *Exerc Sport Sci Rev*. 1976;4:335-374.

28. Ratcliff G. Disturbances of spatial orientation associated with cerebral lesions. In: Potegal M, ed. *Spatial Abilities: Development and Physiological Foundations*. New York, NY: Academic Press Inc; 1982:301-331.

29. Whyte J. Mechanisms of recovery of function following CNS damage. In: Rosenthal M, Griffith ER, Bond, MR, et al, eds. *Rehabilitation of the Adult and Child with Traumatic Brain Injury*. 2nd ed. Philadelphia, Pa: F A Davis Co; 1990:79-88.

30. Goldman PS. Functional development of prefrontal cortex in early life and the problem of neuronal plasticity. *Exp Neurol*. 1971;32:366-387.

31. Goldman PS. The role of experience in recovery of function following orbital prefontal lesions in infant monkeys. *Neuropsychologia*. 1976;14:401-412.

32. Bach-y-Rita P. Brain plasticity as a basis of sensory substitution. *Journal of Neurologic Rehabilitation*. 1987;1:67-72.

33. Brudney J, Korein J, Grynbaum BB, et al. EMG feedback therapy: review of treatment of 114 patients. *Arch Phys Med Rehabil*. 1976;57:55-61.

34. Ayres AJ. Sensory integrative processes and neuropsychological learning disability. *Learning Disorders*. 1968;3:41-58.

35. DeQuiros JB, Schrager OL. *Neuropsychological Fundamentals in Learning Disabilities*. San Rafael, Calif: Academic Therapy Publications; 1978:58-60.

36. Bright T, Bittick K, Fleeman B. Reduction of self-injurious behavior using sensory integration techniques. *Am J Occup Ther*. 1981;35:167-172.

37. Resman MH. Effects of sensory stimulation on eye contact in a profoundly retarded adult. *Am J Occup Ther*. 1981;35:31-35.

38. Bouska MJ, Kauffman NA, Marcus SE. Disorders of the visual perceptual system. In: Umphred DA, ed. *Neurologic Rehabilitation*. St. Louis, Mo: C V Mosby Co; 1985:552-585.

39. Montgomery PC. Assessment and treatment of the child with mental retardation. *Phys Ther*. 1981;61:1265-1272.

40. Farber S. *Neurorehabilitation: A multisensory Approach*. Philadelphia, Pa: W B Saunders Co; 1982.

41. Vlvisaker M, Chorazy JL, Cohen SB, et al. Rehabilitative assessment following head injury in children. In: Rosenthal M, Griffith ER, Bond, ME, et al, eds. *Rehabilitation of the Adult and Child with Traumatic Brain Injury*. 2nd ed. Philadelphia, Pa: F A Davis Co; 1990:572-573.

42. Reisman JE, Hanscher B. *Sensory Integration for Adults with Developmental Disabilities*. Hugo, Minn: PDP Press Inc; 1990.

43. Miller L. *Miller Assessment for Preschoolers*. Littleton, Colo: The Foundation for Knowledge in Development; 1982.

44. DeGangi GA, Berk RA. Psychometric analysis of the test of sensory integration. *Physical and Occupational Therapy in Pediatrics*. 1983;3:43-60.

45. Kirk S, McCarthy J, Kirk W. *Illinois Test of Psycholinguistic Abilities*. Rev ed. Urbana, Ill: University of Illinois Press; 1968.

46. Gardner MF. *Test of Visual Perceptual Skills (Non-motor)*. Seattle, Wash: Special Child Publications; 1982.

47. Colarusso RP, Hammill DP. *Motor Free Visual Perception Test*. Novato, Calif: Academic Therapy Publications; 1972.

48. Ayres AJ. *Sensory Intergration and Praxis Test*. Los Angeles, Calif: Western Psychological Services; 1989.

49. Golden C, Purisch A, Hammeke T. *Luria-Nebraska Neuropsychological Battery: Forms I and II*. Los Angeles, Calif: Western Psychological Services; 1985.

50. Benton AL, Hamsher K deS, Varney NR, et al. *Contributions to Neuropsychological Assessment: A Clinical Manual.* New York, NY: Oxford University Press Inc; 1983.

51. Reitan R, Wolfson D. *The Halstead-Reitan Test Battery: Theory and Clinical Interpretation.* Tuscon, Ariz: Neuropsychology Press; 1985.

52. Shumway-Cook A, Horak FB. Assessing the influence of sensory interaction on balance. *Phys Ther.* 1986;66:1548-1550.

53. Ayres AJ. *Sensory Integration and Learning Disorders.* Los Angeles, Calif: Western Psychological Services; 1972.

54. Ayres AJ. *Sensory Integration and the Child.* Los Angeles, Calif: Western Psychological Services; 1979.

Chapter 19

Psychological Growth as a Determinant of Motor Development

Elizabeth L. Leonard, PhD, PT
Affiliate Staff Scientist
Section of Child Neurology
Division of Neurology
and
Division of Neurobiology
Barrow Neurological Institute
St. Joseph's Hospital and Medical Center
Phoenix, AZ 85013

The past three decades have marked a resurgence in infant study, and during the last decade, major interest has been rekindled in studying motor development. The theoretical models used in physical therapy for evaluating and treating neurological disorders in children were born during the decades of the 1920s to the 1940s when experimental neurophysiology, rehabilitation, and scientific study of children were in their own infancy. New antibiotics were developed, and a vaccine for poliomyelitis was discovered. Over the past quarter century, when physical therapists first convened to discuss therapeutic approaches based on this research, much has changed. Our major change has resulted in mandated educational programs for children with disabilities, requiring physical therapy services to optimize their education. Another development has been a significant research effort dedicated to studying the impact that early experience has on learning. These separate but interrelated areas have significant import for the directing and executing programs for children with neurologic disorders, during a period of major technological and political change. The purpose of this chapter is to review research illustrating how perceptual, cognitive, and motor systems interconnect during infant development. In recent years, infancy research has illuminated several aspects about early development that show clearly simultaneous development and integration of emerging systems across developmental domains. These interdomain influences have been ignored largely in traditional theories of motor development. In particular, the influence of cognitive factors on motor development will be discussed in detail.

The neurophysiological approaches to therapeutic exercise introduced in the l960s have reached maturity, and we have witnessed the growth of physical therapy as a health profession. Despite advances, challenges lying before us are formidable because little scientific research has validated the clinical efficacy of these approaches for children with central nervous system (CNS) disorders, although the approaches have been used widely in clinics.[1,2] Procedures used in pediatric physical therapy have especially been vulnerable to scientific scrutiny.[3,4] This criticism has not only forced us to assume a "defensive posture" but has also provided the impetus to push forward the boundaries of scientific inquiry to improve the lives of children with neurologic disorders.

The neurophysiological approaches to therapeutic exercise discussed and disseminated as part of the NUSTEP conference[5] were influenced strongly by views of CNS physiology described originally by the early experimentalneurophysiologists including Magnus,[6] Sherrington,[7] and, later, Peiper.[8] Their research described changes in neural functioning, principally in animals with progressively sectioned rostral lesions, by examining neural changes in behavior at each lesioned section. Applied to children and adults with CNS pathology, resulting neurological symptoms were treated therapeutically with models developed from this corpus of research. The concept of a hierarchical system of CNS reflex organization that could modify movement dysfunction by altering kinesthetic and proprioceptive inputs through exercise derived from this work.

The impact of this research on physical therapy treatment procedures has been significant, but we have begun to search for other factors contributing to motor development besides the role of reflex function in motor behavior. There appears to be consensus among physical therapists engaged in motor science research that models based on research on infrahuman species and neurologically compromised adults may not be efficacious therapeutically because they use a dated understanding of CNS neurophysiology. Touwen[9] stated that neural behavior observed in mature lesioned animals and neurologically impaired adults may resemble reactions seen in young infants, but these behaviors reflect superficial similarities rather than real differences. He questioned whether it was scientifically or therapeutically appropriate to use such comparisons to understand neuropathology resulting from childhood brain injury. Clearly, there is a need to enhance our understanding of motor function by formulating new postulates that rely on contemporary research. Krebs and Harris[10] have challenged us to put aside existing theories and move forward.

After a four decade hiatus, motor development is no longer a dormant area of infancy research studied predominantly by one discipline. Biomechanical, neurological, developmental, and neurobiological components of motor function including development of infant perception, learning, and memory are investigated actively. Interdisciplinary study is carving out new areas of fruitful investigation in motor and cognitive science. Physical therapists share a rapprochement in their interest in motor development with psychologists, motor scientists, anthropologists, linguists, and other neuroscientists. Motor development shares an interest with the study of infant perception, cognition, motivation, and learning, all of which have contributed to this renaissance in the study of motor development.

Resurgence in the scientific study of children has prompted re-examination of many different theories developed before the infancy explosion of recent decades. Motor development theory, as proposed initially by Gesell[11] and McGraw,[12] has not been the only theory questioned. Contemporary child development research has also questioned psychological studies at variance with prevailing theories for evaluating and treating children with neurologic disorders; this questioning includes the concept of sensorimotor development. Technological advances such as magnetic resonance imaging, positron emission tomography, neonatal extracorporal membrane oxygenation, and new experimental and statistical methods have profoundly influenced the research and clinical study of children with neurologic disorders. Examination of our theoretical body of knowledge is essential to determine whether physical therapy should continue to embrace present evaluation and treatment approaches or modify them based on experimental research rather than anecdotal observations. We are at a major juncture, with profound implications for professional education, clinical practice, and scientific credibility.

Barr and Zelazo[13] identified fundamental assumptions questioning foundations of knowledge in the light of contemporary infancy research. Researchers and clinicians must decide whether the experimental evidence is sufficiently powerful to compel changes in physical therapy education and clinical practice.

Reflective clinicians would be unencumbered by encrusted beliefs or vested interests but vexed by the case that didn't fit, or the prediction that did not turn out as expected. Clinicians must now be interested in changing behaviors that provide a better fit with experience or helped solve a paradox in their understanding of a clinical problem.[13(p6)]

It is no longer acceptable for physical therapists to say it works so I will use that clinically, we must also be asking how and discovering why.

COGNITIVE INFLUENCE ON MOTOR DEVELOPMENT

James[14] described the newborn's world as existing as a "blooming, buzzing confusion." The notion of the infant as a bundle of reflexes, reliant totally on a caregiver and incapable of self-directed activity, is no longer tenable. The view of infants as "competent" in the sense that they control their environment through movement and action from the earliest days of life has replaced the view of the human infant as a helpless being.

During the first year, over one of the briefest periods within the human life span and a period of rapid developmental change, the infant's motor repertoire changes dramatically as he locomotes bipedally, develops the capacity to use tools such as a spoon, ceases nursing and learns to drink from a cup, and holds a crayon adaptively. These motor skills acquired during the first year illustrate rapid progression of gross and fine motor abilities during infancy. The accomplishments of the infant reflected in this progression of milestones is not restricted to the motor domain. During this same period of time, the infant's vocalizations change from idiosyncratic sounds to the articulated language of his parents, and his development of cognitive representation is reflected in his demonstrated capacity to think symbolically.[15] These profound changes are orchestrated by an interaction between the infant and his environment and do not occur in a vacuum. Although physical therapists have been interested in sensorimotor development, the notion that psychological mechanisms guide changes in motor, cognitive, linguistic, and social domains has not generally been acknowledged. Indeed, the role that cognition plays in understanding the evolution of motor behavior has largely been ignored.

A maturational model has dominated the study of motor development since it was originally proposed by Gesell[11] and McGraw[12] over half a century ago. These scientists painstakingly described motor behavior according to an age-defined chronology where new behaviors were seen as milestones within motor ontogeny. Gesell's[11] premise stated that motor behavior emerged in a hierarchically ordered, invariant sequence dependent on cortical maturation dictated by a genetic blueprint of CNS maturation. This was a continuously elaborated endogenous process beginning with conception and proceeding in ordered stages. Each stage represented a higher level attained by CNS maturation but devoid of environmental influences. Implicitly, the premise assumed that CNS changes produced behavioral change. It was never a theoretical consideration that developmental patterns could be influenced environmentally or that infant behavior was learned through organismic-environmental interaction. New research has shown unequivocally that the environment effects developing perceptual and organ systems and exerts powerful influences on the trajectories of development. The infant learns to construct meaningful representations of his world. Knowledge does not unfold spontaneously.

How does the infant come to know his world? According to Newell and Barclay,[16] knowledge involves accumulation of information about specific events, tasks, situations, and attunements from the environment. From a metacognitive perspective, an infant acquires knowledge about his own psychological, social, and physical behavior through purposeful environmental interaction. Newell and Barclay[16] stated that this involves an awareness of one's actions for mediating different task demands.

Although maturation is one contributor to motor development, constitutional, environmental, learning, and experiential factors also shape, pace, and constrain development of motor behavior. The evaluation of normal and abnormal development implores us to consider several assumptions about motor development to formulate a perspective on the evolution of human motor ontogeny.

Prechtl[17] stated that infant neurological assessment techniques are useful only when they can provide useful diagnostic and prognostic information about the vulnerability of the neonatal brain to insult. A coherent assessment system is multidimensional and multifactorial and includes both neurological and behavioral evaluation. Prechtl[17] adopted a neo-classical position and stated that the concept of newborn reflex organization is antiquated and should be replaced by a systems perspective reflecting the neonate's capacity to initiate and regulate neural activity through information processing, learning, and environmental adaptation.

RELATING COGNITIVE, DEVELOPMENTAL, AND MOTOR THEORIES

Wolff[18] described different models explaining developmental ontogeny. One model, termed *maturationism,* stated that intrinsic timetables control the course of ontogeny, where experience can initiate but not induce function. The role of maturational theories of motor development has had asignificant impact on the development of systems for therapeutic remediation and is illustrated most clearly by neurodevelopmental therapy.[19] Wolff[18] also described an epigenetic-constructivist-interactionist model that incorporates the role of heredity and epigenetic influences on behavioral development. In this model, the interactionist component reflects the position that biology and experience are different facets of a unitary developmental process. The constructivist component illustrates how ontogenetic transformations can be shaped by morphological, physiological, and behavioral properties genetically or environmentally present in a developing organism. Antecedent organismic conditions are incorporated by later developing structures and functions. Stages are integrated successively until they converge at maturity.

Motor development was assumed to be highly canalized function directed toward specific end states by intrinsic mechanisms. Epigenesis describes how, during development, biology and experience interact to account for developmental change.[20] Continuous and reciprocal epigenetic interactions between the child and his environment incorporate perceptual and cognitive processes as developmental covariants. The interdigitation of intrinsic, extrinsic, and environmental factors is acknowledged to be important in influencing developmental change in a dynamical systems model but has not been a component of a maturational model.

Kagan et al[21] illustrated how developmental processes change at different rates over time. During childhood, psychological structures are formed as a result of individual processes that are syntonic and yoked. The correlation between two emerging abilities may but need not imply a common underlying structure. A close temporal emergence between certain abilities during particular periods of growth may reflect a common source.

Fischer[22,23] used the term *interval synchrony* to describe the emergence of two or more new developmental abilities between a relatively limited time interval. For example, if one uses the criteria of wariness to document the onset of stranger anxiety, both Zelazo and Leonard[24] and Bowlby[25] have the onset of stranger anxiety at a chronological age of about 9 months. This is concordant with the onset of unsupported sitting. Even though these two behaviors appear to be yoked temporally, they do not appear to share a common developmental pathway.[21] There are examples where interval synchrony illustrates a common underlying developmental phenomena. Zelazo[26] and Zelazo and Leonard[24] described how the onset of independent locomotion, expressive language, and functional object use coincided developmentally and met criteria for optimal level and interval synchrony in Fischer's[22,23] stage theory of cognitive development.

Zelazo[26] proposed that the basis for the interdomain emergence of these new skills was due to a fundamental change in the speed of information processing, leading to the capacity to generate two associations rapidly that formed a necessary but not sufficient condition for the expression of these diverse behaviors. A compelling basis for this view is the relatively brief period in development, between 11 to 14 months of age, when these changes occur. These developments are so pervasive as to constitute a genuine transformation: a true metamorphosis in cognitive development. Moreover, Zelazo and Leonard[24] stated that although mental and motor development may proceed synchronously, they need not, as is the case in some infants with motor retardation who are cognitively intact.

Although physical therapists have acknowledged that motor development proceeds in stages according to a maturational timetable, they have not recognized that cognitive factors play an instrumental role in orchestrating changes in motor behavior. Covariation in the rate of growth in related psychological dimensions forms sequences with regular relationships between structure, function, and action. Psychological structures produced by childhood experiences undergo dynamic transformations and are consolidated and reconstructed over time. Organisms never stop developing, but rates of change will vary over time; where there is slow or little change among sets of critical variables, growth is said to be stable.[21]

SENSORIMOTOR DEVELOPMENT AND DEVELOPMENTAL ASSESSMENT

Interest in finding predictability in forecasting developmental function lead early infancy-researchers to explore whether or not developmental diagnosis was possible, based on the premise that development was linear or near linear.[27-29] If the characteristics of a particular developmental state at Time 1 was stable, development could be predicted at another point in time. There was a hope that when infant tests were developed originally, they would have predictive as well as discriminant validity. Finding stability in motor and psychological development from infancy through early childhood certainly would have made developmental diagnosis a more exact science.

Tests such as the Bayley Scales of Infant Development,[30] Denver Developmental Screening Test,[31] and Gesell Developmental Schedules[32] confound assessment of motor and mental abilities, making developmental prediction from infancy unreliable when these measures are used.[33-36] Bayley[30] acknowledged that the Mental scale could not predict future mental behavior; this fact was verified empirically later by Hanzig.[27] Critical examination of Mental scale items reveals that the requirements necessary to pass test criterion requires, in many cases, reliance on motor performance.[36,37] For example, on the Bayley Mental scale at age 2.6 months the infant is required to raise his arms in anticipation of being lifted by his mother. This measure of early social referencing requires a motor action to infer a cognitive operation and exemplifies the motor confound on the Mental scale. If a baby with muscle hypotonia or hypertonia cannot elevate his arms because of muscle weakness or spasticity, are we to infer from the absence of arm lifting that he does not anticipate the contingent relation between maternal proximity and the desire to be held? Items that require overt motor actions to infer cognitive abilities by requiring the infant to stack cubes or place objects into containers are even more obvious examples of how infant tests rely on motor function to determine a diagnostic impression of mental ability and illustrate clearly the confounding of cognitive assessment.

An information processing model of cognitive development bypasses this sensory-motor confound and measures more directly the development of psychological structures used for encoding, storing, and retrieving information.[33-36] These procedures use infant attention to measure rates of habituation and dishabituation to visual and auditory stimuli used to construct mental schemata. These procedures measure infant attention and rates at which mental representations for repeated visual and auditory stimuli are created. Information processing research has demonstrated that central processing measured in newborns and young infants appears to predict later intelligence, whereas prediction of IQ from traditional infant tests has been poor.[27-29]

Static and dynamic stimuli both are used to measure formation of mental schemata in neonates through toddlers. Dependent measures using static visual stimuli record visual fixation to stimuli such as bull's eyes and checkerboards. Dynamic stimuli create events that unfold over a period of seconds to maintain attention in older infants who become bored with static presentations.[33-36]

Zelazo and colleagues[38] measured habituation, recovery, and dishabituation of newborn head turning to speech stimuli and showed discriminant and predictive validity for neurologically intact and impaired infants. They demonstrated that this head-turning procedure provided diagnostic information that was useful clinically for evaluating neonatal mental behavior independent of a motor confound. Cohen and Parmelee[39] demonstrated significant correlations between newborn and infant visual processing when they compared preterm infants at term conceptional age and at age 5 years. Correlations between .40 and .61 were reported by Lewis and Brooks-Gunn[40] with a visual habituation paradigm measured in 12-week- old infants and the Bayley Mental scale at age 2 years. Fagan and McGrath[41] used a visual recognition memory task and found correlations of .37 and .57 during midinfancy and vocabulary tests administered at ages 4 and 7 years. In normal 3-month-old infants, visual in-

formation processing procedures have yielded modest correlations with mental ability at school entry.[39]

Perceptual and cognitive infant research has shown that information is encoded and can be recalled, illustrating the infant's early capacity for learning. Nonretarded motor-impaired infants may suffer from a competence-performance problem. They may have the necessary cognitive competence to acquire visual and auditory schemata but be limited by virtue of motor impairment from expressing that knowledge when tests requiring sensorimotor skills are used. Information processing procedures appear to permit a more accurate assessment of mental ability in motor impaired infants by eliminating motor performance as an outcome measure.

Piaget's[42] concept of sensorimotor intelligence postulated that psychological structures, termed *structures d'essemble*, were constructed by repeating sensorimotor schemes and that intelligence, the ability to think symbolically, did not develop until the end of the sensorimotor period. Piagetian theory has been contested by recent infant cognitive research.

Clinically used infant tests are correlated so poorly with later intellectual development that there is no predictive validity, although there may concurrent validity dependent on the measure used. Discriminant and predictive validity improve inversely with degree of CNS pathology, but in the absence of severe neurologic disturbance, the correlation to later development is weak.[27] The more severely impaired the infant, the greater the likelihood that correlations between measures obtained during infancy and early childhood will be significant, although modest at best. A significant diagnostic dilemma exists because measures confounding infant assessment are the clinical indices used to evaluate development in children with neurological disorders. Zelazo[34] demonstrated that motor performance measures tested on commonly used infant tests can convey a clinical impression that a child with motor impairment is mentally retarded when he may have normal intelligence. He pointed out how the twin assumption that motor delay conveyed mental retardation or that motor precocity predicted mental superiority persisted for many years in pediatric literature.

Kagan[43] demonstrated that infants are capable of forming schemata, or internal representations of mental events, that can be seen or heard independent of motor output. Kagan[43] acknowledged that the infant's instrumental adaptation to the environment could be influenced by motor facility, but that this was not necessary for establishing cognitive structures. Children can acquire cognitive representations of events through observation, a fact illustrated by cerebral palsied children who have normal mentation yet may lack any volitional control of movement.

Motor activity requires increased attention and improves the likelihood that infants pay particular notice to certain salient features, but motoric manipulation is subordinate to schemata formation. Rather, CNS maturation delimits the range of behaviors that can be expressed at particular points during development.[44]

Professionals responsible for interpreting traditional tests must understand that misinterpretation can not only result in misdiagnosis but also convey wrong information to parents challenged in rearing developmentally impaired children. Performance on conventional infant-tests can yield a misimpression that children are intellectually impaired when neuromotor dysfunction limits gross and fine motor performance. Information processing procedures bypass the motor system for acquiring information based on performance criteria requiring a motoric response. More studies are required to gain an increased appreciation of how developing psychological structures influence motor development.

Development of new research paradigms that improve diagnostic acumen through more explicitly defining motor, cognitive, and emotional factors subserving development will advance the science of development diagnosis. Using specific tests that do not confound assessment of motor, cognitive, and social behavior will improve the clinical utility and the discriminant and predictive validity of infant tests.

The clinical application of kinematic analysis of movement has shown great promise for furthering understanding of normal and aberrant motor development during infancy and childhood.[45-48] Kinematic procedures measure motor behavior directly and are largely independent of cognitive confounds. Scientists using kinematics to describe normal and abnormal motor behavior are modifying traditional views of infant motor development just as developmental psychologists using information processing procedures have modified traditional views of infant cognition. It is likely that the concept of sensorimotor intelligence will require modification as new diagnostic procedures that are specific for assessing motor and cognitive abilities are developed further.

NONLINEARITY IN PSYCHOLOGICAL AND MOTOR DEVELOPMENT

Stage theory has been used to explain motor and psychological development. The role that developmental sequences have played in evaluation and treatment planning for developmentally impaired children is unquestioned. Developmental sequences of motor behaviors have had a major role in the intervention procedures used in neurodevelopmental therapy,[19] Rood,[49] and proprioceptive neuromuscular facilitation.[50]

Stage theories of psychological development are represented by the work of S. Freud,[51] A. Freud,[52] Erikson,[53] and Piaget.[42] An assumption of stage theory is that invariant sequences are formed, with hierarchical relationships defining transitions from one stage to another. In motor development theory,[11] according to the principle of cephalocaudal development, an infant must crawl before he walks; in psychoanalytic theory, an infant can develop substantial psychological autonomy before totally resolving issues in separation.[54] Stage theory assumes that children must master the developmental tasks of each stage before progressing to the next set of developmental skills. However, crawling has not been shown empirically to be a necessary prerequisite for bipedal locomotion, nor has resolving separation anxiety been a prerequisite for establishing mastery over other psychological developments acquired during infancy.

Several research examples have illustrated how the presumed invariance of cephalocaudal development has not been shown to be a necessary condition for motor development. A maturational model has not accounted adequately for individual differences or cultural variability in the rate

and sequence in which motor behavior develops.[15,55,56] Moreover, cultural and environmental factors have been shown to shape the trajectory of motor behavior to a greater degree than has generally been acknowledged.[57,58]

Piaget[42] proposed that cognition developed from the child's interaction with the environment and that cognitive growth emerged through the complementary processes of assimilation and accommodation. The infant assimilated information through action with the environment. Accommodation described the process by which information was incorporated to induce psychological change. During the sensorimotor period, which extends from birth to age 2 years, infants pass through six stages, beginning with organization of reflex responses and progressing to development of symbolic representation. Initially, this involves exercise of sensorimotor schemes resulting from elaboration of primitive reflexive responses. Separate schemes for sucking, grasping, and other motor sequences are incorporated increasingly into more sophisticated actions as infants combine schemes to attain a goal. Infants were not considered capable of independent thought until the preoperational period, when language and the capacity for symbolic thinking were acquired. This ability developed from the elaboration of sensorimotor activity.

Piaget[42] acknowledged violation of stage invariance and developed the concept of decalage to explain nonsequential development of cognitive abilities where stage invariance existed. A child who developed the capacity to conserve mass before number illustrates an example of decalage.

Mounoud and Bower[59] showed that year-old infants adjusted arm movement and force of hand grasp to weights of different rods placed in their hands and could conserve weight. This ability was not present when infants were tested initially at an age of 7 months. Conservation of weight is a Piagetian task expected to be accomplished during the concrete operational period at a mental age of about 7 years. This unusual demonstration not only illustrates a highly salient example of a vertical decalage, or a between-stage invariance, but also suggests that infants about 1 year old possess the capacity to discern a relationship between size and mass. If infants can discern this relation, then cognitive operations might be functional sooner than has previously been acknowledged.

Bowlby[25] recognized that cognitive processes might not only influence development earlier in infancy than thought before but also influence emotional development. Bowlby[25] illustrated how research from information processing and systems theory is modifying traditional psychoanalytic theory that uses psychic energy and drive-reduction concepts to explain personality development. Importantly, Bowlby[25] noted that awareness and intentionality emerged by the end of the first year and was used in regulation of affect. Bowlby[25] acknowledged a biological readiness for affective mediation that matured near the infant's first birthday. Konner[60] described how cross-cultural universals in psychosocial development, such as social smiling, attachment behavior, and language development, can be attributed to neural and neuroendocrine maturation of cortical structures including corticospinal pathways, basal ganglia, and limbic structures.

Psychological Growth as a Determinant of Motor Development

Zelazo[61] stated that formation of memory engrams produces neural-chemical changes based on experience as the infant calibrates internalized mental events (schemata) with external stimuli. Memory formation is a cognitive phenomenon that has affective components reflecting internal feeling states manifested expressively by behaviors such as smiling or crying. Moreover, the infant experiences a match that is constantly changing in regard to the internalized standard to account for learning. This internal calibration between schemata and experience is fluid and dynamic and allows the infant to process and internalize new information progressively. The yoking of emotions with cognitive behaviors is compatible with the concept of a central executive function for regulating interdomain behaviors.[61]

Recently, Zelazo et al[62] demonstrated that infants 72 hours of age systematically controlled direction of head turning to avoid responding to redundant auditory information, which in this instance was naturally spoken words. Systematic avoidance of redundant sounds implied that infants used a motor response—head turning—to avoid redundancy that produced boredom—an affective response.

Transitions in cognitive development can be observed during play by studying the quality of infant's ability to manipulate toys and discern function relations in how toys are used.[63,64] Zelazo and Kearsley[64] showed that infants between the ages of 9.5 to 15.5 months changed in their ability to manipulate toys from indiscriminate stereotypical activity consisting of mouthing, fingering, waving, or banging to use of toys in goal directed functional activities. The motor competence required to manipulate toys during a 15-minute session of free play was measured by recording the quality of toy manipulation. No differences existed in the physical requirements for manipulating toys for all ages studied. The results showed the changes were in the infant's capacity to alter toy manipulation from nondirected stereotypical to directed functional activity. Leonard and Zelazo[65] found a similar pattern of responses in an age-corrected group of premature infants who, when compared with a normal referent group, discerned functional relations between toys at 15 months but not at 12 months of age. When the premature and normal infants were compared on the Bayley Mental scale at 12 and 15 months of age, their scores were not statistically different.

In the examples cited above, it is likely that neuromotor maturation was not a sufficient condition to account for these changes. The dexterity required to manipulate toys in the play experiments was not very different between ages sampled. The changes cited above demonstrated an evolving motor competence that had as an underlying feature the infant's capacity to understand associative relations. Zelazo[26] proposed that the capacity to generate rapid specific associations constituted a cognitive metamorphosis that allowed infants to generate ideas. This ability appeared toward the end of the first year, between the ages of about 11 to 14 months, when infants appear literally to show the dawn of active thought.[24] The year-old infant appears to have developed the capacity to generate novel ideas. In dynamical systems terminology, this would constitute a *major phase shift* where de novo forms of behavior, in this instance the ability to activate hypotheses,[43] appears for the first time in development. That this ability illustrates interdomain developmental transitions is a compelling reason to argue that the bases for these changes are influenced cognitively. It is at this time that babies begin to speak, spontaneously scribble, and take their first independent steps as they toddle tentatively across the room.[26] Clearly, there are other points in infant development where there are major developmental transitions, but none appear to be as profound as the changes occurring at the end of the first year.

INFANT MOTOR LEARNING AND INSTRUMENTAL RESPONDING

Physical therapists are aware of transitions in motor development that occur at about age 3 months when the so-called primitive reflexes are no longer elicited easily. Transitions in behavior during infancy around certain nodal points were recognized by McCall and associates.[66] Nonlinearity in motor development is reflected in the spurts, plateaus, and regressions seen in changes in motor behavior during the first year.[67,68] Newborns will "walk" if placed upright and inclined forward, a behavior that ceases to exist after the fourth month of life and is replaced by unassisted bipedal locomotion between 9 to 15 months of age. This change in locomotor behavior follows a U-shaped curve and illustrates nonlinearity in motor development.[67]

Zelazo and colleagues[55] performed one of the earliest studies on infant locomotion and demonstrated that the presumed discontinuity in locomotor development could be influenced by opportunities for practice and contingent reinforcement. Stepping could be increased when an innate neuromotor response was transformed through instrumental learning. The presumed invariance of a cephalocaudal progression of motor development has been illustrated in cross-cultural studies that demonstrated the effects of culture and experience on the acquisition of motor behaviors.[67,68]

Zelazo,[69] Leonard,[67] and Zelazo et al[68] argued that infants transform innate motor patterns from the initially appearing "reflexive responses" to the volitionally controlled responses influenced by higher-order control as instrumental control of innate motor patterns is acquired through practice and experience. The infant's ability to activate motor behaviors in response to specific stimuli has been demonstrated for a variety of motor responses including sucking,[70] kicking,[71] stepping,[55,67,69] and head turning.[61] Thus motor behaviors that were previously thought to be under reflex control have been shown, across a variety of motor behaviors, to be shaped by instrumental learning. The ability of infants to transform innate motor patterns into voluntary motor acts challenges some traditional assumptions of neurodevelopmental therapy. Review of recent research argues for a close examination of neurodevelopmental theory to determine whether it is theoretically tenable and therapeutically efficacious.

In a large study of infants with brain injury, Katona[72,73] distinguished between primitive reflexes and elementary neuromotor patterns. He demonstrated that brain damaged infants could learn to activate elementary motor patterns through a therapeutically designed intervention program used to remediate motor dysfunction caused by CNS pathology. Katona[72,73] showed that activation of innate elementary neuromotor patterns could be used to habilitate infants with neurologic deficits, through early training to shape and train motor responses. Zelazo et al,[68] Leonard,[67] and Zelazo et al (N. Zelazo, PhD; unpublished data; 1990) demonstrated that stepping and sitting could be modified through opportunities for practice and contingent reinforcement in normal infants, in infants at risk for cerebral palsy, and in an infant with cystic periventricular leukomalacia. Moreover, in contrast to existing therapeutic procedures used in physical therapy, instrumental learning of motor responses can be acquired in relatively brief training sessions. Zelazo et al[68] illustrated that meaningful changes in motor responses can occur with as little as 12 minutes a day of specific exercises.

Rovee-Collier and Fagan,[71] Rovee-Collier and Hayne,[74] and Ohr et al,[75] in studies with normal infants, demonstrated that infants as young as 12 weeks of age could be conditioned instrumentally to kick, activating a crib mobile. Kicking was reactivated once conditioning trials were terminated by briefly re-exposing infants to the initial training conditions. The studies were designed to investigate the development of memory but not of motor memory in particular. However, the results provide additional evidence that infants encode, store, and retrieve motor memories much earlier in development than acknowledged previously.

SUMMARY AND CONCLUSION

The goal of this review was to draw attention to the increasing body of infant literature illustrating how cognition influences development of motor behavior. It is no longer desirable to continue using neurophysiological approaches of therapeutic exercise without seriously examining the scientific theory that underlies these approaches. Experimental investigations using appropriate control groups are essential to determine clinical efficacy.

The corpus of research reviewed suggests that the maturational theory and the concept of sensorimotor development may require significant modification in light of current investigations. Central influences reflecting higher-order control appear to be present in neonates and are elaborated progressively as maturation enables larger bits of information to be processed and as the storage capacity for memory expands during the first year of life. This relative process for the acquisition of motor behavior occurs gradually as infants gain instrumental control of motor actions and acquire knowledge. Toward the end of the first year, infants can activate and process the ability to perform two motor acts in succession. It is hypothesized that this capacity is accompanied by an increased awareness of the infant's environment.

The therapeutic consequences that derive from this research suggest that the contribution of cognitive factors to the development of motor behavior has been underestimated significantly. Additionally, the heavy reliance of motor performance in traditional tests of infant development may require re-examination if we are to understand more completely how brain pathology influences early development. Both tasks raise significant challenges as we attempt to become more skillful clinicians in our evaluation and treatment of children with neuromotor pathology.

Acknowledgments

Some of the research reported in this review was supported partially by a grant to me from the New Hampshire Developmental Disabilities Council and aided by the Social and Behavioral Science Research Grant, Number 12-236, from the March of Dimes Birth Defects Foundation; I appreciate the support of these agencies. I also thank Philip Zelazo for drawing attention to the central factors that influence development of cognition and motor behavior. Additionally, I appreciate the thoughtful critiques of this chapter that were provided by Stuart Goldman and Philip Zelazo. I accept full responsibility for the views expressed.

References

1. Piper M, Kunos I, Willis D, et al. Early physical therapy on the high risk infant: a randomized control trial. *Pediatrics.* 1986;78:216- 224.
2. Palmer F, Shapiro B, Wachtel R, et al. The effects of physical therapy on cerebral palsy. *N Engl J Med.* 1988;318:803.
3. Denhoff E. Current status of infant stimulation programs for children with developmental disabilities. *Pediatrics.* 1981;67:32-37.
4. Ferry P. On growing new neurons: are early intervention programs effective? *Pediatrics.* 1981;67:38-41.
5. An exploratory and analytical survey of therapeutic exercises: proceedings of Northwestern University Special Therapeutic Exercise Project. *Am J Phys Med.* 1967;46:9-1135.
6. Magnus R. Korperstellung: the experimental basis for theories of vestibular function. *Proceedings of the Royal Society of Medicine [Berlin].* 1924;XXII.
7. Sherrington C. *The Integrative Action of the Nervous System.* New Haven, Conn: Yale University Press; 1947.
8. Peiper A. *Cerebral Function in Infancy and Childhood.* New York, NY: Consultants Bureau; 1961.
9. Touwen B. Primitive reflexes: conceptual or semantic problem? In: Prechtl H, ed. *Continuity of Neuro Functions from Prenatal to Postnatal Life.* Boston, Mass: Blackwell Scientific Publications Inc; 1984:115-125.
10. Krebs D, Harris S. Elements of theory presentation in physical therapy. *Phys Ther.* 1988;68:690-693.
11. Gesell A. *The First Five Years of Life: A Guide to the Study of the Preschool Child.* New York, NY: Harper; 1940.
12. McGraw M. *The Neuromotor Maturation of the Human Infant.* New York, NY: Hafner Publishing Co; 1945.
13. Barr R, Zelazo PR. Do challenges to development compel changes in practice? In: Zelazo PR, Batt R, eds. *Challenges to Developmental Paradigms: Implications for Theory, Assessment, and Treatment.* Hillsdale, NJ: Lawrence Erlbaum Associates Inc; 1989:3-10.
14. James W. *The Principles of Psychology (1880).* New York, NY: Dover Publications Inc; 1960.
15. Zelazo PR. The development of walking: new findings and old assumptions. *Journal of Motor Behavior.* 1983;15:99-137.
16. Newell KM, Barclay CR. Developing knowledge about action. In: Kelso JAS, Clark JE, eds. *The Development of Movement Control and Coordination.* New York, NY: John Wiley & Sons Inc; 1982:175-212.
17. Prechtl H. Assessment methods for the newborn infant: a critical evaluation. In: Stratton P, ed. *Psychobiology of the Human Newborn.* New York, NY: John Wiley & Sons Inc; 1982:21-52.
18. Wolff P. The concept of development: how does it constrain

assessment and therapy? In: Zelazo PR, Barr R, eds. *Challenges to Developmental Paradigms: Implications for Theory, Assessment, and Treatment.* Hillsdale, NJ: Lawrence Erlbaum Associates Inc; 1989:13-28.

19. Bobath B. The very early treatment of cerebral palsy. *Dev Med Child Neurol.* 1967;9:373-390.

20. Wilson R. Synchronies in mental development: an epigenetic perspective. *Science* 1978;202:939.

21. Kagan J. Kearsley R, Zelazo PR. *Infancy: Its Place in Human Development.* Cambridge, Mass: Harvard University Press; 1978.

22. Fisher K. A theory of cognitive development: the control and construction of hierarchies of skills. *Psychol Rev.* 1980;87:477-531.

23. Fisher K. Developmental levels as periods of discontinuity. In: Fisher K, ed. *Levels and Transitions in Children's Development: New Directions in Child Development.* San Francisco, Calif: Jossey-Bass Inc, Publishers; 1983;12:5-19.

24. Zelazo PR, Leonard E. The dawn of active thought. In: Fisher K, ed. *Levels and Transitions in Children's Development: New Directions for Child Development.* San Francisco, Calif: Jossey-Bass Inc, Publishers; 1983;12:37-49.

25. Bowlby J. *A Secure Base: Parent-Child Attachment and Healthy Human Development.* New York, NY: Basic Books Inc, Publishers; 1988.

26. Zelazo PR. The year-old infant: a period of major cognitive change. In: Bever T, ed. *Regressions in Development: Basic Phenomena and Theoretical Alternatives.* Hillsdale, NJ: Lawrence Erlbaum Associates Inc; 1982:45-77.

27. Honzig MP. Measuring mental abilities in infancy: the value and limitations. In: Lewis M, ed. *Origins of Intelligence.* New York, NY: Plenum Publishing Corp; 1983:67-105.

28. McCall R. The development of intellectual functioning in infancy and the prediction of later IQ. In: Osofosky J, ed. *The Handbook of Infant Development.* New York, NY: John Wiley & Sons Inc; 1979:707-741.

29. Stott L, Ball R. Infant and preschool mental tests: review and evaluation. *Monogr Soc Res Child Dev.* 1965;30.

30. Bayley N. *Manual for the Bayley Scales of Infant Development.* New York, NY: The Psychological Corporation; 1969.

31. Frankenberg W, Dodds J. *The Denver Developmental Screening Test.* Denver, Colo: University of Colorado Medical Center; 1968.

32. Knobloch H, Malone A, Stevens R. *Manual of Developmental Diagnosis: The Administration and Interpretation of the Revised Gesell and Amatruda Developmental and Neurological Examination.* New York, NY: Harper & Row, Publishers Inc; 1980.

33. Zelazo PR. An information processing approach to infant-toddler assessment and intervention. In: Fitzgerald HE, Lester BM, Yogman M, eds. *Theory and Research in Behavioral Pediatrics.* 3rd ed. New York, NY: Plenum Publishing Corp; 1986:1-45.

34. Zelazo PR. An information processing approach to infant cognitive assessment. In: Lewis M, Taft L, eds. *Developmental Disabilities: Theory, Assessment, and Intervention.* Jamaica, NY: S P Medical and Scientific Books; 1982:229-255.

35. Zelazo PR. Infant-toddler information processing and the development of expressive ability. In: Zelazo PR, Barr R, eds. *Challenges to Developmental Paradigms: Implications for Theory, Assessment, and Treatment.* Hillsdale, NJ: Lawrence Erlbaum Associates Inc: 1989:93-112.

36. Zelazo PR. An information processing paradigm for infant-toddler mental assessment. In: Vietze P, Vaughan H, eds.

Early Identification of Infants with Developmental Disabilities. San Diego, Calif: Grune & Stratton Inc; 1988:300-317.

37. Leonard E. *Neonatal Neuromotor Abnormalities: Effects on Infant Mental Test Performance.* Boston, Mass: Tufts University; 1986. Dissertation.

38. Zelazo PR, Weiss MJ, Papageorgiou A, LaPlante D. Recovery and dishabituation of sound localization among normal, moderate, and high risk newborns. *Infant Behavior and Development.* 1989;12:321-340.

39. Cohen S, Parmelee A. Prediction of five year Standford-Binet scores in preterm infants. *Child Dev.* 1983;54:1242-1253.

40. Lewis M, Brooks-Gunn J. Visual attention at three months as a predictor of cognitive functioning at two years of age. *Intelligence.* 1981;5:131-140.

41. Fagan J, McGrath S. Infant recognition memory and later intelligence. *Intelligence.* 1981;5:121-130.

42. Piaget J. *The Origins of Intelligence in Children.* New York, NY: International University Press; 1952.

43. Kagan J. Do infants think? *Sci Am.* 1972;226:74-83.

44. Kagan J. Three themes in developmental psychology. In: Lipsitt L, ed. *Development Psychology: The Significance of Infancy.* Hillsdale, NJ: Lawrence Erlbaum Associates Inc; 1976:129-137.

45. Heriza C. Organization of leg movements in preterm infants. *Phys Ther.* 1988;68:1340-1346.

46. Leonard E, Maulucci R, Eliason L. Kinematics of reaching in normal and cerebral palsied infants. Presented at the Seventh International Conference on Infant Studies; April 19-22, 1990; Montreal, Quebec, Canada.

47. Leonard E, Maulucci R, Eliason R. Kinematics and temporal analysis of upper extremity movement in normal and cerebral palsied three year olds. Presented at the 65th Annual Conference of the American Physical Therapy Association; June 24-28, 1990; Anaheim, Calif.

48. Kluzik J, Fetters L, Coryell J. Quantification of control: a preliminary study of effects of neurodevelopmental treatment on reaching in children with spastic cerebral palsy. *Phys Ther.* 1990;70:65-78.

49. Rood M. Neurophysiological mechanisms utilized in the treatment of neuromuscular dysfunction. *Am J Occup Ther.* 1956;10:220-224.

50. Knott M, Voss D. *Proprioceptive Neuromuscular Facilitation.* New York, NY: Harper & Row, Publishers Inc; 1968.

51. Freud S. An outline of psycho-analysis. In: *Standard edition.* London, England: Hogarth Press; 1964;23:141-207.

52. Freud A. *Normality and Pathology in Childhood: Assessments of Development.* Madison, Conn: International Universities Press Inc; 1965.

53. Erikson E. *Childhood and Society.* New York, NY: W W Norton & Co Inc; 1950.

54. Bowlby J. The nature of the child's tie to his mother. *Int J Psychoanal.* 1958;39:350-373.

55. Zelazo PR, Zelazo N, Kolb S. Walking in the newborn. *Science.* 1972;176:314.

56. Leonard E, Zelazo PR. From reflexive to instrumental control; a developmental model of motor learning. Presented at the American Physical Therapy Association/Canadian Physiotherapy Association Joint Conference; June 12-16, 1988; Las Vegas, Nev.

57. Konner M. Maternal care and infant behavior and development among the Kalahari Desert San. In: Lee R, DeVore I, eds. *Kalahari Hunter Gathers.* Cambridge, Mass: Harvard University Press, 1977.

58. Super C. Environmental effects on motor development: the

case of African infant precocity. *Dev Med Child Neurol.* 1976;93:73.

59. Mounoud P, Bower T. Conservation of weight in infants. *Cognition.* 1974;3:29-40.

60. Konner M. Spheres and modes of inquiry; integrative challenges in child development research. In: Zelazo PR, Barr R, eds. *Challenges to Developmental Paradigms: Implications for Theory, Assessment, and Treatment.* Hillsdale, NJ: Lawrence Erlbaum Associates Inc; 1989:227-258.

61. Zelazo PR. Infant-toddler information processing and the development of expressive ability. In: Zelazo PR, Barr R, eds. *Challenges for Developmental Paradigms: Implications for Theory, Assessment, and Treatment.* Hillsdale, NJ: Lawrence Erlbaum Associates Inc; 1989:93-112.

62. Zelazo PR, Weiss M, Tarwuinio N. Habituation and recovery of neonatal orienting to auditory stimuli. In: Weiss MJ, Zelazo PR, eds. *Newborn Attention: Biological Constraints and Environmental Influences.* Norwood, NJ: Ablex Publishing Corp. In press.

63. Fenson L, Kagan J, Kearsley R, Zelazo PR. Developmental progression of manipulative play in the first two years. *Child Dev.* 1976;47:232-236.

64. Zelazo PR, Kearsley R. The emergence of functional play: evidence for a major cognitive transition. *Journal of Applied Developmental Psychology.* 1980;1:95-117.

65. Leonard E, Zelazo PR. Play in developmental evaluation. Poster presented at the Sixth Biennial Meeting of the International Society of Infant Studies: April 21-24, 1988; Washington, DC.

66. McCall RB, Eichorn D, Hogarty PA. Transitions in early mental development. *Monog Soc Res Child Dev.* 1977;42.

67. Leonard E. Early motor development and control: foundations for independent walking. In: Smidt G, ed. *Gait in Rehabilitation.* New York, NY: Churchill Livingstone Inc; 1990:121-140.

68. Zelazo PR, Weiss MJ, Leonard E. The development of unaided walking: the acquisition of higher order control. In: Zelazo PR, Barr R, eds. *Challenges to Developmental Paradigms: Implications for Theory, Assessment, and Treatment.* Hillsdale, NJ: Lawrence Erlbaum Associates Inc; 1989:139-165.

69. Zelazo PR. From reflexive to instrumental behavior. In: Lipsitt L, ed. *Developmental Psychobiology: The Significance of Infancy.* Hillsdale, NJ: Lawrence Erlbaum Associates Inc; 1976:87-104.

70. Lipsitt L, Kaye H. Change in neonatal responses to optimizing and nonoptimizing sucking stimuli. *Psychonomic Science.* 1965;2:221-222.

71. Rovee-Collier C, Fagan J. Extended conditioning and 24 hour retention in infants. *J Exp Child Psychol.* 1976;21:1-11.

72. Katona F. Developmental clinical neurology and neurohabilitation in the secondary prevention of pre- and perinatal injuries of the brain. In: Vietze P, Vaughan H, eds. *Early Identification of Infants with Developmental Disabilities.* San Diego, Calif: Grune & Stratton Inc; 1988:121-144.

73. Katona F. Clinical neurodevelopmental diagnosis and treatment. In: Zelazo PR, Barr R, eds. *Challenges to Developmental Paradigms: Implications for Theory, Assessment, and Treatment.* Hillsdale, NJ: Lawrence Erlbaum Associates Inc; 1989:167-187.

74. Rovee-Collier C, Hayne H. Reactivation of infant memory: implications for cognitive development. *Adv Child Dev Behav.* 1987;20:185-238.

75. Ohr PS, Fagen J, Rovee-Collier C, et al. Amount of training and retention by infants. *Dev Psychobiol.* 1989;22:1, 69-80.

Chapter 20

Motor Control Problems in Parkinson's Disease

Mark W. Rogers, PhD, PT
Assistant Professor
Programs in Physical Therapy
Northwestern University Medical School
Chicago, IL 60611

Individuals with Parkinson's disease (PD) often display a number of sensorimotor deficits that result in an impaired ability to execute functional movements. In the past 20 years, significant progress has been made in our fundamental and clinical understanding of this progressive neuro degenerative disorder.

The primary pathology in PD has generally been recognized to involve the substantia nigra pars compacta region of the midbrain, where dopaminergic neurons degenerate, together with their nigrostriatal fiber tract, resulting in a severe depletion of dopamine in the basal ganglia.[1] It has become apparent, however, that the disease is infinitely more complex, involving changes in a number of brain structures and neurotransmitter systems.[1,2]

Recent developments, such as the discovery that the compound 1-methyl-4- pheynl-1,2,3,6-tetrahydropyridine (MPTP) produces clinical symptoms and perhaps pathologic changes very similar to PD in otherwise healthy adult humans[3,4] and such as the use of tissue transplantation procedures,[5] have generated new and controversial concepts concerning the etiology, pathogenesis, and treatment of PD. An accumulating body of information from a variety of disciplines has also added substantially to our understanding of the alterations in motor control processes that may precipitate movement dysfunction in parkinsonians (PKs) (subjects with parkinsonism).[6-9]

In light of the foregoing, it is striking that significant advances in the physical therapy management of motor control problems in PD have not been forthcoming, despite the complex and puzzling nature of the motor control deficits in such persons[10] and the fact that the specific mechanisms underlying the various disturbances of movement are poorly understood. No new generally acknowledged systematic approaches to the physical therapy evaluation and treatment of PKs have evolved in, at least, several decades.

Our present challenge is to assimilate and incorporate the wealth of existing new information pertaining to PKs' motor deficits so as to evolve new strategies for therapeutic interventions. Moreover, given the ever-expanding opportunities for clinical and laboratory-based research training andimplementation and the development and availability of new biomedical technology, physical therapy must move to the forefront in the effort to examine, quantify, and understand the changes in motor control that accompany PD. It is likely that only through such self-directed and collaborative endeavors will legitimate and effective therapies be established.

ORGANIZATIONAL FRAMEWORK FOR THE CONCEPTUALIZATION OF MOTOR CONTROL PROBLEMS

Before examining the problems of motor control that accompany PD, an organizational framework for conceptualizing movement dysfunction will be presented. The generalized nature of the scheme is such that it may be used for any individual who might present signs of motor disturbances, regardless of etiology.

Several additional features should also be emphasized: 1) an interactive systems perspective of motor control is encouraged rather than a single independent system analysis; 2) a unification of current knowledge is advocated from the disciplines of neuroscience, musculoskeletal physiology and biomechanics, and motor behavior as they may relate to functional clinical assessment categories; and 3) movement control is viewed as a continuum of interactive yet distinguishable stages that may serve as a model for designing evaluation and treatment procedures seeking to identify at which point and how a particular motor control problem may interfere with function.

Overall, the framework might serve as a guidepost for the generation of hypotheses seeking to identify alterations or impairments in specific control factors that may alter functional components of movement. Moreover, it may further lead to testable predictions as to how and where in the continuum of movement a particular motor control problem might disrupt function.

Factors in Motor Control

The evaluation and treatment of motor control problems must include consideration of the neural, musculoskeletal-biomechanical, and behavioral factors that may be contributing to movement dysfunction. The *neural* factors include the structures, pathways, and processes that participate in the control of movement. The *musculoskeletal-biomechanical* factors include the structure and properties of muscles, joints, and soft tissues and the physical laws governing movement. The *behavioral* factors include not only the cognitive, motivational, perceptual, and emotional processes but also the functional outcome of a movement in terms of either solving a motor problem or satisfying a goal in a particular environmental context.

Functional Components of Motor Control

The components of motor control include at least the following functional categories that normally contribute to the execution of purposeful movement: range of motion, muscle tone, sensation, strength, endurance, speed, posture and balance, coordination, adaptive control, cognition, and emotion. Any of the components may be altered as a result of damage to the movement control system and, consequently, may interfere with functional movements. Clinically, we attempt to evaluate the neural, musculoskeletal-biomechanical, and behavioral factors underlying the components and to apply treatment to minimize sources of motor problems, while using strategies to enhance the recovery of movement function.

Stages of Motor Control

Abnormal changes in any of the functional components of motor control may result in a disturbance in an individual's ability to perform functional movements. Such impairments may interfere with motor control at virtually any stage, from the initial state of the system through the outcome of movement. Individuals often appear, however, to have difficulty with particular aspects of a motor act (eg, initiation or accuracy of execution). In attempting to determine where in the movement continuum the altered components may interfere with function, it is useful to analyze purposeful movement by decomposing it into the following functional stages: initial condition (state of system); preparation (response identification, selection, execution); initiation; execution; termination; and outcome.

OVERVIEW OF THE PARKINSONIAN CLINICAL SYNDROME

The clinical syndrome of PD was first described in detail by James Parkinson in 1817 in *An Essay On The Shaking Palsey*.[11] Although PD is usually regarded as a disorder of movement, a complex array of nonmotor abnormalities have also been observed. For example, involvement of the autonomic system may result in orthostatic hypotension; paroxysmal flushing; diaphoresis; thermal regulatory problems; and bladder, sphincter, and sexual disturbances.[12] Sensory symptoms such as aches, pain, numbness, and burning-tingling paresthesias have been reported.[13] The special senses may also be affected in PD and result in visual, olfactory, and vestibular dysfunction.[13-15] A broad range of behavioral abnormalities from severe depression to degenerative dementia have been found for some PKs.[16] The extent to which such nonmotor abnormalities may interact with and contribute to movement dysfunction in PD should be taken into account by the clinician, and a thorough examination of nonmotor as well as sensorimotor and musculoskeletal systems should generally be conducted.

MOTOR SIGNS

While the foregoing systemic, sensory, cognitive, and other nonmotor features of PD may often prove to be disabling, the motor manifestations of the disorder would ap-

pear to be the most important with respect to deficits in functional mobility. In this regard, the major motor signs of PD include tremor at rest, rigidity, hypokinesia, postural and balance difficulties, and disturbances of gait.

Because tremor at rest is usually more of a cosmetic problem than a functional problem,[17] the present discussion will focus on the remaining primary motor signs. In particular, possible factors underlying motor control problems associated with rigidity; hypokinesia; and disturbances of posture, balance, and gait will be examined. It is important to recognize, however, that tremor at rest is but one form of a number of different types of tremor that may be present in the PKs.[18] For instance, action or postural tremors are often present in individuals with PD and may cause significant functional problems.[17,18] Finally, the extent to which the various oculomotor deficits that have been observed in PD[19,20] might contribute to deficits in functional movement should also be considered.

Rigidity

Alterations in muscular tone in Pks may include two related but dissociable disorders.[21] First, there may be an increase in the tonic resting levels of muscular activity as revealed by electromyography (EMG); second, there may be an increased resistance to passive lengthening of muscles that is present equally in all directions of movement (rigidity). The latter is often regularly interrupted by a superimposed tremor at a frequency of 5 to 6 Hz so as to induce a cog-wheeling, ratchety-like tendency during a prolonged stretch.[22] The degree of rigidity is relatively independent of the rate of elongation, but it is sustained for the duration of a maintained stretch.[22]

Joint angular stiffness (torque to joint-angle ratio) has been used as an index of rigidity during passive limb displacement when generated through a servo controlled torque motor at a constant velocity.[23] During such kinds of perturbations, a series of EMG responses typically appears in preactivated muscles.[24] The first response (M1), at latencies of less than 40 ms, is thought to represent a spinally mediated stretch response; the origin of the second, or long-latency component (M2), at latencies of about 100 ms, is controversial.[25]

A consistent finding has generally been normal M1 response amplitudes in the presence of abnormally large long-latency responses, which may contribute to the production of rigidity in PKs.[26-30] Moreover, while the magnitude of the long-latency response in healthy individuals is dependent on such factors as instructional set, stretch velocity, amplitude, and duration, responses in PKs appear to be relatively independent of such factors.[30] Thus the gain (output to input ratio) of the long-latency component in PKs would appear to be relatively fixed, abnormally high, and generally incapable of adapting to changes in response conditions. It is still unresolved, however, whether there is a satisfactory degree of correlation between M2 response amplitudes and quantitative indices of rigidity.[27,28]

In the above connection, both Burke[31] and Marsden[32] have indicated that it is difficult to attribute rigidity in PKs to long-latency stretch responses alone, particularly because the responses are triggered by abrupt perturbations and rigidity is evoked during slow, sustained, tonic stretch. Similarly, the abnormal presence of the shortening reaction (Westphal phenomenon) in a passively shortened muscle in PD also is a tonic response that might contribute to the enhanced stiffness about a joint.[33] Taken together, such findings suggest the possible involvement of tonic stretch and shortening responses in rigidity in PKs.

The extent to which possible changes in the passive mechanical properties of muscles and joints secondary to the effects of the nervous system involvement might contribute to the clinical sign of rigidity has recently been raised.[34,35] Such alterations may not only contribute to increasing resistance to passive lengthening of muscles but also may explain some aspects of flexed posture in PD; it might relate to changes in length-tension relationships in certain muscles.[35]

One should also be aware that the degree of rigidity within a given individual will not necessarily remain constant on a moment-to-moment basis and may vary with changes in the emotional state of the patient.[22] Although rigidity may be reinforced by emotional stress or anxiety,[31] the phenomena kinesia paradoxica results in a transient increase in mobility that is due to a sudden heightening of emotion.[36] Such observations illustrate the influence of behavioral factors on motor control problems in PD.

Although rigidity in PKs has been implicated as a possible contributing element to accompanying problems such as flexed posture,[35] respiratory difficulties,[36] and slowness of movement,[37] the extent to which it directly contributes to movement dysfunction has not been well established.[17,37] In fact, Hallett[17] has suggested that the increased muscular stiffness associated with rigidity might represent a generalized compensatory mechanism for an inability to respond with an appropriate voluntary response to an imposed perturbation. As such, the enhanced stiffness might be used by the motor control system to compensate for the main problem of hypokinesia.

Hypokinesia

Although it is generally acknowledged that hypokinesia (poverty of movement) is the most disabling feature of PD, the term is often used with respect to a broad range of motor control problems. Such deficits in movement function may include the following: 1) lack of spontaneous movement (eg, masked face); 2) delay in initiation; 3) slowness of movement; 4) delay in stopping movement; 5) reduced amplitude (eg, micrographia); 6) inability to sustain repetitive movement; 7) intermittent halting of movement; and 8) difficulty in executing simultaneous or sequential actions. Because the various clinical signs may be dissociated from one anther in some PKs, it is thought that such features may not all be different outcomes of the same motor deficit.[38]

In general, the stricter use of the term hypokinesia will refer to abnormal delays in the time taken to initiate (akinesia) and execute (bradykinesia) an intentional movement.[39] Since the classical studies of Wilson,[40] both akinesia and bradykinesia have generally been regarded as common motor control problems associated with PD. The measurement of reaction time (RT) and movement time (MT) in conjunction with EMG and kinematic recordings during relatively simple single-joint movements and more complex multijoint sequential motor tasks have provided some insights into the alterations in motor control processes associated with hypokinesia.

Akinesia. Although a number of studies[27,39-50] have indicated that the RTs of akinetic PKs are longer and more variable than those of healthy individuals, other reports[51-53] have not found such delays. Such apparently conflicting data have been attributed to the wide range of symptomatology of PKs,[38-42] which presumably reflects both the site and extent of lesion.

In the above connection, it is well known that RT will normally increase for movements that are more complex.[54] The delay in RT as a function of task complexity is thought to reflect differences in central processing associated with the identification of different stimulus inputs and selection of response strategies (ie, motor planning).[54] Thus akinesia in PKs may be demonstrated more markedly for tasks requiring greater planning such as in choice versus simple RT and in tracking versus ballistic types of movement.

In an important study, Evarts et al[38] found that choice reaction time (CRT) was impaired to the same extent as simple RT (SRT) in PKs. The investigators pointed out, however, that the failure to observe a greater prolongation of the CRT versus the SRT condition might have been due to the relatively simple motor task used that consisted of a rapid elbow supination or pronation movement. In this case, subjects were not required to control the precision of amplitude, velocity, or trajectory of movement.

To clarify the above issue, we investigated whether akinesia in PKs may be attributable to a disturbance in central processing related to motor planning.[50] We examined the question by comparing PKs and age-matched healthy subjects while they performed simple ballistic (bRT), simple tracking (tRT), and choice tracking reaction (cRT) ankle plantar movements.

The results indicated that while RTs were prolonged in both groups for each of the tracking movements versus bRT movements, between-group differences were not observed for the bRT or tRT tasks. In contrast, the PKs demonstrated significantly greater cRT and cRT minus bRT difference delays than the normals. These findings suggested that in addition to a delay in actively recruiting motor units to initiate a movement,[55] akinesia in PKs may be due to a central processing problem related to a deficit in motor planning. Furthermore, the results supported and extended the observations of other studies that suggested potentially important interactions between cognitive processing of information and the degree of motor impairment.[56,57]

With respect to motor preparation and movement initiation, other evidence has indicated that at least SRT may be shortened in PKs by the introduction of a warning cue before a reaction stimulus.[45] This finding may have beenindicative of an ability to specify an appropriate motor response in advance of the stimulus to move.[58] In a related study, which contrasted predictable and unpredictable movements of either forefinger, Bloxham et al[58] observed that PKs were unable to use advance information, which was given before the reaction signal, to reduce their RTs. The authors indicated that the results might have been attributable to an inability to maintain the appropriate response in store during the interval between the warning cue and the reaction signal.

A key difference between the latter and former studies was the respective use of simple and choice experimental conditions. Taken together with the findings related to RT and upcoming task complexity, such observations may be indicative of a disturbance in the process of motor preparation that might contribute to abnormal delays in initiating relatively more complex movements in some PKs.

Bradykinesia. It is generally well known that individuals with PD typically move more slowly than healthy subjects of comparable age. Moreover, speed of movement deficits have been shown to involve both proximal and distal segments of the body.[59-62] Bradykinesia in PKs has routinely been quantified by measuring the movement time or the velocity of movement associated with a variety of single-joint and multijoint motor tasks. The various quantitative measurements of speed of movement execution are likely the most consistent and useful indices of hypokinesia in PD.[17,38]

Draper and Johns[63] were among the earliest investigators to quantify speed of movement performance of isolated body segments, using a pronation- supination task. In commenting on speed of movement deficits, they noted that PKs showed an inability to modify their velocity of movement for movements of increased amplitude. Although healthy control subjects showed a close relationship between movement amplitude and peak velocity over a wide range of amplitudes, PKs could barely double their maximum velocity as the amplitudes of movement increased. Thus, there was not only a reduction in speed of movement but also an inability to modify or adapt the velocity to meet the changing requirements of the task.

Another important observation was that the bradykinetic movements appeared discontinuous with several, segmented, small amplitude movements appearing in the velocity records. Although it was suggested that such intermittent pauses might be attributable to action tremor, such interruptions were unidirectional and of a higher frequency than the usual 8 to 9 Hz oscillation of action tremor. Interestingly, the intermittency of motion was smoothed out by adding masses to the handle of the manipulandum to increase the inertial load to be overcome.

At the muscular level, an inability to deliver sufficient neural activity in the initial agonist EMG burst during single-joint ballistic movements has been linked with bradykinesea in PKs.[59] Normally, such movements are characterized by a single triphasic pattern of EMG activity in agonist and antagonist muscles. The first agonist burst presumably provides the impulsive force for the movement, the antagonist activity contributes to decelerating the movement, and the final agonist burst may serve to adjust the finalposition. In bradykinetic subjects, the correct agonist is recruited and the normal agonist-antagonist sequence is preserved, but the amplitude of the first agonist burst is reduced.[59,64] This results in a movement that is insufficient to reach a desired target distance such that a repetitive series of agonist bursts is required to complete a movement. Multiple cycles of EMG bursts have been a common finding among such individuals.

A related finding may be the slow rate of rise of the initial agonist burst observed by Evarts et al[47] for PKs. Further-more, although the movements made by bradykinetic PKs may be slower than healthy subjects, the amplitude and duration of the first EMG burst appears to scale grossly as a function of movement amplitude and resistive load.[64] The chief problem, therefore, appears to reside in an ability to achieve the appropriated absolute level of initial agonist activation in the presence of an apparently intact spatial and temporal structure of agonist-antagonist relationships during such tasks.[64] This may be indicative of a reduction in the descending activation of spinal motoneurons, which is in keeping with the results of single motor unit studies.[55]

The issue of predictive control of ongoing movements has been studied in PD using single joint, visual pursuit tracking tasks over a range of movement velocities.[46,58,65] When a healthy subject performs such tasks using an oscilloscope screen, he or she does so by monitoring the target trace and generating appropriate adjustments in movement so as to match the target after a reaction time interval. With repeated exposures to the same target trajectory, the subject will tend to adopt a strategy to move more in synchrony with, or in advance of, the tracking target according to predictive knowledge of the trajectory.[46]

Flowers[46] has reported that bradykinetic PKs were unable to reduce their tracking error for both time lags and degree of congruence when following a repetitive, known path versus an unpredictable target. He suggested that such individuals lack the ability to use an internalized model of external events to execute a movement but instead must rely on external sensory, especially visual, information for the control of movement. Such a control mode of execution would preclude the use of anticipatory or predictive control and impose lower limits on the maximum speed of movement.

In more recent studies, Bloxham et al[58] and Day et al[65] found that PKs performed similarly to healthy controls by being able to reduce the extent of the lag between the target movements and their own movements as a function of the predictability of the upcoming target. Such findings suggested that PKs might be capable of using predictive motor control strategies for movement execution. As noted by Day et al,[65] however, PKs may not achieve the same gains in precision of ongoing movement execution as control individuals when using predictive action because their disorder impedes fast accurate movements. Thus the advantage of speed associated with prediction may be traded off against the desire to obtain the accuracy of slow corrective movements.

With respect to the apparent discrepancies between the earlier and later studies, Bloxham et al[58] have attributed such differences to the natureof the movement tasks used. Whereas Flowers' protocol required an abrupt reversal in movement direction at a time when the target trace was apparently not visible to subjects, the other investigations used targets that were always in view and of a more continuous nature. The assumption was that the movement to a visual target represented an external trigger that served to reinforce the evolving movement execution. Because clinical observation[66] has indicated that visual cues may augment movement performance in PKs (see below), such a stimulus not maintained by Flowers[46] may have precluded the ability to sustain a predictive motor output.[58]

Further examination of the ability of PKs to adapt their

movements appropriately to different combinations of amplitude and accuracy has been conducted by Sanes and Evarts.[67] Their approach used an experimental method advocated by Fitts,[68] whereby MT was found to vary systematically with changes in target size and distance between targets. Thus movements of different amplitudes may have an equivalent degree of difficulty if the target sizes are modified accordingly. Interestingly, for movements of low difficulty, PKs showed MTs and total number of movements per unit time comparable to control subjects. The performance of PKs worsened appreciably, however, when the index of difficulty increased. Also, movements to smaller targets were performed more slowly, even though the target distance was held constant. One interpretation of the results might be that PKs were unable to modify or adapt their motor responses appropriately to the changing demands of the task.

The above observations have important implications related to whether or not more complex movements involving a sequence of events or multiple segments of the body may result in increased motor control problems for individuals with PD. That this increase may be the case has been suggested by earlier findings of Schwab and colleagues[51] who recorded the following motor problems in PKs: 1) rapid fatigue with repetitive movements, 2) inability to execute simultaneous actions, and 3) inability to execute sequential actions.

More recent investigations have confirmed and extended these observations. In an interesting and potentially important study, Johnels et al[69] examined a complex motor task involving the sequencing of postural changes, locomotion, and manual activities in PKs. A motion analysis system was used to record the kinematics of movement in which subjects lifted a box from the floor, carried the box while stepping forward, and placed it on a shelf located overhead. They were instructed to move the object immediately back to the starting position and repeat the task sequence four times in succession without pausing.

When healthy persons executed the sequence at maximal speeds, the postural, locomotor, and manual phases started quickly with considerable overlap between phases. That is, the locomotion phase would commence before the posture component was terminated, while the manual phase began before the completion of the stepping. In the unmedicated (off) condition, PKs showed prolonged overall movement time and slowing of the different phases. Strikingly, there was a tendency to show discrete separations between movement components, with actual pauses between them. Thus, there appeared to be a change from simultaneous to sequential modes of execution. Moreover, there appeared to be selective disturbances with respect to where in the sequence certain patients would encounter difficulty. It was also found that PKs often improved markedly when movement components were performed in isolation. These findings suggested that such individuals may have an impairment in the ability to coordinate different simultaneous motor tasks into an effective motor behavior.

In reviewing the motor disturbances of PD, Marsden[70] has pointed out that the primary problem would appear to be an inability to combine and execute a series of motor programs that comprise a complex motor plan. It is notable that the work of Benecke et al[71] and Beradelli and colleagues[72] has supported this contention for upper limb movements in much the same manner as Johnels et al.[69] Similar difficulties are also known to accompany such routine movements as rolling[73] or rising from a chair.

When attempting to sort through and reconcile the numerous and diverse features of hypokinesia in PKs, it should be remembered that the potential influence of nonneural factors such as changes in muscle fiber type composition,[74] changes in elastic properties,[35] and musculoskeletal deformities[36] (kyphosis and scoliosis; dystonic hands and feet) might also contribute meaningfully to such problems of motor control.

With respect to the stages of movement presented earlier, these factors would markedly alter at least the initial state of the motor control system such that new solutions may be required to solve movement problems related to functional goals. The extent to which musculoskeletal changes may contribute to the various manifestations of hypokinesia remains to be established. To reiterate an observation made with respect to rigidity, the emotional status of PKs also appears to have a profound influence on all of the motor problems of PD. This apparent relationship would seem to have potentially important implications for behaviorally based investigations and approaches to treatment.

Freezing Phenomenon

There has been accumulating evidence to suggest that the sudden arrestation of particularly rhythmical movements such as stepping (festinating gait), speaking, or writing may be a unique problem of motor control that is a distinct form of hypokinesia apparently not associated with other features of akinesia or bradykinesia.[75,76] The so-called freezing phenomenon has been dissociated from rigidity and tremor and may be observed typically as severe halting on attempting to initiate or execute rhythmic, repetitive movements.[76]

Two lines of evidence have prompted Marabayashi and Nakamara[76] to speculate that freezing may be due to a disturbance of rhythm formation adequate to sustain repetitive movements. First, using a repetitive finger tapping task synchronized to a periodic sound, they observed that when the target frequency surpassed a particular transition frequency (usually at 2.5 and 4 Hz), all PKs who displayed freezing or festination could no longer maintain the required response "and performed a hastened tapping with 5 to 6 Hz, irrespective of signal frequency." In this abnormal, halting transition, correlations among intertap response intervals were random. Second, clinical observation has shown that periodic, particularly visual, stimuli may facilitate movement performance in many PKs.

The importance of visual input to the control of movement in PD (see below) has been recognized widely at least since its documentation by Martin.[66] In one case, the author described a PK who with vision could maintain finger tip to finger tip contact with the experimenter while holding the outstretched arms at shoulder height but with eyes closed was unable to maintain elevation of the arms. More quantitative evaluations have also shown a dissolution of arm movements during a positioning task with and without visual guidance in such individuals.[77]

It may also be of relevance that visual stimuli appear to be critical in eliciting kinesia paradoxica such as when a patient is suddenly thrown a ball and is able to catch it.[78] Such responsiveness may be contrasted with the contention the external stimuli might also be related to both the triggering and the reversal of freezing episodes.[70] On the basis of the visual tracking experiments noted earlier, Bloxham et al[58] have commented that the basal ganglia are particularly involved with the control of movements that are less automatic and not triggered by external stimuli. This point has also been raised by Miller and DeLong[21] who emphasized that the chief motor difficulty in PD is in controlling self-paced movements not requiring visual information.

POSTURE AND BALANCE

The abnormalities of posture (the relative orientation of the body segments to each other during quasistatic and dynamic conditions) and balance (the maintenance of the projected location or trajectory of the body center of mass [CM] within the area defined by the base of support) in PD often include the following: 1) stooped posture; 2) diminished associated reactions, such as arm swing during locomotion; 3) absence of equilibrium and righting responses; and 4) lack of postural fixation of the proximal limb and axial segments during voluntary movements. These features are often accompanied by insecurity while standing or walking, loss of balance, and falls. As noted earlier, a number of musculoskeletal abnormalities (kyphosis, scoliosis, dystonia of hands and feet) often accompany PD and result in limitations in postural control.

External Disturbances

In one of the earliest reports, Martin[79] identified an abnormal lack of righting responses of the head, neck, trunk and a compensatory pelvic shift in PKs who were tilted while seated. This may have been indicative of a vestibular deficit in PD.[15]

A number of recent quantitative studies have also shown changes in the normal EMG or the biomechanical responses or both that presumably underlie balance control during externally applied disturbances to upright stance.[80-84] Traub et al,[80] using an expected upper-limb disturbance in standing PKs, have shown reduced incidence or EMG amplitudes of gastrocnemius muscle responses that normally precede the remote mechanical effects on posture or balance as a result of a localized disturbance of the arm.

During sudden translational movements of a platform upon which subjects stood or sat, Horak et al[81] have noted that PKs used inappropriate muscle responses that were not effectively sequenced under the different test conditions. Also, the EMG response characteristics suggested that PKs might have abnormally used two postural movements simultaneously, resulting in an ineffective correction of imbalance. Such observations again may have been indicative of a generalized inability of PKs to adapt their movements to specific environmental situations.

Using stance support-surface rotational movements that induced ankle dorsiflexion, Dichgans and Diener[82] observed abnormally large long-latency stretch responses in triceps surae muscles in PKs, suggesting an exaggerated gain. Using a similar method, Allum et al[83] detected three major differences between PKs and control subjects: 1) additional EMG activity between short- and long-latency responses of soleus muscle was found in PKs; 2) the functionally useful EMG response components were delayed in PKs; and 3) most importantly, stabilizing ankle torque was reduced and delayed in PKs. Based on a comparison of the PKs' response profiles and those of patients with labyrithine deficiencies, the authors concluded that a vestibular deficit did not appear to underlie the response changes in the PKs; their changes were probably attributable to alterations in somatosensory mediated reactions.

In studying responses to a sudden forward or backward acceleration of a treadmill, Dietz et al[84] found slowed rates of increase and diminished EMG durations in ankle dorsiflexors and plantar flexors for PKs versus age-matched controls. Such responses, which were also generally reduced in amplitude, apparently did not scale appropriately as a function of either the treadmill acceleration or the duration of the applied motion.

Although the foregoing alterations in EMG responses in PKs are difficult to interpret, the finding of Allum et al[83] pertaining to the reduction and delay in corrective ankle torque may have potentially important implications for functional retraining. It may be that the ankle joint torque profile was associated with braking the fall after the external disturbance; such a braking function may be altered in PD.

Intentional Movements

The interactions between postural, balance, and voluntary motor components during the execution of intentional movements in PD has been reviewed recently[85] and will now be discussed briefly. In this connection, Martin[66] has pointed out that the ability of PKs to execute anintentional movement may greatly be enhanced if appropriate postural adjustments are made for the patients or if they consciously control the postural changes that normally occur automatically. For example, an individual who has difficulty rising from a seated position can be assisted by intentionally emphasizing the normally automatic forward movement of the trunk in preparation for standing. Similarly, the inability to initiate a step can be improved if an individual's CM is first shifted for him or her. Martin[66] also observed that such postural changes were not attributable to muscular weakness.

Recent evidence has indicated that so-called anticipatory postural adjustments (APAs) often precede and accompany both expected externally imposed disturbances to a single body segment and internally generated disturbances of posture or balance associated with a voluntary movement.[86-88] In a novel experimental approach, Viallet and colleagues[89] examined the postural responses of the arms during voluntary and imposed limb loading and unloading in PKs. Such unloading of a weight applied at the distal forearm during elbow flexion normally leads to an inhibition in the tonically active brachioradialis muscle, which minimizes the extent of subsequent elbow flexion (ie, postural disturbance) after the unloading. For voluntary unloading, healthy subjects showed an earlier inhibition before the onset of load removal. This inhibition effectively reduced the subsequent elbow displacement to a greater extent than that which followed imposed unloading by an experimenter where the EMG reduction did not occur until after the onset of load reduction. For PKs, the decrease in brachioradialis EMG was less than for controls, especially for voluntary conditions where a comparatively large displacement of the forearm followed the unloading. This alteration was often delayed and resulted in a lack of anticipatory EMG changes, which suggested an impaired interaction between postural and voluntary components of movement.

A well-studied example of anticipatory postural control involves especially rapid shoulder flexion movements made by standing subjects. In such cases, posterior leg and trunk muscles may be activated phasically not only before the onset of movement but also in advance of the primary agonist muscle, the anterior deltoid.[87,88] These early changes in muscle activation have been associated with body segmental movements that presumably served to minimize the disturbance to posture or balance caused by the reactive forces associated with the movement.[88]

Two experimental and clinical observations led us to investigate the control of postural (leg and trunk) and agonist (arm) muscles before rapid arm-flexion movements in standing PKs.[90] First, in standing human beings, postural adjustments preceding rapid voluntary arm movements have been thought to be programmed centrally as part of a total movement synergy. Second, PKs have frequently been shown to manifest abnormal delays in movement initiation and execution and deficits in postural stabilization, all of which have been thought to reflect a disturbance in the central programming of the voluntary task or associated postural adjustments.

Briefly, we examined the EMG responses of the anterior deltoid (AD) of the moving limb and the ipsilateral paraspinal (ES) and contralateral biceps femoris (BF) muscles in nine PKs and age-matched control subjects. Rapid arm-flexion movements were evaluated during simple reaction time and self-paced conditions.

As shown in Figure 20-1, healthy subjects typically demonstrated a phasic burst of EMG activity in BF, followed by or concomitant with bursts in ES and the primary agonist muscle AD. Moreover, the recruitment of postural muscle preceded movement onset for essentially all trials. Although the PKs generally displayed intermuscular response profiles that resembled those of the control subjects (Fig. 20-2A), they activated BF and ES before movement onset in only 82% and 81% (respectively) of the total trials. This lower incidence of postural muscle activation was further exemplified by four of the PKs, who recruited either one or both of the muscles in fewer than 50% of the total trials.

Although the mean EMG onset latencies before movement onset did not differ between groups, the overall premovement EMG durations for postural muscles BF and ES were significantly shorter for PKs versus healthy subjects. Moreover, although normal individuals (Fig. 20-1) and some PKs (Fig. 20-2A) displayed relatively distinct single bursts of EMG activity, several of the PKs produced repetitive EMG bursts (Fig. 20-2B) in the prime mover (as re-

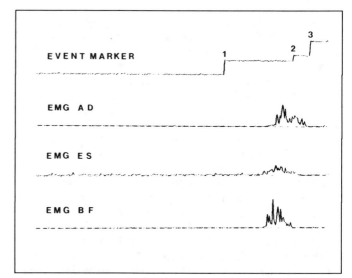

Fig. 20-1. *Representative EMG recordings from anterior deltoid (AD), paraspinal (ES), and biceps femoris (BF) muscles during a visual reaction-time arm flexion movement in a healthy subject. Upper trace is an event marker signifying 1) presentation of a light flash to initiate movement, 2) movement onset as triggered by the release of a microswitch, 3) the end of movement as detected by passage of the arm through a photoelectric beam. Vertical calibration=0.5 mV for EMG traces. Horizontal calibration=200 ms. Reprinted by permission from Rogers et al.[90]*

ported earlier for elbow movements[59]) and in the postural muscles of the lower limb and trunk. Such profiles were never observed for healthy subjects and might be related to abnormally intermittent motor-unit discharge patterns[55] or a manifestation of action or postural tremor.[91]

Although the group mean RTs did not differ between PKs and controls, four of the nine PKs were objectively akinetic, as revealed by their delayed RTs. Further analysis also showed that the same akinetic individuals demonstrated significant delays in the time taken to recruit the prime mover AD and postural muscles BF and ES after the visual reaction signal. Although the delay in EMG recruitment time for the primary agonist muscle in akinetic PKs is well known, similar delays for postural muscle components have, to our knowledge, not been reported.

Overall, the findings indicated that both the postural (leg and trunk) and the primary agonist (arm) muscles may be affected similarly in PD. The results further suggested that both the spatial (lack of recruitment and intermittent EMG bursts) and the temporal (decreased EMG durations and prolonged akinetic recruitment times) features of centrally organized neural command signals may be altered in individuals with PD. These observations have generally been supported by the results of other investigations of postural and movement interactions in PKs.[92,93] Finally, the various changes in EMG response profiles were not uniformly observed across subjects. This observation again underscores the wide range of symptomatology of PKs.

More recently, we have turned our attention to examining the dynamic transition from bipedal to single limb stance that precedes and accompanies both the single-leg flexion movements[94-97] and the initiation of gait.[98-102] An understanding of the normal neuromuscular and biomechanical control processes underlying such tasks is of particular relevance to individuals with PD because they frequently demonstrate an inability to perform the normally automatic transfer of weight support that is a necessary prerequisite to removing a lower limb from the floor.

Briefly, both initiation of gait and single-leg flexion movements have been found to be accompanied by 1) an initial increase in the vertical component (Fz) of the ground reaction force (GRF) before unloading of the stepping of flexing (fl) leg and 2) an initial displacement of the center of pressure toward the fl limb. These observations have led to the proposal that an initial displacement of the body CM toward the fl limb results in an increase in Fz needed to propel the body toward the single stance (st) limb.[98,100] Such a theory of weight transfer has not been supported by direct measurement of the body CM trajectory. Because the GRFs used to quantify changes in stance support reflect both the location and acceleration of the CM,[103] it is possible that the changes observed represented the dynamics of the forthcoming movement.[101]

We examined the GRFs and CM trajectory in the frontal plane in healthy subjects who stood on two separate force platforms and performed single-leg flexion movements over a range of self-selected speeds.[94-97] Three principal findings were obtained. First, an abrupt increase in Fz always preceded the unloading of the fl limb for more rapid speeds, although such early vertical force changes were less commonly found for the slowest movements. Second, the lateral horizontal (Fy) GRFs were always initially exerted in the fl to st limb direction. For more rapid speeds, however, the Fy contribution beneath the fl limb was proportionately greater

(4:1) than the Fyst contribution to the resultant Fy, although Fyfl and Fyst became equivalent during the slow movements. Third, the CM was always displaced directly toward the st limb, regardless of the speed of movement. Thus the early increases in Fzfl were not produced by a shift in the body weight to the fl leg before its removal from the ground.

Overall, the findings suggested that the transfer of the CM laterally for more rapid speeds was generated by a coupling of both an initial increase in the pressure (Fzfl) and frictional (Fyfl) components of the GRF beneath the fl leg. For slower speeds, however, the frictional force contribution beneath the st limb was increased while the frictional and pressure contributions beneath the fl leg were simultaneously reduced. Such speed-related differences in the kinetic profiles likely reflected the requirements necessary for overcoming the inertial force of the body mass during dynamic transitions in stance support. The results also underscore the need to examine the dynamic changes in posture that accompany functional movements.

In a series of related studies we have also examined the momentum profiles of the total body and individual body segments and the resultant joint torques of the lower limbs as a function of speed of ascent during the sit-to-stand transfer.[104-106] A key finding of these investigations was the relative invariance of the dynamic motion of the total body in the horizontal versus the vertical directions as the speed of ascent was progressively increased. Such differences may have been related to the need to maintain balance or regulate the position of the trunk in the parasagittal plane while varying the total body momentum.

We have also observed speed related differences in the amplitude and timing characteristics at the hip, knee, and ankle resultant joint torques. These differences also suggested functional differences associated with the propulsive

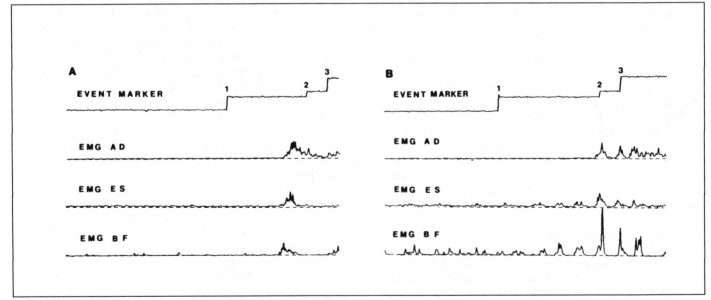

Fig. 20-2. *Representative EMG recordings from respective muscles during a visual reaction-time arm flexion movement (A) in a subject with parkinsonism; (B) showing multiple burst patterns in a subject with parkinsonism. Same caption and calibration as in Fig. 20-1.*

versus the braking phases of the task. Such observations could be relevant to the difficulties displayed by many PKs in attempting to stand from a seated position.

Gait

The characteristic gait of PKs can readily be identified by the slowed velocity; short, shuffling steps; lack of arm swing and rotational movements; festination; and difficulties in starting and stopping. The extent to which such features may be manifestations of the other signs of PD has not been established, although some authors[107] have proposed specific deficits in the neural control of locomotion.

Quantitative assessments[107-112] of PKs' gait have generally revealed the following changes in the normal profiles of kinematic, kinetic, EMG, and temporal-distance factors: 1) smaller range of lower-limb joint angular displacements; 2) generalized lack of extension at the hip and knee and lack of ankle plantar flexion; 3) reduced transverse rotation of the pelvis and thorax; 4) en-bloc movements of the trunk and pelvis; 5) reduction in vertical GRF and sagittal plane horizontal GRF at push-off; 6) possible reversed movements of the ankle joint with abnormal foot-floor contact; 7) reduced foot elevation above the floor; 8) reduced speed with diminished stride length; 9) increased time of double limb support; 10) continuous lower limb muscle activity between cyclical phasic activations; 11) abnormal coactivation of antagonist muscles; and 12) reduced EMG amplitudes.

On the basis of such findings as the lack of knee flexion in early stance, a reversal in the normal phase related movements at the ankles, and a flat foot or forefoot floor contact at stance onset, Forssberg and colleagues[107] have proposed that PKs' gait resembles the locomotion behavior of developing children. They suggested that in addition to possible changes induced by hypokinesia, PKs' gait may be in part attributable to "deficits in the neural circuits controlling plantigrade locomotion."[107]

With respect to stepping initiation that has commonly been associated with episodes of complete movement arrestation in PD,[75] Ingvarsson et al[113] have observed two general categories of impairment. First, the transfer of the body weight laterally required several efforts before the stepping load could be unloaded and advanced. Second, an apparently adequate lateral weight transfer occurred in the presence of a block or delay in the initiation of the stepping cycle.

It may be of relevance that in healthy individuals the transition from stationary standing to walking has been found to be, in part, associated with an abrupt deactivation of tonically active soleus muscles or gastrocnemius muscles or both followed by a phasic recruitment of tibialis anterior muscles (Fig. 20-3).[98-102,114] Such EMG changes have been found to precede the earliest loss of heel contact associated with the actual stepping response by as much as some 500 ms[101,114] and are thought to be associated, respectively, with the onset and reinforcement of the forwardacceleration of the body mass.[101] Thus alterations in ankle muscle activity that likely give rise to characteristic changes in the GRFs beneath the feet would appear to be an important process for overcoming the inertial force of the body mass with respect to the sagittal plane.

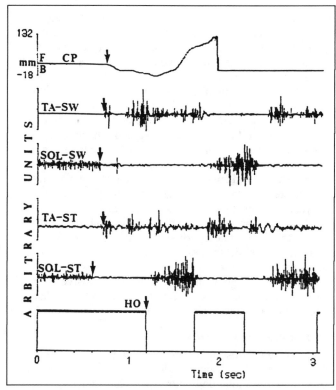

Fig. 20-3. *Representative example of the resultant center of pressure (CP) displacement beneath the feet and EMG recordings from soleus (SOL) and tibialis anterior muscles of the initial swing (SW) and stance (ST) limbs during the initiation of a series of steps in a healthy subject. Arrows indicate the onset of event modification. F=forward; B=backward; HO=onset of earliest reduction in heel-floor contact associated with the first step. Reprinted from Lin.[114]*

We have recently observed that the interval of time by which an associated initial posterior displacement of the center of pressure precedes heel-off of the stepping limb may be extended significantly when healthy subjects performed self-paced versus externally cued stepping initiation at comparable speeds. Such a strategy would presumably allow a longer period of time during which nonmuscular (gravity) forces could assist the body in falling forward before and during the first step. This finding may be relevant to the difficulties displayed by PKs for self-generated as opposed to externally triggered movements (see below).[21]

IMPLICATIONS FOR CLINICAL PRACTICE

In view of the foregoing and other observations and findings, a number of implications for clinical practice will be suggested and discussed.

Classification and Evaluation Schemes

It has become increasingly apparent that the motor syndrome of PKs is a diverse, highly variable, and, at this time, unpredictable symptomatology. The lack of uniformity in the changes in motor control function among PKs underscores the wide range of motor disturbances. For instance, Evarts and colleagues[38] have noted extensive intraindividual and interindividual independence with respect to abnormal delays in initiating and executing movements. Similarly, our own observations[90] and those of others[92] on the diversity of alterations in postural and movement interactions lend additional support to this contention.

In terms of clinical management, such observations point to the need for the development of valid and reliable measurement procedures that could lead to improved classification and identification of patient-specific treatment procedures. Instrumented evaluative protocols designed to quantify the speed, extent, and accuracy of functional movements would appear to be one such promising direction. Moreover, information pertaining to quantitative links between routine clinical measurements (eg, speed of movement, range of motion, strength) and dynamic kinesiological factors that underlie functional movements is vitally needed.[106] Overall, the development of focused evaluation and classification procedures would greatly assist in establishing treatment goals that are not based exclusively on uniform assumptions about the motor control problems that classically have been associated with PD.

Neuromuscular Control

Evidence in support of changes in the normal neural activation profiles of muscles during a variety of upper limb, lower limb, and total body movements has indicated a number of common features among PKs. Such alterations have generally included 1) enhanced level of tonic myoelectric activity at rest, with inability to deactivate neuromuscular activity appropriately; 2) increased time taken to recruit motor units and reduction in motor unit firing frequency; 3) decreased amplitude, scaling, or duration of initial EMG bursts; 4) multiple, intermittent EMG bursts; 5) absence of motor unit recruitment in presumed postural muscle components; and 6) enhanced long-latency stretch response amplitudes.

Although the degree of correspondence between the alterations in any or all of the above neuromuscular control signals and the form and the extent of functional movement problems may often be difficult to interpret as a result of musculomechanical interactions,[115] the factors nevertheless may provide broad directives for generating experimental and treatment related hypotheses. As such, particular problems of motor control in parkinsonism may in part be related variously to the following:

1. Achieving the recruitment threshold of muscular components.
2. Adequately sustaining the activation for muscular elements or modulating (scaling) the amplitudes of responses.
3. Effectively deactivating tonically active muscles to achieve appropriate transitions in posture.
4. Dealing with abnormal delays in the time taken to recruit motor units.

In such cases, therapeutic procedures to augment or diminish neuromuscular activation might be used to facilitate functional movement.

There is also the obvious need to increase and maintain the extensibility and mobility of muscles, joints, and soft-tissues, as has recently been emphasized.[116] In light of the known decrease in type II muscle fibers in PKs,[74] it may also be of value to consider therapeutic approaches that stress more forceful and more rapid muscle-use demands so as to try to engage the principle of training specificity.[117] Such changes in the inherent properties of themusculoskeletal apparatus may potentially have profound effects on the strategies used by an already altered neural control system in effectively generating functional movements.

Task Complexity and Adaptive Movements

Mounting evidence has reinforced the long standing observation that individuals with PD have particular difficulty with movements requiring the sequencing of a number of motor subtasks. Such so-called complex actions (eg, stepping initiation, sit-to-stand, turning while walking, transporting objects, simultaneous goal directed actions) are precisely the type of movements that impair function in PKs. Emphasis on the execution of movements requiring the linkage of a number of sequential or simultaneous control functions would therefore appear to be a potentially important point of focus for therapeutic approaches.

In the above connection, an equally compelling body of information has emphasized the general lack of ability to adapt or scale, adequately, the speed, amplitude, or perhaps the direction of a given movement or motor response in PKs. Thus, it would appear that the direct and explicit use of, at least, a range of complex response speeds, amplitudes, and directions in the context of different environmental configurations and sites might be a potentially useful treatment strategy. Moreover, such emphasis might be implemented most effectively from the earliest stages of therapy because it has become increasingly apparent[97,104-106] that such modifications in control factors may not necessarily be merely scaled versions of a range of speeds or possibly amplitudes. It may also be the case that movements that are slower, of smaller amplitudes, or performed in a limited range of directions would not necessarily represent simpler versions of an identical movement and might possibly be of greater difficulty to certain patients than presumably more challenging faster, larger, and multidirectional movements.

Conditioning Approaches and Instructional Set

An essentially unexplored mode of treatment in PD has been that of behavioral conditioning approaches. Such apparently primitive forms of learning have been shown to influence response variables in organisms ranging from the invertebrate sea snail, Aplysia, through human beings.[118] Thus a potentially powerful tool for influencing motor responses would appear to be available. Clearly, biofeedback approaches have used concepts of conditioning to a limited extent. What would appear to be needed, however, is an expanded application of conditioning principles to specific motor problems of PKs. In essence, we know little of the rules of the various forms of conditioning as they might apply to PD.

It is noteworthy that investigations by Rothwell and associates[119] and Horak et al[120] have also demonstrated a conditioning-like effect on healthy human long-latency stretch responses resembling classical response habituation to repeated stimuli. The extent to which abnormally large gains of stretch responses in PKs might be susceptible to change with conditioningapproaches represents one of a number of possible applications in this area. Similarly, the extent to which instructional set or anticipatory modulation of input-output functions might lead to modifications of motor responses in PD remains to be elucidated.

Intersensory Feedforward Facilitation

If the changes in neuromuscular activation profiles do, in fact, contribute to the various motor problems in PD, then movement function might potentially be enhanced through the use of intersensory facilitation during movement preparation, as suggested by Chan,[121] for single joint movements. For instance, it is well known that in healthy individuals the presentation of an auditory warning stimulus given before or simultaneously with a light-flash reaction signal will reduce visual reaction time.[122] Similarly, the presentation of an electrical cutaneous stimulus applied to one thumb together with an auditory reaction signal that triggers simultaneous bilateral thumb- flexion movements has been found to shorten, substantially, the reaction times resulting from the auditory stimulus presented alone.[123] Such facilitatory effects also have been found to vary with the intensity of the accessory signal.[124] Manipulation in the timing and intensity of visual, auditory, or somatosensory stimuli before movement initiation might be used to affect changes in motor responses of PKs related to recruitment, timing, or amplitude of neuromuscular activation.

A clue to the applicability of this approach can be found in the well- recognized clinical observation described by Martin[66] (and more recently examined by Forssberg et al[107]) that visual markings in the form of bold lines on the ground substantially improve the gait performance of many PKs. This point has been reiterated by other investigators,[75,125] particularly with respect to moving visual stimuli or rhythmical, repetitive cues. Also, many individuals with PD have reported that music appears to enhance their movements. This may be indicative of a similar therapeutic application through the use of acoustic facilitation. For instance, rhythmical auditory cues as basic as those provided by a metronome might be used to precue the sequencing of voluntary attempts to shift the weight of the body either laterally during the initiation of gait (shift-step) or forward and upward when attempting to stand (lean-stand).

Treadmill Facilitation of Gait and Functional Electrical Stimulation

Based on the assumption of the existence of a basic central pattern-generating neural circuitry underlying human locomotion, which may be accessed by supraspinal and peripheral input pathways, recent attempts to retrain walking in adult neurologically impaired patients have been advanced.[126] Given the proposed role of the basal ganglia in contributing to the control of locomotion[127] and the apparent integrity of some spinally mediated responses in PKs,[128] it may be that the multisensory and mechanical effects of treadmill walking could provide a source of augmentation of the gait of PKs. Moreover, such a form of training could potentially be used in conjunction with functional electrical stimulation applied with appropriate spatial and temporal activa-

tion variables or with any of the above intersensory stimuli to enhance locomotor functioning.

If it is true, as it would appear, [99,101,102,114] that the neuro muscular control at the ankle joint is normally critically important to the initiation of stepping (Fig. 20-3) and that PKs do not adequately deactivate tonically active soleus muscles while failing to sequence tibialis anterior muscle activations appropriately, then electrical stimulation of the ankle dorsiflexors might possibly be used for both activating anterior compartment muscles while reciprocally deactivating posterior compartment ankle muscles as a means of inducing anterior postural transitions before stepping. Although such a postulation remains to be examined, it represents but one example of a testable hypothesis generated by merging lines of clinical observation, quantitative findings, and existing therapeutic tools and procedures in the context of functionally relevant motor control problems in PD.

Acknowledgments

I gratefully acknowledge Lois Deming-Hedman, MS, PT, for her constructive comments and for her contributions, along with those of Jane W. Schneider, MS, PT, to the formulation of the concepts in the section on Organizational Framework for the Conceptualization of Motor Control Problems.

References

1. Forno LS. The neuropathology of Parkinson's disease. In: Hefti F, Weiner WJ, eds. *Progress in Parkinson Research*. New York, NY: Plenum Publishing Corp; 1988:11-21.
2. Agid J, Javoy-Agid F, Ruberg M. Biochemistry of neuro transmitters in Parkinson's disease. In: Marsden CD, Fahn S, eds. *Movement Disorders*. Stoneham, Mass: Butterworth Publishers; 1987;2:166-230.
3. Davis GC, Williams AC, Markey SP, et al. Chronic parkinsonism secondary to intravenous injection of merperidine analogues. *Psychiatry Res*. 1979;1:249-254.
4. Langston JW, Ballard P, Tetrud JW, et al. Chronic parkinsonism in humans due to a product of meperidine-analog synthesis. *Science*. 1983;219:979-980.
5. Madrazo I, Drucker-Colin R, Diaz V, et al. Open microsurgical autograft of adrenal medulla to right caudate nucleus in two patients with intractable Parkinson's disease. *N Eng J Med*. 1987;316:831-834.
6. Desmedt JE, ed. *Motor Control Mechanisms in Health and Disease*. New York, NY: Raven Press; 1983.
7. Delwaide PJ, Agnoli A, eds. *Clinical Neurophysiology in Parkinson's Disease*. New York, NY: Elsevier Science Publishing Co Inc; 1985.
8. Yahr MD, Bergmann KJ, eds. *Advances in Neurology: Parkinson's Disease*. New York, NY: Raven Press; 1986;45.
9. Benecke R, Conrad B, Marsden CD, eds. *Motor Disturbances, I*. San Diego, Calif: Academic Press Inc; 1987.
10. Marsden CD. The mysterious motor function of the basal ganglia. *Neurology*. 1982;32:514-539.
11. Parkinson J. *An Essay on the Shaking Palsey*. London, England: Sherwood, Neely, and Jones; 1817.
12. Tanner CM, Goetz CG, Klawans HL. Autonomic nervous system disorders. In: Koller WC, ed. *Handbook of Parkinson's disease*. New York, NY: Marcel Dekker Inc; 1987:145-170.

13. Snider SR, Sandy KR. Sensory dysfunction. In: Koller WC, ed. *Handbook of Parkinson's Disease.* New York, NY: Marcel Dekker Inc; 1987:171-180.

14. Ward CD, Hess WA, Calne DB. Olfactory impairment in Parkinson's disease. *Neurology.* 1983;33:943-946.

15. Reichert WH, Doolittle J, McDowell FM. Vestibular dysfunction in Parkinson's disease. *Neurology.* 1982;32:1133-1138.

16. Mayeux R. Mental state. In: Koller WC, ed. *Handbook of Parkinson's Disease.* New York, NY: Marcel Dekker Inc; 1987:127-144.

17. Hallett M. Quantitative assessment of motor deficiency in Parkinson's disease: ballistic movements. In: Delwaide PJ, Agnoli A, eds. *Clinical Neurophysiology in Parkinsonism.* New York, NY: Elsevier Science Publishing Co Inc; 1985:139-161.

18. Young RR. Tremor in Parkinson's disease. In: Delwaide PJ, Agnoli A, eds. *Clinical Neurophysiology in Parkinsonism.* New York, NY: Elsevier Science Publishing Co Inc; 1985:139-161.

19. DeJong JD, Melvill-Jones G. Akinesia, hypokinesia, and bradykinesia in the oculomotor system of patients with Parkinson's disease. *Exp Neurol.* 1971;32:58-68.

20. White OB, Saint-Cyr JA, Sharpe JA. Ocular motor deficits in Parkinson's disease: I. The horizontal vestibulo-ocular reflex and its regulation. *Brain.* 1983;106:555-570.

21. Miller WC, DeLong MR. Parkinsonian symptomatology: an anatomical and physiological analysis. *Ann NY Acad Sci.* 1988;515:287-302.

22. Delwaide PJ, Gonce M. Pathophysiology of Parkinson's signs. In: Jankovic J, Tolosa E, eds. *Parkinson's Disease and Movement Disorders.* Baltimore, Md: Urban & Schwarzenberg Inc; 1988:59-73.

23. Mortimer JA, Webster DD. Evidence for a quantitative association between EMG stretch responses and Parkinsonian rigidity. *Brain Res.* 1979;162:169-173.

24. Hammond PH. Involuntary activity in biceps following the sudden application of velocity to the abducted forearm. *J Physiol (Lond).* 1954;127:17-18.

25. Evarts EV, Hagbarth KE, Tatton WG, et al. Group discussion on long-loop reflexes: their origin and significance. In: Delwaide PJ, Agnoli A, eds. *Clinical Neurophysiology in Parkinsonian.* New York, NY: Elsevier Science Publishing Co Inc; 1985:163-172.

26. Tatton WG, Lee RG. Evidence for abnormal long-loop reflexes in Parkinsonian patients. *Brain Res.* 1975;100:671-676.

27. Chan CWY, Kearney RE, Melvill-Jones G. Tibialis anterior response to sudden ankle displacements in normal and Parkinsonian subjects. *Brain Res.* 1979;173:303-313.

28. Beradelli A, Sabra A, Hallett M. Physiological mechanisms of rigidity in Parkinson's disease. *J Neurol Neurosurg Psychiatry.* 1983;46:45-53.

29. Rothwell JC, Obeso JA, Traub MM, et al. The behavior of the long-latency stretch reflex in patients with Parkinson's disease. *J Neurol Neurosurg Psychiatry.* 1983;46:35-44.

30. Lee RG, Murphy JT, Tatton WG. Long-latency myotatic reflexes in man: mechanisms, functional significance, and changes in patients with Parkinson's disease and hemiplegia. In: Desmedt JE, ed. *Motor Control Mechanisms in Health and Disease.* New York, NY: Raven Press; 1983:489-507.

31. Burke D. Pathophysiological aspects of rigidity and dystonia. In: Benecke R, Conrad B, Marsden CD, eds. *Motor Disturbances, I.* San Diego, Calif: Academic Press Inc; 1987:87-100.

32. Marsden CD. Summary part II: rigidity/dystonia. In: Benecke R, Conrad B, Marsden CD, eds. *Motor Disturbances, I.* San Diego, Calif: Academic Press Inc; 1987:145-152.

33. Andrews CJ, Burke D, Lance JW. The response to muscle stretch and shortening in Parkinsonian rigidity. *Brain.* 1972;95:795-812.

34. Dietz V, Quintern J, Berger W. Electrophysiological studies of gait in spasticity and rigidity: evidence that altered mechanical properties of muscle contributes to hypertonia. *Brain.* 1981;104:431-449.

35. Watts RL, Wiegrer AW, Young RR. Elastic properties of muscles measured at the elbow in man: II. patients with Parkinsonian rigidity. *J Neurol Neurosurg Psychiatry.* 1986;49:1177-1181.

36. Jankovic J. Pathophysiology and clinical assessment of motor symptoms in Parkinson's disease. In: Koller WC, ed. *Handbook of Parkinson's disease.* New York, NY: Marcel Dekker Inc; 1987:99-126.

37. Buchthal F, Fernandez-Ballesteros ML. Electromyographic study of the muscles of the upper arm and shoulder during walking in patients with Parkinson's disease. *Brain.* 1965;88:875-896.

38. Evarts EV, Teravainen H, Calne DB. Reaction time in Parkinson's disease. *Brain.* 1981;104:167-186.

39. Angel RW, Alston W, Higgins JR. Control of movement in Parkinson's disease. *Brain.* 1970;93:1-14.

40. Wilson SAK. Some disorders of motility and of muscle tone, with special reference to the corpus striatum. *Lancet.* 1925;2:1-10.

41. Barbeau A, Degroot JA. The problem of measurement in akinesia. *J Neurosurg.* 1966;24:331-334.

42. Weisendanger M, Schreider P, Villoez JP. Electromyographic analysis of rapid volitional movement. *Am J Phys Med.* 1969;48:17-24.

43. Cassell K, Stern GA. A computerized tracking technique for the assessment of Parkinsonian motor disabilities. *Brain.* 1973;96:815-826.

44. Velasco F, Velasco M. A quantitative evaluation of the effects of L-dopa on Parkinson's disease. *Neuropharmacology.* 1973;12:89-99.

45. Heilman KM, Bowers D, Watson RT, et al. Reaction times in Parkinson's disease. *Arch Neurol.* 1976;33:139-140.

46. Flowers K. Visual closed-loop and open-loop characteristics of voluntary movement in patients with Parkinsonism and intention tremor. *Brain.* 1976;99:269-310.

47. Evarts EV, Teravainen HT, Beuchert DE, et al. Pathophysiology of motor performance in Parkinson's disease. In: Fuxe K, Calne DB, eds. *Dopaminergic Ergot Derivations and Motor Function.* New York, NY: Pergamon Press Inc; 1979:45-59.

48. Teravainen HT, Calne DB. Assessment of hypokinesia in Parkinsonism. *J Neural Transm.* 1981;51:149-159.

49. Chan CWY. Could Parkinsonian akinesia be attributable to a disturbance in the motor preparatory process? *Brain Res.* 1986;386:183-196.

50. Rogers MW, Chan CWY. Motor planning is impaired in Parkinson's disease. *Brain Res.* 1988;438:271-276.

51. Schwab RS, Chafetz ME, Walker S. Control of two simultaneous voluntary motor acts in normals and in Parkinsonism. *AMA Archives of Neurology.* 1954;72:591-598.

52. King HE. Defective psychomotor movement in Parkinson's disease: exploratory observations. *Percept Mot Skills.* 1959;9:326.

53. Talland GA. Manual skills in Parkinson's disease. *Geriatrics.* 1963;18:613-620.

54. Schmidt RA. *Motor Control and Learning*. Champaign, Ill: Human Kinetics Publishers Inc; 1988:80-88.

55. Milner-Brown HS, Fisher MA, Weiner WJ. Electrical properties of motor units in Parkinsonism an a possible relationship with bradykinesia. *J Neurol Neurosurg Psychiatry*. 1979;42:35-41.

56. Stern Y, Mayeux R, Rosen J, Ilson J. Perceptual motor dysfunction in Parkinson's disease: a deficit in sequential and predictive voluntary movement. *J Neurol Neurosurg Psychiatry*. 1983;46:145-151.

57. Brown RG, Marsden CD. Internal versus external cues and the control of attention in parkinson's disease. *Brain*. 1988;111:323-345.

58. Bloxham CA, Mindel TA, Frith CD. Initiation and execution of predictable and unpredictable movements in Parkinson's disease. *Brain*. 1984;107:371-384.

59. Hallett M, Knoshbin S. A physiological mechanism of bradykinesia. *Brain*. 1980;103:301-314.

60. Beradelli A, Rothwell JC, Day BL, Marsden CD. Movements not involved in posture are abnormal in Parkinson's disease. *Neurosci Lett*. 1984;47:47-50.

61. Weinrich M, Koch K, Garcia F, et al. Axial versus distal motor impairment in Parkinson's disease. *Neurology*. 1988;38:540-545.

62. Shimizu N, Naito M, Yoshida M. Eye-head coordination in patients with Parkinsonism and cerebellar ataxia. *J Neurol Neurosurg Psychiatry*. 1981;44:509-515.

63. Draper IT, Johns RJ. The disordered movement in Parkinsonism and the effect of drug treatment. *Bulletin of The Johns Hopkins Hospital*. 1964;115:465-480.

64. Beradelli A, Rothwell JC, Dick JP, et al. Scaling the size of the first agonist EMG burst during rapid movements in patients with Parkinson's disease. *J Neurol Neurosurg Psychiatry*. 1986;49:1273-1279.

65. Day BL, Dick JPR, Marsden CD. Patients with Parkinson's disease can employ a predictive motor strategy. *J Neurol Neurosurg Psychiatry*. 1984;47:1299-1306.

66. Martin JP. *The Basal Ganglia and Posture*. London, England: Pitman Publishing Ltd;1967.

67. Sanes JN, Evarts EV. Psychomotor performance in Parkinson's disease. In: Delwaide PJ, Agnoli A, eds. *Clinical Neurophysiology in Parkinsonism*. New York, NY: Elsevier Science Publishing Co Inc; 1985:117- 132.

68. Fitts PM. The information capacity of the human motor system in controlling the amplitude of the movement. *J Exp Psychol*. 1954;47:381- 391.

69. Johnels B, Ingvarsson P, Rydgren U, et al. Measuring motor function in Parkinson's disease. In: Benecke R, Conrad B, Marsden CD, eds. *Motor Disturbances, I*. San Diego, Calif: Academic Press Inc; 1987:131- 144.

70. Marsden CD. Defects of movement in Parkinson's disease. In: Delwaide PJ, Agnoli A, eds. *Clinical Neurophysiology in Parkinsonism*. New York, NY: Elsevier Science Publishing Co Inc; 1985:108-115.

71. Benecke R, Rothwell JC, Dick JP, et al. Performance of simultaneous movements in Parkinson's disease. *Brain*. 1986;109:739-757.

72. Beradelli A, Accornero N, Argenta M, et al. Fast complex arm movements in Parkinson's disease. *J Neurol Neurosurg Psychiatry*. 1986;49:1146-1149.

73. Lakke JP. Axial apraxia in Parkinson's disease. *J Neurol Sci*. 1985;69:37-46.

74. Edstrom L. Selective changes in the sizes of red and white muscle fibers in upper motor neuron lesions and Parkinsonism. *J Neurol Sci*. 1970;11:535-550.

75. Stern GM, Lander CM, Lees AJ. Akinetic freezing and trick movements in Parkinson's disease. *J Neurol Transm (Suppl)*. 1980;16:137- 141.

76. Narabayashi H, Nakamura R. Clinical neurophysiology of freezing in Parkinsonism. In: Delwaide PJ, Agnoli A, eds. *Clinical Neurophysiology in Parkinsonism*. New York, NY: Elsevier Science Publishing Co Inc; 1985:50-77.

77. Cooke JD, Brown JD, Brooks VB. Increased dependence on visual information for movement control in patients with Parkinson's disease. *Can J Neural Sci*. 1978;5:413-415.

78. Denny-Brown D. Clinical symtomatology of diseases of the basal ganglia. In: Vinken PJ, Brayn GW, eds. *Handbook of Clinical Neurology*. Amsterdam, The Netherlands: North Holland; 1968;6:136. Cited by Bloxham CA, Mindel TA, Frith CD. Initiation and execution of predictable and unpredictable movements in Parkinson's Disease. *Brain*. 1984;107:371-384.

79. Martin JP: Tilting reactions and disorders of the basal ganglia. *Brain*. 1965;88:855-874.

80. Traub MM, Rothwell JC, Marsden CD. Anticipatory postural reflexes in Parkinson's disease and other akinetic-rigid syndromes and in cerebellar ataxia. *Brain*. 1980;103:393-412.

81. Horak FB, Nashner LM, Nutt JG. Postural instability in Parkinson's disease: motor coordination and sensory organization. *Society for Neuroscience Abstracts*. 1984;10:634.

82. Dichgans J, Diener HC. The use of short-and long-latency reflex testing in leg muscles of neurological patients. In: Stuppler A, Weindl A, eds. *Clinical Aspects of Sensory Motor Integration*. New York, NY: Springer-Verlag New York Inc; 1987:165-174.

83. Allum JHJ, Keshner EA, Honegger F, et al. Disturbance of posture in patients in Parkinson's disease. In: Amblard B, Bertha A, Clarse F, eds. *Posture and Gait: Development, Adaptation, and Modulation*. New York, NY: Elsevier Science Publishing Co Inc; 1988:245-271.

84. Dietz V, Berger W, Horstmann G. Corrective responses to disturbances of stance and gait in parkinson's disease: impaired function of spinal reflexes. In: Amblard B, Berthoz A, Clarac F, eds. *Posture and Gait: Development, Adaptation, and Modulation*. New York, NY: Elsevier Science Publishing Co Inc; 1988:259-271.

85. Rogers MW. Control of posture and balance during voluntary movements in Parkinson's disease. In: Duncan PW, ed. *Balance*. Alexandria, Va: American Physical Therapy Association; 1990:79-86.

86. Marsden CD, Merton PA, Morton HP. Human postural responses. *Brain*. 1981;104:513-534.

87. Belen'kii VY, Gurfinkel VS, Pal'stev YI. Elements of control of voluntary movement. *Biophysics*. 1967;12:135-141.

88. Bouisset S, Zattara M. A sequence of postural movements precedes voluntary movement. *Neurosci Lett*. 1981;22:263-270.

89. Viallet F, Massion J, Massarino R, et al. Performance of bimanual load-lifting task by parkinsonian subjects. *J Neurol Neurosurg Psychiatry*. 1978;50:1274-1283.

90. Rogers MW, Kukulka CG, Soderberg GL. Postural adjustments preceding rapid arm movements in Parkinsonian subjects. *Neurosci Lett*. 1987;75:246-251.

91. Lance JW, Schwab RS, Peterson EA. Action tremor and the cogwheel phenomenon in Parkinson's disease. *Brain*. 1963;86:95-110.

92. Dick JPR, Rothwell JC, Berardelli A, et al. Associated postu-

ral adjustments in Parkinson's disease. *J Neurol Neurosurg Psychiatry*. 1986;49:1378-1385.

93. Bazalgette D, Zattara M, Bathien N, et al. Postural adjustments associated with rapid voluntary arm movements in patients with Parkinson's disease. In: Yahr MD, Bergmann KJ, eds. *Advances in Neurology*. New York, NY: Raven Press; 1986;45:371-374.

94. Rogers MW, Pai YC. Postural transitions accompanying rapid leg flexion movements in standing subjects. *Phys Ther*. 1988;68:802. Abstract.

95. Rogers MW, Pai YC. Dynamic transfer of body mass from bipedal to single limb stance. In: Proceedings of the Twelfth International Congress of Biomechanics; June 26-30, 1989; Los Angeles Calif. Page 172.

96. Rogers MW, Pai YC. Postural transitions from bipedal to single limb stance support. In: Abstracts of the Sixth International Symposium on Motor Control; July 3-7, 1989; Albena, Bulgaria. Page 152.

97. Rogers MW, Pai YC. Dynamic transitions in stance support accompanying leg flexion movements in man. *Exp Brain Res*. 1990;81:398- 402.

98. Carlsoo S. The initiation of walking. *Acta Anat (Basel)*. 1966;65:1-9.

99. Herman R, Cook T, Cozzens B. Control of postural reactions in man: the initiation of gait. In: Herman RM, Grillner S, Stein PS, et al, eds. *Neural Control of Locomotion*. New York, NY: Plenum Publishing Corp; 1976:363-388.

100. Mann RA, Hagy JL, White V, et al. The initiation of gait. *J Bone Joint Surg [Am]*. 1979;61:232-239.

101. Breniere Y, Do MC, Sanchez J. A biomechanical study of the gait initiation process. *Journal de Medecine Nucleaire et Biophysique*. 1981.

102. Rogers MW, Lin SI. Temporal characteristics of ankle muscle activity during the initiation of stepping in humans. *Society for Neuroscience Abstracts*. 1989;15:1202.

103. Gurfinkel VS. Physical foundations of stabilography. *Agressologie*. 1973;14:9-14.

104. Pai YC, Rogers MW. Control of body mass transfer as a function of speed of ascent in sit-to-stand. *Med Sci Sports Exer*. 1990;22:378-384.

105. Pai YC, Rogers MW. Segmental contributions to total body momentum in sit-to-stand. *Med Sci Sports Exer*. In press.

106. Pai YC, Rogers MW. Speed variation and resultant joint torques during sit-to-stand. *Arch Phys Med Rehabil*. In press.

107. Forssberg H, Johnels B, Steg G. Is Parkinsonian gait caused by a regression to an immature walking pattern? In: Hassler RG, Christ JF, eds. *Advances in Neurology*. New York, NY: Raven Press. 1984;40:375-379.

108. Knutsson E. An analysis of Parkinsonian gait. *Brain*. 1972;95:475-486.

109. Murray MP, Sepic SB, Gardner GM, et al. Walking patterns of men with Parkinsonism. *Am J Phys Med*. 1978;57:278-294.

110. Knutsson E, Martensson A. Posture and gait in Parkinsonian patients. In: Bles W, Brandt T, eds. *Disorders of Posture and Gait*. New York, NY: Elsevier Science Publishing Co Inc; 1986:217-229.

111. Koozekanani SH, Balmaseda MT, Fatehi MT, et al. Ground reaction forces during ambulation in parkinsonism: pilot study. *Arch Phys Med Rehabil*. 1987;68:28-30.

112. Delwaide PJ, Delmotte PH. Comparison of normal senile gait with parkinsonian gait. In: Calne DB, Comi G, Crippa D, et al, eds. *Parkinsonism and Aging*. New York, NY: Raven Press. 1989:229-237.

113. Ingvarsson PE, Johnels B, Steg G. Dissolution of motor program coordination in Parkinson's disease. In: Grillner S, Stein PG, Stuart DG, et al, eds. *Neurobiology of Vertebrate Locomotion*. New York, NY: Macmillan Publishing Co; 1986:105-118.

114. Lin SI. *The Effects of Instructional Set on the Timing of Ankle Muscle Recruitment During Gait Initiation*. Evanston, Ill: Northwestern University; 1990. Thesis.

115. Winter DA. Concerning the scientific basis for the diagnosis of pathological gait and for rehabilitation protocols. *Physiotherapy Canada*. 1985;37:245-252.

116. Schenkman M, Butler RB. A model for multisystem evaluation treatment of individuals with Parkinson's disease. *Phys Ther*. 1989;69:932-943.

117. Enoka RM. *Neuromechanical Basis of Kinesiology*. Champaign, Ill: Human Kinetics Publishers Inc; 1989:214.

118. Kandel E. Cellular mechanisms of learning and the biological basis of individuality. In: Kandel ER, Schwartz JH, eds. *Principles of Neural Science*. New York, NY: Elsevier Science Publishing Co Inc; 1985:816-833.

119. Rothwell JC, Day BL, Berardelli A, et al. Habituation and conditioning of human long latency stretch-reflex. *Exp Brain Res*. 1986;63:197-204.

120. Horak FB, Diener HC, Nashner LM. Influence of central set on human postural responses. *J Neurophysiol*. 1989;62:841-853.

121. Chan CWY. Could parkinsonian akinesia be attributable to a distance in the motor preparatory process? *Brain Res*. 1986;386:183-196.

122. Nickerson RS. Intersensory facilitation of reaction time: energy summation of preparation enhancement? *Psychol Rev*. 1973;80:489-509.

123. Day BL, Rothwell JC, Marsden CD. Interaction between the long latency stretch reflex and voluntary electromyographic activity prior to a rapid voluntary motor reaction. *Brain Res*. 1983;270:55-62.

124. Stoffels EJ, Van Der Molen MW, Keuss PJG. Intersensory facilitation and inhibition: immediate arousal and location effects of auditory noise on visual choice reaction time. *Acta Psychol (Amst)*. 1985;58:45-62.

125. Deeke L. Cerebral potentials related to voluntary actions: parkinsonian and normal subjects. In: Delwaide PJ, Agnoli A, eds. *Clinical Neurophysiology in Parkinsonism*. New York, NY: Elsevier Science Publishing Co Inc; 1985:90-105.

126. Barbeau H, Wainberg M, Finch L. Description and application of a system for locomotor rehabilitation. *Med Biol Eng Comput*. 1987;25:341- 344.

127. Garcia-Rill E. The basal ganglia and the locomotor regions. *Brain Research Reviews*. 1986;11:47-63.

128. Delwaide PJ. Are there modifications in spinal cord functions of parkinsonian patients? In: Delwaide PJ, Agnoli A, eds. *Clinical Neurophysiology in Parkinsonism*. New York, NY: Elsevier Science Publishing Co Inc; 1985:20-32.

Chapter 21

Stroke: Physical Therapy Assessment and Treatment

Pamela W. Duncan, MA, PT
Associate Professor
Graduate Program in Physical Therapy
Senior Fellow in the Center for Aging
and Human Resources
Duke University
Durham, NC 27710

As I reflect on the current issues in stroke rehabilitation, I am reminded of a parable told by Lamm[1]: "An Admiral in the United States Navy was on the high seas and all of a sudden a little blip showed up on the radar screen. The admiral told the Ensign, 'Tell that ship to change its course 15 degrees.' The words came back on the radio, 'You change your course 15 degrees.' The admiral said, 'Tell that ship that we're the US Navy and to change its course 15 degrees.' The words came back on the radio, 'You change your course 15 degrees.' The admiral himself got on the radio and said, 'I am an Admiral in the US Navy. Change your course 15 degrees.' The words came back, 'You change your course 15 degrees—I am a lighthouse.'" There are several lighthouses in the practice of neurological physical therapy. The first lighthouse is the current information from the motor control and motor learning literature that is challenging some of our theoretical assumptions. The second lighthouse is the health care system in which we are delivering our services. The purpose of this chapter is to discuss the implications of these "lighthouses" for stroke rehabilitation.

Stroke is the third leading cause of death in the United States and a major source of disability.[2] Once the initial period of high mortality is over, survival is good, with 50% of patients with strokes alive in 7 years.[3,4] Five-year survival rates have increased 16%.[4] A very recent study of survival following stroke among patients in five North Carolina counties revealed that for all strokes the 1-year survival rate increased from 49% between 1970 and 1973 to 62% between 1979 and 1980.[5] Because of variations in subject populations, time to follow-up, and methods of assessment it is difficult to estimate precisely the level of disability among survivors. Estimates of dependence in some aspects of activities of daily living range from 30% to 60%.[6] A recent study of function in a New Zealand population-based cohort of 680 patients with strokes revealed that of those who survived 6 months, 65% of them continued to have motor deficits.[7] The cost of care and the loss of earnings as a result of stroke have been estimated to be 7.5 to 11.2 billion dollars a year.[8] Stroke, therefore, is a major social and economic burden.

This burden will continue to increase because of the improved survival from stroke and the growing size of the elderly population.

Stroke rehabilitation is a health service often provided in hopes of decreasing the disability[2] and the social and economic costs associated with this disability. Rehabilitation in general is an expanding service. Currently, rehabilitation services are excluded from Medicare prospectivepayment systems. Between 1984 and 1985, the number of rehabilitation hospitals excluded from prospective payment rose 106%, and the number of excluded rehabilitation units within hospitals increased 155%.[9] Many survivors of stroke receive expensive and intensive rehabilitation in an attempt to improve functional independence and motor recovery. Current concerns about allocation of health care services and cost-effectiveness, however, have challenged us to analyze critically our methods of assessing and treating stroke.

ASSESSMENT OF MOTOR AND FUNCTIONAL DISABILITY

If health planning is to be effective and we attempt to evaluate the effects of our stroke rehabilitation programs, we must have two things. First, we must have good operational definitions and a conceptual framework of the rehabilitation process.[10] Second, we must have a good understanding of the natural history of stroke.[11] The World Health Organization (WHO) has recommended a classification of illness that describes the level of illness we are trying to influence.[12] From the WHO classification, any illness can be considered at four levels:

1. Pathology: The underlying disease or diagnosis. In stroke, the pathology may be due to thrombosis, emboli, or hemorrhage.
2. Impairment: The immediate physiological consequences, or signs and symptoms. Some of the common impairments after stroke are paresis, loss of selective motor control, abnormal tone, sensory impairments, and perceptual disorders.
3. Disability: The functional consequences, or the abilities lost. Examples of disabilities after stroke are impairments

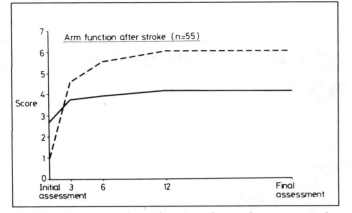

Fig. 21-1. *Recovery of arm function after stroke. – – – – is the median, —— the mean. (Reprinted from Skilbeck et al,[19] with permission.)*

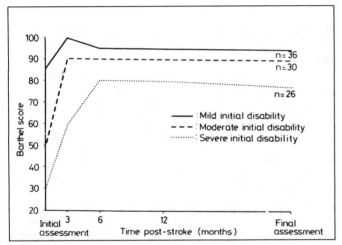

Fig. 21-2. *Median Barthel Index scores for survivors in three groups. (Reprinted from Wade et al,[15] with permission.)*

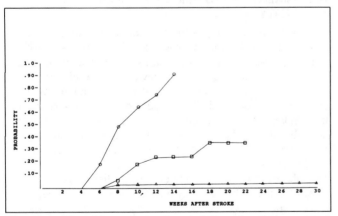

Fig. 21-3. *Life-table analysis of probability of walking ≥ 150 ft without assistance. ○, patients with motor deficit only (n = 27); □, patients with motor deficits plus somatic sensory deficit (n = 32); △, patients with motor deficit plus somatic sensory deficit plus homonymous visual deficit (n = 32). (Reprinted from Reding and Potes,[28] with permission of the American Heart Association, Inc.*

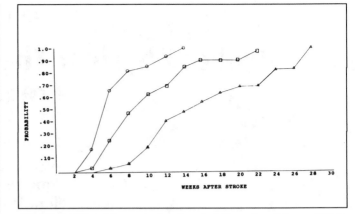

Fig. 21-4. *Life-table analysis of probability of walking ≥150 ft with assistance. ○, patients with motor deficit only (n = 27); □, patients with motor deficit plus somatic sensory deficit (n = 32); △, patients with motor deficit plus somatic sensory deficit plus homonymous visual deficit (n = 32). (Reprinted from Reding and Potes,[28] with permission of the American Heart Association, Inc.)*

in activities of daily living: feeding, dressing, transfers, and walking.
4. Handicap: The social and societal consequences, or freedoms lost. The handicap refers to a patient's inability to maintain social and family relationships, to a loss of vocation or leisure activities, and to impaired life space.

This WHO classification helps the therapist determine which level or levels of the illness she is trying to influence.

We need a good natural history to allow us to identify which patients should receive specific interventions and to provide us a basis for comparing spontaneous recovery with recovery that is due to intervention. Many patients who survive stroke experience some level of spontaneous recovery. This recovery can be either marginal or dramatic. In 1954, Twitchell was the first person to attempt to describe the sequence and time course of recovery from varying degrees of hemiplegia.[13] More recently, however, many investigators have described recovery at the level of disability in many different populations. Probably the one research group that has done the most to describe the natural history of disability secondary to stroke is Wade and his colleagues.[14-19] In analysis of recovery of arm function in 92 patients over 2 years, Wade et al[15] concluded statistically significant improvement is observed for only 3 months (Fig. 21-1). A similar analysis of activities of daily living revealed that the majority of recovery also occurs within 3 months (Fig. 21-2). The general consensus of these and other studies is that in most patients spontaneous improvement is complete within 6 months, and in fact, most of the recovery occurs within the first 6 to 12 weeks. However, if the patient experiences very severe motor deficits, recovery of function is minimal and protracted. An interesting side point, however, is that in a study of recovery in severely disabled strokes, Andrews et al[20] demonstrated that these were the patients who received the most physical therapy services, yet 47% of them demonstrated no functional gains.

Factors that have been shown to be associated with poor functional recovery include prior history of stroke, ini-

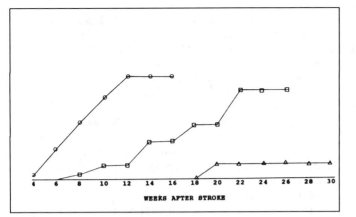

Fig. 21-5. *Life-table analysis of probability of reaching Barthel Index score of ≥95. ○, patients with motor deficit only (n = 27); □, patients with motor deficit plus somatic sensory deficit (n = 32); △, patients with motor deficit plus somatic sensory deficit plus homonymous visual deficit (n = 32). (Reprinted from Reding and Potes,[28] with permission of the American Heart Association, Inc.)*

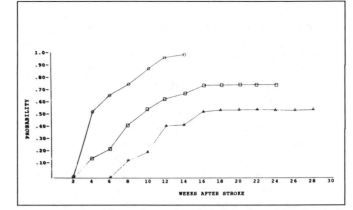

Fig. 21-6. *Life-table analysis of probability of reaching Barthel Index score of ≥60. ○, patients with motor deficit only (n = 27); □, patients with motor deficit plus somatic sensory deficit (n = 32); △, patients with motor deficit plus somatic sensory deficit plus homonymous visual deficit (n = 32). (Reprinted from Reding and Potes,[28] with permission of the American Heart Association, Inc.)*

tial motor deficit, loss of sitting balance, sensory deficits, visual-spatial deficits, cognitive deficits, and urinary and bowel incontinence.[7,21-27] There is a lot of controversy about the effects of age on recovery. In many studies, age appears to be a predictor; however, if one considers that older people have more severe strokes, age loses importance as a predictor of function.

An important and incompletely answered question in stroke recovery is, - "What is the relationship between impairments and functional outcomes?" One of the most recent and important investigations that has attempted to answer this question was produced by Reding and Potes.[28] They classified 95 consecutive patients admitted to Burke Rehabilitation Hospital with initial strokes into those with 1) motor deficits only; 2) motor and sensory deficits; and 3) motor, sensory, and visual deficits. Using life-table analysis, they analyzed the probability of achieving certain outcomes: 1) walking 150 feet without assistance (Fig. 21-3), 2) walking 150 feet with assistance (Fig. 21-4), 3) reaching a Barthel ADL Index 95 (Fig. 21-5), and 4) reaching a Barthel ADL Index 60 (Fig. 21-6). Their results demonstrated that as the number of impairments increased, the probability of higher level function is extremely low and the recovery is very protracted. This type of analysis is critical for the future rehabilitation of stroke because it allows us to begin to categorize patients into certain subgroups and provides us a scientific basis for establishing the type and intensity of interventions. In addition, the life-table analysis used in this study is an important statistical tool that should be incorporated into stroke research.[29] This statistical method allows us to analyze not only the probability of achieving an outcome but also how long it takes to reach the outcome. This type of analysis could be useful in helping us compare spontaneous recovery with recovery resulting from interventions.

At this time, we have knowledge of the recovery from the disability secondary to stroke, but we need more longitudinal studies of recovery from the specificphysical impairments (ie, balance, volitional movements, force control,

perception). Recently, several colleagues and I analyzed the relationships of recovery of movement at the shoulder with pain in the shoulder. In a prospective cohort study of 144 patients with strokes, we observed that if shoulder external rotation does not occur with shoulder flexion or abduction the patient increases his chance of having a painful shoulder 19 times.[30] Again, detailed analysis of recovery from impairments will help us more realistically establish therapeutic programs and compare spontaneous recovery of impairments with recovery resulting from interventions.

To improve how we measure recovery of impairment and disability and measure the effectiveness of our intervention we must use clinical measures that are well characterized. These measures must be reliable, valid, and sensitive to change. Our traditional assessments of patients with strokes have relied on qualitative and nonstandardized measures. Of course, we are not the only health care providers having problems in assessing these patients. In a recent review of clinical trials reported in *Stroke,* Asplund[31] reported that of 28 publications produced between 1984 and 1985, no single neuro logical assessment was used more than once in these publications, and only a few of the authors reported climimetric qualities of validity and reliability. There are, however, at least three assessments of functional motor recovery that are well-established clinical measures: 1) Fugl-Meyer assessment,[32] 2) Motor Assessment Scale,[33] and 3) Modified Motor Assessment Scale.[34]

The Fugl-Meyer assessment includes five areas: upper extremity motor function, lower extremity motor function, sensation, range of motion, and balance. A three-point scale is applied to each item: 0=the function cannot be performed, 1=the function is partially performed, and 3=the function is fully performed. The Fugl-Meyer assessment is valid, reliable, and sensitive to change.[35-39]

The Motor Assessment Scale developed by Carr and Shepherd[33] measures motor and functional abilities. This assessment consists of nine items: supine to sidelying, supine to sitting over side of bed, balanced sitting, sitting to standing, walking, upper arm function, hand movement, advanced hand activities, and general tonus. Each item is rated on a seven-point scale. Reliability measures and some measure of validity have been established.[37,40]

Recently, Lindmark and Hamrin[34] modified the Fugl-Meyer assessment to develop the Motor Capacity Assessment. This new assessment measures upper extremity motor function, lower extremity motor function, mobility skills (roll, sit, stand, and walk), balance, sensation, range of motion, and pain. Both the involved and noninvolved sides are tested. Most items are scored on a four-point ordinal scale: 0=activity cannot be performed, 1=can perform the activity with much help, 2=can perform the activity with little help, and 3=can perform activity independently. Walking is graded on a seven-point scale. This new measure has established reliability.[34] Validation of this instrument is currently being tested. A potential advantage of this assessment is that it tests both the involved and noninvolved sides.

The most ubiquitous and well-established functional outcome measure in stroke is the Barthel Index.[41] The Barthel Index is a measure at the level of the disability. It assesses 10 very basic functions: bowel, bladder, grooming, toilet use, feeding, transfer, mobility, dressing, stairs, and bathing. An appropriate criticism of the Barthel Index is that it is not useful in high functioning stroke patients. It asks, Did the patient improve in basic activities of daily living? It is not, nor should it be, a measure of slight changes. The current stroke assessments are by no means perfect, but we must accept the responsibility of using the best available measures to monitor the impact of disability from stroke on society, provide the basis for prognosis, and evaluate the effects of recovery and intervention.

EVALUATION OF IMPAIRMENTS

Now I would like to switch the focus from assessment of motor and functional disability to the evaluation of impairments, or motor control deficits, after stroke. In disability assessment we are establishing if the patient can or cannot perform certain movements of functions; in evaluation we are asking ourselves what are the impairments that are causing the functional limitations. As practicing physical therapists, we have certain assumptions about the relationship between impairment and disability. For example, a common assumption in stroke is that the movement deficits we observe are not caused by primary weakness, or inability to produce force, but rather they are due to spasticity and loss of selective motor control. An example of how we may draw conclusions about the relationship between impairment and movement deficits may be provided by the following patient example. As the patient with a stroke attempts to flex her knee, she flexes her hip. As therapists, we may prematurely decide that the observed motor behavior is due to the stereotypical flexion synergy of stroke. Subsequently, we attempt to inhibit or prevent hip flexion as the patient flexes her hip. Yet, is this correct? All of us who have worked with orthopedic patients after prolonged immobilization of their knees know that the patients have very weak hamstring muscles so when they attempt to flex their knees they flex their hips. They do this to enhance the biomechanical advantage by placing the hamstring muscles, which are two-joint muscles,

on stretch across the hip. If we prevent the hip from flexing with knee flexion, the patient is at a tremendous disadvantage. Likewise in stroke, before we assume that the observed motor deficit is due to the "flexion" synergy, we should determine if the patient has weakness, or poor force control, of the hamstrings. There is sufficient evidence from the literature that suggests that weakness, or insufficient force control, is a primary problem after stroke. Previous investigators have reported the following changes after stroke that could contribute to force control deficits, or weakness. (For a review, see Dourbomnais and Vanden Noven[42] and Duncan and Badke.[43])

1. Motorneurons changes:
   Decrease in number of motor units.
   Altered recruitment order of motor units.
   Impaired frequency of firing of motor units.
2. Nerve changes:
   Decrease in peripheral nerve conduction.
3. Muscle changes:
   Changes in morphology and contractile properties.
   Changes in mechanical properties of muscles.

Differentiation between which impairment or combination of impairments is contributing to abnormal movement is a difficult task. The movement deficits after stroke are a reflection of the complexity of motor control. To delineate more clearly the role of certain impairments and their interrelationships in stroke, Susan Attermeier, Mary Beth Badke, and I have developed a model for analyzing the motor control deficits after stroke.[43] This model is based on the systems theory of motor control. In establishing the conceptual model, we used the analogy suggested by Gelfand[44] that "movement is a language"(Fig. 21-7). The first prerequisite for language is to have a concept. The conceptual basis for movement comes from our cognition, perception, and motivation. How does the patient perceive, or interpret, his environment? Does the patient understand the task goal? Can he problem solve? Is he motivated? If the perception of the task is impaired, the patient will never appear to organize or execute

Fig. 21-7. *Model for assessing abnormal motor control.*

MOVEMENT IS A LANGUAGE

CONCEPT - LETTERS - WORDS - VOCABULARY

CONCEPT	PERCEPTION - COGNITION MOTIVATION
LETTERS	ROM - STRENGTH TONE - SENSATION
WORDS	POSTURE SYNERGIES MOVEMENT
VOCABULARY	ADAPTABILITY/FLEXIBILITY

the movement patterns appropriately. For example, we may observe that a patient is leaning forward and standing in plantar flexion, demonstrating increased extensor tone in the lower extremity. We may immediately try to modify either the tone or the range of motion; however, these movements may be compensating strategies for the patient. His perception of vertical may be forward, and therefore, if this is the case, his observed motor behaviors are appropriate. In essence, the movement may not look right to us but it is right for the patient.

Once the movement concept is understood, the motor task is planned; if the letters are present, words can be developed. The "letters" of the language are range of motion, biomechanical alignment, muscle tone, strength (force control), and sensation. These are the things that the central nervous system (CNS) has to work with to produce the motor behavior. Altered letters will change the expression and efficiency of the motor behavior, but these alterations alone will not necessarily change the organization and sequence of movement patterns. For example, abnormal tone is one of the most salient features of stroke. Yet, if we "normalize tone we do not necessarily normalize movement." Tone is the gain for the system. A good analogy for understanding this concept is to compare tone to the volume dial on a radio. By turning the dial you alter the expression (volume), but you do not change the program that is being heard; so be it in CNS damage.

Every movement is constructed from the contraction of muscles, but there are potentially thousands of combinations of muscle contractions that produce unique and purposeful movements. Functionally related patterns of muscle contractions are called synergies. In applying Gelfand's analogy, the synergies are the words of our movement vocabulary. The synergies are an expression of motor programs. The CNS programs the muscles as to which ones are going to contract, when, in what sequence, and with what force.

Finally, we are fluent in language only if we have developed a vocabulary of words. The vocabulary of the movement language includes activation of selected synergies that are characterized by adaptability, efficiency, and accuracy. It is the individual's ability to create adaptive behavior (eg, vary tasks, vary speed, vary environmental factors) that makes movement functional in a variety of contexts.

Table 21-1. *Correlation Between Tone and Movement*

Tone	Movement
1. Flaccid	No movement
2. Minimal spasticity	
3. Moderate-severe spasticity	Posturing of extremities
4. Spasticity decreases	More selective motor control
5. Minimal or no spasticity	More normal and selective control, increased speed and coordination

Patients with strokes have language deficits. The model presented is a tool for specifically identifying the impairments that are contributing to the movement disorders. As such, the model will assist us in establishing organized and realistic treatment programs.

The process we use to interpret this model must be very systematic. As Kay Shepard suggested at this conference (see Shepard in this volume), we must 1) observe the movement deficit, 2) identify all possible causes of the movement deficit, 3) generate a conceptual hypothesis, 4) generate an operational hypothesis, and 5) test the hypothesis.

As Shepard stated, the difference between a conceptual hypothesis and an operational hypothesis is that an operational hypothesis is testable. When establishing an operational hypothesis, methods of measuring the impairments and the movement deficits must be incorporated. Obviously, this is where we are having some problems in neurological physical therapy: we have not developed well-established measurement tools. For example, how do we reliably and validly measure either muscle tone or muscle strength?

Another potential problem in interpreting this model is that when we observe impairments that vary simultaneously we may immediately assume cause-and-effect relationships. For example, since reading Signe Brunnstrom,[45] clinicians have observed a parallel between tone and movement in stroke patients (Tab. 21-1). Because these two symptoms covary some clinicians have assumed cause and effect. This is not necessarily true. Both abnormal tone and impaired movements are symptoms reflecting the severity of the CNS damage; one of the impairments may or may not cause another.

Differentially diagnosing the motor control deficits after stroke is indeed a complex task. However, with more understanding of motor control theory and better measurements of impairment of disability we may begin to "get the big picture." Only until we adequately diagnose the causes of the deficits can we select the appropriate therapeutic technique and strategies.

THERAPEUTIC MODELS

Our therapeutic approaches to stroke rehabilitation have been based on the following three major models:

Compensatory Model

This model emphasizes activities of daily living that make the patient more independent in meeting his basic needs. The goal is to improve function rather than to enhance motor recovery or alter the impairment. The therapist teaches the patient to compensate for his motor deficits and adapts either the conditions or the environment so that the patient can function with ease and independence. As therapists, we have often avoided the compensatory approach in fear that this would impair recovery and contribute to learned nonuse of the impaired side. Some patients, however, have such severe deficits that the compensatory approach is all we have to offer.

Facilitation Model

The primary goals of the therapeutic approaches based

on the facilitation model are to enhance motor recovery after stroke and to minimize compensatory strategies. In fact, a major assumption of the facilitation model is that teaching of compensatory strategies will limit motor recovery. The three primary facilitation approaches are as follows:

Brunnstrom. Recovery of stroke is an orderly process in which several stages can specifically be identified. Recovery proceeds from stereotypical synergies to more selective motor control. The therapist should facilitate the basic synergies with sensory cues, associated reactions, and reflexes.[45]

Bobath. The stereotypical synergies are pathological, unwanted manifestations of spasticity. A primary goal of therapeutic intervention is to normalize tone to prevent the stereotypical movement patterns. Another goal is to facilitate symmetrical posture and normal postural responses.[46]

Proprioceptive neuromuscular facilitation. Sensory cues, which are a variety of techniques that incorporate specific muscle contractions, resistance, directions of movement, and patterns of movements, are used to facilitate motor recovery. Additionally, a developmental sequence of activities is used for progression.[47]

As Gordon[48] has discussed, some common assumptions underlie the approaches based on the facilitation model.
1. The brain controls movements but not muscles. All the facilitation approaches assume that CNS lesions lead to disordered patterns of movement rather than simply paralysis or weakness and that the abnormal movement patterns result from the lesion itself rather than occur as compensation for the lesion.
2. Sensory stimulation will facilitate and help organize the correct movement patterns.
3. Abnormal patterns of movement are a result of lack of inhibitory control from higher centers.
4. The primary source of motor control deficits are from abnormal neuro physiology rather than from any biomechanical or muscle factors.

Some of us have become discontent with different aspects of the facilitation models for several reasons. First, the theoretical assumptions underlying the facilitation model are not consistent with our current knowledge of normal and abnormal motor control. Second, we have become dissatisfied with our outcomes. We may have been able to normalize tone, but our normalizing tone did not normalize movement; we may have been able to facilitate a movement pattern, but when the patient attempted to move there was very little carry over to more complex tasks.[48]

Motor Control Model

This third model of therapeutic intervention is relatively new and incorporates current theories of motor control and principles of motor learning. A major tenet of the motor control model is that motor control is an extremely complex interaction of the CNS, musculoskeletal system, and biomechanics.[48] The CNS has an uncanny ability to perceive and predict what is necessary for motor performance. It programs the movement, and the program is executed through an intact musculoskeletal and biomechanical system.[49] Movement is not sensory driven, but rather sensory information is used as feedback to compare the intended movement with the actual movement.[49] Another important concept of

this theory is that motor control is task specific. Each movement is organized based on the specific conditions of the task, and if one practices under one condition it does not necessarily carry over to another. The motor control approach does not emphasize learning movement patterns but rather solving the motor problem.[50] Part of relearning motor skills is that rather than the patient being able to perform every movement perfectly he must develop the ability to detect errors in his movements and to self-correct. Finally, the motor control approach incorporates current theory of motor learning as previously described by Winstein.[51]

Treatment Approaches

Obviously, the theoretical model we accept determines how we treat the patient. Take for example a frequent therapeutic goal in stroke rehabilitation to increase weight shift to the involved leg. Table 21-2 compares the differences in the treatment strategies of a therapist using the facilitation model as compared with one using the motor control model.

Of course, the important question is, "Is one model of therapeutic intervention more effective than another?" At this time, seven studies have reported comparing the effectiveness of different therapeutic interventions (Tab. 21-3).[52-58] Because of the strongly contrasting rationales for treatment, one would expect differences in relative efficacy among the different therapeutic interventions. Although in all of these studies the patients improved, there was no significant differences in the improvements among the different interventions strategies. The safest conclusion we can reach

Table 21-2. *Comparison of Treatment Strategies Using Different Models for Goal of Weight Shift to the Involved Leg*

Facilitation Model	Model Control Model
Prerequisites: normal tone, inhibit reflexes or stereotypical synergies, facilitate equilibrium	Prerequisites: range of motion, biomechanical alignment, force control, ability to detect error
Sequence of activities: bridging, sit to stand, stand, walk	Selecting activities: uses the ideas of task specificity (ie, if goal is to improve weight shift in standing, then practice standing; if it is to improve weight shift in walking, then practice walking)
Use facilitation cues to get weight shift; hands on, compression, resistance, etc	Select goal directed tasks that require patient to order and sequence weight shift (ie, reaching)
Goal is to get "normal" movement, and the therapist corrects the patient if he is wrong	Movement does not have to be "normal," patient can make mistakes. The goal is to develop error detection and let the patient self-correct

Table 21-3. *Studies to Determine if One Model of the Therapeutic Intervention Is More Effective Than Another*

1. Bobath versus Brunnstrom
   Wagenaar et al[52] 1990
2. Sensorimotor Integration Treatment versus Functional Treatment
   Jongbloed et al[53] 1989
3. Electromyographic Biofeedback versus Bobath
   Basmajian et al[54] 1987
4. Neuromuscular Re-education versus Functional Treatment
   Lord and Hill[55] 1986
5. Functional versus Bobath versus Proprioceptive Neuromuscular Facilitation
   Dickstein et al[56] 1987
6. Facilitation versus Functional Treatment
   Logigan et al[57] 1983
7. Facilitation versus Functional Treatment
   Stern et al[58] 1970

at this time is that therapeutic interventions are not detrimental to patient outcomes, but on the other hand, there is not sufficient evidence that one therapeutic intervention is superior to another. In fact, in a recent controversy in *Neurology Series* our colleagues in neurology challenged us: "There is no evidence that current rehabilitation methods affect the natural recovery of motor, sensory, coordination, or visual deficit following stroke. They do allow the patient to cope with residual deficits more effectively and with greater independence."[59]

Efficacy and Effectiveness of Models

We may believe, especially after reading the proceedings of this II STEP conference, that we need to re-evaluate our theoretical models for evaluating and treating patients with strokes; maybe the motor control model has a lot to offer. However, we will be making the same mistakes that we have made in the past if we accept the motor control model as the truth. Not one clinical study has evaluated the efficacy or the effectiveness of this model in neuro logical rehabilitation. We must initiate controlled clinical trials that will assess if the motor recovery after stroke is enhanced by this therapeutic intervention. Some of the methodological problems that we face in designing such studies to evaluate stroke rehabilitation are as follows:

Selection of subjects. Patients with strokes are not a homogeneous group; they demonstrate different potentials for recovery.[14,21,26-28] In previous study designs, patients with strokes have not been stratified on any preestablished basis of probability of improvement. In fact, several researchers have demonstrated that the patients who recover the least are the ones who get the most intensive therapy.[20,60] Only occasionally have some researchers restricted their subjects to those who are the most likely to recover. Subject eligibility criteria should be guided by the principle of selecting subjects most likely to benefit from rehabilitation.[61]

Variability in rehabilitation potential. Patients with

strokes differ in their ability to recover and improve function after stroke. Stroke is a disease of the elderly. Many elderly patients have comorbid diseases as well as cognitive and physical impairments that affect the prognosis for recovery. These comorbid factors must be considered when investigating the effectiveness of stroke rehabilitation.

Classification of neurological deficits. It seems to me that to evaluate stroke rehabilitation programs effectively, subjects should not only be classified on the basis of potential for recovery but also be classified on the basis of the underlying neurological deficit. There are several problems, however, in the classification of site and size of lesions. Investigators have found poor correlation between the artery shown by angiography to be occluded and the results of the computed tomography.[62] Categorization by lesion location is hampered by the fact that patients may have multiple lesions and various degrees of cortical and subcortical extensions.[63] In addition, lesion size is more correlated with neurological deficits than is lesion location.[64] Reding and Potes[28] suggest that the problems of misclassifying patients on the basis of the neuroanatomical deficits can be eliminated by categorizing patients on their clinical deficits (motor, somatosensory, and visual-field deficits).

Spontaneous recovery versus recovery resulting from intervention. Many patients with strokes who survive stroke experience some level of spontaneous recovery. This recovery can be marginal or dramatic and has been demonstrated by several independent investigators to be completed within 6 months of stroke onset.[13-19] Because most rehabilitation programs occur within this period of spontaneous recovery, it is difficult to establish if the recovery is due to the intervention or to spontaneous recovery. If it were ethical or feasible to restrict intervention to after the 6-month spontaneous recovery phase, the improvements may be slight because of limiting intervention to a time when the effects of intervention may not be optimal.

Measuring outcomes. One of the major obstacles to investigating effectiveness of stroke rehabilitation programs is selection of valid and reliable outcome measures. The most frequent outcome measures used have included mortality, length of hospitalization, institutionalization, cost of illness, neurological assessments, and activities of daily living. Many of the current outcome measures do not have established test characteristics of reliability, validity, and sensitivity to changes.

Variability in rehabilitation programs. One of the biggest obstacles to evaluating stroke rehabilitation programs is a lack of consensus on therapeutic interventions. As I have discussed, there are at least three models of therapeutic interventions. There is no consensus among therapists as to the "best" approach. Additionally, not only is the intervention between stroke and commencement of rehabilitation variable but also the duration and frequency of intervention.

Study design. The "gold standard" for assessing effectiveness of stroke rehabilitation programs is the randomized clinical trial with patients matched for age, sex, side of stroke, comorbidity, and other factors that predict outcome. One half of the patients would be randomized for intervention and the other half would be deprived of intervention. Because rehabilitation is an accepted, albeit not proven health service for stroke, ethical considerations preclude such a design.[59] Studies of rehabilitation outcomes, therefore, have compared the effect of specific types of intervention with less focused interventions.[45,46]

However, these methodological issues are not the primary barrier to scientific investigation of the effectiveness of stroke rehabilitation. As Back-y- Rita[65] states, "The most serious barriers are the absence of scientific rehabilitation role models and an understanding of the need of theory as a basis of practice." We now have available to us the theoretical models and a better understanding of the research methodological issues that will help us critically evaluate our roles. Thus we have come to a time that we have the potential for answering whether specific physical therapy interventions influence motor recovery. Our first goal is to establish efficacy rather than effectiveness of therapeutic inventory. In efficacy research, the intervention is clearly defined and administered to patients with any one type of disability, reducing variability of outcome and concentrating on those who get optional type, duration, and frequency of rehabilitation.[66,67] In contrast, effectiveness studies would analyze the benefits of therapy on all those who receive it.[66,67] Because stroke is such a variable disease and most patients with strokes have comorbid factors and physical impairments, it is very unlikely that we will ever establish the effectiveness of stroke rehabilitation in enhancing motor recovery of all patients.

Efficacy studies should be initiated. To do this, we must carefully select and classify patients and their neurological deficits. Second, we must specify the type and frequency of interventions and control for the timing of the interventions. Our research design should include only valid and reliable measures of impairments and disabilities. Life-table analysis may help us differentiate between recovery that is due to spontaneous recovery and due to interventions. Randomized trials of therapeutic interventions may be difficult, but I suggest we explore randomizing select patients with strokes, after rehabilitation, into two groups for 1) continuation of intensive therapeutic interventions to enhance motor recovery or 2) discontinuation of therapy.

CONCLUSIONS

Stroke is a very complex disease with severe consequences. Not all patients have the same probability of achieving motor recovery. We must take an active role in identifying those patients who may benefit from aggressive therapy designed to change the impairments. Other patients may benefit from intervention to minimize the disability and handicap. We must evaluate the efficacy of our intervention, and last but not least, we must continually evaluate our theoretical assumptions. Finally, our value in the health care system will be established if we affect the disability level and quit promising more than we can deliver.

References

1. Lamm RD. Columbus and Copernicus. Presented at the 65th Annual Conference of the American Physical Therapy Association; June 24, 1990; Anaheim, Calif.
2. Garraway M, Akhtr AJ. Theory and practice of stroke rehabilitation. *Recent Advances in Geriatric Medicine*. 1978;1:7-20.
3. Matsumoto N, Whisnant JP, Kurkand LT, Okazaki H. Natural history of stroke in Rochester, Minnesota: 1955-1969. *Stroke*. 1973;4:20-29.
4. Garraway WM, Whisnant JP, Drury I. The changing pattern of survival following stroke. *Stroke*. 1983;14:699-703.
5. Howard G, Toole JF, Becker C, et al. Changes in survival following stroke in five North Carolina counties observed during two different periods. *Stroke*. 1989;20:345-350.
6. Dombovy ML, Basford JR, Whisnant JP, Bergstralh EJ. Disability and use of rehabilitation services following stroke in Rochester, Minnesota: 1975-1979. *Stroke*. 1987;18:830-836.
7. Bonita R, Beaglehole R. Recovery of motor function after stroke. *Stroke*. 1988;19:1497-1500.
8. Feigenson JS. Stroke rehabilitation: effectiveness, benefits, and cost; some practical considerations. *Stroke*. 1979;10:1-4.
9. Wallace C. More study needed before revising rehab payment system. *Modern Health Care*. 1988;1:25-26.
10. Wade DT. Designing district disability services: the Oxford experience. *Clinical Rehabilitation*. 1990;4:147-158.
11. Basmajian JV. The winter of our discontent: breaking intolerable time locks for stroke survivors. *Arch Phys Med Rehabil*. 1989;70:92-94.
12. *International Classification of Impairments Disability and Handicaps*. Geneva, Switzerland: World Health Organization; 1980.
13. Twitchell TE. Sensory factors in purposive movement. *J Neurophysiol*. 1954;17:239-254.
14. Wade DT, Wood VA, Jewer RL. Recovery after stroke: the first three months. *J Neurol Neurosurg Psychiatry*. 1985;48:7-13.
15. Wade DT, Langton-Hewer R, Skilbeck CE, et al. The hemiplegic arm after stroke: measurement and recovery. *J Neurol Neurosurg Psychiatry*. 1983;46:521-524.
16. Wade DT, Hewer RL. Motor loss and swallowing difficulty after stroke: frequency, recovery and prognosis. *Acta Neurol Scand*. 1987;76:50-54.
17. Wade DT, Skilbeck CE, Hewer RL. Predicting Barthel ADL Score at 6 months after an acute stroke. *Arch Phys Med Rehabil*. 1983;64:24-28.
18. Parker JM, Wade DT, Hewer RL. Loss of arm function after stroke: measurement, frequency, and recovery. *International Rehabilitation Medicine* 1986;8:69-73.
19. Skilbeck CE, Wade DT, Hewer RL, et al. Recovery after stroke. *J Neurol Neurosurg Psychiatry*. 1983;46:5-8.
20. Andrews K, Brocklehurst JC, Richards B, et al. The recovery of the severely disabled stroke patient. *Rheumatism and Rehabilitation*. 1982;21:225-230.
21. Jongbloed L. Prediction of function after stroke: a critical review. *Stroke*. 1986;17:765-777.
22. Sandin KJ, Smith BS. The measure of balance in sitting in stroke rehabilitation prognosis. *Stroke*. 1990;21:82-86.
23. Shah S, Vanclay F, Cooper B. Predicting discharge status at commencement of stroke rehabilitation. *Stroke*. 1989;20:766-769.
24. Olson TS. Arm and leg paresis as outcome predictors in stroke rehabilitation. *Stroke*. 1990;21:247-251.
25. Loewen SC, Anderson BA. Predictors of stroke outcome using objective measurement scales. *Stroke*. 1990;21:78-81.
26. Dove HG, Schneider KC, Wallace JD. Evaluating and predicting outcome of acute cerebral vascular accident. *Stroke*. 1984;15:858-864.
27. Heinemann AW, Roth EJ, Cichowsli K, Betts H. Multivariate analysis of improvement and outcome following stroke rehabilitation. *Arch Neurol*. 1987;44:1167-1172.

28. Reding MJ, Potes E. Rehabilitation outcome following initial unilateral hemispheric stroke: life table analysis approach. *Stroke.* 1988;19:1354-1358.

29. Rimm A, Harty A, Kalbflisch J, et al. *Basic Biostatistics in Medicine and Epidemiology.* Norwalk, Conn: Appleton-Century-Crofts; 1980.

30. Mathisen L, Berquist K. *A Prospective Study of Hemiplegic Shoulder Pain.* Durham, NC: Duke University; 1990. Thesis.

31. Asplund K. Clinimetrics in stroke research. *Stroke.* 1987;18:530-531.

32. Fulg-Meyer AR, Jaasko L. The post-stroke hemiplegic patient method for evaluation of physical performance. *Scand J Rehabil Med.* 1975;7:13-31.

33. Carr JH, Shepherd RB, Nordholm L, et al. Investigation of new motor assessment scale for stroke patients. *Phys Ther.* 1985;65:175-180.

34. Lindmark B, Hamrin E. Evaluation of functional capacity after stroke as a basis for active intervention. *Scand J Rehabil Med.* 1988;20:103-109.

35. Duncan PW, Propst M, Nelson S. Reliability of the Fugl-Meyer assessment of sensorimotor recovery following stroke. *Phys Ther.* 1983;63:1606-1610.

36. Fugl-Meyer AR. Effect of rehabilitation in hemiplegic as reflected in relation between motor recovery and ADL function. In: Proceedings of IRMA; 1976; Mexico City, Mexico. Abstract, p 683.

37. Poole JL, Whitney SL. Motor assessment scale for stroke patients: concurrent validity and interrater reliability. *Arch Phys Med Rehabil.* 1988;69:195-197.

38. DeWeerdt WJG, Harrison MA. Measuring recovery of arm-hand function in stroke patients. *Physiotherapy Canada.* 1985;37:65-70.

39. Dettmann MA, Linder MT, Sepic S. Relationships among walking performance, postural stability, and functional assessments. *American Journal of Rehabilitation Medicine.* 1987;66:77-90.

40. Loewen SC, Anderson BA. Reliability of the Modified Motor Assessment Scale and the Barthel Index. *Phys Ther.* 1988;68:1077-1081.

41. Mahoney FI, Barthel DW. Functional evaluation: the Barthel Index. *Md State Med J.* 1965;14:61-65.

42. Dourbonnais D, Vanden Noven S. Weakness in patients with hemiparesis. *Am J Occup Ther.* 1989;43:313-319.

43. Duncan PW, Badke MB. *Stroke Rehabilitation: Recovery of Motor Control.* Chicago, Ill: Year Book Medical Publishers Inc; 1987.

44. Gelford IM, ed. *Models of Structural-Functional Organization of Certain Biological Systems.* Cambridge, Mass: The MIT Press; 1971: 329-345.

45. Brunnstrom S. *Movement Therapy in Hemiplegic.* New York, NY: Harper & Row, Publishers Inc; 1990.

46. Bobath B. *Adult Hemiplegia: Evaluation and Treatment.* London, England: William Heinemann Medical Books Ltd; 1978.

47. Voss D, Ionta M, Myers BJ. *Proprioceptive Neuromuscular Facilitation.* Philadelphia, Pa: Harper & Row, Publishers Inc; 1985.

48. Gordon J. Assumptions underlying physical therapy intervention: theoretical and historical perspectives. In: Carr J, Shephard RB, Gordon J, et al, eds. *Movement Science: Foundations for Physical Therapy in Rehabilitation.* Rockville, Md: Aspen Publishers Inc; 1987:1-30.

49. Brooks V. *The Neural Basis of Motor Control.* New York, NY: Oxford University Press; 1986.

50. Carr JH, Shephard R, Gordon J, et al. *Movement Science: Foundations for Physical Therapy in Rehabilitation.* Rockville, Md: Aspen Publishers Inc; 1987.

51. Winstein CJ. Motor learning considerations in stroke rehabilitation. In: Duncan DW, Badke MB. *Stroke Rehabilitation: Recovery of Motor Control.* Chicago, Ill: Year Book Medical Publishers Inc: 1987.

52. Wagenaar RC, Meijer OG, Piet CW, et al. The functional recovery of stroke: a comparison between neuro-developmental treatment and the Brunnstrom method. *Scand J Rehabil Med.* 1990;22:1-8.

53. Jongbloed L, Stacey S, Brighton C. Stroke rehabilitation: sensorimotor integrative treatment versus functional treatment. *Am J Occup Ther.* 1989;43:391-397.

54. Basmajian JV, Gowland CA, Finlayson AJ, et al. Stroke treatment: comparison of integrated behavioral-physical therapy vs traditional therapy programs. *Arch Phys Med Rehabil.* 1987;68:267-272.

55. Lord JB, Hill K. Neuromuscular reeducation versus traditional programs for stroke rehabilitation. *Arch Phys Med Rehabil.* 1986;67:88-91.

56. Dickstein R, Hocharman S, Pillar T, et al. Stroke rehabilitation: three exercise therapy approaches. *Phys Ther.* 1986;66:1233-1238.

57. Logigan MK, Samuels MA, Falconer J. Clinical exercise trial for stroke patients. *Arch Phys Med Rehabil.* 1983;64:364-367.

58. Stern PH, McDowell F, Miller JM. Effects of facilitation exercise techniques in stroke rehabilitation. *Arch Phys Med Rehabil.* 1970;51:526-531.

59. Reding MJ, McDowell FH. Focused stroke rehabilitation programs improve outcome. *Arch Neurol.* 1989;46:700-701.

60. Brocklehurst JC, Andrews K, Richards B, et al. How much physical therapy for patients with stroke? *Br Med J.* 1978;1:1307-1310.

61. Gresham GE. Stroke outcome research. *Stroke.* 1986;17:358-360.

62. Lincoln NB, Blackburn M, Ellis S, Jackson J. An investigation of factors affecting progress of patients on a stroke unit. *J Neurol Neurosurg Psychiatry.* 1989;53:493-496.

63. Knopman D, Rubens A. The validity of computed tomographic scan findings for the localization of cerebral function. *Arch Neurol.* 1986;43:328-332.

64. Hertanu J, Demopoulos J, Yang W. Stroke rehabilitation: correlation and prognostic value of computerized tomography and sequential functional assessments. *Arch Phys Med Rehabil.* 1984;65:505-507.

65. Bach-y-Rita P. Theory-based neuro rehabilitation. *Arch Phys Med Rehabil.* 1989;70:162.

66. Barer DH, Ebrahim SB, Mitchell JRA. The pragmatic approach to stroke trial design. *Neuroepidemiology.* 1988;7:1-12.

67. Brook RH, Lohr K. Efficacy, effectiveness, variations and quality. *Med Care.* 1985;23:710-720.

Chapter 22

Cerebral Palsy: Contemporary Treatment Concepts

Linda Fetters, PhD, PT
Assistant Professor
Department of Physical Therapy
Sargent College of Allied Health Professions
Boston University
Boston, MA 02215

The task of this meeting is at once formidable yet exciting. Each of the presenters and participants recognizes the need for substantial change in the approach to rehabilitation of people with neurological problems manifesting as difficulty with movement, particularly functional movement. I will stress functional movement throughout my presentation because I believe it is an aspect of physical therapy that may have been undertaught in our academic programs, if not underemphasized in the clinic. As Landau[1] suggested, no one comes into the clinic complaining of spasticity; they complain about the inability to accomplish movement tasks in their everyday life. Thus lack of functional abilities brings people to physical therapy, and I believe our central goal must be to assist these individuals in their quest for independence and function. Although no one would disagree with this noble goal, I believe we have not fully incorporated the concept of function into therapeutic exercise in the clinic or into outcome measures for clinical research.

Cerebral palsy (CP) is a category of disability including individuals with sensorimotor disorder. The anatomical area, degree of disability, and associated problems vary. Nelson[2] compares the term CP to the term mental retardation in that there are many different types and causes of the problem. We probably do not know what causes most cases of CP. Analyses by Ellenberg and Nelson[3] of data from the Collaborative Perinatal Project of the National Institute of Neurological and Communicative Disorders and Stroke suggest that despite the advent of improvements in obstetrical and neonatal care, there has been an inconsistent decrease in the frequency of cerebral palsy during the past 20 years. Cerebral palsy was evident in 189 of the 45,559 children followed to age 7 years in the Perinatal project, or approximately 0.4% of this sample. In attempting to understand the etiology of CP, Nelson and Ellenberg offer these insights:

Many of the current hypotheses concerning the causes of cerebral palsy have changed little in general outline, despite elaboration in detail, in the 145 years since the disorder first came to medical attention. Meanwhile, there has been explosive growth in the developmental neurosciences in recent years, revealing enormously complex interactions among components of the developing nervous system, and showing that interference in theseinteractions can result in derangement of the intricately orchestrated developmental program of the brain. This study indicates that a large proportion of cases of cerebral palsy remains unexplained. New contributions to explanation may come about as advances in the understanding of brain development and maldevelopment are translated from the basic to the clinical neurosciences. Much of what is considered known about the origins of cerebral palsy may warrant reevaluation.[3(p86)]

And just as what is considered known about the origins of CP may warrant re- evaluation, I believe that treatment for CP also warrants a re-evaluation. Some of our assumptions need to be re-examined. And to improve the motor competence of patients with CP, we need to develop and test new assumptions, focus on the attainment of functional motor outcomes, and use creative methods for measuring these functional outcomes. The new assumptions and methods must be formulated from current research and thinking in motor control and motor learning and from work in psychology and other behavioral sciences.

PREVIOUS ASSUMPTIONS AND NEW THOUGHTS

Muscle Tone and Movement

One assumption common to the neurophysiologic approaches to CP is that aberrant muscle tone is responsible for the decrease in normal movement patterns associated with CP.[4] If normal muscle tone is achieved, it is assumed that normal movement will follow. Research support exists for the emergence of improved patterns of muscle activation after a decrease in spasticity; however, these studies have used electromyographic records from single-joint movement as opposed to functional movement as outcome measures.[5,6] But research support also exists for the opposing view: a decrease in spasticity is not followed by improvement in movement.[1,7] Although debate will continue, the important point here is that fundamental to the argument is a definition of muscle tone and its aberrations such as spasticity.

Muscle tone continues to be an elusive concept to define, and clinical assessment of muscle tone has been unreliable (and I would suggest invalid).[8] Clinical spasticity has many suggested etiologies including increase in stretch reflexes, decrease in higher center control, and spread of cutaneous excitation to motor neuron pools beyond the desired site.[9-11] Important work in the area of dorsal root stimulation in CP offers new explanations for spasticity.[12] The research was conducted in preparation for dorsal rhizotomy. Stimulation of dorsal roots at thresholds that should have stimulated monosynaptic pathways elicited marked polysynaptic patterns. There appeared to be an overexcitation of nervous pathways from a given sensory input. These authors identified two patterns of abnormal muscle irradiation.

The first pattern involved bilateral hip adductor contraction. Stimulation at 1 Hz caused the ipsilateral hip adductors to contract, whereas at 50 Hz bilateral contraction of hip adductors occurred, which is a very familiar pattern in CP. The second pattern was the triple flexion response. Stimulation at 1 Hz caused a single muscle group in the lower extremities to contract, whereas stimulation at 50 Hz caused contractions of hip flexors, hamstrings, and tibialis anterior muscles, forming the triple flexion response. The quadriceps femoris muscle responded monosynaptically at 1 Hz, but when the stimulation frequency was raised to 50 Hz, polysynaptic activity occurred in the tibialis anterior, hamstrings, and biceps brachii muscles. Thus a triple flexion response occurred simultaneously in the lower limb and in the elbow flexors. This too is a familiar pattern in cerebral palsy. An important point is that normal human response to this type of dorsal root stimulation is activation of the monosynaptic pathways at the lower frequencies followed by inhibition of these pathways at increasing frequencies. Polysynaptic activation does not usually occur. The important therapeutic point is that sensory stimulation appears to be abnormally translated to muscle activation.

These authors also directly related the muscle irradiation patterns to the patterns of clinical spasticity that were evident preoperatively in each of these patients. That is, the pattern of muscular irradiation that was evident upon dorsal root stimulation was precisely the pattern of spasticity that had been noted clinically before surgery.

This finding is indeed important and thought provoking research. I am not certain what the direct clinical applications are at this time, but I believe at least a few points should guide us clinically. First, we might view spasticity as an abnormal reaction to sensation. Even normal sensory experience may provoke an atypical response. Patients may need to learn to isolate motor output in response to overexcitation of neural pathways. Learning may take place using many of the neurophysiologic approaches we have already developed. In addition, we should be fully exploiting the biofeedback paradigms available to assist patients in isolating functional movement groups. Second, the lack of presynaptic inhibition, which might be responsible for these aberrant responses, might be amenable to various drugs.[12] Our close collaboration in studies using medication and physical therapy may yield exciting new clinical results.

In addition to conceptualizing spasticity as the presence of aberrant mechanism, spasticity may also be conceptualized as the absence of the movement patterns necessary for efficient species-specific movement. The clinical problem becomes not the presence of spasticity but the lack of more functional movement patterns. There is growing evidence that children with CP and patients with other types of movement dysfunction have difficulty with force generation in many muscle groups.[7,10] We may observe and evaluate the spasticity, but the problem is more about what we do *not* evaluate; that is, the lack of proper force generation for movement. Spasticity in this case might be viewed as an adaptive response to allow the patient to generate adequate, albeit often overadequate, forces to produce a movement.

An example from the gait literature may illustrate this point. The stride frequency and stride length adopted by normal subjects for walking at a constant speed results in minimized metabolic cost.[13] The optimal frequency can be predicted as the resonant frequency of a harmonic oscillator.[14] A system oscillating at resonance requires the least amount of force to maintain the oscillation, which would otherwise stop as a result of damping and viscous properties. In walking, for example, muscular effort is required to maintain the gait cycle to counteract the tendency for braking forces, joint friction, and gravity to cause the cycle to stop. Thus the population of normal walkers seems to be sensitive to the oscillatory properties of their limbs that in turn will lead to a minimal metabolic cost.

A system that does not oscillate at resonance also is unstable. For example, when a top spins at high frequencies it maintains a stable trajectory. As the frequency of the top decreases it begins to wobble. When subjects were directed to walk at lower than preferred frequencies, they often reported feeling "off-balance" and even used the term "unstable." Instability in walking will lead to an increase in the need for accessory muscular input to stabilize and prevent falling. The resulting instability of the system might result in the increased need for accessory musculature and the spasticity often associated with CP gait. Thus spasticity might be an adaptive response to the instability caused by low stride frequency and not the cause of the decreased stride frequency.

The biomechanical, efficiency, and muscle tissue changes that occur during the lifetime of a child with CP suggest that CP is not a static problem as previously described, but it is a problem that changes as the child matures and develops strategies for coping with the world with systems that are dysfunctional. The notion that cerebral palsy is only a neurological problem needs modification. The historical approaches to therapy involving muscle strengthening may need to be rethought and revised in light of the research documenting muscle tissue changes resulting in loss of muscle fiber, particularly type II fibers that assist in providing tonic holding contractions.[15-17] If the peripheral structures are incapable of generating sufficient force, then it may not matter what we believe we are affecting centrally. Weakness may indeed be an important factor in the movement deficit in the child with CP, a problem that may need attention very early in the therapeutic course.

Primary Reflexes

The assumption that muscle tone is a prerequisite for normal movement has been coupled with a second assumption: primary reflexes, if retained past certain periods in development, actually prevent the development of more normal movement patterns from developing.[18,19] We often assess reflexes in relation to what they indicate about the integrity of the nervous system.[20] We make the additional assumption that persistent reflexes may in some way interfere with the expression of more mature movement patterns. Primary reflexes such as automatic walking, asymmetrical tonic neck reflex, and newborn sucking have been described as ontogenetic adaptions.[21] This term suggests that reflexes are viewed as movement patterns that serve specific needs for the human infant at a particular time in development. Rather than viewing retained primary reflexes as the "culprits," we may view them as expressions of movement toward species-specific goals when no other movement patterns are available. This new notion acknowledges the human drive to move and the utilization of whatever patterns of movement are available. The lack of expression of more maturemovement patterns is due most probably to many difficulties but not to the presence of primitive reflexes. In all likelihood, inhibiting primitive reflexes will not facilitate the appearance of mature responses unless concomitant motor learning of more functional behaviors occurs.

The assessment of primary reflexive status is most useful in sorting out the question of adaptations. The assessment and treatment of functional patterns of movement both in quantity and quality is the most important task of the developmental therapist. To the end that primary reflexes are adaptive responses, we should evaluate and, perhaps under some conditions, promote their use. When more mature patterns of movement are absent, we need to create "affordances" within the environment that precipitate the movement that will enable the greatest functional movement. The use of reflexes to promote movement has been advocated by some neurophysiologic approaches, but it is not commonly accepted in the treatment of CP.

Let me summarize the main points by making the following suggestions:

Suggestion 1: Physical therapists should discontinue the assessment of the phenomenon referred to as muscle tone and concentrate on assessing functional movement.

Suggestion 2: The atypical patterns attributed to spasticity may be viewed as an overreaction to sensory stimulation. Patients need to learn to isolate movement patterns in response to this overstimulation.

Suggestion 3: Primitive reflexes should be viewed as species-specific movement patterns that function in the absence of alternative patterns to accomplish functional movement.

Improvement of Functional Abilities

The conceptual basis for my emphasis on functional movement was derived from the work of J. and E. Gibson.[22-24] They developed an approach to understanding the human organism, called "ecological psychology." The concept of affordance is fundamental to this approach and provides a conceptual basis for developmental therapy.

The term *affordance* was created by the psychologist J. Gibson.[22] It names a concept that links humans to their environment. It may seem an obvious link, that of person and place, but in psychology it has been a unique way of conceptualizing human action. The more behaviorist notion of a passive human organism being stimulated by the environment has given way to the concept that human action is a function of environmental affordances. Instead of the dichotomy of the actor and the environment for action, the concept of affordance suggests that the two are linked. Separation of the two isartificial just as the dichotomy of sensory and motor systems may be artificial.[21] Gibson defines affordance as follows:

> The affordances of the environment are what it offers the animal, what it provides or furnishes, either for good or ill. The verb to afford is found in the dictionary, but the noun affordance is not. I have made it up. I mean by it something that refers to both the environment and the animal in a way that no existing term does. It implies the complementarity of the animal and the environment. [22(p127)]

The original work in ecological psychology and the concept of affordance has been applied to development by E. Gibson, a developmental psychologist.[24] She suggests that infants spend the first year of life exploring and defining the affordances in their world. That is, infants reveal the properties of objects and the environment and the relationship between themselves and the physical world. They discover how they can act on the world and the consequences of those actions. These may sound like ideas similar to those of Piaget,[25] Brunner,[26] or other developmentalists, but there is uniqueness in the ecological approach. The uniqueness is in the environment's elicitation of action from the infant. The infant is constrained to act in ways that are precipitated from the environment. Greenough's concept of an experience-expectant process is similar in this regard in that the organism has a genetic endowment that is then further elaborated through environmental interaction.[27] The infant is organized for specific affordances in the world. For example, there is evidence that the newborn has depth perception, suggesting that the visual system is organized at birth to perceive a three-dimensional world (3-D); the infant will take advantage of the 3-D world it is exposed to after birth.[28-30] This 3-D world is not constructed with experience. In this way, the infant and environment are attuned to each other from the start.

A classic example of an affordance in the animal world is that of the herring gull. Gulls are born organized to peck at a red spot. This may seem like a splinter skill except that adult gulls have a red spot on their bills. A peck from "junior" is a sign for the adult gulls to open their bill and offer the food content of the bill to their offspring. The affordance in the gull world is the organization between the baby gull's inborn ability to peck at red spots and the adult's coloring and feeding behavior—a useful fit.

Infants spend the first year in what E. Gibson refers to as *exploration,* a common and useful term. She describes the infant as an active participant in the world and not as a passive creature who is acted upon. "We don't simply see, we look. The visual system is a motor system as well as a sensory one. When we seek information in the optic array, the head turns, the eyes turn to fixate, the lens accommodates to focus . . . ."[24(p5)]

The sensory and motor systems converge around the united function of providing the infant with knowledge about the world. Why is this important for physical therapy? Or perhaps more importantly, have we not understood this all along? In any case, the concept is important in that an entire approach to psychology acknowledges that the environment is critical in eliciting the type of action (movement if you will) that is adaptive. The environment constrains the action. We exploit this principle each time we put a toy on a chair to encourage a child to kneel or to increase hip extension. As developmental therapists, I believe we have figured out that to work with children (who of course do not always follow oral instructions) we need to create environments that elicit opportunities for normal, or at least preferred, movement patterns. We know how differently a child may move in the clinic versus the home environment, and as a consequence, we often observe or treat children in their homes. Finnie[31] was instrumental in developing the therapeutic ideas of the Bobaths[4] for use in home and school environments, thus increasing the ecological validity of the neurodevelopmental treatment approach. We construct affordances in the environments of children with disabilities to elicit the type of movement that is functional for exploration. Children will not often continue activities unless these activities allow for exploration and knowledge gathering, two key aspects of the ecological approach.

Knowledge of ecological psychology is important for at least two reasons. First, it provides a theoretical foundation that has been lacking for developmental therapy. Second, it reminds us that movement is always linked to sensation and exploration. If we work toward movement for its own sake, forgetting the context in which it must and will take place, we are not likely to help children become more functional.

The ecological approach to psychology and the concept of affordance provide a dynamic perspective of the child-environment interaction, with the child viewed as an active participant in a world for which the human organism is uniquely organized. When disorganization occurs within the child or the environment, both are affected. Thus the child with sensorimotor problems develops unique and perhaps atypical relationships with the environment. These relationships may still serve the exploratory needs of the child; however, children may use patterns of movement that are atypical or potentially harmful in the long term. Therapists can assist children and families in providing an ecology for movement that supports functional movement while diminishing atypical movement that may hamper function in the long term. Children will persist in exploring their environment regardless of the type of movement used. An example of this is the use of "W" sitting; that is, sitting with the legs folded back so that the heels touch the buttocks. Therapists who have tried to discourage this type of sitting soon realize what they are up against. The child with poor sitting balance still wants to explore objects and the world. This exploratory behavior is master, and whatever stable posture is available will be used. Often, W sitting affords the most stable posture and will constantly be used during exploration. The posture is not the focus for the child, only a means to an end—exploratory ability. For therapists, the sitting position may be the focus. We may want to discourage the hamstring tightness that may be facilitated in this position, but we need to

refocus on the utility of the position. Unless exploratory behavior can continue, any new sitting posture will quickly be abandoned; thus the achievement of a new sitting posture must facilitate exploration. Creating a game that requires "ring" sitting may provide the necessary incentive. Knocking over containers of water with the knees from a ring sitting positionmay create the necessary enthusiasm to sustain the posture. A remote sensor can be attached to a computer and the sensor hit with the knees to activate a game. These may seem elaborate and contrived methods, but if change is to occur the new patterns must incorporate the behaviors that will drive movement, exploration, and knowledge gathering. Encouraging movement means facilitating these behaviors.

The goals of the therapist and family might include increasing the exploratory experiences of the child (something we already do), and in addition, we might encourage and practice modeling exploration for children with sensorimotor problems.[32] If a child has difficulty exploring cause and effect relationships because of lack of exploratory interest or an inability to carry out the necessary motor acts to explore, then a cause-effect demonstration might be useful. Dropping a cup of water off the tray for an infant might seem like promoting anarchy, but if the infant cannot perform the act or never thought to try, why not spill some water to elicit the effect? Watching family members, particularly siblings, explore materials and relationships between their actions and the world provides much needed exploratory material to infants with sensorimotor impairment. Note that the movement itself is important, but the consequences of the movement are equally so, not only to provide for perceptual and cognitive development but also to provide further motivation for movement and exploration of the world.

This concept of fit in the world is important. The human organism comes to the world organized to experience certain of its aspects. If the infant is deficient in some of the typical organization, such as poor motor organization, the environment will provide very different affordances to this infant. I am making the assumption that all humans have what I refer to as species-specific movement; that is, movement that is shared by all other humans. For instance, the drive to stand and walk could be described as a species-specific movement. If a child is born with this species-specific movement drive but does not have the coordination of muscles to perform the action normally, the result is movement toward the species-specific goal (eg, standing) but with atypical movement patterns. The affordances within the environment may elicit the motivation to stand, but the movement result is not accomplishing the goal. In this situation, therapists can rearrange the environment, thus creating affordances that will yield the desired movement. Before this rearranging, or rather in conjunction with this, we may need to work with the child on components of movement. We can put a toy on a chair to elicit pull to stand, but if the child is too weak or has decreased range of hip motion, the action may not be possible. What then? We need to work on the component skills and then elicit these components in a functional movement sequence. The component skills, however, will best be elicited by exploiting the characteristics of the environment that elicit movement. For instance, the child with decreased hip extension and poor strength in the hip extensor muscle might work on kicking in the prone position in the bathtub. It would be fun (it makes a sufficient mess) and stirs up the bubble bath. Encouraging a child to lie prone on a mat and extend the hip might in principle elicit the same goal, but there would be little in that environment to elicit the action naturally. The bath is an ecologically valid stimulus for the desired action, but the mat activities are not.

The use of therapeutic balls in treatment offers another example. We often move the ball under the child or with the child to stimulate balance and righting reactions. This is a somewhat artificial mechanism for eliciting these responses. We might design a more ecologically valid intervention by eliciting these reactions through the child's self-initiated movement rather than by moving the child on the ball. Creating games in which the child must move may cause balance and righting reactions to occur without conscious effort in the context of normally occurring action.

Although we often may need to work on the components of functional movement, we always exploit the affordances within the environment that will naturally or automatically elicit movement. Parents are the natural resources to develop ecologically valid treatment; they frequently offer creative, practical suggestions, and they can implement these suggestions on a daily basis. Effective treatment must not only include parents, but the family-child environment must be the vehicle for change.

Movement Variables to Use in the Future

I would like to conclude this morning by suggesting what might be useful movement variables to assess and improve with individuals with CP. Historically, CP has been defined and categorized by the parts of the body involved and the nature of the muscle tone.[33] Diagnoses such as spastic quadriplegia, diplegia, or hemiplegia, however, ignore the fundamental aspects of movement that may be disordered.[34] Research of CP has typically been conducted by grouping subjects according to topographical description. One subject with spastic diplegia, however, may have a very different set of movement problems from another subject with the same diagnosis. Grouping subjects, especially for study and for selecting appropriate treatment, by the use of more fundamental movement variables leads to a clearer understanding of the effects of intervention on particular aspects of movement. Variables might include the following:
1. The ability to generate adequate speed.
2. The generation and maintenance of adequate force production and the timing of the sequences of force production.
3. The ability to generate adequate frequencies of movements at constant speeds.

Only the combined research efforts of clinical and research physical therapists will define what the clinically relevant variables are.

CONCLUSION

We are at an important time in the development of treatment strategies for patients with movement disorders. The traditional neurophysiologic approaches to treatment need to be examined in terms of the basic assumptions and treatment ideas. Current knowledge from motor control, motor learning, psychology, and many of the basic and behavioral sciences needs to be blended into our patient practices. It is critical to develop assumptions based on empirical evidence and to test these assumptions. In addition, treatment strategies need empirical evidence if they are to continue to be used in practice and taught to new generations of therapists. A sound basis for treatment of movement disorders will evolve only as a scientific basis is empirically developed.

Acknowledgment

Portions of this chapter appeared in my lesson in *In Touch Home Study Course: Topics in Pediatrics* and are reprinted here with permission from the American Physical Therapy Association.

References

1. Landau WM. Spasticity: the fable of a neurological demon and the emperor's new therapy. *Arch Neurol.* 1974;31:217-219.
2. Nelson KB. What proportion of cerebral palsy is related to birth asphyxia? *Pediatrics.* 1989;112:572-573. Editor's Column.
3. Nelson KB, Ellenberg JH. Antecedents of cerebral palsy: multivariate analysis of risk. *N Eng J Med.* 1986;315:81-86.
4. Bobath K. *A Neurophysiological Basis for the Treatment of Cerebral Palsy.* Philadelphia, Pa: J B Lippincott Co; 1980.
5. Gottlieb GL, Corcos DM, Agarwal GC. Organizing principles for single-joint movements: I. A speed-insensitive strategy. *J Neurophysiol.* 1989;62:342-357.
6. Latash ML, Penn RD, Corcos DM, Gottlieb GL. Intrathecal baclofen unmasks residual voluntary motor control in spasticity. *J Neurosurg.* In press.
7. Sahrmann SA, Norton BJ. The relationship of voluntary movement to spasticity in the upper motor neuron syndrome. *Ann Neurol.* 1977;2:460-465.
8. Harris SR, Haley SM, Tada WL, et al. Item reliability of the Movement Assessment of Infants. *Physical and Occupational Therapy in Pediatrics.* 1986;6:21-39.
9. Corcos DM, Gottlieb GL, Penn RD, et al. Movement deficits caused by hyperexcitable stretch reflexes in spastic humans, *Brain.* 1986;109:1043-1058.
10. Young RY, Wiegner AW. Spasticity. *Clinical Orthopedics and Related Research.* 1987;219:50-62.
11. Feldman RG, Young RR, Koella WP. *Spasticity: Disordered Motor Control Yearbook.* Chicago, Ill: Medical Specialty; 1980.
12. Barplat-Romana G, Davis R. Neurophysiological mechanisms in abnormal reflex activities in cerebral palsy and spinal spasticity. *J Neurol Neurosurg Psychiatry.* 1980;43:333-342.
13. Pierrynowski MR, Winter DA, Norman RW. Transfers of mechanical energy within the total body and mechanical efficiency during treadmill walking. *Ergonomics.* 1980;23:147-156.
14. Holt KG, Hamill J, Andres RO. The force driven harmonic oscillator as a model for human locomotion. *Human Movement Science.* In press.
15. Castle ME, Reymond TA, Schneider M. Pathology of spastic muscle in cerebral palsy. *Clin Orthop.* 1979;142:223-233.

16. Rose SJ, Rothstein JM. Muscle mutability: I. General concepts and adaptations to altered patterns of use. *Phys Ther*. 1982;62:1773-1787.
17. Gossman MR, Sahrmann SA, Rose SJ. Review of length-associated changes in muscle. *Phys Ther*. 1982;62:1799-1808.
18. Milani-Comparetti A, Giodoni EA. Pattern analysis of motor development and its disorders. *Dev Med Child Neurol*. 1967;9:625-630.
19. Capute AJ, Accardo PJ, Vinning EP, et al. *Primitive Reflex Profile*. Baltimore, Md: University Park Press; 1977.
20. Peiper A. *Cerebral Function in Infancy and Childhood*. New York, NY: Consultants Bureau; 1963.
21. Oppenheim RW. Ontogenetic adaptations and retrogressive processes in the development of the nervous system and behavior: neuroembryological perspective. In: Connolly K, Prechtl HFR, eds. *Maturation and Development: Biological and Psychological Perspectives*. Philadelphia, Pa: J B Lippincott Co; 1981.
22. Gibson JJ. *The Ecological Approach to Visual Perception*. Boston, Mass: Houghton Mifflin Co; 1979.
23. Gibson JJ. *The Senses Considered as Perceptual Systems*. Boston, Mass; Houghton Mifflin Co; 1966.
24. Gibson EJ. Exploratory behavior in the development of perceiving, acting, and the acquiring of knowledge. *Ann Rev Psychol*. 1988;39:1-41.
25. Piaget J. *The Origin of Intelligence*. New York, NY: International Universities Press Inc; 1952.
26. Bruner J. Organization of early skilled action. *Child Dev*. 1973;44:1-11.
27. Greenough WT. Enduring brain effects of differential experience and training. In: Rosenweig MR, Bennet EL, eds. *Neural Mechanisms of Learning and Memory*. Cambridge, Mass: The MIT Press; 1976.
28. Bower TGR. Object perception in infants. *Perception*. 1972;1:15-30.
29. Bower TGR, Broughton J, Moore MK. Infant responses to approaching objects: an indicator of response to distal variables. *Perception and Psychophysics*. 1971;9:193-196.
30. Dodwell PC, Muir D, DiFranco D. Infant perception of visually presented objects. *Science*. 1979;203:1138-1139.
31. Finnie N. *Handling the Young Cerebral Palsied Child at Home*. New York, NY: E P Dutton; 1970.
32. Fetters L. Object permanence development in children with cerebral palsy. *Phys Ther*. 1981;61:327-333.
33. Bax MCO. Terminology and classification in cerebral palsy. *Dev Med Child Neurol*. 1964;6:295-297.
34. Fetters L. A paradigm shift for measurement and treatment in cerebral palsy. *Phys Ther*. In press.

Chapter 23

Motor Attainments in Down Syndrome

Alice M. Shea, ScD, PT
Associate for Research and Continuing Education
Department of Physical Therapy
The Children's Hospital
Boston, MA 02115

My name is Paige Calvin. I have done a lot of things in my life. These things are most important to me: my family, my friends and my work . . . . Someday, I want to be independent, live with my friends and go to work every day . . . .[1]

Paige Calvin, a young woman with
Down syndrome

Down syndrome has recently been defined as a "congenital disorder caused by trisomy of the 21st chromosome in which the affected person has mild to moderate mental retardation, short stature and a flattened facial profile."[2] Dr. J. Langdon Down, one of the first to describe the syndrome in 1866, used the term *Mongolian* to describe these individuals because of his belief that their physical characteristics indicated membership in an ethnic group, a conclusion that was later disproved by anthropologists.[3] In 1959, after scientists had devised techniques to visualize chromosomes, Lejeune and associates[4] found an additional chromosome 21 in the cells of a child with Down syndrome, leading to the term *Trisomy 21*, which is used to describe the most common form of the disorder.

The incidence of Down syndrome in the United States is one in 800 to 1000 births, with about 5000 of these infants born yearly.[5] Older mothers are more likely to give birth to an infant with Down syndrome, but because of the use of prenatal diagnosis by women in this age group the mean age of mothers of children with Down syndrome has been decreasing in recent years. The extra chromosome is of maternal origin in most instances; however, current information indicates paternal origin in 20% to 30% of Down syndrome births.[6]

Recent advances in molecular biology and in other areas have broadened our knowledge of the components of this syndrome, although the etiology is still undetermined. The last two decades have brought deinstitutionalization of individuals with mental retardation, public school integration of these students, and early intervention and preschool programs for these infants and children. All of these factors have combined to bring physical therapists into contact with both children and adults with Down syndrome in increasing numbers. This chapter will focus on some features of the syndrome that have relevance for assessment and treatment by the physical therapist; studies of motor control, motor learning and motor development; assessment; and intervention and treatment efficacy.

FEATURES OF THE SYNDROME

A great variability exists in expression of the characteristics of Down syndrome. Although some features are seen in most individuals, other manifestations are noted in only a proportion of individuals.[7]

Hypoplasia

Hypoplasia is seen in a number of the malformations found in Down syndrome. Total head growth is diminished, with anteroposterior diameter more deficient than biparietal diameter (ie, microbrachycephaly).[8] This pattern results in midface hypoplasia with epicanthal folds, upward slanting palpebral fissures, flattened nasal bridge, and protrusion of the tongue (Fig. 23-1). These are the phenotypic features of individuals with Down syndrome; however, not all individuals with Down syndrome have all of these features.[9]

Linear growth retardation, which begins in the first year of life, is another indication of hypoplasia.[10,11] Present day deficiencies in growth are less than those reported in earlier studies of institutionalized children.[12,13] Growth of the trunk is relatively greater than growth of the extremities, with the hands and feet being short and broad. Growth studies have also indicated a tendency to become overweight, which begins in the second year of life and continues into adolescence.[10,11] The etiology of this condition is not known, although hypoactivity and body proportions (elongation of the trunk relative to the extremities) have been suggested as possible reasons.

Hypoplasia has also been noted in the lungs of individuals with Down syndrome at various ages. This hypoplasia takes the form of inadequate alveolarization of the terminal lung units distal to the respiratory bronchioles, accompanied by alveolar enlargement with a marked deficiency in total alveolar number and a comparable reduction in the total cross-sectional area of the vascular bed. The latter may also be associated with the development of pulmonary hypertension in Down syndrome.[14]

Musculoskeletal Anomalies

Growth and development of hard tissue in Down syndrome is generally retarded, and as in other areas, variability is increased. Retardation in skeletal maturation is most often seen in the first 6 to 8 years of life, after which more normal

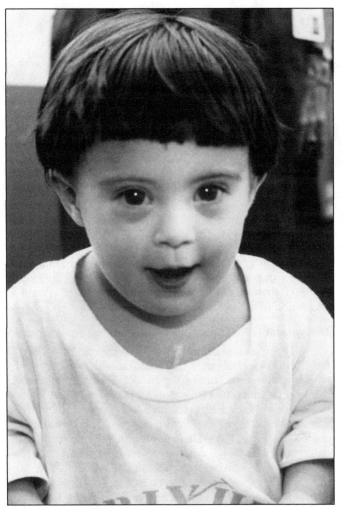

Fig. 23-1. *Child with Down syndrome.*

rates prevail; at puberty, skeletal maturation is less deficient than in early childhood. [13,15]

In addition to the retardation in growth of the cranium mentioned previously, the palate has been reported to be narrow and short in almost 100% of individuals with Down syndrome. There may be rib anomalies, and in most individuals, there are decreased acetabular and iliac angles. [16] There is not an increased incidence of congenital hip dislocation, although some authors have reported an increased incidence of later subluxations and dislocations. [17] Instability of the patellofemoral joint may occur in 4% to 8% of the individuals, but it is rarely considered disabling, although surgery may be required. [18] Other conditions such as scoliosis occur more frequently in Down syndrome populations, but moderate to severe curves are not more frequent than in other groups. Abnormalities of the feet such as metatarsus primus varus, hallux valgus, pes planus, and hindfoot valgus are commonly seen in Down syndrome. Their relationship to posture and gait has not been established. A report of an anatomical study of muscles in Down syndrome, with a sample of five specimens, indicated absence of muscles—some finger and wrist flexors and the psoas minor—to a greater degree than would be expected in a normal population. A finding specific to Down syndrome was lack of differentiation of midface musculature. [19]

Hyperflexibility of joints that is due to ligamentous laxity is frequently described, but it has not been subjected to measurement in Down syndrome except for a study by Dummer. [20] He measured trunk motions and found that school-age children with Down syndrome were more flexible in flexion and rotation of the spine than other children with mental retardation. Pueschel et al[21,22] postulated an intrinsic deficit of connective tissue as a basis for hyperflexibility, using evidence of abnormal protein structure of tendons of these children.

A skeletal abnormality that has been a subject of much discussion in recent years is that of atlantoaxial instability, found in 12% to 20% of persons with Down syndrome and thought to be related to increased laxity of the transverse ligaments between the atlas and odontoid. Only 1% to 2% have symptoms (ie, pyramidal tract signs, abnormal gait, head tilt) and require spinal fusion. Children with asymptomatic instability usually do not require surgery but should not engage in contact sports, somersaults, diving, trampoline exercise, or other activities that could lead to cervical spine injury. [23] Radiographs are recommended at age 2 years and periodically in childhood and adolescence for diagnosis.

Congenital Heart Disease

Congenital heart disease occurs in about 40% of individuals with Down syndrome. The survival of children at 1 year of age who do not have heart disease in 85% in contrast with 60% who have congenital heart malformations. Survival is affected by severity of the defect. Advances in surgical techniques have resulted in approximately 75% survival after repair of endocardial cushion defect, the most common and severe defect, and higher survival for patients with ventricular septal defects. [24] These defects are hemodynamically significant, and following successful surgery, improvement occurs in symptoms and in growth, the latter being more deficient in children with congenital heart disease. [10,11]

Nervous System

Growth and development. Another indication of hypoplasia in Down syndrome is brain weight reduction to 76% of normal, with brain stem and cerebellum reduced to 66% of normal. [25] The middle lobes of the cerebellum have particularly been noted to be reduced in size. [26] The reduction in brain weight and the aforementioned reduction in head circumference are thought to result from postnatal curtailment of growth and maturation of the brain, occurring in infancy and early childhood. [27] There have been reports of narrowed superior temporal gyri, which are often bilateral, and also a reduction of secondary sulci, giving a simplicity of convolutional pattern. [28]

A microscopic abnormality found in the cerebral cortex is a paucity of small neurons, thought to result from curtailment of a single cell type, probably the aspinous stellate. [26,27] This disturbance in the development of neurons probably occurs in the early prenatal and, to a lesser degree, perinatal and postnatal periods of brain maturation. [29,30]

Another neuropathological finding in Down syndrome

relates to morphology of dendrites. Abnormalities include abnormally thin, short spines and a slight reduction in their numbers, occurring from the newborn period on.[31,32] The latter was postulated because no abnormalities of morphology were found in preterm infants with Down syndrome, but after birth, the number of spines seemed to reach a plateau and the dendrites lacked growth.[28]

Other abnormalities. Wisniewski et al[30] investigated synaptic density in the visual cortex and found it to be 1% to 28% lower in subjects with Down syndrome than in age-matched control subjects from birth onward. Other findings in the same study included decreased length of synapses in comparison with controls and reduced average surface area of synaptic contact. Such abnormalities may reduce the efficiency of synaptic transmission.

Scott and co-workers[28] observed dorsal root ganglion neurons in culture from individuals with Down syndrome and compared them with those of a control group with regard to electric membrane properties. Results indicated that the Down syndrome neurons were electrically abnormal, with after-hyperpolarization reduced, membrane time constant increased, and threshold rheobasic depolarization reduced. These and other differences were explained by hypothesizing an underlying membrane deficit in potassium ion permeability.

Myelination. There is agreement that myelination in fetuses and newborns with Down syndrome is not delayed, but one study indicated delay in 26% of tissue specimens of individuals between 2 months and 6 years of age, with delay observed in only 8% of control cases. The myelination delayaffected tracts with late beginnings and slow cycles of myelination, mainly the associated and intercortical fibers of the frontotemporal lobes. The delay seemed also to be related to systemic diseases (eg, congenital heart disease) occurring during the time of myelination. In some cases, where developmental information was available, a correlation was found between developmental and myelination delay (no details given of methodology involved).[33] Kemper,[27] in contrast, observed that myelination was on schedule not only at birth but also in early childhood, but he did not comment on a possible relationship with health or systemic illness.

Premature aging. The pallor of myelin staining, an age-related change that normally appears in about the eighth decade in fiber systems of the corona radiate, appears in the second decade in Down syndrome and may be an indicator of premature aging.[34] Other signs include perivascular mineral deposits in the first decade and spinal plaques, neurofibrillary tangles, gyral atrophy, and ventricular dilatation in the second decade. The spinal plaques and neurofibrillary tangles are comparable to those found in Alzheimer's disease in the sixth and seventh decades.[34] Clinical deterioration occurs in approximately one third of all older individuals with Down syndrome, many of whom, however, have spent all of their lives in institutions. Most older individuals with Down syndrome do not show evidence of the progressive dementia of Alzheimer's disease. It may be that the distribution pattern as opposed to the density of senile plaques and neurofibrillary tangles is important to the development of dementia. Kemper[27,34] postulated that the distribution pattern in Down syndrome is an extreme example of an age-related rather than dementia-related distribution pattern.

Possible consequences of neural abnormalities. Courchesne,[35] in a variety of studies of event-related brain potentials, has suggested some consequences of the previously described neural abnormalities. He concluded that spatiotemporal patterns of excitatory postsynaptic potentials may be abnormal because of reduced presynaptic and postsynaptic lengths and widths and also that their effectiveness may be reduced. Courchesne suggested the following:

> Abnormal structural features in Down syndrome such as dysgenesis of dendritic spines or small cortical cell types must necessarily produce abnormal initial neural configurations from which functional neural activity makes cell, axonal, and synaptic selection. These selections from abnormal configurations result in distorted structure and function and ultimately in behavioral expression.[35]

MOVEMENT IN DOWN SYNDROME

Down syndrome affects all areas of development. Studies of cognitive and language development have been prominent in the literature.[36,37] Motor achievements have received increasing attention in the last two decades. The chromosomal disorder affects movement not only through its effects on the nervous system but also through its effects on physical growth and development and on a variety of body systems.

Early Development

Motor development progresses more slowly in Down syndrome than in the normal situation, but there is a good deal of variability in attainment of early motor milestones and in later performance of motor skills (Tab. 23-1).[38] Several factors have been implicated as sources of this variability. First is home rearing as contrasted with institutional rearing. Institutional living, which had been the mode for many infants, children, and adults with Down syndrome until 1970, was associated with greater deficits in all areas of development.[39] In addition, recent improvements in health care services also may be a factor in developmental progress. Moderate to severe congenital heart disease has been associated with greater delays in early gross motor development (Tab. 23-2).[40] Present day corrective surgery, which is being done earlier, may be having some effect on these delays. Degree of hypotonia, as measured by amount of resistance to

Table 23-1. *Variability in motor milestones* [a]

	Average	Range
Sitting alone	10 months	6 to 28 months
Creeping	15 months	9 to 27 months
Standing	20 months	11 to 42 months
Walking	24 months	12 to 65 months

[a] From Pueschel.[38]

Table 23-2. *Median Age of Attainment of Gross Motor Skills by Cardiac Status* [a]

Gross Motor Skills	Age (in months) of Attainment	
	With and Without Mild CHD	With Moderate or Severe CHD
Sitting	9.6	15.0
Reciprocal creeping	19.4	22.3
Standing with support	14.0	21.5
Walking independently	25.0	32.2

[a] From Zausmer and Shea. [40]

passive motion, also has been noted to relate to motor progress and to progress in other areas of development.[41] As will be noted in a later part of this chapter, some questions have been raised as to the nature of what is being termed hypotonia because of recent findings in the area of motor control research. Variation in movement and in posture seems to be related to ligamentous laxity in some joints as well as to decreased strength and ability to activate musculature. For some children, movement is slow and quantity of movement is reduced. This slowness has been attributed to hypotonia and to increased reaction time, which has been documented in studies of adults with Down syndrome.[42] Prolonged reaction time, in turn, has been postulated to be due to hypotonia and to deficits in collating and integrating information (eg, visual, proprioceptive, auditory) across modalities.[43] These factors would undoubtedly also affect skill acquisition.

Delayed dissolution of primitive reflexes and slow emergence of righting and equilibrium reactions have been noted.[44] The relationship of equilibrium reactions to motor milestones has been found to be similar to that of normal children.[45] In addition, the latency of response found in Down syndrome may add to the problems in stability that are seen. Infants can frequently maintain postures, but they have difficulty with the weight- shifting and rotational movements (eg, movement between sitting and prone) that accompany transitions.[46] Infants with Down syndrome who spend a good deal of their waking time in the supine position in their early months (sometimes because of breathing difficulty or digestive problems) have a limited repertoire of movement experiences. They may also exhibit some hypersensitivity about their hands and knees, possibly because of lack of the tactile contact normally occurring in the prone position. Infants with Down syndrome seem more likely to have this hypersensitivity than normal children who spend more time in the supine position; therefore, other factors may be involved.

Gait

Clinical observations of walking in Down syndrome indicate much variability in patterns and in age of achievement of independent walking.

Two studies using film analysis are available on gait

patterns of children with Down syndrome.[47,48] In the first, 7-year-old children were evaluated and a wide range of walking patterns was noted. Total amplitude of movement at the knee and ankle; angle of the hip, knee, and ankle at foot strike; and angle of the hip at toe-off were all indicative of immature patterns. A mature heel-toe mechanism was generally absent and replaced by a flat footed contact. There was reduced ankle flexion during toe-off and reduced extension on push-off, with a stepping kind of gait and out-toeing of the feet.[47]

The second study examined gait patterns of ten 5-year-old children with Down syndrome and compared them with those of a chronological age-matched group of children without handicaps.[48] Findings for the children with Down syndrome included smaller average step length (thought to be related to their short limb length and to knee flexion at foot contact), a reduced time of single limb support, and an increased time of double limb support (considered to be related to instability). The increased flexion of the hip and knee at support phase was considered to be an attempt to lower the center of gravity to compensate for instability. More individual variation occurred in the patterns of ankle flexion and extension than in the patterns of movement at the hip and knee joints. Children with Down syndrome began their extension phase earlier and began their period of support with the foot in a flatter, or more extended, position. As would be expected, delays occurred in the change in direction of ankle motion at push-off and swing phase. The authors suggested that this pattern may be due weakness of the posterior muscles of the calf or to abnormal neuromuscular control of that segment. They emphasized the variability in patterns by using the example of two of the children with Down syndrome, one of whom had a pattern that was very deviant from the normal and the other had a pattern that more closely approximated that of the control group.[48]

Later Motor Performance

Motor performance in later childhood, adolescence, and adulthood has received less attention than has been given to infancy and early childhood. Henderson et al[49] administered the Cratty Gross Motor Test to a group of children with Down syndrome who were between 7 and 14 years of age and compared their performance with that of a group of controls matched for mental age and chronological age. The results showed that the children with Down syndrome had consistently lower scores than did the matched control children, particularly in those tasks involving agility and balance. Connolly and Michael[50] compared the scores of 7- to 11-year-old children with Down syndrome with those of a mental and chronological age-matched group of children on the Bruininks-Oseretsky Test of Motor Proficiency. The group with Down syndrome was found to have significantly lower scores in running speed, balance, strength, and visual motor control. I studied a group of 11- to 14-year-old children, using the Peabody Gross Motor Developmental Scales.[51] Bestperformances were on the receipt and propulsion (ball playing) subscales, with balance being the area of greatest difficulty, particularly static balance.

Giving further support to the previous studies, Le Blanc et al[52] gave static and dynamic balance tests to 25 children with Down syndrome whose mean age was 12 years and compared their performance with that of a group of 25 subjects matched for chronological age and IQ. The children with Down syndrome had higher dynamic but lower static balance scores than those of the other children, a finding similar to results in my study.

Deceleration of Development

Deceleration of developmental rate in Down syndrome has been reported in a number of studies, and attempts have been made to relate this deceleration to the previously described Alzheimer-like changes. Carr,[53] however, who followed a group of individuals with Down syndrome from infancy to adulthood, has questioned this interpretation. She did find deceleration of both mental and motor development from 6 months to 4 years of age, with a more gradual decline from 4 to 11 years of age and a steady progress from 11 to 21 years of age. Carr[53] suggested that this apparent decline in rate of development could be attributed, in part, to the nature of behaviors tested in early life in contrast to the complex nature of items on later assessments. Two other studies that looked at motor development between 6 and 24 months and 6 and 36 months, respectively, noted declines in motor scores.[36,54] The declines were attributed to the delays in independent sitting and walking that affected performance on subsequent scale items. Studies have also documented performance on early mental scales to be superior to motor scale performance.[36,55]

Strength and Endurance

The previous research has indicated there may be strength deficits in children with Down syndrome. A few studies have been done. Grip strength was assessed using dynamometer measurements of children 4 to 17 years of age.[56] The results were compared with measurements of normal children in the same age range. Strength was found to improve with age in both groups, with the normal group having significantly greater strength.

Three groups of children and adolescents with Down syndrome, 6 to 10 years, 10 to 15 years, and 15 to 19 years, were compared with age-matched individuals with mental retardation.[20] Cybex® performance of elbow flexion and extension and bicycle performance with resistance were used as strength measures. Older and younger comparison groups were stronger on the elbow extension test than children with Down syndrome, but there was not a consistent pattern on these measures except for better bicycle performance in the 10- to 14-year-old Down syndrome group. No reliability information was reported.

In another study, the contribution of plantar flexion force versus hypermobility to the posture of heels-down squatting assumed by some children with Down syndrome was measured.[57] Force was shown to be a more important determinant, with balance being a possible interacting factor.

Strength and endurance were studied in two groups of Norwegian males with Down syndrome with mean ages of 14 and 25 years. With a regular training program, both groups showed improvement in both trunk strength and endurance. The older group showed the greatest improvement, with weight loss occurring as well. Disruption of the training program resulted in a regression in physical fitness, indicating that long-term benefits required continuous training.

There is, then, some evidence for reduced muscle strength in Down syndrome, but studies have only been of relatively small numbers of individuals, with no information given for the most part on reliability of measures. There is no normative data, which will ultimately be necessary, given the variability within Down syndrome.

Muscle Tone

Although low muscle tone is described as characteristic of individuals with Down syndrome, very few attempts have been made to do any kind of measurement other than use scales describing resistance to passive motion. One other method has been palpation of leg and arm muscles by evaluators who were trained to compare the subject's muscle consistency with that of rolls of foam of graduated firmness held in the examiner's other hand.[56] In this study, all three groups of children with Down syndrome had lower muscle tone than the age-matched controls who were normal children.

Davis and associates, in two studies,[59,60] examined the notion of hypotonia in Down syndrome, from a motor control perspective. In the first, they analyzed the invariant characteristic of Asatryan and Feldman, which is a curve on a graph of joint torque versus joint angle.[59] Their task required the subjects (Down syndrome between 14 and 21 years and age-matched normals) to maintain a steady joint angle against an external load. Torque was changed by partial unloading in order to obtain torque-by-length functions at three separate initial joint angles. In the first part of the experiment the subjects were told not to intervene when unloading occurred; in the second part they were told to tense their muscles before the unloading. The results indicated that both groups exhibited systematic torque-by-length functions. Subjects with Down syndrome exhibited underdamped motions in comparison with the normal group, as shown by differences in the slope of torque by angle functions in the second part of the experiment. The authors concluded that resting stiffness was the same for subjects with Down syndrome and for normals, but that subjects with Down syndrome were less capable of voluntarily increasing the stiffness level and exhibited an underdamped muscle-joint system. The authors suggested that stiffness and damping could be considered to be sensitive indices of hypotonia.

The follow-up study examined the question of whether stiffness might be subject to training effects (ie, if stiffness would change following anincrease in muscular strength).[60] Subjects with Down syndrome were compared with other individuals with mental retardation and with normal subjects. There was an 8-week weight-training program using free weights, with pretesting and posttesting using a cable tensiometer of isometric strength of elbow flexors. The before and after measures of maximum voluntary contraction (MVC) showed increases for only half of the subjects. The MVC was higher for the nonhandicapped subjects than for the other groups, who did not have significantly different results. Torque and integrated electromyographic (IEMG) measures from the elbow flexor muscle group were recorded simultaneously during the MVC and the step loading of weights. Stiffness was measured by using the slope of torque-by-IEMG magnitude function obtained from step loadings. These measures were not significantly different for the three groups nor were there changes after training. The authors noted a weakness of the study, namely training with isotonic contractions and testing with isometric ones. They believed that the question of strength training affecting stiffness was not answered, but that results reiterated a lack of significant differences in muscle stiffness among the three groups. Significant differences did exist in the magnitude of the maximum torque and EMG measures rather than in their relationship. The subjects also had difficulty in maintaining a constant force against resistance, suggesting that they may have had difficulty in activating their muscles.

Postural Control

Because of the identified cerebellar hypoplasia and the previously mentioned balance deficits, there has been interest in postural control mechanisms in Down syndrome. Delays in emergence of equilibrium reactions had previously been identified, but the deficits in balance had not been examined from a motor control perspective until the research of Shumway-Cook and Woollacott,[61] published in 1985. They compared children with Down syndrome in two age groups (1 to 3 years and 4 to 6 years) with a group of normal children of the same chronological age. They used displacements of a mechanical platform with the children in standing position and measured electromyograms from leg musculature. As reported in other studies, onset latencies of responses in children with Down syndrome were significantly slower than those of the normal children and resulted in increased body sway. Postural responses to loss of balance were slow and considered inefficient for maintaining stability, and their adaptation to changing environmental contexts was attenuated.

Myotatic reflexes in response to platform perturbations were present at latencies comparable to those of normal children, leading to the conclusion that hypotonia per se is not the reason for the balance deficit in Down syndrome. The delays found in long-latency postural responses were considered more significant because these delays are characteristic of cerebellar lesions.

Sensory Factors

The sensory factors in movements in Down syndrome have been examined in a number of different contexts in different age groups. A study of an asymmetrical pointing task and its relationship to ability to point straightahead, with vision eliminated after completing the task, indicated that children with Down syndrome had more difficulty than control groups in making straight ahead judgments after asymmetrical pointing.[62] The authors suggested that the asymmetrical pointing produced kinesthetic after-effects that disrupted the subjects' spatial frame of reference. The authors suggested that training emphasizing the use of proprioceptive reafferent feedback, in this case movements in the same direction, may be beneficial in Down syndrome.

Tasks requiring the use of both proprioceptive and visual reference systems, such as drawing and copying, also have been found deficient in Down syndrome.[63] One interpretation is that children with Down syndrome have difficulty with integration of information across modalities, such as in this case of visual and proprioceptive systems. And performance of tracking and tapping tasks have been found deficient, suggesting that children with Down syndrome were relying on feedback rather than the development of motor programs for these tasks.[64]

Additionally, because verbal abilities are an area of difficulty for children with Down syndrome, auditory processing has been studied extensively and has been found to be consistently more deficient than visual task performance.[65]

Experiments have also been done with the so-called moving room in an effort to look at visual and mechanical-vestibular proprioception. Results of one study indicated that when infants with Down syndrome had gained experience in a posture such as sitting they were able to maintain stability in a situation where the walls moved and the floor on which they were sitting remained still.[66] In the newly acquired posture of standing, they were not able to tolerate this discrepancy and would fall more frequently than a group of normal infants with similar experience in standing. The results indicated that the infants with Down syndrome were in need of visual cues for a longer period than the normal infants. The authors postulated that infants with Down syndrome may require a higher level of vestibular input before a discrepancy arises, with information from the surround, and that vestibular input may enhance this link.

Effgen,[67] in an expanded version of the previous research, studied infants with Down syndrome who could sit but not stand. She added the factor of tilting the room so there was an additional condition of nonvisual somatosensory vestibular input. As in the previous study, the infants with Down syndrome did not respond to the room moving away from them, but they did show responses to the tilting of the room, with some improvement in the level of responses between the first and third trials, possibly indicating learning.

PHYSICAL THERAPY MANAGEMENT

In Down syndrome, given the motor deficits, the variability in manifestations, and the variability between individuals in their motor attainments, there are clearly many areas of interest to physical therapists.

The physical therapy literature deals mainly with assessment and treatment in infancy and preschool years, with very little mention of treatment beyond that point.[46,50,54,68-81] This emphasis mirrors current practice where the majority of involvement is with infants and toddlers, with much less contact in later childhood and adult life.[82]

The following section will describe some aspects of physical therapy management, related research on efficacy of intervention, and some considerations for the future.

ASSESSMENT

History

History taking provides an excellent opportunity for interaction with parents or other caretakers. Listening carefully to their questions is of great importance in order to respond to them to the fullest extent possible. Without their information the most detailed assessment will be inadequate. In addition, parents are an excellent source of information both about their individual children and about Down syndrome in general. As a preparation for assessment, the account of progress to the current status is very pertinent, including the presence of congenital heart disease, recent acute illness, or any other condition that might relate to motor performance (eg, hypothyroidism). History taking also provides an opportunity to observe the postures and spontaneous movement of the child and to estimate the appropriate developmental level to begin testing. The former is particularly important in Down syndrome because of the variability in the amount and the quality of movement. In the case of the infant, positioning and handling by the parent is of interest. Later, as for all children, information about primary caretaker(s) and about the child's interactions with siblings and other children in physical activities is very useful, both in understanding the child and in program planning.

Tests

Tests of motor development and motor skills can provide a framework for understanding the infant or child's level of competency in motor activities. Assessment in infancy and childhood has included a variety of developmental tests such as the Gesell examination,[83] the Bayley scales,[84] the Peabody Developmental Motor Scales,[85] and the Movement Assessment of Infants (MAI).[86] The Peabody has the advantage of recent norms and a relatively broad range of items that allows follow-up of children into school-age (despite its limitations as noted in a recent publication[87]). Another positive feature is that its subgroups allow descriptions of abilities in several areas. The MAI, despite its age limitations, has the advantage of looking at several components of movement in addition to development in the first year of life. The Gesell includes both gross and fine motor skills, as the Peabody does, and also adaptive behavior, even though it has a more limited age range.[88]

In interpreting the results of developmental tests to parents or others, several precautions should be considered:
1. The specific limitations of the individual tests.
2. The limitations of infant testing in terms of its predictive value.
3. The fact that there is no normative or natural history data for infants or children with Down syndrome.
4. Progress will not be distributed evenly across skill areas because of motor deficits in Down syndrome; therefore, scoring will be affected.

Additionally, too much emphasis on specific developmental ages, which may not be valid, may cause disappointment to parents when later testing results in relatively lower scores, in part because of the complexity of items.

Other Components

Because of the deficits mentioned earlier, it is important to include the assessment of some of the components of posture and movement such as postural alignment, resistance to passive movement, response to sensory stimuli, joint range of motion, strength, and postural responses. Reliability and validity of specific instruments for these measurements in Down syndrome have not been reported, and be-

Table 23-3. *Range of Attainment of Self-help Skills* [a]

	Average	Range
Finger feeding	12 months	8 to 28 months
Using spoon and fork	20 months	12 to 40 months
Toilet Training	48 months	28 to 90 months
Dressing	58 months	38 to 98 months

[a] From Pueschel. [38]

cause standards are not available for normal children, interpretation is based on clinical judgment. The analysis of the interaction of these components and their relationship to test results is also based on clinical judgment.

Assessment of independence in activities of daily living should be included either as part of the test (eg, the Gesell) or as part of a functional assessment. Parents should be aware of the wide range of milestones (Tab. 23-3). The physical therapist is frequently the member of the team who observes and reports the actual performance of the child rather than the teamneeding to use questionnaire results. Thus the therapist is able to comment on the assessment's adequacy and give advice to parents about appropriate short-term objectives based on actual performance.

INTERVENTION

Parent Education

Any plan for intervention with the child is dependent on the degree to which our findings and explanations of them are in accord with the parents' own view of the child. This is particularly true in later childhood and adolescence. In the early months of life, it is very important to reinforce the parents' judgment and their conclusions, to the extent that this is possible, thus reaffirming their acceptance of the infant and their own nuturing abilities. By adding to their knowledge of Down syndrome, we are able to have a more lasting influence on the everyday life of the infant or child, whether or not he or she has regular treatment. We are contributing to the ability of the parents to be advocates for their children by giving them accurate information or, in some instances, by referring them to appropriate sources, including reading materials.[89-91]

If possible, we would like to see parents as early in the infants life as they are comfortable with seeing us so we can help them sort through the variety of information they are receiving about movement, some of which may not be accurate. They may not be ready to absorb a great deal of material, but they are ready for information about positioning and handling this infant, who may feel as if he will slip from their hands. Some parents, not necessarily the experienced ones, will perform extremely well on their own, demonstrating how to give the infant enough support so that he is stable but not more than he needs so that he can begin to try to support himself. Reinforcing the activities the parents are already doing, including tactile, visual, and vestibular input, also is very important. One of the most rewarding aspects of care of infants with Down syndrome for parents and therapists is the child's responsiveness to a variety of sensory stimuli. Despite the paucity of facial expression in some of these children, parents quickly become attuned to recognizing signs of over-stimulation.

One of the areas where physical therapists can be most helpful is in clarifying the differences between motor and cognitive development. Even though a developmental relationship does exist, parents benefit from understanding that even though a child's early motor milestones are relatively slow, this does not necessarily translate into a more retarded mental development, a prevailing concern of many parents.[36,54,55]

Treatment

From the results of the assessment, a decision can be made about providing direct treatment. Making projections about the progress of an infant or childon the basis of one assessment is unwise, both because of the variability of developmental rate in Down syndrome and because of the aforementioned lack of natural history data. The rationale for providing direct treatment is based on the occurrence of specific problems in posture or movement that appear to be interfering with developmental progress. In some instances, such as when development is progressing well with appropriate and functional patterns of posture and movement, monitoring by the physical therapist on a periodic basis may be all that is needed. Anticipatory guidance can be given to the parents, at the time of assessment, about expectations for the next stages of development and about appropriate play materials, activities, and environmental adaptations.

When treatment is indicated, objectives may include the following, which have been outlined previously.[92]

1. To promote optimal patterns of posture and movement. Techniques may involve use of sensory stimuli including tactile, vestibular, and proprioceptive input to increase muscle tone of the trunk and extremities and to promote stability. Because one study[58] has indicated that strength can be improved in Down syndrome, appropriate strengthening activities can be included, starting at a relatively young age, in instances where weakness is apparent. Rotational movements between the trunk and extremities also are facilitated to increase stability and to foster transitional movements such as between sitting and the prone position. After the child is walking independently, emphasis is on balance, both static and dynamic, including walking on a variety of surfaces, walking over obstacles, and climbing stairs.

2. To prevent the development of deviant postures and movement patterns. The physical therapist gives the child a range of experiences of functional postures and movement, particularly those that some infants and children might be reluctant to assume without assistance or motivation, such as weight- shifting in the prone position (Fig. 23-2) and sitting with a narrow base (Fig. 23-3). The therapist works on head and trunk control to prevent the development of abnormal compensatory head and trunk postures.

3. To facilitate movement experiences for which the infant or child shows readiness but does not seek out, such as walking without support, handling increased textures of food, finger feeding, or spoon feeding. The physical therapist may approach these areas from a sensorimotor or a behavioral perspective or from a combination of both.

4. To learn about the infant or child's approach to motor learning and state of readiness for developmental

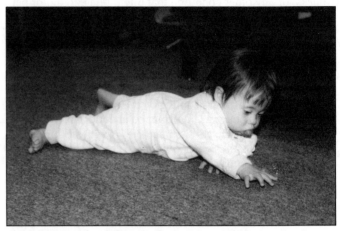

Fig. 23-2. *Weight-shifting in the prone position.*

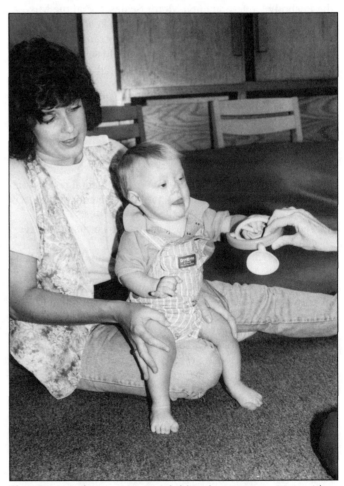

Fig. 23-3. *Mother positioning child in the sitting position with a narrow base.*

Table 23-4. *Down Syndrome (DS) Intervention Studies that Included Physical Therapy*

Study	N		Duration	Disciplines Intervening	Outcome Measure
	Age		Frequency	Type of Intervention	Outcome
1a. Connolly and Russell (1976) [69]	All DS 40 (variable treatment)	53 (controls)	½-d, 10 wk	Several disciplines	Developmental tests
	0-3 y		3 times/y	Intensive sensori-motor stimulation	Significantly higher scores in treatment group
1b. Connolly et al Follow-up (1980) [72]	20 (treatment)	53 (controls)	. . .	. . .	Developmental tests Intelligence tests
	3.2-6.3y		. . .	. . .	Significantly higher scores in treatment group
2. Kantner et al (1976) [70]	3 (normal) Randomized treatment and control	4 (with DS)	2 wk	PT	Inhibition of post-rotary nystagmus
	6-24 mo		10 sessions/d	Vestibular stimulation	1 child with DS in treatment group approximated normal value
3. Piper and Bless (1980) [74]	All DS 21 (treatment)	16 (controls)	6 mo	Several disciplines	Griffiths scale
	X̄ age 9.3 mo		1 hr biweekly	Transdisciplinary sensori-motor	No significant difference between groups
4. Harris (1981) [75]	All DS 10 (treatment)	10 (controls)	9 wk	PT	Bayley, Peabody, treatment objectives
	2.5-21.5 mo		40 min 3 times/wk	Neurodevelopmental treatment	No significant difference in developmental tests, treatment group better performance on treatment objectives
5. Lydic et al (1985) [78]	All DS 9 (treatment)	9 (controls)	12 wk	PT	Peabody, MAI
	4-10 mo		3 times/wk	Vestibular stimulation	No differences between groups
6. Purdy et al (1987) [80]	5 (with DS)		28-54 d	PT-Parents	Tongue posture
	21-31 mo (single subject design)		daily	2 behavior modification 3 oral motor Rx for tongue protrusion	Some indications of improvement each method
7. Sellers and Capt (1989)[81]	1 (with DS)		12 d	PT	Transitional movements and reciprocal crawling
	18 mo (single subject)		Use of restraint for specific periods	Abduction restraint and NDT	Carry over in prone position to sit and prone pivot

motor skills and to communicate this information to his or her parents. Many children are visual learners[65] and respond well to demonstrations of activities. Complex verbal commands will often have a very negative effect because of the auditory processing problems present in Down syndrome.[37] Parents will sometimes spend a good deal of time on activities like walking, which the child may not be ready for, and need the benefit of learning from the physical therapist about preliminary activities that will lead in that direction.

5. To foster independence in movement and self-care within the limits of safety of the child and others. Stair climbing is an example of an important activity, both functionally and in terms of strength and balance, that should be practiced and encouraged within safe limits with supervision.

6. To provide suggestions for carry over of treatment objectives to school and family life in ways that are enjoyable for both the child and the family. Siblings have important roles in providing visual stimulation, such as opportunities for games of ball and other activities. The physical therapist may demonstrate what the child is ready for and the family can carry on from there. The therapist may also be involved in seating arrangements for good posture in school.

Efficacy of Treatment

Physical therapists have participated in a number of studies examining the effects of intervention in Down syndrome (Tab.23-4). Most of these studies have looked at the effect of intervention on developmental milestones and motor test scores. As can be seen on the table, only four of the studies have examined specific effects of treatment on posture or movement.

To look at the effect of treatment on motor milestones, if in fact such an effect exists, relatively large numbers of subjects would be needed—larger than any of the previous studies—because of the variability within Down syndrome and the need for control of factors such as congenital heart disease, gender, and socioeconomic status. I suggest that we look at factors such as strength measurements and biomechanical variables (eg, the configuration of the pelvis in relation to unilateral balance) and that we gather some longitudinal data about development of movement in Down syndrome from infancy through childhood. All of the above would help us become more confident in developing our treatment approaches and in making decisions about when treatment is necessary. Even though clinicians may not be participants in motor control research, they may still provide the questions leading to studies that are relevant to clinical problems. We need to explore some of the sources of variability in Down syndrome such as why some children can ride bicycles and some cannot. Is it simply a question of balance? Is it practice combined with motivation? Or is it all of these factors along with others that are yet unknown? Given the balance problem described in several studies, is it possible for us to improve balance in any way?

CONCLUSION

Our knowledge of children and adults with Down syndrome is at a very early stage of development, providing us with many opportunities. The role of physical therapists, both in studying motor performance and in working with these individuals and their families, also is at a very early stage but with much promise for the future.

References

1. Calvin P. These things are most important. In: Pueschel SM, Tingey C, Rynders JE, et al, eds. *New Perspectives on Down Syndrome*. Baltimore, Md: Paul H Brookes Publishing Co; 1987:xvii.
2. Crocker AC. The words we use. *Down Syndrome News*. 1989;13:113, 124.
3. Down JLH. Observations on an ethnic classification of idiots. *London Hospital Clinical Lectures and Reports*. 1866;3:259-262.
4. Lejeune J, Gautier M, Turpin R. Les chromosomes humains en culture de tissus. *Comptes Rendus de Seances de L'Acadamie des Sciences*. 1959;248:602-603.
5. Huether C. Demographic projections for Down syndrome. In: Pueschel SM, Tingey C, Rynders JE, et al, eds. *New Perspectives on Down Syndrome*. Baltimore, Md: Paul H Brookes Publishing Co; 1987:105-112.
6. Hassald T, Chiu D, Yamane JA. Parental origin of autosomal trisomies. *Ann Hum Genet*. 1984;48:129-144.
7. Levinson A, Freedman A, Stamps F. Variability in Mongolism. *Pediatrics*. 1955;16:43-53.
8. Kurnit DM, Neve RL. Inborn errors of morphogenesis in Down syndrome. In: Pueschel SM, Tingey C, Rynders JE, et al, eds. *New Perspectives on Down Syndrome*. Baltimore, Md: Paul H Brookes Publishing Co; 1987:81-91.
9. Roche AF. The cranium in Mongolism. *Acta Neurologica*. 1966;42:62-78.
10. Cronk CE. Growth of children with Down's syndrome: birth to age 3 years. *Pediatrics*. 1978;61:564-568.
11. Cronk CE, Crocker AC, Pueschel SM, et al. Growth charts for children with Down syndrome: 1 month to 18 years of age. *Pediatrics*. 1988;81:102-110.
12. Rarick GL, Seefeldt V. Observations from longitudinal data on growth in stature and sitting height of children with Down syndrome. *J Ment Defic Res*. 1974;18:63-78.
13. Barden HS. Growth and development of selected hard tissues in Down syndrome: a review. *Hum Biol*. 1983;55:539-576.
14. Cooney TP, Thurlbeck W. Pulmonary hypoplasia in Down's syndrome. *N Engl J Med*. 1982;307:1170-1173.
15. Roche AF. Skeletal maturation and elongation in Down' disease (Mongolism). *Eugenics Review*. 1967;59:11-21.
16. Caffey J, Ross S. Pelvic bones in infantile mongolism. *American Journal of Roentgenology*. 1958;80:408-467.
17. Diamond LS, Lyne D, Sigman B. Orthopedic disorders in patients with Down syndrome. *Orthop Clin North Am*. 1981;12:57-71.
18. Dugdale TW, Renshaw TS. Instability of the patellofemoral joint in Down syndrome. *J Bone Joint Surg [Am]*. 1986;68:405-413.
19. Bersu ET. Anatomical analysis of the developmental effects of aneuploidy in man: the Down syndrome. *American Journal of Medical Genetics*. 1980;5:399-420.
20. Dummer GM. Strength and flexibility in Down's children. In: *AAHPER Research Consortium Papers: Movement Studies*. Washington, DC: The American Association for Health, Physical Education and Recreation; 1978;1(bk 3).
21. Pueschel SM. Health concerns in persons with Down Syndrome. In: Pueschel SM, Tingey C, Rynders JE, et al, eds. *New Perspectives on Down Syndrome*. Baltimore, Md: Paul H Brookes Publishing Co; 1987:113-133.

22. Pueschel SM, Scola PH, Perry CD, Pezzulo JC. Atlantoaxial instability in children with Down syndrome. *Pediatr Radiol.* 1981;10:129-132.

23. American Academy of Pediatrics, Committee on Sports Medicine: atlantoaxial instability in Down syndrome. *Pediatrics.* 1984;74:152-153.

24. Spicer RL. Cardiovascular disease in Down syndrome. *Pediatr Clin North Am.* 1984;31:1331-1343.

25. Crome L, Cowie V, Slater E. A statistical note on cerebellar and brain stem weight in mongolism. *J Ment Defic Res.* 1966;10:69-72.

26. Zellweger H. Down syndrome. In: Vinken PJ, Bruyn GW, eds. *Handbook of Clinical Neurology.* Amsterdam, The Netherlands: North-Holland; 1977;31(pt2):367-469.

27. Kemper TL. Neuropathology of Down syndrome. In: Nadel L, ed. *The Psychobiology of Down Syndrome.* Cambridge, Mass: The MIT Press; 1988:269-289.

28. Scott BS, Becker LE, Petit TL. Neurobiology of Down's syndrome. *Prog Neurobiol.* 1983;21:199-237.

29. Ross MH, Galaburda AM, Kemper TL. Down's syndrome: is there a decreased population of neurons? *Neurology.* 1984;34:909-916.

30. Wisniewski KE, Laure-Kamionowska M, Connell F, Wen GY. Neuronal density and synaptogenesis in the post-natal stage of brain maturation in Down syndrome. In: Epstein CJ, ed. *The Neurobiology of Down Syndrome.* New York, NY: Raven Press; 1986:29-44.

31. Marin-Padilla M. Pyramidal cell abnormalities in a child with Down syndrome: a Golgi study. *J Comp Neurol.* 1976;167:63-82.

32. Takashima S, Becker LE, Armstrong DL, Chan F. Abnormal neuronal development in the visual cortex of the human fetus and infant with Down syndrome: a quantitative and qualitative Golgi study. *Brain Res.* 1981;225:1-21.

33. Wisniewski KE, Schmidt-Sidor B. Postnatal delay of myelin formation in brains from Down syndrome infants and children. *Clin Neuropathol.* 1989;8:55-62.

34. Kemper TL. Neuroanatomical and neuropathological changes with aging. In: Albert ML, ed. *The Clinical Neurology of Aging.* New York, NY: Oxford University Press Inc; 1984:9-52.

35. Courchesne E. Physianatomical considerations in Down syndrome. In: Nadel L, ed. *The Psychobiology of Down Syndrome.* Cambridge, Mass: The MIT Press; 1988:291-313.

36. Schnell RR. Psychomotor development. In: Pueschel SM, ed. *The Young Child with Down Syndrome.* New York, NY: Human Sciences Press Inc; 1984:207-226.

37. Miller JM. Language and communication characteristics of children with Down syndrome. In: Pueschel SM, Tingey C, Rynders JE, et al, eds. *New Perspectives on Down Syndrome.* Baltimore, Md: Paul H Brookes Publishing Co; 1987:233-268.

38. Pueschel SM. The child with Down syndrome. In: Levine MD, Carey W, Crocker AC, Gross RT. *Developmental-Behavioral Pediatrics.* Philadelphia, Pa: W B Saunders Co; 1983:353-362.

39. Centerwall SA, Centerwall WR. A study of children with Mongolism reared in the home compared with those reared away from home. *Pediatrics.* 1960;25:678-685.

40. Zausmer EF, Shea AM. Motor development. In: Pueschel SM, ed. *The Young Child with Down Syndrome.* New York, NY: Human Sciences Press Inc; 1984:143-226.

41. Reed RB, Pueschel SM, Schnell RR, Cronk CE. Interrelationships of biological, environmental and competency variables in young children with Down syndrome. *Applied Research in Mental Retardation.* 1980;1:161-174.

42. Berkson G. An analysis of reaction time in normal and mentally deficient young men: I, II, and III. *J Ment Defic Res.* 1960;4:51-77.

43. Anwar F. Motor function in Down's syndrome. In: Ellis N, ed. *International Review of Research in Mental Retardation.* San Diego, Calif: Academic Press Inc; 1981;10:107-138.

44. Cowie VA. *A Study of the Early Development of Mongols.* New York, NY: Pergamon Press Inc; 1970.

45. Haley SM. Postural reactions in infants with Down syndrome. *Phys Ther.* 1986;66:17-22.

46. Lydic JS, Steele C. Assessment of the quality of sitting and gait patterns in children with Down's syndrome. *Phys Ther.* 1979;59:1489-1494.

47. Parker AW, Bronks R. Gait of children with Down syndrome. *Arch Phys Med Rehabil.* 1980;61:345-351.

48. Parker AW, Bronks R, Snyder CW. Walking patterns in Down's syndrome. *J Ment Defic Res.* 1986;30:317-330.

49. Henderson SE, Morris J, Ray S. Performance of Down syndrome and other retarded children on the Cratty Gross Motor Test. *Am J Ment Defic.* 1981;85:416-424.

50. Connolly BH, Michael BT. Performance of retarded children with and without Down syndrome on the Bruininks Oseretsky Test of Motor Proficiency. *Phys Ther.* 1986;66:344-348.

51. Shea AM. *Motor Development in Down Syndrome.* Cambridge, Mass: Harvard University; 1987. Dissertation.

52. Le Blanc D, French R, Shultz B. Static and synamic balance skills of trainable children with Down syndrome. *Percept Mot Skills.* 1977;45:641-642.

53. Carr J. Six weeks to twenty one years old: a longitudinal study of children with Down's syndrome and their families. *J Child Psychol Psychiatry.* 1988;29:401-431.

54. Piper MC, Gosselin A, Gendron M, et al. Developmental profile of Down's syndrome infants receiving early intervention. *Child: Care, Health and Development.* 1986;12:183-194.

55. Harris SR. Relationship of mental and motor development in Down's syndrome infants. *Physical & Occupational Therapy in Pediatrics.* 1981;1:12-18.

56. Morris AF, Vaughn SE, Vaccaro P. Measurements of neuromuscular tone and strength in Down syndrome children. *J Ment Defic Res.* 1982;26:41-46.

57. MacNeill-Shea SH, Mezzomo JM. Relationship of ankle strength and hypermobility to squatting skills of children with Down syndrome. *Phys Ther.* 1985;65:1658-1661.

58. Skrobak-Kaczynski J, Varick T. Physical fitness and trainability of young male patients with Down syndrome. In: Berg K, Ericksson BO, eds. *Children and Exercise, IX.* Baltimore, Md: University Park Press; 1980;10.

59. Davis WE, Kelso JAS. Analysis of invariant characteristics in the motor control of Down's syndrome and normal subjects. *Journal of Motor Behavior.* 1982;14:194-212.

60. Davis WE, Sinning WE. Muscle stiffness in Down syndrome and other mentally handicapped subjects: a research note. *Journal of Motor Behavior.* 1987;19:130-144.

61. Shumway-Cook A, Woollacott M. Dynamics of postural control in the child with Down syndrome. *Phys Ther.* 1985;65:1315-1322.

62. Anwar F, Hermelin B. Kinaesthetic movement after-effects in children with Down's syndrome. *J Ment Defic Res.* 1979;23:287-297.

63. Henderson SE, Morris J, Frith U. The motor deficit in Down's syndrome children: a problem of timing? *J Child Psychol Psychiatry.* 1981;22:233-245.

64. Frith U, Frith C. Specific motor disabilities in Down syndrome. *J Child Psychol Psychiatry*. 1974;15:293-301.

65. Rohr A, Burr DB. Etiological differences in patterns of psycholinguistic development of IQ 30 to 60. *Am J Ment Defic*. 1978;82:549-553.

66. Butterworth G, Cicchetti. Visual calibration of posture in normal and motor retarded Down's syndrome infants. *Perception*. 1978;7:513-525.

67. Effgen SK. *An Analysis of the Effects of Visual and Somatosensory-vestibular Input on the Postural Reactions of Infants Having Down Syndrome*. Atlanta, Ga: Georgia State University; 1984. Dissertation.

68. Zausmer EF, Pueschel SM, Shea AM. A sensory-motor stimulation program for the young child with Down's syndrome: a preliminary report. *MCH Exchange*. 1972;11:1-4.

69. Connolly B, Russell FF. Interdisciplinary early intervention program. *Phys Ther*. 1976;60:1405-1408.

70. Kantner RM, Clark DL, Allen LC, et al. Effects of vestibular stimulation on nystagmus response and motor performance in the developmentally delayed infant. *Phys Ther*. 1976;56:414-421.

71. York-Moore R. Physiotherapy management of Down's syndrome. *Physiotherapy*. 1976;62:16-18.

72. Connolly B, Morgan S, Russell FF, et al. Early intervention with Down syndrome: follow-up report. *Phys Ther*. 1980;60:1405-1408.

73. Harris SR. Transdisciplinary therapy model for the infant with Down's syndrome. *Phys Ther*. 1980;60:420-423.

74. Piper M, Pless IB. Early intervention for infants with Down syndrome: a controlled trial. *Pediatrics*. 1980;67:463-470.

75. Harris SR. Effects of neurodevelopmental therapy on motor performance of infants with Down's syndrome. *Dev Med Child Neurol*. 1981;23:477-483.

76. Connolly B, Morgan S, Russell F. Evaluation of children with Down syndrome who participated in an early intervention program. *Phys Ther*. 1984;64:1515-1519.

77. Harris SR. Down syndrome. In: Campbell SK, ed. *Pediatric Neurologic Physical Therapy*. New York, NY: Churchill Livingstone Inc; 1984.

78. Lydic JS, Windsor MM, Short MA, et al. Effects of controlled rotary vestibular stimulation on the motor performance of infants with Down syndrome. *Physical & Occupational Therapy in Pediatrics*. 1985;5:93-118.

79. Rast MM, Harris SR. Motor control in infants with Down syndrome. *Dev Med Child Neurol*. 1985;27:682-685.

80. Purdy AH, Deitz J, Harris SR. Efficacy of two treatment approaches to reduce tongue protrusion of children with Down syndrome. *Dev Med Child Neurol*. 1987;29:461-467.

81. Sellers JS, Capt B. Use of abduction restraint in facilitating selected motor patterns in a child with Down syndrome: a case report. *Physical & Occupational Therapy in Pediatrics*. 1989;9:63-68.

82. Shea AM, Reed RB. Physical activities and programs of 11 to 14 year old children with Down syndrome. Poster Presentation at Combined Sections Meeting, Section on Pediatrics, American Physical Therapy Association; February 3, 1990; New Orleans, La.

83. Knobloch H, Stevens F, Malone AF. *Manual of Developmental Diagnosis: The Administration and Interpretation of the Revised Gesell and Amatruda Developmental and Neurological Examination*. New York, NY: Harper & Row, Publishers Inc; 1980.

84. Bayley N. *The Bayley Scales of Infant Development*. New York, NY: The Psychological Corporation; 1969.

85. Folio R, Fewell R. *Peabody Developmental Motor Scales*. Allen, Tex: DLM Teaching Resources; 1983.

86. Chandler LS, Andrews MS, Swanson MW. *Movement Assessment of Infants: A Manual*. Rolling Bay, Wash: L S Chandler; 1980.

87. Hinderer KA, Richardson PK, Atwater SW. Clinical implications of the Peabody Developmental Motor Scales: a constructive review. *Physical & Occupational Therapy in Pediatrics*. 1989;9:81-106.

88. Eipper DS, Azen SP. A comparison of two developmental instruments in evaluating children with Down's syndrome. *Phys Ther*. 1978;58:1066-1069.

89. Stray-Gundersen K, ed. *Babies with Down Syndrome: A New Parents Guide*. Kensington, Md: Woodbine House; 1986.

90. Hanson MJ. *Teaching the Infant with Down Syndrome: A Guide for Parents and Professionals*. Austin, Tex: Pro-Ed; 1987.

91. Pueschel SM. *A Parent's Guide to Down Syndrome: Toward A Better Future*. Baltimore, Md: Paul H Brookes Publishing Co; 1990.

92. Shea AM. Growth and development in Down syndrome in infancy and early childhood: implications for the physical therapist. In: Campbell SK, Carter RE, eds. *In Touch Self-Study Courses: Topics in Pediatrics, Lesson 5*. Alexandria, Va: American Physical Therapy Association; 1990.

Chapter 24

Head Trauma in Children: Application to Assessment and Treatment of Patients with Neurological Disorders or Dysfunction

Stephen M. Haley, PhD, PT*
Mary Jo Baryza, MS, PT
Marybeth Troy, MS, OTR/L
Cheri Geckler, PhD
Sandra Schoenberg, OTR/L
Medical Rehabilitation Research and Training Center
Rehabilitation and Childhood Trauma
Department of Rehabilitation Medicine
Tufts University School of Medicine
New England Medical Center Hospitals
Boston, MA 02111-1901

Infants and children who have experienced a traumatic head injury provide unique challenges for physical therapists. Assessment and treatment strategies for the child and family must remain grounded within a developmental framework. New models of motor control and learning need to be incorporated into physical therapy practice to refine and update current assessment and treatment approaches for childhood head injury. Unlike infants and children with congenital neurological deficits, children who suffer a traumatic head injury are likely to have experienced a relatively normal course of motor development before the injury. Physical therapy treatment is simultaneously directed toward the recovery of motor control processes that had previously been learned and the development of the capacity of the child to return to a normal developmental course. Factors such as the extent of cognitive recovery, the return to age-appropriate behavioral and social competence, and the ability of the child to participate in an active physical therapy program have a major impact on the eventual recovery of motor control and function.

The objectives of this chapter are to provide a broad overview of the epidemiology and motor control deficits seen in children with traumatic head injury and to describe three areas of physical therapy management of children with traumatic head injury that exemplify the application of a motor control and learning perspective. These three areas of focus are 1) assessment of the recovery of early motor function and the relationship of that recovery to cognitive and behavioral recovery, 2) motor assessment of children using a skill acquisition approach, and 3) application of a computer-based assessment and training workstation centered on the assessment and training of postural stability and reaching.

EPIDEMIOLOGY AND MOTOR CONTROL DEFICITS

About 1 million children sustain a traumatic head injury each year in the United States. [1] Over one fourth of all the severe head injuries that lead to disabilities occur in children and adolescents. [2] Head injuries are the leading cause of disability in children. [3] Fortunately, only a relatively small percentage of head injuries are fatal (5%-10%). Of the nonfatal head injuries, about 50% to 75% are serious enough to receive medical attention. Of those who receive medical care, 30% to 50% are hospitalized at least overnight for observation. About 5% to 10% of children with head injuries who are hospitalized have temporary or permanent neurological sequelae [1]

The children who have identifiable motor deficits and are referred to physical therapy for treatment are likely to be among the most severely injured children. By most accounts, physical and motor deficits often are considered less pervasive and common than long-term behavioral and cognitive deficits. [4] However, even children with minor head injuries are at risk to develop motor control and motor performance problems that can potentially affect their age appropriate functioning. Recent follow-up studies indicate that the extent of developmental and motor control deficits may have been underestimated as a result of the lack of sensitive outcome measures in many early outcome studies. [5]

The mechanisms and types of head injuries are quite different in children than adults. [6] Even within pediatric age groups, injury mechanisms differ widely. Below the age of 1

---

* Presenter of this paper at the II STEP conference.

year, falls are the most common injury mechanism. Unfortunately, a large percentage of children who are victims of child abuse are less than 1 year of age.[7] During the toddler and preschool period, falls continue to be the most frequent mechanism of injury, but pedestrian and motor vehicle accidents also are relatively frequent. During the early school years, falls become less prevalent, and pedestrian and bicycle accidents are more prominent. In early adolescence, motor vehicle accidents become more common, as are sports related accidents and penetrating accidents (knifings, gunshot wounds). In later adolescents, motor vehicle accidents are the most common mechanism of head injury. Sports related accidents and assaults are also more common at this age than in earlier age groups.

The vast majority of head injuries in children and adolescents are closed head injuries involving mechanical impact to the brain with or without skull fracture. Closed head injuries typically produce a general deterioration in all aspects of functioning; differential effects may be noted depending on the location, extent, and type of injury. Penetrating injuries are less common, especially in young children, and frequently have focal effects such as hemiparesis and sensory field or visual field losses.[8]

A number of factors are related to the severity of injury and eventual physical and motor sequelae. Initial injury severity is judged by presence and length of loss of consciousness; cerebral symptoms such as vomiting, dizziness, lethargy, or nausea indicating concussion; presence of skull fracture; and severity of neural damage. A severe head injury is often characterized by concussion with loss of consciousness greater than 30 minutes, depressed or compound skull fracture, or other symptoms of serious injury such as aphasia or posttraumatic psychosis.[9]

Injuries to neural tissue may be a result of the immediate damage from the impact or from secondary or reactive processes after the injury or from both.[10] Immediate damage is the result of skull fractures, intracranial hemorrhage with subsequent hematoma development, cerebral contusions and tears, brain stem lesions, shearing (tissue sliding against each other), and cerebral edema. Secondary reactions to trauma include the development of intracranial pressure (particularly important in children), ischemic brain damage, and the development of circulatory disorders that are due to trauma.

Unfortunately, little is known about the relationship between the location and extent of neural damage and their effect on motor function. This is especially true in closed head injuries in which damage is often diffuse. Recently, there has been speculation that the motor system may be more vulnerable to damage after closed head injury than other developmental domains. This may be true because 1) motor functions are controlled by highly specialized tissue in the cerebral cortex that is topographically organized and that has functions that may not easily be replaced by other tissue and 2) closed head injuries appear to affect, disproportionally, subcortical white matter involved in motor function.[11]

Another important consideration in the appearance of motor sequelae is the developmental timing of the injury. It now appears that, in general, injuries to infants and very young children have a more severe effect, particularly on the motor system, than injuries to older children.[11,12] Motor abilities that are in the process of rapid developmental change may be the most vulnerable; interference may be in the form of loss of developmental potential rather than loss of function.[13] During infancy, the brain is undergoing rapid growth, and even the most basic motor systems are experiencing development. Head injuries during early critical periods could alter the basic ability of the infant to learn fundamental motor skills. Traumatic head injuries in toddlers could interfere with the important process of developing independent mobility. Head injuries in the preschool years may interfere with more complex areas of motor functioning, including visual-motor and perceptual skills. Injuries during the school-age period may be most detrimental to the development of sports skills and perceptual-motor abilities. Even during the adolescent period, the brain is going through a rapid developmental change and reorganization, enabling the young adult to develop abstract abilities in solving difficult motor planning tasks. Much more research is needed to understand the effect of the developmental timing of injury on the eventual motor outcome and how we might incorporate this factor into physical therapy prognosis and management.

Although we most often think of traumatic head injuries in children as isolated events, physical therapists must keep in mind the importance of the effects of extracranial injuries in the overall physical therapy management plan. Children with head injuries frequently are victims of extracranial injuries that seriously interfere with motor function. Spinal cord and brachial plexus injuries, fractures, dislocations, and internal organ injuries are associated commonly with pediatric head injury.[14] The presence of multiple trauma dramatically increases the incidence of motor impairments at hospital discharge and follow-up.[15] Physical therapists should recognize that not all motor dysfunction may be neurologically based from the effects of the head injury alone.

Children with severe head injuries (initial Glasgow Coma Scale[16] less than or equal to 8) frequently demonstrate significant motor sequelae. Children with severe head injuries have a high incidence of spasticity and ataxia,[17] delayed motor milestones, abnormal gross- and fine-motor function,[18,19] visual-motor deficits, and motor deficits in speeded performance.[20,21] Even children with minor head injuries (Glasgow Coma Scale greater than 12; loss of consciousness less than 20 minutes) have been reported to have visual-motor and fine-motor deficits[22] and a decrease in age appropriate play and physical activity.[23] Although motor deficits have been noted in numerous outcome studies, methodological and measurement issues preclude generalizing the above findings. Additional studies by physical therapists using standardized motor measures are needed to understand the processes of motor recovery and the physical therapy treatment factors that promote return to age-appropriate motor function.

APPLICATIONS TO MOTOR CONTROL AND MOTOR LEARNING

Three areas have been chosen to demonstrate the application of motor control and motor learning theory to the physical therapy assessment and treatment of children with traumatic head injuries. Although these are not the only possible areas of these concepts, they do represent the authors' current attempts to incorporate these ideas into clinical research and practice.

Recovery of Early Motor Function

Very little is known regarding the effect of cognitive and behavioral status of the child on rate and extent of motor recovery after traumatic head injury. Of primary interest to physical therapists is how children regain motor function that was present before the injury and how children continue to develop new motor skills throughout development. Unfortunately, no published motor instruments have been developed to chart the motor recovery of pediatric head injury, and little antidotal data are available. The Levels of Cognitive Functioning Scale[24] are the most commonly used indicators of cognitive and behavioral recovery in children and adults. A pediatric version has been developed,[25] but it has not been used extensively, so the eight-point adult scale is often used for children. The focus of physical therapy intervention is very different as cognitive and behavioral recovery proceeds. Table 24-1 summarizes how the physical therapy focus may change as the cognitive and the behavioral levels improve.

An important framework of recent motor control and learning theory is that the motor system has inherent self-organizing capabilities. It is presumed that this self-organizing ability requires active involvement in the attainment of new motor learning. Yet, most children who are in the early stages of recovery after head injury go through periods of confusion, agitation, amnesia, and disorientation. A number of authors have described characteristic child behaviors at the various cognitive recovery levels.[9,25,26] During the first four cognitive levels, a child develops, at best, a vague awareness of external stimuli and sources of discomfort. Toward Level IV (confused, agitated), the child may have agitated, nonpurposeful movement but lacks motor planning ability or goal directed behavior. It is unlikely that much can be done from a motor learning perspective to enhance motor skills or activity level during Levels I through IV. However, it would be important in future natural history studies to document the amount of motor return that occurs and to relate it to preinjury levels of function, injury severity, and the rate of moving through the cognitive recovery levels.

During Levels V through VIII, the child is increasingly able to become an active participant in the process of motor recovery. What motor learning, feedback, and practice principles are most appropriate as cognitive recovery proceeds? At Level V, the child is able to follow simple commands fairly consistently and is able to perform previously learned tasks when structured for him or her such as brushing teeth. The child may be able to accomplish feeding within a structured situation and begin to participate in developmentally appropriate activities of daily living with verbal and physical assistance. During Level VI, the child is able to follow one-step commands consistently and begins to show carry over from previously learned skills but still has difficulty with carry over with new learning. Attempts to refine motor control is more effective at Level VI because attention and compliance with activities are improved. At Level VII, the child knows the general sequence of daily activities, can initiate purposeful activity with some structure, and can accomplish or direct developmentally appropriate self-care activities, possibly needing supervision for safety purposes. At this stage, the physical therapist often can work on finer levels of motor control. At Level VIII, the child demonstrates carry over for new learning, is able to initiate and carry out

Table 24-1. *Physical Therapy Treatment Focus at Cognitive Recovery Levels*

Cognitive Level		Physical Therapy Focus
Level I	No responses to stimulation	Maintain flexibility
Level II	Generalized response to stimulation	Increase activity as tolerated
Level III	Localized response to stimulation	Stimulation to reduce coma
Level IV	Confused, agitated behavior	Monitor positioning and alignment
Level V	Confused, inappropriate, nonagitated behavior	Initiate self-care training Begin mobility training Initial evaluation of motor control deficits Relearning of previously mastered motor skills
Level VI	Confused, appropriate behavior	Encourage increased therapy involvement Train adaptive and functional activities Further evaluate motor control deficits
Level VII	Automatic, appropriate behavior	Stimulate interest in preinjury activities Self-protection training in mobility Improve speed and proficiency in motor activities Emphasize functional performance
Level VIII	Purposeful, appropriate behavior	Develop activity, fitness, and endurance program Monitor mobility, activities of daily living, and activity progress Provide child and family sense of control over motor skill program and future goal

purposeful activities within physical and developmental capabilities, and is able to regulate safety and social appropriateness limits that were learned before the injury. Not only must the physical therapist adapt treatment focus and expectations in response to the child's cognitive and behavioral status, but he or she must also effectively adapt and apply principles of motor learning, practice, and schedules of feedback to facilitate maximal gain.

Motor recovery of the child after traumatic head injury provides the therapist with the unique challenge of incorporating considerations of preinjury cognitive development, cognitive and behavioral recovery level, motor learning principles, and motor control goals into an integrated physical therapy treatment plan. A first step that must be undertaken is to develop natural history studies that record preinjury status and track simultaneous behavioral, cognitive, and motor recovery so that important relationships among these behavioral domains can be understood. Future motor learning studies should be developed for children at different cognitive stages to determine the most effective motor learning principles at each cognitive recovery stage.

Motor Assessment Using a Skills Acquisition Framework

Assessment strategies must take into account a number of important characteristics of the child with head injury. In early recovery stages, strategies may include testing arousal and sensation, identifying the cognitive recovery level, and assessing preinjury functioning in order to establish realistic goals. It is clear that many children who sustain injuries are not part of a normal population. There is a disproportionate number who have already existing motor performance and behavioral problems before injury.[27]

Three content areas that are particularly important to stress in an evaluation are visual-motor problems, praxis, and speed of movement. Screening and assessment of perceptual- and visual-motor problems are important because deficits in visual relations and spatial relations are common in the child with brain injury. Deficits in praxis (motor planning) should be assessed by observations of the child in transitional movements, by comparisons of performance on familiar and unfamiliar motor tasks, and by use of standardized testing. In a criterion-related sample of 10 children with traumatic brain injury who were administered the Ayres Sensory Integration and Praxis Test,[28] praxis was the most common and severe deficit associated with traumatic brain injury. Deficits in speed of movement of children after severe and minor head injury also have been a consistent finding in the literature. Speed of movement is particularly affected during sequencing activities and when sorting and organizing items are involved.

For infants and young children, use of developmental motor testing is important to examine the age appropriateness of recovering motor milestones. Bagnato and Neisworth[12,29] have done the most work in this area regarding the demonstration of a consistent model for the developmental follow-up of children after head injuries.

Assessment of adaptive motor function is a crucial area for routine assessment because it is essential to correlate performance and motor control deficits seen in the clinic with the actual adaptive motor problems children experience

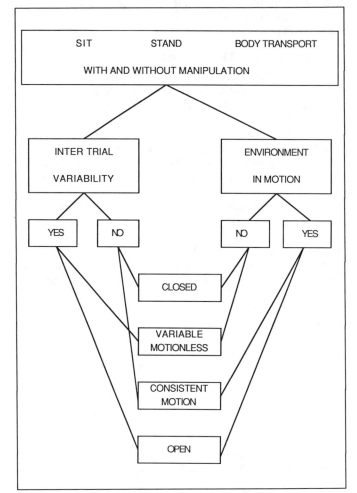

Fig. 24-1. *Skill acquisition taxonomy for use with pediatric head injury (adapted from Gentile[35]).*

in their home and school environments. In our experience, the motor control and performance deficits often underestimate the actual adaptive problems. This frequently is due to behavior problems and a lack of initiation to act rather than to a purely motor phenomenon. For children with minor injuries, it is important to assess their social activity level and leisure and recreational activities. We have used a new instrument called the Pediatric Evaluation of Disability Inventory[30] to assess adaptive behavior in infants and young children and the Scales of Independent Behavior[31] for school-aged children and adolescents. For a more comprehensive discussion, a number of sources provide an excellent overview of assessment principles and clinical and standardized measures for the child and adolescent with head injury.[4,32-34]

Results of specific items on standardized tests and clinical evaluations and reports of performance by caregivers of the child can effectively be arranged and interpreted within a motor skill acquisition framework. Gentile[35] has developed a taxonomy of tasks in the development of skilled motor behavior. We have adapted her system by considering sitting and standing balance along with body transport as common functional positions used during activities (Fig. 24-1). Postural security in these positions and the corresponding activities are likely to be affected by brain injury. When describing motor performance, Gentile considers manipulation (present or absent) as a critical factor in the task analysis. Does the person need to stabilize the body and execute reach-grasp as opposed to nearly maintaining stability without performing upper or lower extremity activity?

The taxonomy identifies two task categories that help to clarify motor performance. These include intertrial variability, present or absent, and the regulatory environmental condition, stationary or in motion. With these considerations in mind, Gentile[35] developed the taxonomy of motor tasks describing conditions: 1) Closed tasks (intertrial variability absent, environment stationary are the least demanding; performance remains consistent over time and may be learned through practice and knowledge of results. 2) Variable motionless tasks (intertrial variability present, environment stationary) require a problem-solving approach to motor learning. 3) Consistent motor tasks (intertrial variability absent, environment in motion) increases postural demands because of the judgment required before executing a motion. 4) Open tasks (intertrial variability present, environment in motion) remain the most challenging because of the unpredictability of the activity. See Table 24-2 for a listing of functional tasks that are examples of different levels of the taxonomy.

In addition to the above definition, the task analysis also includes information regarding the pacing or timing of the activity. In closed and variable motionless tasks where the environment is stable, the timing of the movement is directed by the performer. These movements are considered self-paced. Consistent motion and open tasks involve the performer meeting the demands of a moving object or environment and therefore are externally paced.

Children with head injury often have difficulty learning new motor tasks. Gentile[35] states that learning a new skill involves comparing the actual result of a particular movement with the intended result. To do this, both pieces of information must be kept in short-term memory, a difficult task for many children with head injuries. Tasks that have intertrial variability are the most difficult to learn because each variation must be learned separately and stored for later retrieval. Children with head injuries have the most difficulty learning open tasks and usually less difficulty learning closed tasks. Relative difficulty in learning consistent motion and variable motionless tasks depend on the degree of impairment in timing ability versus short-term memory ability.

For children with head injuries, we have also found it useful to distinguish across task requirements: 1) discrete skill, one that has a definite beginning and end; 2) continuous skill, one in which movement flows and has no recognizable beginning and end; 3) serial task, one in which a series of distinct elements forms a complete response and the order of the elements are important; and 4) speed of movement task, one in which the task demand of speed is an important requirement. We have found that tasks that are serial in nature and have a speed requirement are generally much more difficult for children after head injury than other tasks. In addition, serial movement tasks require the use of short-term memory to sequence the activity. When the speed of an activity needs to be increased, then the timing becomes exter-

nally paced instead of self-paced. Speed of movement may be altered by problems with postural stability, proximal control, dexterity, cognitive and perceptual processing, visual or postural praxis, or combinations of the above deficits.

The application of the skills acquisition framework for assessment and treatment planning will be demonstrated with a case example.

Case Description. Shawn was a healthy 5-year-old boy before he sustained a head injury during a sledding accident when his sled hit a tree. He had a brief episode of loss of consciousness at the scene; however, he walked home. About 15 to 20 minutes later he complained of severe headache, was vomiting, and became unresponsive. He was diagnosed with a left epiduralhematoma, which was evacuated at the trauma center. Shawn showed decerebrate posturing throughout the first 10 days of his hospitalization. He remained in a coma for 4 days and required mechanical ventilation for 12 days. A magnetic resonance imaging at 8-days postinjury revealed brain stem hemorrhages, internal capsule damage, and left temporal contusion. Strong spasticity was present in both lower extremities. Ankle range of motion was a problem from the start because medical problems made positioning difficult. Shawn started to use his left side purposefully on day 12 and to sit with support on day 15. Progress in the motor area was hampered by spasticity, agitation, and behavior outbursts. On day 22, Shawn started to use his right upper extremity spontaneously. By day 39, he started to walk in the parallel bars with support. By day 46, he was able to come-to-stand using a walker. By day 80, he was walking with supervision in a posterior walker. Shawn was discharged home on day 133 with the ability to ambulate about 40 feet using a posterior walker with ankle-foot orthoses. Shawn is now 15 months postinjury and 6½ years old. He is completing kindergarten and is receiving physical therapy and occupational therapy twice weekly at a local outpatient facility.

Table 24-3 summarizes a series of standardized test results from Shawn at 15 months post-head injury that highlights specific deficit areas. Note that Shawn is below age-appropriate function in many motor performance and adaptive areas. Table 24-4 presents major strengths and weaknesses when results of the clinical evaluation, including the standardized tests, are compiled into a skill acquisition framework. It shows that Shawn has difficulty when he needs to stabilize his body and manipulate the environment at the same time. As the postural requirements increase from sitting to body transport, the complexity of tasks he can perform are seen to decrease. Shawn has most success with the closed tasks and only limited success with open tasks. When he is sitting on a stable surface, he has almost age-equivalent skills; however, he has difficulty when things are externally paced. The one open task he can perform under body transport conditions (walking in a crowded hallway at school) is successful only because he uses a walker at school. This walker provides a stable environment within which Shawn can operate.

Results of the standardized testing battery (including tests such as the Bruininks-Oseretsky Test of Motor Proficiency[36] and the Tufts Assessment of Motor Performance[37]) provide a comprehensive and detailed analysis of Shawn's

Table 24-2. *Examples of Activities Based on the Skill Acquisition Taxonomy*

Task Category		Stationary	Motion
I.	Sitting stability no manipulation	a) Sit on one chair b) Sit on a variety of chairs	c) Sit on rocking toy d) Sit on moving wheelchair
II.	Sitting stability with manipulation	a) Sit, put on shoes b) Sit, use computer	c) Sit, place objects on conveyor belt d) Sit, play video game
III.	Standing stability no manipulation	a) Stand and talk b) Stand on a variety of surfaces	c) Stand on escalator d) Stand and wait to cross busy street
IV.	Standing stability with manipulation	a) Stand and open a door b) Stand and throw a variety of balls at target	c) Stand and touch swinging ball (Bruininks Test) d) Stand and kick a moving ball
V.	Body transport no manipulation	a) Walk down an empty hallway b) Run obstacle course	c) Walk on treadmill d) Walk on a moving train
VI.	Body transport with manipulation	a) Walk, carry an object b) Walk, carrying a variety of objects	c) Ride bicycle d) Run and kick a ball

a) = closed task; b) = variable motion task; c) = consistent motion task; and d = open task.

Table 24-3. *Summary of Deficit Areas from Standardized Testing of a Child 15 Months Post-Head Injury*

Test	Domain	Comments
Bruininks-Oseretsky Test of Motor Proficiency[36]	Response speed Upper limb coordination Visual-motor control Running speed and agility Balance Strength Bilateral coordinaton	Below 2 SD Below 2 SD Below 1 SD Below 2 SD Below 2 SD Below 2 SD Below 1 SD
Scales of Independent Behavior[31]	Motor skills Social and communication Personal living skills	Below 2 SD Below 1 SD Below 2 SD
Temporal-distance Measures of gait[a]	Cadence Stride length	110 steps/min (slow for age) 70 cm (short for age)
Tufts Assesment of Motor Performance[37]	Timing	Activities of daily living, mobility skills slow for age
Isometric force[b]	Upper extremity	Weak force production in elbow extensors, shoulder abductors, bilateral grip
	Lower extremity	Weak force production in hip and knee extensors
Sensory Ingegration and Praxis Test[28]	Manual form perception Graphesthesia Localization of tactile stimuli Postural praxis Oral praxis Standing and walking balance	Below 2 SD Below 2 SD Below 1 SD Below 1 SD Below 2 SD Below 2 SD

[a] Temporal-Distance Gait System, Human Performance Technology, East Setauket, NY.
[b] Force Evaluation Testing System, Hogan Health Industries, Draper, UT.

Table 24-4. *Strengths and Weakness of Case when Arranged into a Skill Acquisition Framework*

Task Category	Strengths	Weakness
I. Sitting stability no manipulation	a) Sit on side of the bed c) Sit on a moving bus	
II. Sitting stability with manipulation	a) Cuts food with a knife and fork c) Play video games	d) Catch falling objects (response speed)
III. Standing stability no manipulation	a) Stands on even surface for 5 minutes b) Stand on uneven surface	c) Stand on one foot
IV. Standing stability with manipulation	a) Push elevator button a) Throw ball	c) Catch ball d) Kick moving ball from standing
V. Body transport no manipulation	a) Walks in home d) Walk in crowded hallway (with walker)	a) Walk balance beam d) Walk on moving train
VI. Body transport with manipulation	a) Carry large ball a) Ride big wheel	b) Shuttle run d) Carry glass of water d) Run and kick ball

a) = closed task; b) = variable motion task; c) = consistent motion task; and d) = open task.

performance in relationship to age expectations; however, the results do not help directly with treatment planning. Arranging the results of the evaluation into a skill acquisition framework provides the physical therapist with essential information about basic stability and transport and manipulation abilities. This approach has enabled us to develop more relevant and timely treatment plans. In Shawn's case, therapy should concentrate on using his cognitive and verbal skills to teach Shawn pacing techniques so he can more quickly perform activities of daily living and can start to anticipate timing for the externally paced tasks. In addition, the therapist needs to gradate carefully the postural requirements of each task so Shawn can increase movements under different conditions of postural stability.

Computer-based Assessment and Training Workstation

Two of the most important functional skills for children are the ability to maintain postural stability in a sitting and standing position and to reach and manipulate. Although there has recently been strong interest in theevaluation and documentation of standing balance, evaluation systems have failed to incorporate the assessment of postural stability and reaching as a unified functional task. This failure has been supported traditionally by the inclusion of reaching and balance items in separate domains in many standardized tests. From a motor control framework, postural stability differs according to the requirements of the specific reaching or manipulation task demand, yet we know very little about the interactions between postural stability and reaching. How does a reaching-task demand in a sitting or standing position affect postural stability? To what extent does changing posture alter the performance ability of reaching or manipulation tasks? What are the differences between children after head injury and healthy children in patterns of stability during reaching tasks?

Many of the children that have motor control deficits after traumatic head injury exhibit deficits in postural stability when attempting specific reaching or manipulation tasks. Gentile's[35] taxonomy of skill acquisition provides the basic framework for developing tasks that incorporate both a postural stability and a manipulation requirement.

The computer-based assessment and training workstation that is currently being developed at our center is a modification of a system to measure perceptual- motor behavior.[38] The workstation is composed of pressure sensors that have four channels to record sitting and standing pressure changes (anterior- posterior and laterally (Fig. 24-2). The system also includes a touch- sensor screen, two electromyographic recording electrodes, and a touch plate for the recording of start time for the reaching tasks. A number of reaching tasks can be designed for the computer screen, including stationary targets, moving targets and, complex and simulated moving backgrounds. Both the accuracy and timing of the reach and touch and the pattern of postural sway during the reach can be recorded.

This system is in its initial stage of development; however, it provides an example of an assessment procedure that was developed with a motor control framework. Furthermore, we intend to examine the applicability of the system to enhance motor learning. We are very interested in the potential of the system for the training of postural stability when reaching or manipulation tasks are imposed. The computer system appears to provide a modality that is developmentally acceptable to young children, that is motivating and challenging to encourage repeated practice, and that provides a variety of feedback schedules for effective motor learning and retention.

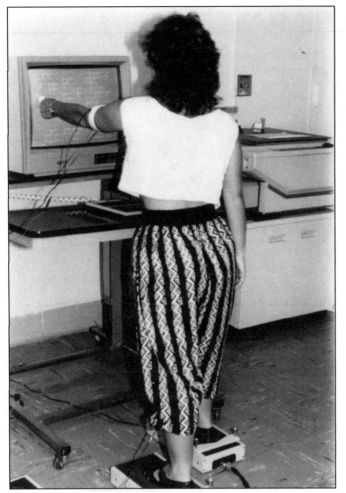

Fig. 24-2. *Subject being tested on computer-based workstation system that simultaneously records reaching performance (speed and accuracy) and postural stability (change in center of pressure).*

Many questions remain unanswered regarding the effectiveness of a computer system for effective motor learning and retention of functional tasks in children. Can therapists devise tasks similar enough to daily functional tasks to ensure carry over of learning? Which feedback schedules best promote retention of the new skill? Can we divide functional tasks into components, and if so, how do we recognize the relevant components of a functional task? How do we know when to cease practice on a computer-based training system and to begin practice on the actual functional task? Are the learning principles that have been formulated through research on healthy adults applicable to children with neurological deficits after traumatic head injury?

It has become clear from the II STEP conference that applications of new concepts of motor control and learning must be initiated and tested by physical therapists. Reliance on other professionals to provide evidence for the application of motor control and learning principles in physical therapy assessment and treatment are misguided. Physical therapists have the available patient population, interest, and professional and clinical responsibility to discover, develop,

and disseminate motor learning principles that are effective and that have empirical support in patient populations.

SUMMARY

This chapter described selected motor deficits common in childhood head trauma and provided three examples of how motor control and learning principles could be applied to physical therapy practice in the assessment and treatment of pediatric head injury. We discussed 1) motor learning at early stages of recovery, 2) assessment using a motor skill acquisition framework, and 3) motor assessment and training using a computer workstation that combines postural stability and reaching as an integrated functional task. Future clinical and research endeavors in these areas must not only propose certain applications of motor control and learning approaches but also provide data to support the importance of these approaches in physical therapy practice.

Acknowledgment

This chapter was supported in part by Grant No. H133B80009 from the National Institute on Disability and Rehabilitation Research, United States Department of Education.

References

1. Goldstein FC, Levin HS. Epidemiology of pediatric closed head injury: incidence, clinical characteristics, and risk factors. *Journal of Learning Disabilities*. 1987;20:518-525.

2. Kraus JR, Fife D, Cox P, et al. Indicence, severity and external causes of pediatric brain injury. *Am J Dis Child*. 1986;140:687-693.

3. Annegers JF. The edpidemiology of head trauma in children. In: Shapiro K, ed. *Pediatric Head Trauma*. Mount Kisco, NY: Futura Publishing Co Inc; 1983.

4. Ylvisaker M, Chorazy AJ, Cohen SB, et al. Rehabilitation assessment following head injury in children. In: Rosenthal M, Griffith ER, Bond MR, Miller JD, eds. *Rehabilitation of the Adult and Child with Traumatic Brain Injury*. Philadelphia, Pa; F A Davis Co; 1990.

5. Bagnato SJ, Feldman H. Closed head injury in infants and preschool children: research and practice issues. *Infants and Young Children*. 1989;2:1-13.

6. Ward JD. Pediatric head injuries: special considerations. In: Becker DP, Gudeman SK, eds. *Textbook of Head Injury*. Philadelphia, Pa: W B Saunders Co; 1989.

7. Kahn-D'Angelo L. Serious head injury during the first year of life. *Physical & Occupational Therapy in Pediatrics*. 1990;9:49-61.

8. Grafman J, Salazar A. Methodological considerations relevant to the comparison of recovery from penetrating and closed head injuries. In: Levin HS, Grafman J, Eisenberg HM, eds. *Neurobehavioral Recovery from Head Injury*. New York, NY: Oxford University Press Inc; 1987.

9. Lehr. E. Measurement and process of recovery. In: Lehr E, ed. *Psychological Management of Traumatic Brain Injuries in Children and Adolescents*. Rockville, Md: Aspen Publishers Inc; 1990.

10. Jellinger K. The neuropathology of pediatric head injuries. In: Shapiro K, ed. *Pediatric Head Trauma*. Mount Kisco, NY: Futura Publishing Co Inc; 1983.

11. Ewing-Cobbs L, Miner ME, Fletcher JM, Levin HS. Intellectual, motor, and language sequelae following closed head in-

jury in infants and preschoolers. *J Pediatr Psychol.* 1989;9:72-89.

12. Bagnato SJ, Neisworth JT. Neurodevelopmental outcomes of early brain injury: follow-up of fourteen case studies. *Topics in Early Childhood Special Education.* 1989;9:72-89.

13. Sattler JM. Assessment of brain damage. In: Sattler JM. *Assessment of Children.* 3rd ed. San Diego, Calif: Jerome M. Sattler, Publisher; 1988.

14. Hoffer MM, Garrett A, Brink J, et al. The orthopaedic management of brain-injured children. *J Bone Joint Surg [Am].* 1971;53:567-577.

15. Mayer T, Walker ML. Shasha I, et al. Effect of multiple trauma on outcome of pediatric patients with neurologic injuries. *Child's Brain.* 1981;8:189-197.

16. Teasdale G, Jennett B. Assessment of comas and impaired consciousness: a practical scale. *Lancet.* 1974;2:81-84.

17. Brink JD. Recovery of motor and intellectual function in children sustaining severe head injuries. *Dev Med Child Neurol.* 1970;12:565-571.

18. Eiben CF, Anderson TP, Tockman L, et al. Functional outcome of closed head injury in children and young adults. *Arch Phys Med Rehabil.* 1984;65:168-170.

19. Kriel RL, Krach LE, Sheehan M. Pediatric closed head injury: outcome following prolonged unconsciousness. *Arch Phys Med Rehabil.* 1988;69:678-681.

20. Chadwick O, Rutter M, Schaffer D, Shrout PE. A prospective study of children with head injuries: IV. Specific cognitive deficits. *Journal of Clinical Neuropsychology.* 1984;3:101-120.

21. Bauden HN, Knights RM, Winogran W. Speeded performance following head injury in children. *J Clin Exp Neuropsychol.* 1985;7:39-54.

22. Levin HS, Ewing-Cobbs L, Fletcher J. Neurobehavioral outcome of mild head injury in children. In: Levin HS, Eisenberg HM, Benton AL. *Mild Head Injury.* New York, NY: Oxford University Press Inc; 1989.

23. Casey R, Ludwig S, McCormack MC. Morbidity following minor head trauma in children. *Pediatrics.* 1986;78:497-502.

24. Hagen C. Malikmus D, Durham P. Levels of cognitive functioning. Rehabilitation of the head injured adult: comprehensive physical management. Downey, Calif: Professional Staff Association of Rancho Los Amigos Hospital, Inc; 1979.

25. Kenner S. *Pediatric Brain Injury Cognitive Recovery Scale.*

Research ed. Elizabethtown, Pa: University Hospital and Rehabilitation Center; 1984.

26. Reilly AN, Lutz MM, Spiegler B, Lynn P. Head trauma in children: the stages to cognitive recovery. *Matern Child Nurs J.* 1987;12:405-412.

27. Bijur P, Golding J, Haslum M, Kurzon M. Behavioral predictors of injury in school-age children. *Am J Dis Child.* 1988;142:1307-1312.

28. Ayres AJ. *Sensory Integration and Praxis Tests Manual.* Los Angeles, Calif: Western Psychological Services; 1989.

29. Bagnato SJ, Neisworth JT. Efficacy of inter-disciplinary assessment and treatment for infants and preschoolers with congenital and acquired brain injury. *Analysis and Intervention in Developmental Disabilities.* 1985;5:107-128.

30. Feldman AB, Haley SM, Coryell J. Concurrent and construct validity of the Pediatric Evaluation of Disability Inventory. *Phys Ther.* In press.

31. Bruininks RH, Woodcock RW, Hill BK, Weatherman RF. *Scales of Independent Behavior.* Allen, Tex: DLM Teaching Resources; 1985.

32. Blaskey J. Head trauma. In: Campbell SK, ed. *Pediatric Neurologic Physical Therapy.* New York, NY: Churchill Livingstone Inc; 1984.

33. Perrin JCS. Head Injury. In: Molnar GF, ed. *Pediatric Rehabilitation.* Baltimore, Md: Williams & Wilkins; 1985.

34. Haley SM, Cioffi MI, Lewin JE, Baryza MJ. Motor dysfunction in childhood and adolescents after traumatic brain injury. *Journal of Head Trauma Rehabilitation.* In press.

35. Gentile AM. Skill acquisition: action, movement, and neuromotor processes. In: Carr JH, Shepherd RB, eds. *Movement Science: Foundations for Physical Therapy in Rehabilitation.* Rockville, Md: Aspen Publishers Inc; 1987.

36. Bruininks RH. *Bruininks-Oseretsky Test of Motor Proficiency.* Circle Pines, Minn: American Guidance Service; 1978.

37. Gans BM, Haley SM, Hollenborg SC, et al. Description and interobserver reliability of the Tufts Assessment of Motor Performance. *Am J Phys Med Rehabil.* 1988;67:202-210.

38. Maulucci RA, Eckhouse RH. A workstation for quantifying perceptive-motor behavior. In: Davis R, Kondraske GV, Tourtellatte WW, Syndulko K, eds. *Physical Medicine and Rehabilitation State of the Art Reviews: Quantifying Neurologic Performance.* Philadelphia, Pa: Hanley & Belfus Inc; 1989;3:chap 2.

Chapter 25

Head Trauma in Adults: Problems, Assessment, and Treatment

Patricia Leahy, MS, PT, NCS
Assistant Professor
Department of Physical Therapy
Philadelphia College of Pharmacy and Science
Philadelphia, PA 19104

The purpose of this chapter is to examine the management of adult patients with head trauma as it relates to the overall topic of contemporary concepts of motor control. A number of earlier chapters relate to this topic, from different theories of motor control to the recovery process and maximizing function. Although it is too soon to integrate all that was presented at this conference into this chapter, I will attempt to discuss the contents of other chapters as it relates to this one.

In this chapter, I will discuss the assessment and management of patients with moderate and severe head injuries. Although mild head injuries can have devastating effects, these tend to be limited to the areas of attention and cognition, without motor control deficits. Therefore, the following discussion is aimed at the problems, assessments, and management of patients with moderate and severe head injury.

PATHOPHYSIOLOGY

In discussing the pathophysiology of head injury, it is necessary to differentiate between *primary damage* and *secondary effects*. Primary damage is a direct result of the trauma to the brain. Secondary effects occur after the accident as a result of metabolic and physiologic events. Both help to determine a patient's eventual status.

Primary Damage

Depending on the nature, direction, and magnitude of forces, primary damage may be of any or all of the following types:

1. Diffuse axonal injury (DAI). This is a widely scattered shearing of axons within their myelin sheaths.[1] It is not intense in any one location, but the cumulative effect is dramatic.[2] Basically, the patient has a series of disconnection syndromes among the brain stem, the cortical centers, and the structures in between. Because much of the gray matter is spared, we sometimes see "islands" of ability, even in very involved patients. This type of injury occurs only in the axons of the cortical cells in less severe injuries and proceeds in a centripetal (downward and inward) direction with increasing severity of injury. The most severely injured patients have lesions in subcortical structures including the basal ganglia, the midbrain, and the brain stem.

If DAI exists alone, without superimposed focal damage, the neurologic profile is fairly typical. The patient is deeply comatose from the time of injury, and initial abnormal motor function consists of extensor posturing of bilateral upper and lower extremities, which occurs spontaneously or in response to painful stimulation.

2. Contusions-lacerations. These focal injuries occur as a result of impact between the head and the external environment (such as a windshield) or with impact of the brain on the skull. These lesions are often superimposed on DAI, particularly in high velocity accidents such as motor vehicle accidents. In low velocity accidents, such as falls, significant disability may result from the focal lesions, with less severe DAI. The most commonly involved sites of focal injury are the anterior and inferior surfaces of the frontal and temporal lobes. Because this is the area of the cortex that involves limbic function, it is reasonable to relate many of the commonly seen deficits in motivation and initiation to these focal lesions.

3. Penetrating wounds. With gun shot wounds or missile injuries, the pattern of injury and resultant deficits rely on the course of the bullet. Because this is not the typical type of adult head injury, it will not be discussed in detail.

Secondary Effects

Energy requirements of the brain are extremely high. In normal individuals, blood flow to the brain accounts for 1/5 of the resting cardiac output, and oxygen consumption by the brain accounts for 1/6 of the whole body oxygen consumption. This is rather dramatic when you consider that the brain typically makes up just 1/50 of the total body weight. Because of these large demands and because there is no capacity for storage of energy-rich substrate in the brain, the supply of oxygen and glucose must be constant.

Unfortunately after severe head injury, the following conditions frequently occur, all of which decrease the energy supply to the brain, causing secondary brain damage:

1. Edema. Because the brain is enclosed in a rigid cavity, edema may lead to increased intracranial pressure, with devastating effects. When pressure effects occur within the cranial cavity, "shifts" of brain tissue may occur, with the brain tissue being pushed from areas of high pressure to

areasof lower pressure. There are several common shifts that occur and I will mention them briefly because of the relevance of the involved anatomy to commonly seen dysfunction. The cingulate gyrus (part of the limbic system) herniates under the falx cerebri, which is the rigid dural fold that separates the two cerebral hemispheres. Limbic system involvement will be discussed later as a major concern in managing patients with head injury. The medial portion of the temporal lobe or lobes may herniate through the gap between the midbrain and the free edge of the tentorium cerebelli (the expansion of the dura that separates the posterior fossa from the underlying structures). When this occurs, damage to long descending axons causes initial motor dysfunction that worsens to loss of consciousness as the ascending reticular activating system is unable to assert its influence on higher centers. However, if the DAI was severe to begin with, the patient will be in a comatose state already, making this shift difficult to diagnose. The last type of herniation involves the downward displacement of the brain stem through the foramen magnum, usually resulting in death.

2. Hypoxia. This may be of intracranial or extracranial origin. Causes include airway obstruction, aspiration, crush injuries to the chest, or arterial hypotension resulting from massive blood loss (often from an undiagnosed visceral injury).

3. Intracranial hemorrhaging. Because this may be delayed, it must be monitored for carefully, even in minor head injury. A bleed may cause pressure effects, as discussed above.

4. Intracranial infection. This is likely to occur any time the dura is breached, either as a direct result of the trauma or as the result of surgery or catheter placement.

5. Posttraumatic epilepsy. Early seizures increase the demand for oxygen and glucose.

6. Acute hydrocephalus. Early hydrocephalus results from the inability of the cerebral venous sinus system to clear the large amount of blood that may result from trauma. The ventricular system expands at the expense of brain tissue. This is not a common occurrence, but is very important to recognize if it does occur because ventriculoperitoneal shunting can remedy the problem.

In addition to the primary and secondary brain damage, there are often associated injuries that may affect a patient's outcome. These include fractured limbs, spinal cord injuries, brachial plexus injuries, abdominal injuries, and amputations.

Crucial to understanding the management of patients with traumatic brain injury is an appreciation for the marked variability among patients. Differences exist in premorbid status (age, cognitive ability, behavioral disorders including substance abuse and depression, educational andoccupational history, and past medical history); in the type and location of the brain injury (diffuse versus focal versus diffuse with superimposed focal); in the severity of the lesion; and in the support systems available to the patient (family dynamics, community support, financial status, health care options). All of these factors interact to affect the likelihood of a good recovery, and all must be considered in the management of the patient.

MEASUREMENT OF PERFORMANCE

Assessment of a patient with traumatic brain injury is a complex process requiring the expertise of a highly skilled team of professionals. For the purposes of this chapter, the measurement process is described briefly so that the comprehensiveness of the evaluation can be appreciated and discussed. For a full description of patient evaluation, see Rosenthal et al.[3]

The Glasgow Coma Scale (GCS) is used to determine level of consciousness and to infer the severity of injury. It has been tested for interrater reliability and shown to have a high degree of agreement.[4] This test involves three subtests: eye opening, motor response, and verbal response. The total score ranges from 3 to 15, with patients that score above 12 considered to have minor head injuries; those who score between 9 and 12 considered to have moderate injuries; and those with scores of 8 or under designated as comatose with severe head injury. Coma is defined as a state in which there is no eye opening (even to pain), failure to obey commands, and inability to utter recognizable words. This is in contrast to the persistent vegetative state, in which the patient opens his or her eyes and has normal sleep-wake cycles but cannot interact meaningfully with the environment.

The motor response subtest of the GCS is a powerful predictor of short term outcome. Of patients with a GCS score of 8 or less either 6 hours after injury or after a lucid period, approximately 50% will die.[5]

The Glasgow Outcome Scale has been expanded from its original three categories to eight. The categories are dead, vegetative, and two levels each of severely and moderately disabled and good recovery. This scale is used primarily for research purposes so that outcome can be quantified. In a reliability study with two raters and 150 subjects, agreement was high ($r = .95$).[6]

The Rancho Los Amigos Level of Cognitive Functioning (LOCF) is a descriptive scale that outlines predictable recovery of gross cognitive and behavioral performance in patients with traumatic brain injury (Tab. 25-1).[7] It does not address specific cognitive deficits, but it is useful for communication purposes and in general treatment planning.

Neuropsychological testing involves the evaluation of cerebral functions through the administration of standardized tests or procedures. It focuses on cognitive and perceptual-motor performance with specific tests for many functions, including memory. Because neuropsychological testing can identify strengths and weaknesses that can be helpful in designing a treatment program,physical therapists can benefit from an understanding of the results and implications of neuropsychological testing. However, patients' actual performance of functional tasks may conflict with testing results, in which case the actual functional performance is the more important measure.

Speech and language assessment examines communication effectiveness. Evaluation of communication is complex because there are many nonlinguistic cognitive functions that are important components of communication. Speech and language pathologists try to determine whether the patient's confused language is representative of confused thinking (cognitive problems); or clear thinking is being misrepresented by confused language (language problems); or,

Table 25-1. *Rancho Los Amigos Level of Cognitive Functioning*[a]

I.   No Response: Unresponsive to any stimulus.

II.   Generalized Response: Limited, inconsistent, nonpurposeful responses, often only to pain.

III. Localized Response: Purposeful responses; may follow simple commands; may focus on presented object.

IV. Confused, Agitated: Heightened state of activity; confusion, disorientation; aggressive behavior; unable to do self-care; unaware of present events; agitation appears related to internal confuson.

V.   Confused, Inappropriate: Nonagitated; appears alert; responds to commands, distractable; does not conentrate on task; agitated only in response to external stimuli; verbally inappropriate; does not learn new information.

VI. Confused, Appropriate: Good directed behavior, but needs cuing; can relearn old skills such as activities of daily living; serious memory problems; some awareness of self and others.

VII. Automatic, Appropriate: Appears appropriate, oriented; frequently robot-like in daily routine; minimal or absent confusion; shallow recall; increased awareness of self, interaction in environment; lacks insight into condition; decreased judgment and problem solving; lacks realistic planning for future.

VIII. Purposeful, Appropriate: alert, oriented; recalls and integrates past events; learns new activities and can continue without supervision; independent in home and living skills; capable of driving; defects in stress tolerance, abstract reasoning persist; many function at reduced levels in society.

[a] Reprinted with permission of the Professional Staff Association, Rancho Los Amigos Hospital.

as is often the case, is some combination of both. Physical therapists can learn a great deal by working with skilled speech pathologists but should be aware that physical therapists also can contribute to the speech and language assessment by relating how the patient communicates in physical therapy.

Visual-perceptual testing is often performed by occupational therapists. Some patients may need formal neuro-ophthomalogic evaluations. Areas of concern include the following: double vision, altered depth perception, blurred vision, tracking difficulties, inability to localize, body scheme deficits, spatial relation problems, and topographical disorientation. Attempting to involve a patient in a physical therapy program without an appreciation of such deficits would be frustrating and inefficient, for both the patient and the therapist.

Behavior analysis is needed when the patient demonstrates socially unacceptable behavior. Such an assessment requires evaluation of the brain (for temporal lobe seizures), the body (for sources of discomfort that the patient may be unable to localize), the person's history (how did the patient deal with stress premorbidly?), and the environment. Based on the patient's level of cognitive function, approaches to behavior management include manipulation of the environment, physical management such as placement in a locked unit, medical management, behavior modification treatment, or counseling.

Physical evaluation will be mentioned only briefly because this is an area familiar to physical therapists. Assessment of a patient with traumatic brain injury would include evaluation of passive range of motion and resistance to passive movement, spontaneous movement, response to stimulation, volitional movement, and functional activities. Commonly seen movement problems include general deconditioning, unilateral or bilateral hemiparesis, ataxia, apraxia, balance and coordination deficits, and associated injuries.

COGNITIVE-PHYSICAL COMBINATIONS

Each patient is unique, but given the tremendous number of possible constellations of deficits, it is useful to develop categories so that you can place patients into some type of framework. To learn from your experiences with patients, it is necessary to determine what similarities exist among patients. In the terminology of dynamical action, I am suggesting that it ishelpful to "compress the degrees of freedom," making a "high- dimensional system" into a "low-dimensional system." The following categorization is a method that I have developed to organize my patients. I believe that it helps me to practice efficiently and to learn from my experiences because I have a framework from which to practice. As pointed out by Shepard and Winstein earlier in this volume, models need not be accurate, just useful.

I think of my patients as fitting into one of three cognitive levels: low, mid, or high. Generally, low level patients are in LOCF stages I-III; mid level are in stages IV-VI; and high level are in stages VII-VIII.

I then assign them to one of three physical levels: severely impaired, moderately impaired, or minimally impaired. In general terms, severely impaired means dependent for most daily living skills (as a result of physical disability); moderately impaired either means ambulatory with assistance or an assistive device or means functional in a wheelchair; and minimally impaired means independent but with high level balance and coordination deficits.

By combining these two pieces of information, I can quickly estimate the patient's level of function and based on my experience, start to formulate some assumptions. For example: 1) A patient who is low level cognitively and minimally impaired physically is likely to be an acutely ill patient with a fairly positive prognosis. Although this patient is dependent because of a low level of consciousness, signs of severe motor involvement such as extreme extensor tone are not present. In my experience, patients with loss of consciousness who do not have severe motor symptoms tend to improve significantly. 2) A patient with high level cognitive function but with severe physical disability will need extensive adaptive equipment so that he or she can interact with the environment to the best of his or her ability. It is extremely important to evaluate this type of patient carefully because communication deficits may make it difficult to realize the high level of cognition at which the patient functions. 3) A final example is the patient who has mid level cognitive skills and is only minimally impaired physically. For this type of patient, it is very important that family and caregivers understand the patient's deficits. Because the patient functions well from a physical standpoint, expectations may be unrealistic in regard to such factors as family responsibility and return to work.

My use of this model has allowed me to integrate, more readily, cognitive performance into my goal setting. I have found that it appears to be the cognitive status, more than anything else, that determines whether or not the patient will be able to return to a functional role in society. Advances in assistive technology have made it easier to substitute for physical disabilities. For example, computerized environmental control units can be used by individuals with very little motor function to manipulate the world around them. It is possible to turn lights on and off, answer the phone, and change the television channel, through eye movement alone. However, attempts to compensate for cognitive function are still in experimental stages and not available for practical use. Most individuals with cognitive dysfunction rely on their families for supervision and assistance. Patients with very low cognitive functioning (Rancho levels I-III) may require assistance that is unrealistic to expect from most families, necessitating placement in long term care facilities.

It is beyond the scope of this chapter to explore all of the different management strategies for patients with various levels of ability. For a more thorough discussion of management issues in general, see *Neurology Report*.[8]

ISSUES OF INTEREST TO MOVEMENT SCIENTISTS

Motivation

As physical therapists, we focus primarily on the motor system. It is important for us to consider that normal behavior requires the involvement of three major systems: sensory, motor, and motivation.[9] Brooks[10] simplifies this by referring to just two systems: limbic and nonlimbic. I emphasize this because I think that dysfunction of the limbic system plays a significant role in the unique disorders that we see in adults with traumatic brain injury and that research efforts need to be directed to this area.

Earlier in this volume, Craik states that the requirements of movement include deciding to move; initiating, maintaining, and stopping the movement; maintaining equilibrium throughout movement; and adapting the movement. We see deficits in all of these components in patients with traumatic brain injury. I would like to focus attention on the decision to move. Many patients with brain injury who *can* move, *do not* move. They lack the perceived need to move. Before we can assess a patient's problem solving abilities, we must know whether he or she perceives a problem and is motivated to solve it. For these patients, we need research into the motivational components of movement.

It appears that the limbic system continues to play a role throughout a movement, especially when the movement is goal directed. Studies have shown that areas of the limbic system (specifically the cingulate gyri) become active during the recognition of errors. Patients with brain injury who lack insight into their own performance may be displaying dysfunction of the limbic system.

Automaticity

We have all experienced the frustration of working with a patient who is able to improve his performance simply by maintaining attention. The patient himself may be able to verbalize what needs to be done to correct a movement and then correct the movement, but only while focusing attention on the movement. He may be unable to carry out the activity in a more automatic nature while thinking about another activity. Research in this area needs to focus on determining the most effective treatment techniques. Much of current clinical practice is performed in a cognitive mode. The carryover into functional ability has not been investigated. In developing studies to examine questions such as this, it is essential to look at retention, not simply performance. As studies on normals have shown, the conclusions can be extremely different.[11]

Application of Motor Learning Principles

A great deal has been learned about how people with intact central nervous systems learn motor skills. It is possible to derive specific guidelines about conditions of practice, provision of feedback, and task analysis and selection. However, it seems rash to think that we can apply these principles to individuals with brain injury. Given the attentional, information processing, and memory disorders of these patients, we may need to make major modifications to the way in which the principles are applied. As an example, consider the provision of feedback. It seems that the long-held belief that immediate feedback is ideal is not true. Studies have shown that a slight delay between a movement and the feedback is beneficial.[11] It has been postulated that this allows the individual time to process internal feedback and compare it with the extrinsic feedback. But does this apply to patients with brain injury? For those with significant processing delays, a longer delay might be beneficial. For those with attentional disorders, it might not be accurate to assume that they are processing their internal feedback and preparing to compare it with the feedback we give them. Further questions arise for patients with severe learning disabilities: How can we help them pay attention to the effects of their movements, both internal and external, and learn from the experience?

Research with Patients with Brain Injury

To answer the above questions, research is needed. Why is it so difficult to accomplish clinical research with the head injury population? First of all, as beginning researchers we are taught to eliminate variability in all aspects of the study except for the independent variable. That is, to conclude that a specific intervention is responsible for any change seen in a patient it is important that no "confounding" variables are present. We need to know that the change was brought about by the manipulation of the one independent variable and nothing else. To do this, we have traditionally used group-comparison designs.

The use of group-comparison designs requires that large numbers of subjects with similar characteristics are available for random assignment to either a control group or an experimental group. When working with head injury survivors, this design often becomes a monumental task. By virtue of the extreme variability in the location, severity, and extent of injury, it is difficult to find large numbers of patients with similar characteristics. This is especially true if attempting to investigate patients with both significant motor *and* cognitive involvement.

To work around this difficulty, I have two suggestions. First, I think that clinicians routinely "group" patients with brain injury. I think thereare models in the minds of master clinicians that have not been externalized and studied. Careful analysis of decision-making strategies may allow us to test some methods of categorizing patients with movement disorders. As an example, I offer the Brooks' model of movement analysis that involves four components: an underlying motivational scale, a motor plan, a motor program, and the execution. Perhaps patients can be grouped according to their deficits in these four components of movement. This is just one example of how we can start to make categories of movement problems to facilitate research.

My second suggestion is to use single subject research design. The major components of these designs are the sequential application, withdrawal, or variation of the intervention and the use of frequent and repeated outcome measures. Although one single-subject experiment gives information about just one patient, a series of single subject designs allows us to look for trends and provides important information for planning improved group design experiments.

Another consideration in the design of research is that the complexity of the problems encountered in brain injury should encourage interdisciplinary research. This approach makes use of the knowledge and tools of many fields of study and prevents the proverbial "re-creating the wheel."

PRIORITIES

In closing, I would like to emphasize the need for caution in setting goals for patients with brain injury. In discussing abnormal motor control at this conference, Craik emphasized the need for a "gold standard." In other words, to what should we compare our patient's attempts at movement? Generally, we compare the patient's movement to "normal" movement. But Craik cautioned that in order for that to be a valid comparison, the only difference between the individual being tested and the individuals making up the norms should be the injury. As we know, this is often not the case. Craik's

suggestion was that it would perhaps be more appropriate to use the individual patient's standards.

In the case of brain injury, I think this is a very important consideration. In following patients with head injuries for many years, it becomes apparent that physical symptoms become less and less stressful to patients and families and that social and psychological problems become more and more important.[12] Loneliness and social isolation are considered to be the most devastating problems. The standard to which we compare our patients should be those patients who have successfully reintegrated into society and are leading satisfying lives. As we well know, this often relates very little to quality of movement.

References

1. Adams JH, Mitchell DE, Graham DI, Doule D. Diffuse brain damage of immediate impact type. *Brain*. 1977;100:489-502.
2. Miller JD, Pentland B, Berrol S. Early evaluation and management. In: Rosenthal M, Griffith E, Bond M, et al, eds. *Rehabilitation of the Adult and Child with Traumatic Brain Injury*. Philadelphia, Pa: F A Davis Co; 1990:24.
3. Rosenthal M, Griffith E, Bond M, Miller JD, eds. *Rehabilitation of the Adult and Child with Traumatic Brain Injury*. Phildelphia, Pa: F A Davis Co; 1990.
4. Teasdale G, Knill-Jones K, Vander Sande JP. Observer variability in assessing impaired consciousness and coma. *J Neurol Neurosurg Psychiatry*. 1978;41:603-610.
5. Bond MR. Standardized Methods of Assessing and Predicting Outcome. In: Rosenthal M, Griffith E, Bond M, et al, eds. *Rehabilitation of the Adult and Child with Traumatic Brain Injury*. Philadelphia, Pa: F A Davis Co; 1990:64.
6. Jennett B, Snoek J, Bond MR, Brooks N. Disability after severe head injury: observations on the use of the Glasgow Outcome Scale. *J Neurol Neurosurg Psychiatry*. 1981;44:285-293.
7. *Rehabilitation of the Head Injured Adult: Comprehensive Physical Management*. Downey, Calif: Professional Staff Association, Rancho Los Amigos Hospsital Inc; 1979.
8. *Neurology Report*. Alexandria, Va: Neurology Section, American Physical Therapy Association; 1990;14(1).
9. Kelly JP. Principles of the functional and anatomical organization of the nervous system. In: Kandel ER, Schwartz JH, eds. *Principles of Neural Science*. 2nd ed. New York, NY: Elsevier Science Publishing Co Inc; 1985:215-216.
10. Brooks VB. *Neural Basis of Motor Control*. New York, NY: Oxford University Press Inc; 1986.
11. Schmidt RA. *Motor Control and Learning: A Behavioral Emphasis*. Champaign, Ill: Human Kinetics Publishers Inc; 1982.
12. Brooks N. *Closed Head Injury: Psychological, Social and Family Consequences*. New York, NY: Oxford University Press Inc; 1984.

Chapter 26

Functional Abilities in Context

Susan R. Harris, PhD, PT, FAPTA
Associate Professor
School of Rehabilitation Medicine
University of British Columbia
Vancouver, B.C. Canada V6T 2B5

With the increased emphasis on accountability in health care, as required by accrediting agencies, third party payers, and health care consumers, physical therapists must strive to provide functional outcome goals for their clients. Many of the classic therapeutic exercise approaches developed for individuals with neurologic disorders have been oriented toward qualitative changes, such as normalization of muscle tone or improvement in gait symmetry, with little regard for the functional significance of those changes. Only recently have we begun to read and hear about the importance of physical therapists setting functional outcomes for clients recovering from central nervous system (CNS) injuries.[1,2]

This chapter will discuss the importance of promoting functional abilities for our clients with neurologic disorders in the context of their natural environments. The processes of developing functionally oriented goals and measuring functional changes as a result of treatment will be described. Involvement of the client and her or his caregivers in setting goals will be highlighted. The use of adaptive devices and equipment to accomplish functional goals will be discussed, and the need to generalize functional goals across different environmental settings will be presented. Examples from recent research literature will be used to clarify the points being addressed, with primary emphasis on individuals from two different patient populations: cerebral palsy (CP) and stroke.

FUNCTIONALLY ORIENTED REHABILITATION: A LITERATURE REVIEW

Whereas functional outcomes have been a focus of adult rehabilitation for clients with CNS injuries during the past two decades,[3-8] only recently has the attainment of quantitative functional outcomes been stressed by physical therapists in the treatment of pediatric clients.[9-11] The Bobaths, originators and leading proponents of the neurodevelopmental treatment (NDT) approach, have emphasized in recent literature the importance of a more functional and task-analytical approach to treatment of the child with cerebral palsy:

Treatment now incorporates systematic preparation for specific functions, and we realize the need for thorough analysis of each task we try to prepare the child to perform. We relate this analysis to the assessment of the individual child, finding out what interferes with or what is missing from each part of the task. We aim at treating the child in "functional

situations," ie, those in which they live at home or at school, to ensure that the tasks are carried over into daily life.[12(p9)]

Despite this new emphasis on measuring functional outcomes as a result of treatment for children with CP, a recent review article examining the efficacy of physical therapy for children with CP suggests that investigators have been remiss in including functional outcome measures in their evaluation of treatment effectiveness, at least in group experimental research. In their review of nine group-comparison studies between 1973 and 1988 that evaluated the efficiency of physical therapy for children with CP, Tirosh and Rabino[13] reported that the outcome measures used included gross motor milestones, neurologic status, mental development, and range of motion. None of the studies cited reported the use of specific functional outcome measures such as independence in self-help skills or the ability to use powered mobility or augmentative communication devices.

The development of functionally oriented treatment goals must be the responsibility not only of physical therapist researchers but also of clinicians working daily with children and adults with CNS disorders. The purpose of this chapter is to provide guidelines for the development of functional treatment goals by describing behavioral strategies and methodologies for measuring change as a result of treatment for individuals in our clinical settings. In addition to outlining these strategies, examples of recently published studies will be included to highlight the use of single- subject research designs in measuring functional changes within individuals.

DEVELOPMENT OF FUNCTIONALLY ORIENTED TREATMENT GOALS

The first step in the development of functionally oriented treatment goals is to learn to define operationally the behaviors in need of change. In their classic article on evaluating treatment effectiveness in CP, Martin and Epstein[14] emphasized the importance of behavioral analysis as the cornerstone of single subject methodology. They stress that therapists must select a target behavior that is both observable and quantifiable through direct observation. The behavior must be well defined in operational terms so that two or more observers can reliably agree on its occurrence or nonoccurrence (interrater reliability).

Equally important to the clear, operational definition

of outcome behaviors is the assurance that the treatment goals are appropriate for the individualclient. Edgar[15] has outlined four decision making points in determining content priorities for goals and objectives in special education settings. These have been modified slightly by me to reflect the development of content priorities for both children and adults with CNS disorders.

The first decision making point is to establish the *current functioning level* of the client. This can be accomplished through standardized developmental assessments, such as the Bayley Scales of Infant Development,[16] or measures of functional status, such as the Barthel Index.[17] However, these assessments should be accompanied by individualized measures that are important to the client and her or his family, such as the amount of time required to transfer safely from wheelchair to bed or the degree of assistance required to complete a meal.

The second decision making point in determining content priorities for goals and objectives is to assess *specific physical limitations* that may interfere with the attainment of certain goals.[15] Examples of physical limitations that may preclude attainment of specific goals might include the presence of contractures or deformities or the presence of sensory deficits such as vision, hearing, or proprioceptive impairments.

The *age of the client or the time elapsed since onset of the CNS injury* is the third decision making point that must be considered in developing appropriate treatment goals. Goals may be more developmentally or maturationally based for the very young child or the adult who has recently sustained a CNS injury, but they still are functionally oriented. It is important to remember that goals can be both developmentally appropriate and functionally relevant. However, as the Bobaths have noted recently, less emphasis should be placed on following a "lock-step" developmental sequence, particularly if it interferes with the attainment of functional outcomes:

> However, we soon found that it was not enough—indeed it was wrong— to try to follow the normal developmental sequence too closely. We had made the child rigidly go through the stage of rolling over, side-sitting, kneeling, kneel-standing, half-kneeling, crawling and then finally standing; one stage after the other. But that sequence is not followed faithfully by normal children.[12(p9)]

Thus for children and adults who have reached a plateau in their developmental or maturational progress postinjury the emphasis must be placed predominantly on the attainment of goals with functional significance. As Edgar[15] has noted, the fourth and final decision making point in determining content priorities for goals and objectives is, in fact, the *functionality of theskills*. As was mandated by the Education for All Handicapped Children Act (Public Law 94-142),[18] which was passed in 1975, physical therapy goals in special education settings "must have some underlying functional significance that leads to enhancement of the student's independence."[19(p296)] In addition, working toward the functional goals has gained renewed emphasis in the treatment of adults with strokes[7,8] and in the rehabilitation of individuals with traumatic brain injuries.[2]

Whereas overall treatment goals tend to be more global and long-term in their scope, they are a necessary prerequisite for the development of short-term, measurable treatment objectives, or target behaviors. Once the content priorities of the long-term goals have been established, the next step is to formulate several short-term treatment objectives for each of the long-term goals. These objectives should directly relate back to the more general, long- term goals and should be ordered sequentially so that the attainment of each step will lead the client closer to the accomplishment of the long-term goal. In this manner, short-term objectives represent behavioral statements of client performance.[19]

FORMULATING SPECIFIC THERAPY OBJECTIVES

The development of measurable therapy objectives, or target behaviors, is the next step in documenting functional changes as a result of treatment. O'Neill and Harris[19(p296)] have outlined four components of individualized, behavioral objectives:
1. *Who* is the student or patient for whom the objective is written?
2. *What* is the movement or behavior to be accomplished?
3. *Under what conditions* will the behavior occur?
4. What is the *criterion* for success?

In developing a specific therapy objective, the who in the objective statement must represent client rather than therapist performance. The what must represent a movement or behavior that is observable, repeatable,and has a definite beginning and end.[20] Under what conditions could include "specific activities of the therapist, equipment necessary for completion of the task, antecedent events, or environmental factors."[19] And finally, the criterion for success will represent how well the client is expected to perform in completing the desired objective. For example, performance may be measured in term of duration or latency of the response or frequency of the behavior.

An example of a long-term goal and sequentially ordered short-term objectives for a client with CNS injury might be as follows:

Goal: Ms. Smith will increase her independence in transfer skills.

Objective 1: With verbal cues from her therapist, Ms. Smith will transfer from her wheelchair to the hospital bed within 90 seconds for 3 consecutive days.

Objective 2: With verbal cues from her husband, Ms. Smith will transfer independently from her wheelchair to her bed at home within 60 seconds for 3 consecutive days.

Objective 3: Ms. Smith will transfer independently from her wheelchair to her bed at home within 60 seconds for 3 consecutive days.

These three short-term objectives represent increasing levels of independence, decreasing levels of time or duration of the activity, and generalizing the objectives to the natural (home) environment. To ensure that the behavior is consistent and learned, the client must perform the activity for 3 consecutive days before moving on to the next objective.

INVOLVEMENT OF THE CLIENT AND CAREGIVERS IN SETTING GOALS

During the past decade, increasing emphasis has been placed on including the client and her or his caregivers in the development of long-term goals and short-term objectives. Clinical decision making about the importance and priority of specific goals should not rest unilaterally with the client's physical therapist but should reflect input from the client herself, her family, and other significant caregivers.

As part of the initial assessment, the physical therapist should query both the client and her caregivers about what goals are important to them as part of the client's rehabilitation. Although clients and their caregivers may not have the background or training to develop individualized behavioral objectives, they typically have preconceived ideas about what aspects of their rehabilitation are important to them. It is then up to the therapist to develop these ideas into formal statements of goals and objectives.

In my own clinical experience in working with infants having developmental disabilities and with their families, the parents' goals have been exactly in line with the goals I would have set for the child myself based on my own assessment and expertise.

MEASURING FUNCTIONAL CHANGE AS A RESULT OF TREATMENT

As health care providers, we have an ethical responsibility to our clients and their caregivers to document that the treatment strategies we are using are efficacious in improving the client's ability to function. Only through systematic measurement of functional outcome behaviors is it possible to document reliably such changes. Wolery[21] has outlined four important reasons for including measurement as part of the therapy process:

1. To develop a scientific base for therapy.
2. To increase the efficiency of treatment programs.
3. To make decisions about how to change therapy.
4. To be accountable to clients, their caregivers, other team members, and others in general.

As discussed previously, the first step in documenting functional change as a result of treatment is to set measurable therapy goals and objectives based on input from the client and her caregivers. To demonstrate that changes in client performance are due to the implementation of specific treatment strategies, it is then necessary to proceed to the next step, the systematic introduction and withdrawal of the intervention strategies. A clinically feasible method for evaluating the effects of a specific treatment strategy on client outcome behaviors is the single-subject research design.[22]

Such designs have gained increasing use in the research literature for documenting functional recovery from stroke[8] and the effects of specific treatment strategies in the rehabilitation of children with CP.[11,23-25].

In setting up single subject designs, Ottenbacher has outlined six steps for observing and recording client behavior.[26] The first step is to determine the setting in which the behavior or performance will be observed and recorded. Ideally, this observation will occur in the natural setting, such as the client's home, work environment, or classroom setting. Measuring performance in the natural setting will en-

sure that there is carry over of functional skills performed initially in a more controlled clinical setting. The multiple baseline design across settings is an ideal design for measuring generalization of acquired functional skills across several different environments.

The second step is to decide on the method to collect data. Ottenbacher[26] described four different methods that are appropriate for use by physical or occupational therapists. The first is *event recording*, defined as a tally of "each occurrence of a defined response throughout an observation session."[26(p70)] For example, Laskas and colleagues[23] measured the number of times that a young child with CP attained heel contact during rising to standing both under baseline and treatment conditions. A second data collection method is *duration recording,* or "the length of occurrence of a response."[26(p71)] Harris and Riffle[24] measured the duration of independent standing, both with and without tone-reducing ankle-foot orthoses, for a preschool child with CP.

A third data collection method is *rate recording,* or "the frequency of a behavior divided by the time frame in which it occurred."[26(p71)] An example might be the number of independent bites of food taken by a client with head injury during a 20-minute meal. The fourth method described by Ottenbacher was *time sampling,* which was defined as "the state of a behavior at specific moments or intervals in time."[26(p71)] In a single-subject withdrawal design (A-B-A), Purdy and colleagues[27] used time sampling to measure tongue protrusion in children with Down syndrome, during both baseline and treatment conditions.

Ottenbacher's[26] third step in observing and recording behavior is to determine the period of time that the behavior will be observed and measured. Because most single subject designs begin with a baseline, or no-treatment condition, it is ideal to collect data until a stable pattern emerges. This may take as short a time as several hours to as long a time as several weeks,[26] but it does not necessitate that *no* treatment be provided during this time. Baseline does not require the absence of any treatment but rather the absence of a specific treatment that is being introduced to effect a specific change, such as the introduction of tone- reducing ankle-foot orthoses in the Harris and Riffle study.[24] Once a stable baseline pattern has emerged, the specific intervention strategy can be introduced to study its effect on the outcome behavior.

The fourth step, as outlined by Ottenbacher,[26] is to observe and record client behavior. A careful operational definition of the behavior to be measured will help to ensure that the data can be collected in a reliable manner. Interrater reliability can be established during a pilot phase of the study and should be checked periodically throughout each phase of the study. Development of a data-recording form will help in the collection of reliable and consistent data.[26]

The fifth step is to record and plot the data collected.[26] Data can be plotted on a simple line or bar graph of on a Standard Behavior Chart.[28]

The sixth and final step in observing and recording behavior is to continue measurement and recording procedures until requirements of the design have been satisfied.[26] Even the least sophisticated of the single subject designs, the simple baseline, or AB design,[14] requires that a minimum of three data points be collected during each phase. Data must be plotted and analyzed as they are collected, using either visual analysis or statistical procedures.[29]

Ottenbacher[26] concludes his description of the six steps for observing and recording behavior by stressing the importance of collecting accurate measurements throughout all phases of the design: "The analysis and interpretation of the data collected can only be as good as the method of observation and recording that was used to collect the data." Readers who wish to learn more about single-subject research designs are referred to Ottenbacher's[26] excellent data on strategies for evaluating clinical change and the recent descriptive article by Gonella.[22] Such designs are clearly gaining increased usage for studying the effects of different types of treatment strategies on functional recovery patterns in clients with CNS lesions.[8,30]

USE OF ADAPTIVE EQUIPMENT TO ACCOMPLISH FUNCTIONAL GOALS

As we begin to let go of the belief that we can actually "normalize" muscle tone, reflexes, and movement patterns in our clients with CNS deficits, it is becoming increasingly important to examine the use of adaptive equipment to aid in obtaining functional outcomes such as independence in self-help skills, communication, and mobility.[30] Our colleagues in special education, psychology, and occupational therapy have been far more involved in documenting functional outcomes through the use of adaptive equipment,[31-33] but physical therapists have begun to join in those efforts as well.[34] A recently published single subject study conducted by an interdisciplinary team of investigators, including occupational therapists, a special educator, and a physical therapist, will be summarized to exemplify an evaluation of the efficacy of adaptive equipment in increasing functional independence.

Using a single-subject withdrawal design (A-B-A), Einset and colleagues[35] examined the efficacy of a mechanical feeding device in increasing feeding independence in four adults with CP. Subjects ranged in age from 24-28 years, had diagnoses of spastic or athetoid or mixed quadriplegia, and were severely impaired in their fine motor skills. The Winsford Feeder was the device used as the independent variable because it required only head movements for use and had been used successfully by adults with quadriplegia secondary to spinal cord injury.

Four functional outcome measures were used to evaluate the efficacy of the Winsford Feeder: 1) the amount of time needed to eat a meal, 2) the amount of staff time needed to assist in feeding, 3) the percentage of the meal eaten, and 4) the clients' impressions about the usefulness of the feeder. Interobserver reliability was collected twice during each phase of the study for staff time required and length of the meal. Percentage agreement between the primary investigator and an independent observer ranged from 91.5% to 99.0% for these two outcome measures.

One finding that was consistent across all four of the subjects was that the electric feeder decreased the percentage of meal eaten, possibly as a result of the fixed range of motion of the feeder and its inability to adapt to small pieces of food as compared with the variability with which the aides could feed the subjects.[35] For two of the subjects the feeder appeared to increase the length of the meal, and for a third subject a training effect apparently occurred as indicated by a downward trend in length of the meal. Two subjects (Subjects 1 and 4) showed a clear decrease in the need for staff time.

Based on results of a questionnaire administered at the completion of the study, all four of the subjects thought that the device allowed more independence in eating, but only two stated that they would like to continue to use the feeder on a regular basis. Three of the four subjects suggested design modifications to increase the functionality of the feeder. Subject 1's data for the three primary outcome measures appear in Figures 26-1 to 26-3.

This study provides a perfect example of the use of single subject designs for evaluating the effects of an adaptive

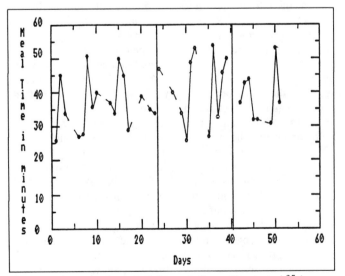

Fig. 26-1. *Length of meal: Subject 1. From Einset et al,[35] by permission.*

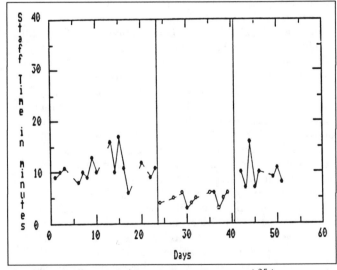

Fig. 26-2. *Staff time: Subject 1. From Einset et al,[35] by permission.*

equipment device on functional outcome measures. The four clients involved had volunteered to serve as subjects and were queried as to their feelings about the usefulness of the device, thus involving them in future setting of goals. In addition, they provided problem- oriented suggestions for improving the design of the feeding device. And finally, the authors attended to cost-benefit analysis, an extremely important issue in light of today's emphasis on accountability in health care:

> The issue of decreasing staff time was one of the initial concerns of the authors because it is a function of physical independence and because it is an important consideration in cost-benefit analysis. Had staff time beendramatically reduced by the use of the feeder, it would have appeared to be a more economically feasible product. As it stands, the electric feeder is a very expensive device and may not increase the independence of a person with cerebral palsy.[35(p50)]

GENERALIZING FUNCTIONAL GOALS ACROSS DIFFERENT ENVIRONMENTAL SETTINGS

For skills to be truly functional, they must be generalizable across different environmental settings in which the client lives, works, and plays. Held[36(p174)] has suggested that we not only should work toward daily functional tasks with our clients, but that ultimately we also "should take our patients beyond simply activities of daily living to activities relevant to occupation and recreation." Recent pediatric research has suggested that therapy integrated into the classroom setting may be just as effective as therapy occurring in a more isolated setting, such as a therapy room or a section of the gymnasium, and that the integrated model was preferred by the teaching staff.[37]

Whereas previously we had thought of recreational activities, such as therapeutic swimming or horseback riding, as adjuncts to traditional therapy, consensus now exists among pediatric physical therapists that activities such as NDT-based therapeutic horseback riding[38] have been shown

to be efficacious in decreasing hypertonus and improving functional posture for children with CP.[39]

An ideal single subject design for measuring generalizability across settings is the multiple baseline design across settings.[22,26] Baseline data for a specific functional outcome behavior are collected on a single client in at least three different settings. Once a stable baseline emerges in the primary setting, the treatment is introduced within that setting, but baseline conditions are maintained in the other two settings. Once stability of the data occur during the treatment phase in the first setting, the intervention is introduced in the second setting, and so forth.

A hypothetical example of a multiple baseline design across settings appears in Figure 26-4. The adult client with posthead-injury is an inpatient in a rehabilitation unit; the specific treatment strategy is the use of sequenced activity cards outlining transfer techniques from the wheelchair to another chair.[2] Baseline data are collected on the duration of time taken to transfer from the wheelchair to a chair in the clinic area, the lounge area, and the dining area. It is important to reiterate that baseline does not necessarily mean the absence of any treatment. This client is continuing to get traditional therapeutic exercise to work on weight-shifting and balance during transfer activities, but the new intervention strategy to be added is the sequenced activity cards that the client will be responsible for organizing before the transfer activity.[2]

Baseline data on the duration of time taken to transfer from wheelchair to chair are collected across all three settings (Fig. 26-4). Once a stable baseline is obtained in the clinic area, the use of the sequenced activitycards is introduced in this setting, but baseline conditions continue in the other two settings (dining and lounge areas). As can be seen in Figure 26-4, all three baselines are relatively stable, but the introduction of the intervention produces a downward trend in the time taken to transfer from wheelchair to chair in each of the three settings, thus suggesting that the use of the

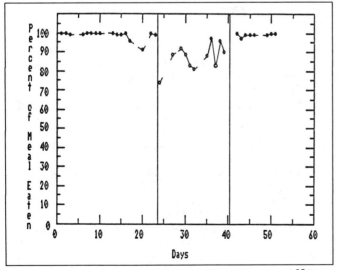

Fig. 26-3. *Percentage eaten: Subject 1. From Einset et al,[35] by permission.*

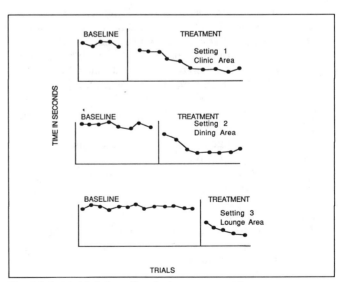

Fig. 26-4. *Multiple baseline design across settings.*

sequenced activity cards is efficacious in decreasing transfer time.

Although this was a hypothetical example based on actual clinical treatment strategies,[2] this would be a relatively simple and functionally relevant study to carry out. Even more important would eventually be to assess the generalizability of transfer skills into the home and community environments once the client was discharged.

SUMMARY AND CONCLUSIONS

The goal of this chapter has been to discuss the importance of promoting functional abilities for our clients with neurologic disorders in the context of their natural environments. Processes for developing functionally oriented goals and objectives have been described, and steps for measuring functional changes as a result of treatment have been presented. The importance of involving the client and her or his caregivers in the goal setting and of using adaptive devices to accomplish functional goals has been highlighted. Finally, the need to generalize functional goals across different environmental settings has been stressed.

In his recent discussion of physical therapists' dissatisfaction with the facilitation approach to treatment, Gordon has stressed the failure of this approach to provide opportunities for function to carry over into daily activities.

Unfortunately, facilitation approaches have not directly confronted the problem of how to achieve functional carry-over. Too often there is simply the assumption that the treatments we perform will somehow mysteriously translate into functional improvement for the patient . . . . The apparent contradiction between facilitation of normal movement and independent function in daily activities has been a major factor in producing disillusionment among therapists, especially as we are increasingly faced with the requirements to discharge patients earlier.[40(pp10-11)]

As we enter the next decade, we must direct our efforts toward evaluating change in our clients through systematic and reliable measurement of functional outcome behaviors. As Gordon[40(p11)] has suggested, "The next advance must be to combine training of normal movement patterns with emphasis on their use during functional activities." It seems appropriate to conclude this chapter with six functional goals for physical therapists for the decade of the 1990s:
1. To develop functional outcome measures for all of our clients.
2. To involve clients and their caregivers in the development of those functional goals.
3. To measure change as a result of treatment through single subject and group-comparison designs.
4. To modify treatment plans based on continuous analysis of outcome measures.
5. To assess the generalizability of functional goals across different environmental settings.
6. To use adaptive devices, powered mobility, and augmentative communication technology in attempting to effect functional changes in our clients.

References

1. Duncan PW, Badke MB. Measurement of motor performance and functional abilities following stroke. In: Duncan PW, Badke MB, eds. *Stroke Rehabilitation: The Recovery of Motor Control.* Chicago, Ill: Year Book Medical Publishers Inc; 1987:199-221.
2. Black KS, Barton LA. Setting functional outcomes for inpatient brain injury rehabilitation: a justification for motor learning treatment strategies. Presented at the Combined Sections Meeting of the American Physical Therapy Association; February 3, 1990; New Orleans, La.
3. Stern PH, McDowell F, Miller JM, et al. Effects of facilitation exercise techniques in stroke rehabilitation. *Arch Phys Med Rehabil.* 1970;51:526-531.
4. Loggian MK, Samuels MA, Falconer J. Clinical exercise trial for stroke patients. *Arch Phys Med Rehabil.* 1983;64:364-367.
5. Dickstein R, Hocherman S, Pillar T, et al. Stroke rehabilitation: three exercise therapy approaches. *Phys Ther.* 1986;66:1233-1238.
6. Lord JP, Hall K. Neuromuscular reeducation versus traditional programs for stroke rehabilitation. *Arch Phys Med Rehabil.* 1986;67:88-91.
7. Basmajian JV, Gowland CA, Finlayson AJ, et al. Stroke treatment: comparison of integrated behavioral-physical therapy vs traditional physical therapy programs. *Arch Phys Med Rehabil.* 1987;68:267-272.
8. Wagenaar RC, Meijer OG, van Wieringen PCW, et al. The functional recovery of stroke: a comparison between neurodevelopmental treatment and the Brunnstrom method. *Scand J Rehabil Med.* 1990;22:1-8.
9. Scrutton D: Introduction. In: Scrutton D, ed. *Management of the Motor Disorders of Children with Cerebral Palsy.* Philadelphia, Pa: J B Lippincott Co; 1984:1-5.
10. Harris SR. Efficacy of physical therapy in promoting family functioning and functional independence for children with cerebral palsy. *Pediatric Physical Therapy.* In press.
11. Kluzik JA, Fetters L, Coryell J. Quantification of control: a preliminary study of effects of neurodevelopmental treatment on reaching in children with cerebral palsy. *Phys Ther.* 1990;70:65-76.
12. Bobath K, Bobath B. The neuro-developmental treatment. In: Scrutton D, ed. *Management of the Motor Disorders of Children with Cerebral Palsy.* Philadelphia, Pa: J B Lippincott Co; 1984:6-18.
13. Tirosh E, Rabino S. Physiotherapy for children with cerebral palsy. *Am J Dis Child.* 1989;143:552-555.
14. Martin, JE, Epstein LH. Evaluating treatment effectiveness in cerebral palsy: single-subject designs. *Phys Ther.* 1976;56:285-294.
15. Edgar E. Individual education plans. In: Haring NG, ed. *The Experimental Education Unit Training Program: An Inservice Program for Personnel Serving the Severely Handicapped.* Seattle, Wash: Unviversity of Washington Press; 1977:239-258.
16. Bayley N. *Bayley Scales of Infant Development.* New York, NY: Psychological Corporation; 1969.
17. Mahoney FI, Barthel DW. Functional evaluation: the Barthel Index. *Md Med J.* 1965;14:61-65.
18. Education for All Handicpped Children Act, Public Law 94-142. US Congress, Senate: 94th Congress, first session; 1975.
19. O'Neill DL, Harris SR. Developing goals and objectives for handicapped children. *Phys Ther.* 1982;62:295-298.
20. White OR, Haring NG. *Exceptional Teaching: A Multimedia*

Training Package. Columbus, Ohio: Charles E. Merrill Publishing Co; 1976:22.

21. Wolery M. Rationale for measurement in therapy. In: Harris SR, Wolery M. *Introduction to Single Subject Research Design*. Presented at 39th Annual Meeting of the American Academy for Cerebral Palsy and Developmental Medicine; October 4, 1985; Seattle, Wash.

22. Gonella C. Single-subject experimental paradigm as a clinical decision tool. *Phys Ther*. 1989;69:601-609.

23. Laskas CA, Mullen SL, Nelson DL, et al. Enhancement of two motor functions of the lower extremity in a child with spastic quadriplegia. *Phys Ther*. 1985;65:11-16.

24. Harris SR, Riffle K. Effects of inhibitive ankle-foot orthoses on standing balance in a child with cerebral palsy. *Phys Ther*. 1986;66:663-667.

25. Hinderer KA, Harris SR, Purdy AH, et al. Effects of "tone-reducing" vs. standard plaster-casts on gait improvement of children with cerebral palsy. *Dev Med Child Neurol*. 1988;30:370-377.

26. Ottenbacher KJ. *Evaluating Clinical Change: Strategies for Occupational and Physical Therapists*. Baltimore, Md: Williams & Wilkins; 1986.

27. Purdy AH, Dietz JC, Harris SR. Efficacy of two treatment approaches to reduce tongue protrusion of children with Down syndrome. *Dev Med Child Neurol*. 1987;29:469-476.

28. White OR, Haring NG. *Exceptional Teaching*. 2nd ed. Columbus, Ohio; Charles E. Merrill Publishing Co; 1980.

29. Wolery M, Harris SR. Interpreting results of single-subject research designs. *Phys Ther*. 1982;62:445-452.

30. Harris SR. Early intervention: does developmental therapy make a difference? *Topics in Early Childhood Special Education*. Winter 1988;7:20-32.

31. Butler C. Effects of powered mobility on self-initiated behaviors of very young children with locomotor disability. *Dev Med Child Neurol*. 1986;28:325-332.

32. Tarnowski KJ, Drabman RS. Increasing the communicator usage skills of a cerebral palsied adolescent. *J Pediatr Psychol*. 1986;11:573-581.

33. Everson JM, Goodwyn R. A comparison of the use of adaptive microswitches by students with cerebral palsy. *Am J Occup Ther*. 1987;41:739-744.

34. Hulme JB, Shaver J, Acher S, et al. Effects of adaptive seating devices on the eating and drinking of children with multiple handicaps. *Am J Occup Ther*. 1987;41:81-89.

35. Einset K, Deitz J, Billingsley F, et al. The electric feeder: an efficacy study. *Occupational Therapy Journal of Research*. January 1989;9:38-52.

36. Held JM. Recovery of function after brain damage: theoretical implications for therapeutic intervention. In: Carr JH, Shepherd RB, Gordon J, et al, eds. *Movement Science: Foundations for Physical Therapy in Rehabilitation*. Rockville, Md: Aspen Publishers Inc; 1987:155-177.

37. Cole K, Harris SR, Eland SF, et al. Comparison of two service delivery models: in-class vs. out-of-class therapy approaches. *Pedicatric Physical Therapy*. 1989;1:49-54.

38. Bertoti DB. Effect of therapeutic horseback riding on posture in children with cerebral palsy. *Phys Ther*. 1988;68:1505-1512.

39. Campbell SK, Consensus conference on efficacy of physical therapy in the management of cerebral palsy: introduction. *Pediatric Physical Therapy*. In press.

40. Gordon J. Assumptions underlying physical therapy intervention: theoretical and historical perspectives. In: Carr JH, Shepherd RB, Gordon J, et al, eds. *Movement Science: Foundations for Physical Therapy in Rehabilitation*. Rockville, Md: Aspen Publishers Inc; 1987:1-30.

Chapter 27

Action Steps: Recommendations for After the Conference

Ann F. VanSant, PhD, PT
Associate Professor
Department of Physical Therapy
College of Allied Health Professions
Temple University
Philadelphia, PA 19140

It is hard to believe that the II STEP conference is drawing to a close. This has been a very stimulating and exciting experience for all of us. After an intensive week of presentations, it is now time to focus on the actions that should result from this meeting. Like the original NUSTEP, the first action that will result from this conference is the process of publishing the proceedings.

The speakers have prepared manuscripts summarizing their talks. Those manuscripts will become the chapters of the proceedings. The first and possibly the most important action step is therefore already underway. We are pleased that the publication should be available early in 1991.

The impact of NUSTEP on physical therapy can largely be attributed to the use of the proceedings as a text for a generation of therapists. That written record was the source of shared concepts among clinicians and educators, and it provided rich hypotheses for physical therapy research. The chapters were read and reread. They generated scholarly interchange among therapists.

Those of us who were fortunate enough to have attended this II STEP program have gathered many new ideas. Now it is time to reflect on what we have heard and to begin to think about the effect of our exposure to the diverse theoretical viewpoints that were presented. Sitting back, putting up one's feet, and relaxing a bit should be high on the order of priorities. Time to reflect helps put ideas into perspective. Take some time to think about what you have heard here, examine the ideas, play with the concepts, and learn the language in which they are expressed. That process needs to go on not only while you are alone with your thoughts but also through the sharing of ideas with others. Discuss with a friend what you have learned, and sort through your ideas alone. Reformulate patient problems and questions using these new theories, and check out your ideas with a colleague.

Remember that in the new science we are discovering that pattern arises from apparent chaos. Order and patterns, or trends, will emerge from seemingly chaotic thoughts and images. The joy of discovery of new ways of thinking and explaining natural phenomena is part of science.

Dr. Duane Roller, the curator of the History of Science Collection here at the University of Oklahoma's library, spoke with members of this conference's planning committee and toured us through the rare books of that collection. He shared his philosophy in building this internationally recognized library. He collected everything he could and discarded nothing. Many seemingly outdated ideas in science circle around again. There is a lesson for us in his philosophy. Do not think that you must discard all that you currently know as a basis for your practice; rather, realize that the knowledge you currently possess can be reexamined from a new perspective. Traditional theories have served us well, but sometimes they are inadequate explanations of patient behavior. When they are inadequate, try new theory. Remember, theories are tools for understanding, devices that help explain the patient behaviors we encounter and that predict how we can help others change their behavior. Sometimes theories are useful, sometimes they are not.

After reflecting and thinking, there is another action step that each of us can take. That step is to read. We can learn so much by reading and rereading articles and books. Follow-up on an area that interests you by reading the background materials that the speakers used to formulate their ideas. This effort will bring a deeper and more thorough understanding of the speaker's perspective. Our increased professionalism brings increased responsibility to keep abreast of new ideas and to incorporate research findings into our professional body of knowledge. Keeping abreast of new ideas is not accomplished just by attending continuing or graduate education courses. Our own professional development depends on reading.

We have come to this meeting as clinicians, educators, and researchers. There are steps each of us can take in these professional roles. To those in clinical practice, I would say that sometimes it is hard to face major changes in thinking because we may have just mastered what is suddenly called traditional thinking or because we are so experienced in using traditional theories that we mistake them as fact. For example, it is often hard to regroup and remember that words like "reflex" and "tone" are theoretical ideas, not real things. It is equally hard to rethink the concept of a reflex if it is so newly learned or so well understood that it seems common sense. Nonetheless, it should be both challenging and comforting to know that there are always new ways to explain things, new ideas to conquer, and new theories to understand. Our professional world is not a boring place. When new ways of thinking emerge, there can be questioning of both the old and the new. Take risks with your new ideas. Do not stand still with your ideas; try them out. Our knowledge grows from such dynamic episodes. Our skills also grow. For me, skills are more than physical competence. Advanced thinking and problem solving abilities are among the best skills we own.

One step that can be taken as you return to the clinic is to share what you gained with your colleagues. Provide in-service education for those who were unable to attend. There is no better way to understand, question, and master ideas than to have to teach them to others. Also share your excitement and thoughts with your colleagues. Try to examine how your current theoretical perspectives are influencing what you select to evaluate, how you interpret your findings, and how you plan treatment. Theory strongly influences each of these fundamental clinical processes.[1] Try out new theoretical perspectives. I had much experience in the clinic trying out the theories of Rood,[2] Brunnstrom,[3] and Bobath.[4] Being able to switch from one theoretical explanation to another was both challenging and beneficial. Initially, I understood some theories better than others and therefore was more comfortable using those in my clinical practice; however, I soon developed a working knowledge of each theory. This knowledge allowed me to engage in wonderful discussions and debate with my colleagues. We shared patient problems and explored each other's approach to clinical problem solving. Eventually, I was able to change theoretical models when confronted with a problem that was resistant to solution. The intellectual stimulation of debate and discussion of theory and research lead to advanced understanding and increased levels of skill in clinical practice. This ability comes only if you try to understand the other side of the coin, the other way of framing a question, the other way of thinking. The clinic is an exciting place to learn and share experiences with colleagues, so as a first step, share your II STEP experiences there and debate the issues and begin to try out these ideas with patient problems.

Educators contemplating the next step face the question, "Should I redo my whole course syllabus?" This conference was designed specifically for academic and clinical educators. Many individuals have been aware of the vast changes in theory that are underfoot, but they have been somewhat perplexed with how to include this new information into entry-level course work and how to provide clinical experiences that incorporate new theory. Where do you begin?

Acquainting students with hierarchical and systems control theories is a useful first step for educators. One valuable resource in my teaching has been an article by Davis.[5] The article provides a relatively simple overview of traditional hierarchies with their associated principles of motor control; it contrasts these concepts with equally basic concepts of a system of control and its associated principles. I particularly emphasize the role of feedback and its effect on a control hierarchy[1] when I teach these ideas. I assure that the students' concepts of hierarchical and systems of control are well developed and clearly differentiated. It is important for students to understand both hierarchical and systems theory at this point in time because we are preparing them to function now and in the future. Hierarchies and systems are the language of today, but different control models may evolve with time. What is important and what endures is to help students identify the theory that underlies their thinking. I provide many examples of how theoretical models influence clinical practice. The students are able to grasp the notions quickly, but need consistent practice to identify those basic theoretical assumptions that are influencing their own thinking. In teaching evaluation and treatment planning skills, I require students to switch from one theory to another to solve the same problem. When students ask questions about treatment that involve what I would do, I remind them that what I do depends on what I think. We then work through to the doing stage by first adopting a theoretical framework that is appropriate for the patient problem. We judge the appropriateness of the theoretical framework by seeing if its assumptions are met before we begin to apply it. On examinations, I often ask students to solve clinical problems from a variety of theoretical perspectives. I believe having an understanding of more than one theory and having the ability to switch theories is critical to successful clinical practice. Overtly sharing our assumptions and theoretical perspectives is extremely important both in the classroom and in the clinic. Of course, we learn from our students. Their quick grasp of ideas and ability to put them to use is often amazing. Some things that take us inordinate amounts of time to fathom are theirs to understand in an instant. This ability is likely because they do not carry the excess baggage of devotion to theories that years of experience tend to impart. The content of our courses should constantly change with time, but the enduring examples of how to think, reason, and problemsolve as a physical therapist should be our primary concern as both clinical and academic educators.

Researchers, just as clinicians, can take action by re-examining the theoretical assumptions on which their works are based. This does not mean that they should abandon their current research efforts or the theory from which the questions grew. Data collected under one theoretical umbrella, however, can be reinterpreted under a different set of theoretical assumptions. Re-examination of data from a different perspective often enriches the research effort. For my work in life-span development, for example, I had to rethink the traditional theory of neuromotor development that proposes maturity as the end point of development. Systems theory provided explanations of age-related change during maturity that were not a part of the traditional thinking about neuromotor development. Dynamical systems theory, as represented at this conference by Heriza (see Heriza, this volume), has also opened a new way for me to think about my data. I am now asking questions about a different array of variables that might effect age- related change in motor behavior; new understandings are beginning to emerge.

The excitement and intellectual curiosity shared as a result of this conference should ensure our continued professional growth. I expect a great number of action steps not only by those who attended this conference but also by those who will benefit when we share our ideas and experience personally and through the published conference proceedings.

References

1. VanSant AF. Concepts of neural organization and movement. In: Connolly BH, Montgomery PC, eds. *Therapeutic Exercise in Developmental Disabilities*. Chattanooga, Tenn: Chattanooga Corporation, 1987:1-8.
2. Stockmeyer SS. An interpretation of the approach of Rood to the treatment of neuromuscular dysfunction. *Am J Phys Med*. 1967;46:900-956.
3. Brunnstrom S. *Movement Therapy in Hemiplegia*. New York, NY: Harper & Row, Publishers Inc; 1970.
4. Bobath K, Bobath B. Cerebral palsy: 1. Diagnosis and assessment of cerebral palsy. In: Pearson PH, Williams CE, eds. *Physical Therapy Services in the Developmental Disabilities*. Springfield, Ill: Charles C Thomas, Publisher; 1972:31-113.
5. Davis WJ. Organizational concepts in the central motor networks of invertebrates. In: Herman RL, Grillner S, Stein PSG, et al, eds. *Advances in Behavioral Biology: Neural Control of Locomotion*. New York, NY: Plenum Publishing Corp; 1976:265-292.

Chapter 28

Past, Present, and Future: The II STEP Conference

Mary Lou Barnes, EdD, PT
Professor
Department of Physical Therapy
Georgia State University
Atlanta, GA 30303

In all probability, the enormity of what has taken place during this conference has not yet struck any of us full force. Even so, I believe that the impact of this meeting on our thinking and actions will exceed that of any other single event in our professional history. This is the first week-long conference ever held in which the majority of the topics were presented by physical therapists dealing with sophisticated research studies conducted by physical therapists. If you like thrills, try contrasting that fact with the details of the original 4-week NUSTEP conference. Were you to do so, you would note that the scientific basis of most of the information disseminated there was borrowed from and presented by members of other disciplines.

Pediatric and neurologic specialists in physical therapy certainly have taken one giant, distinguishing step during these 8 days. I am thrilled to have been invited here to witness this event and to share my perspective as the closing speaker for this II STEP conference.

Almost a year ago, I received a letter from a good friend of mine in which she described the state of flux within our professional discipline. She wrote, "Lately in my professional experience, the process of making decisions has been a risk-taking venture. I have operated as a physical therapist with basic concepts of evaluation and treatment of my patients. My therapy, I believed, enhanced movement in my patients. Now, new concepts are present and my comfortable assumptions are being challenged. These new concepts do not exactly fit with my traditional thoughts. What do I do? My brain is in chaos."

My mind immediately centered on Tom Peters, coauthor of *In Search of Excellence* and *A Passion for Excellence*, who now has a book entitled *Thriving on Chaos*. In the Preface to the latter book, Peters describes the difficulty he had in arriving at an appropriate title for it. He stated that "the word chaos was easy because the situation with which he was dealing was chaotic. The word thriving was almost a given. Who would argue with thriving? The problem was with the prepositions *amidst* versus *on*."[1] Should the book be entitled "Thriving Amidst Chaos" or "Thriving on Chaos?" Peters stated that to thrive amidst chaos means to cope or come to grips with it, to succeed in spite of it. Peters did not like coming to grips with something because that is a reactive approach. The true objective, he said, is to take the chaos as a given and learn to thrive on it. Peters be-

lieves that "the winners of tomorrow will deal proactively with chaos today."[1]

Perhaps one of the problems of our profession is that we have always wanted to come to grips with patient problems and we wanted to do so in an orderly, organized way. We apparently believe, as did Longfellow when he wrote in his poem *Psalm of Life*, that

> *Not enjoyment, and not sorrow,*
> *Is our destined end or way;*
> *But to act, that each tomorrow*
> *Find us farther than today.*
> —Longfellow

To find ourselves farther than our yesterdays we have traditionally come to grips with our inability to know just what to do with our patients largely by two methods. Some of the great names in our brief history did it by an observational method. And although it was certainly intelligent observation, it was without the benefits of the skills and technology of today. For instance, the belief that an infant's early movements are random was espoused by those skilled in observation. Even those who had film or videotape technology at their disposal and who studied tapes in slow motion arrived at the same conclusion. Movements are random. But Esther Thelen, with a different approach and technological analysis, observed that the movements of the neonate are highly organized and predictable.

Our pioneers observed normal movement in order to determine just how to design activities for those who lost or never had the ability to move normally. Margaret Knott and Dorothy Voss are examples of therapists who carefully observed movement. From their observations and the work of Dr. Herman Kabat we have proprioceptive neuromuscular facilitation (PNF) as a method of patient treatment involving therapeutic exercise. And for them, each tomorrow found them farther than today for many, many years.

The second method we have traditionally used to cope with patient problems and to design treatment regimens was to study the literature. It seems almost blasphemous for anyone from the hallowed hall of academe to imply that we could have gotten into trouble by reviewing the literature. By again using PNF as a model, however, we may begin to see the ramifications of that practice.

At the NUSTEP conference of July 1966, Dorothy

Voss[2] used these words in describing the contribution of Dr. Kabat. She said, "In developing the techniques of the method, Kabat relied upon his knowledge of the physiology of Sherrington."[2] The work of others that she referred to as providing Kabat with supportive evidence for the method included, but were not limitedto, Gellhorn on proprioception and cortically induced movement; Coghill, McGraw, and Gesell on development of motor behavior and patterned movement; Hellebrandt on mass movement patterns elicited during exercise in the overload zone; and Pavlov on mechanisms of learning and formation of habit patterns. Kabat thus considered three basic areas: neurophysiology, motor behavior, and motor learning.[2]

Surely Dr. Kabat should not be faulted for using the minds and works of one awesome group of giants in their fields in formulating his neurotherapeutic treatment methods. Because he did, so many of us were able to act that each tomorrow found us farther than today.

In the book *Reflex and Vestibular Aspects of Motor Development, Motor Control and Motor Learning*,[3] there is an interesting discussion on the works of McGraw and Gesell as related to motor development. The authors describe just what can happen when individuals make their own interpretations and apply the results of the research that is not directly related to their own special interests. The authors point out that "while therapists may be well aware of the observations of McGraw and Gesell, we are not at all familiar with the purposes and goals of their research and the scientific context in which these two scientists worked.[3]

Both McGraw and Gesell were attempting to study mental development. Because movement is the easiest early change to monitor in infants, the two researchers studied movement as a way of gaining insight into the mental processes taking place during that period of human development. "Neither of them meant their exquisite descriptions of movement to be an end in themselves. They both sought to answer the fundamental question of whether the sources of developmental change were maturational or experiential and to discuss the relationship between structure and function in generating developmental change."[3]

To gather their data they manipulated the children physically by strapping them into chairs if the babies could not sit alone, and they pulled the children to sitting or standing positions to study movement reactions in those positions. They were not looking at how an infant got into a particular position but rather what the infant did once in that position.

Thus McGraw's research was not intended as a rigid guide to motor development through the description of milestones and phases of motor behavior. Other individuals picked up on her work and used it for that purpose and have further extended these descriptions to form a guide for intervention with the child who is developmentally disabled. And we have even extended the rules of development to govern treatment of adult patients with neurological defects.[3]

We have assumed a cause-effect relationship between one developmental "stage" and another. It may be true that the development of one stage is dependent on its predecessor, but that is not always true; we do not know which stages must evolve from another. Certainly, research now being done by physical therapists and developmental theorists suggest that these assumptions are not always correct.

Margaret Knott, Dorothy Voss, Margaret Rood, Signe Brunstrom, Berta Bobath and "other pioneers in neurologic treatment were quite up-to-date for their time and they provided the profession with a new maturity and considerable progress from the traditional treatments in vogue at the time. We owe them a great debt for their courage and insight."[3] They immersed themselves in the literature and spent countless hours observing movement behaviors in devising neurologic principles on which their treatment regimens were based.

And, taking a little license with Longfellow;

[The professional lives of these great women remind us;]
 We can make our lives sublime,
And, departing, leave behind us
 Footprints on the sands of time.

Oh how very, very much we owe them for their footprints.

One of the results of all the work done by these searching, observing minds had another side to it, however, and that was that we made apostles of them. Some of them were elevated to a position approaching the deity. And then we developed what might be called "discipleships." We have the "PNFers," the "NDTers," the "Roodists," and a host of other sincere, dedicated therapists bent on thriving amidst the chaos these great ladies handed us. We disciples insisted on coming to grips with the chaos. We categorized it, we ordered it, we molded it into a perfect solution for the problems of our patients.

From these therapists we received numerous principles of motor development. Inherent in some of those principles were the notions that "normal motor development proceeds in a cervicocaudal and proximodistal direction" or that "early motor behavior is dominated by reflex activity while maturemotor behavior is reinforced or supported by postural reflexes."[2] It was believed that the adult patient needs to "recapitulate" the developmental sequence in order to master functional activity all over again. We learned that many sensory cues, not all of which are proprioceptive, would be helpful in facilitating movement.[2] We learned all that and much, much more.

We reacted to the chaos resulting from the development of all these "principles of treatment" by adding our own interpretations to them. And unfortunately, in many, perhaps in most, of our educational programs we taught one or more of these concepts of treatment as though they were of biblical origin. Some of you may recall that the document produced from the proceedings of the original NUSTEP conference became a bible for some therapists, professors, and students because it contained some of the principles of treatment and some interpretations of those principles. It seemed as large as some pulpit bibles, and parts were also written in parables. For some of us it also required a concordance for more perfect understanding.

We in academe reacted as we did despite the fact that any good teacher is well aware that learning is fostered by first creating chaos in the mind of the learners. They must be

Contemporary Management of Motor Problems

shaken loose from preconceived biases. We must muddle their minds, and in so doing, we create a climate in which the learner thrives on change and innovation. We create mass confusion and then facilitate learning by showing the learner how to operate in a given climate by thriving *on* the chaos thus created. To do otherwise is to ensure adequate performance while stifling learning. And the same should be true in the way we teach our patients.

By failing to behave as good teachers are wont to do, we have created a whole host of disciples of the disciples. Everything has been neatly packaged and all of the round therapists have been fit into round holes. (We left all the square ones in orthopedics, which is totally unrelated to therapeutic exercise of course). We truly believed that by so doing, each tomorrow would surely find us farther than today.

And we got rid of the chaos. We got rid of it to the extent that when I phoned a well-known physical therapist in an attempt to persuade her to write a chapter on therapeutic exercise for a book I was coediting, she said she could not possibly do that. She went on to say that she knew of only one therapist in the country who could write intelligently on most of the approaches to therapeutic exercise. One therapist. We must have had 60,000 physical therapists within our profession at that time. Were we ever categorized?

And then slowly, slowly came the dawning. Something wonderful began to happen. My sense is that my first awareness of imminent chaos among the disciples occurred at a national conference of our organization during which I was comfortably seated at an afternoon session and quite prepared to nap, write a card to my children, or gossip with my neighbors as befit the occasion. Suddenly I awoke with a start. Something important was going on here. A physical therapist was interpreting research that was directly applicable to physical therapy. And the physical therapist was interpreting research done by that physical therapist.

I looked around me and discovered that all the disciples were hunched over their legal tablets, madly scribbling away. The Roodists were writing, the NDTers were writing, and even the integration therapists were writing. A PNFer paled and a Brunstromite passed out. And I thought, Oh Lord help me! The first commandment from my apostle, which was that "development proceeds from cranial to caudal," was destroyed. And the second, "movement proceeds from proximal to distal"; the fifth, "we move from mobility, to stability, to controlled mobility, to skill"; and the eighth, my beloved "vestibular system is responsible for balance and coordination" were all cast aside.

Ah chaos. We had just gotten therapeutic exercise all straightened out and now we have the beginning of a totally chaotic situation once again. Almost a decade later, however, most of the disciples have survived the disintegration of our commandments that were etched in stone. We have even managed to begin to live without "muscle tone."

Several years ago the editors of the book entitled *Physical Therapy* decided that we just could not permit any of the 76 contributing authors to use the term muscle tone or tone of anything for that matter. Well, chaos is too mild a term to use for what happened. There was great moaning, breast beating, and gnashing of teeth. But the authors' re-

vised text, which was necessary to get around the use of the word tone, was some of the clearest, most descriptive, and most beautifully written in the book.

So it is a fact that we are doing very well thriving on chaos. And our new breed of research therapists have certainly handed us plenty of it this week. My only fear is that some of the disciple may still reside within us. We must each guard against the tendency to place a new Moses on the mountain where new commandments may again be etched in stone. We must also guard against the tendency to throw out the proverbial baby with the bath water. It would be foolhardy to even think that we must discard all we know of the work of McGraw, Gesell, Knott and Voss, Bobath, Brunstrom, Rood, and others of their class. If nothing else we must keep some of the techniques these people developed.

They may have been wrong as to why their techniques worked, or we may have been wrong in our interpretation of their work, but many of the tools they left us are effective. So rather than discarding them it behooves us to prove their efficacy and to search for the answers as to why the techniques work and should be retained. I am not one who would suggest that we discard everything we now use in treatment regimens that have not had their neurophysiologic basis statistically proven. I do strongly urge that we get on with research that will help us to establish the efficacy of what we do.

Had we established the effectiveness of our ministrations before attempting to promote direct access or patient access, the change would likely have become a fait accompli virtually overnight. As it is, we cannot convince some of our peers of the correctness of our actions let alone others in the medical and scientific communities.

For example, some physical therapists can be amused so easily by the seeming mysticism underlying some of the claims made for the restorative powers of craniosacral therapy or somatoemotional release. These same therapists are not amused, however, when someone suggests that they are rushing off to become certified in the mysticism of NDT. Before the NDTers in the crowd start throwing things, I would like to ask that each of you reach out and touch the person sitting next to you. Now, in all likelihood you have just touched an individual who also has practiced professional mysticism. And we will remain shrouded in mysticism until facts are established by research.

It is wonderful to be able to develop certain principles of exercise or movement that are predicated on research that was carried out to establish truth relative to those movements. But let us not then use certain of the principles to the exclusion of all others. Let us never again arrive at principles tangentially from a point that has not been validated by research, preferably that which has been replicated. The ability to observe that which is going on around us is a wonderful talent to have and to use. But research must be done on these observations to establish validity for whatever purposes we might propose for them.

Let us forever keep in mind the specificity of movement and exercise. For example, standing balance is not something directly derived from creeping and crawling activities. In fact, even standing balance and balance while walking appear to be relatively unrelated tasks. We must learn not to extend automatically the results of research on one body part or activity to another area or activity.

Good research must be supported strongly in the decade of the 1990s. There is nothing else that will do as much for the profession and for the patients for whom all of us exist. Research, however, will do little good if the findings are not disseminated appropriately. The most appropriate way to disseminate findings is through the medium of well-written English language, even if it a bit Americanized.

And let us write in the manner of all truly good writers. They seldom use esoteric, uncommon, or contrived terms when simple, familiar, and reasonable terms words will suffice. If the idea is to generate understanding, acceptance, and application of new principles by clinical practitioners who are not researchers, then it is necessary to speak to them. The use of contrived terms tends to place new knowledge in some mystical category and may temporarily generate for the author the illusion of sophistication and profundity.

Let me give you an example of just what I mean. In recently reviewing a research article, I ran across this sentence: "A biped standing perfectly erect is in a state of metastable equilibrium with respect to gravity." Now most of you may be able to paraphrase that sentence perfectly. I could not. A biped standing perfectly erect. What is that? Never having been around many gorillas I cannot attest to their ability to stand perfectly erect, and I have not seen many humans ever do it.

And what is a biped? And what is wrong with bipeds when their equilibrium is metastable? I could not find out by looking in the APTA's favorite *Random House Dictionary*, and my gargantuan *Webster's Unabridged Dictionary* did not contain such a word. Finally, I found it in a medical dictionary. It comes from the Greek word "meta," meaning change, and the Latin word "stabilis," meaning stable; it is used in the disciplines of chemistry and physics. It means marked by a slight margin of stability.[4] And biped, according to *Webster's Unabridged Dictionary*, means "an animal having only two feet, as man."[5]

After consulting with a learned colleague for a lengthy period of time on the vignette of meaning we were to infer from the words "a slight margin of stability," we concluded that we could remain in the scientific community were we to interpret that sentence about bipeds and peculiar equilibrium to wit: "a human can maintain stability within a few degrees of postural sway while standing perfectly erect." Now what is wrong with that? Perhaps it does not sound scientific.

Unfortunately, I went from that author to another and was immediately confronted with this sentence: "The infant, therefore, has two concurrent dynamical states: the immediate topology of movement and the longer term trajectory of ontogeny." I will not bore you with the circumlocution I and my learned colleagues developed for you on that one. It is a fact that in this particular case the terms are neither misused nor contrived. Rather, they are strung together such that unfamiliarity with one of the terms will confuse the learner. Two unfamiliar terms in the same sentence may well bury the message.

Let me hasten to add that both the authors quoted above had messages of great import for all therapists everywhere. But all therapists everywhere will never receive those messages unless and until they are translated for the average bipedal mind. And let us be clear that the therapists in this hall do not have average bipedal minds. You are far above that stage.

Let me also hasten to add that it is perfectly proper for scientists, such as many of our speakers this past week, to talk among themselves in any kind of terms that make dialog succinct. But it is neither proper nor wise for those of us who should go forth from II STEP and spread the word to use all of the scientific language and jargon knowing that the message may be lost on the receiver. Is it not enough that we must master English and the semantics of the medical professions? Do we have to borrow from the language of chemistry, physics, biology, computer technology, archaeology, and all the other "ologies?"

In closing, I would like for you to return with me to the letter from my friend as I read her closing remarks to me. She wrote, "As I have muddled through these thoughts over the past several years, the 'old' and the 'new' are merging. I am moving toward stability with new concepts of movement control, development, and learning. My theoretical insights are now on a different level than they were when I began the process, and I hope my students and patients will benefit from my risk taking."

As we depart from this wonderfully enlightening conference, may the old and the new be merging in us all. May we have some stability with our concepts. Nothing cut in stone, just some small measure of comforting stability. Surely, all of our insights are now on a different level, and all students and patients will certainly benefit from our risk taking, for ultimately out of chaos comes truth if we will only let it.

Longfellow concluded his *Psalm of Life* with a most appropriate parting thought, as to just how we may *all* leave footprints on the sands of time when he wrote:

> *Let us then be up and doing,*
> *With a heart for any fate;*
> *Still achieving, still pursuing,*
> *Learn to labor and to wait.*
> —Longfellow

References

1. Peters T. *Thriving on Chaos*. New York, NY: Alfred A. Knopf; 1987.
2. Voss D. Proprioceptive neuromuscular facilitation. *Am J Phys Med*. 1967;46:838-898.
3. Barnes MR, Crutchfield CA, Heriza CB, Herdman SJ. *Reflex and Vestibular Aspects of Motor Control, Motor Development and Motor Learning*. Atlanta, Ga; Stokesville Publishing Co; 1990.
4. *Taber's Cyclopedic Medical Dictionary*. Philadelphia, Pa: F A Davis Co; 1981.
5. *Webster's New Universal Unabridged Dictionary*. New York, NY: Simon & Schuster Inc; 1979.

Chapter 29

Committees and Participants

COMMITTEES

Conference Planning Committee

Susan Attermeier, MA, PT
Pam Duncan, MA, PT
Martha Feretti, MPH, PT
Susan Harris, PhD, PT
Carolyn Heriza, EdD, PT
Rose Myers, PhD, PT
Patricia Montgomery,
  PhD, PT, Treasurer
Becky Porter, MS, PT,
  Secretary
Deborah Shefrin, MS, PT
Ellen Spake, MS, PT,
  Co-Chair
Darcy Umphred, PhD, PT
Ann VanSant, PhD, PT,
  Co-Chair
Carolee Winstein, PhD, PT

Financial Planning Committee

Patricia Montgomery,
  PhD, PT, Chair
Barbara Connolly, EdD,
  PT
Suzann Campbell, PhD, PT
Susan Effgen, PhD, PT

Program Committee

Carolyn Heriza, EdD, PT,
  Chair
Susan Attermeier, MA, PT
Susan Herdman, PhD, PT
Harry Knecht, EdD, PT
Roberta Newton, PhD, PT
Darcy Umphred, PhD, PT
Carolee Winstein, PhD, PT
Suzann Campbell, PhD, PT

Program Subcommittee for Case Studies, Panel Discussions, and Small Groups

Susan Attermeier, MA,
  PT, Chair
Sally Atwater, MPT, PT
Kathy Black, MS, PT
Lois Deming Hedman,
  MS, PT

Local Arrangements

Ellen Spake, MS, PT,
  Chair
Martha Feretti, MPH, PT
Patricia Montgomery,
  PhD, PT
Rebecca Porter, MS, PT

Exhibit Hall

Susan Harris, PhD, PT

PARTICIPANTS

Wendy Abrahms
Cara Adams
Susan Adler
Leslie Allison
Nancy Appel
Fran Arkusinski
Edith Aston-McCrimmon
Susan Attermeier
Sally Atwater
Emilie Aubert
Nancy Austin
Mary Beth Badke
Ray Edmond Balangue
Susan Barker
Mary Lou Barnes
Robert Bartlett
Melinda Bartscherer
Claire Bassile
Phyllis Beck
Andrea Behrman
Peggy Belmont
Jodell Bender
Susan Bennett
Sue Begmeier
Donna Bernhardt
Delva Bethune
Kristen Birkmeier
Kristie Bjornson
Kathy Black
Cathleen Blatchly
Patricia Blau Nina
  Bloomfield
Connie Anne Blow
Amy Bodkin
Carol Boeker
Connie Bogard
Joanell Bohmert
Diane Borello-France
Jeannie Boucher
Nancy Bower

Laura Brantly
Jeanette Brasseur
Catarina Broberg
Kathryn Brown
Barbara Brucker
Jan Bruckner
Christopher Buneo
Kay Burgess
Carole Burnett
Fran Bussert
Terry Butler
Nancy Byl
Bernice Calvert
Monica Calvert
Suzann Campbell
Judy Canfield
Heather Carling-Smith
Judy Carmick
Blanche Carpenter
Donna Cech
Jane Cedar
Pauline Cerasoli Corinne
  Chan
Lynette Chandler
Ann Charrette
Charlotte Chatto
Diane Cherry
Holly Cintas
Jo Clelland
Nancy Clopton
Lynn Colby
Barbara Connolly
Geri Connor
Carol Coogler
Deborah Cooke
Jane Copeland
Suzy Cornbleet
Mary Pat Corrigan
Jean Crago
Rebecca Craik
Marggie Cramer
Susan Cromwell
Carolyn Crutchfield
Catherine Curtis
Bazilia Da'Silva
Susan Daleiden
Ruth Dannenbaum
Ken Davis
Jody Delehanty
Jennifer Delp
Gerard DeMauro
Teresa (Tara) Denham

Betty Denton Mary
  Deusterhaus-Minor
Judith Deutsch
Judith Dewane
Carol Dichter
Rebecca Didat
Kathy Dieruf
Jean DiMarino
Nancy Dragotta
Stephanie Duggins
Pamela Duncan
Blanche DuPont
Mary Dutton
Mary Jean Dzialga
Elaine Eckel
Peggy Edwards
Scott Edwards
Susan Effgen
Nancy Ehn
David Eisman
Donna El-din
Donna Eliason
Mark Eliason
Sally Emerson
James Eng
Alice Engelhardt
Robert Eskew
Janet Evans
Sandra Falck
Barbara Fenner
Martha Feretti
Linda Fetters Kate
  Finkbeiner
Beth Fisher
Carolyn Fiterman
Susan Flannery
Jan Foster
Debra Fox
Martha Frank
Susan Freed
Gertrude Freeman
Donna Fry-Welch
David Fukumoto
Kenda Fuller
Julie Gahimer
Jody Gandy
Jayne Garland
Elizabeth Garner
Meryl Gersh
Joan Gertz
Kathleen Gill
Carol Giuliani

Marie Goodwin
Carolyn Gowland
Lise Gray
Melissa Gray
Mary Hagen
Patti Halcarz
Steven Haley
Barbara Hanley
Martha Hann
Paul Hansen
Kimberly Harbst
Susan Harris
Meredith Harris
Patricia Harris
Cathy Harrow
Ruth Hausheer
Tammy Hebert
Lois Hedman
Jean Held
Judy Hembree
Carolyn Heriza
Denyse Herrmann
Rosaline Hickenbottom
Jean Hiebert
Julie High
Nancy Hochreiter
Elizabeth Hockey
Maureen Holden
Martha Holmes
Ken Holt
Fay Horak
Melissa Horton
Nancy Howard
Lisa Huber
Mary Hunt
Sharon Huntoon
Denise Hutchins
Caryn Ito
Osa Jackson
Richard Johnson
Elaine Johnson-Siekmann
Gary Kamen
Maryann Kantmann
Sandra Kaplan
M. Ann Karas
Randi Karpinski
Janis Kathrein
Linda Kaufman
Regina Kaufman
Mary Keehn
Kathleen Kelly
Margaret Kelly
Emily Keshner
Joanne King
Naomi
   Kirshenbaum-Cohen
Laura Klassen
Anne Kloos
Philip Koch
Linda Kopriva

Kristin Krosschell
Virginia Kurtz
Barbara Lammert
Jennifer Lander
Cathy Larson
Anne Lea
Patricia Leahy
Judith Leikauskas
Carol Leiper
Elaine Leonard
Elizabeth Leonard
Timothy Leslie
Arlean Levine
Sandra Levine
Annabel Lewis
Jill Liebhaber
Hendrika Lietz
Kathye Light
Deborah Litwack
Steven Lockard
Pam Lubker
Marianne Lukan
Lydia Lum
Marilyn MacKay-Lyons
Betty McNeill
Michael Majsak
Marie-Louise Mangold
Michael Maninang
Sandy Marder-Lokken
Tink Martin
Jeanne McCoy
LeAnn McCrary
Karen McCulloch
Irene McEwen
Julia McFann
Nancy McGibbon
Brian McKiernan
Michelle McLay
Amy McMillan
Marsha Melnick
Polly Menendez
Kathy Mercuris
Alma Merians
Jane Merrill
Barb Miller
Deborah Miller
Ellen Miller
Maureen Mitchell
Julie Monahan
Sally Monroe
Patricia Montgomery
Robert Morgan
Betty-Lynn Morrice
David Morris
Karen Mueller
Rose Myers
Pauline Navarro
Lee Nelson
Roberta Newton
Nancy Nicholson

Virginia Nieland
Mary Nishimoto
Amy Nordon
Anita Nunn
Sharon Nuzik
Deborah O'Rourke
Susan O'Sullivan
Joan Oates
Stephanie Ombry
Carmen Otto
Averell Overby
Stephanie Overholt
Jill Owen
Peggy Owen
Karen Ozga
Robert Palisano
Carol Paskewitz
Susan Perry
Joyce Phelps
Lee Philips
Beth Phillips
Scot Phillips
Karen Pittman
Patricia Pohl
Beth Pomwith
Becky Porter
Cynthia Potter
Charlotte Powell
Beth Provost
Priscilla Raasch-Mason
Sandra Radtka
Patricia Ramo
Shirley Randolph
Inge Reaviel
Susan Rehr
Cindy Renk
Elizabeth Revelj
Pamela Reynolds
Lynne Rezabek
Randy Richter
Rose Marie Rine
Lisa Riolo-Quinn
Cynthia Rivers
Bonnie Robinson
Deirdre Robinson
Maria Rodriquez
Mark Rogers
Penni Romero
Gay Rosenberg
Joanna Ross
Sandy Ross
Sharon Russo
Martin Rutz
Louise Rutz-LaPitz
Paul Sabourin
Patricia Sachon
Monica Safranek
Susan Sandvik
Julie Sanford
Sandra Sarnacki

Cecelia Sartor-Glittenberg
Dale Scalise-Smith
Judith Schank
Susan Scheer
Mary Schmidt
Richard Schmidt
Jane Schneider
Karin Schumacher
Roberta "Pug" Schwertner
Glenn Scudder
Lesta Searles
Marjane Selleck
Sara Shapiro
Nancy Sharby
Sharon Shaw
Alice Shea
Kay Shepard
Linda Simpson
Caren Sizemore
Mary Slavin
Marcia Smith
Patricia Smith
Tammy Sosolik
Teresa Southard
Ellen Spake
Lisa Stajduhar
Barbara Stanerson
Chloe Stannard
Vicki Stemmons
Jennifer Stith
Judith Stoecker
Kathryn Stokes
Sheila Stratman
Mary Surls
Laurie Swanson
Anne Sweeney
Jane Taniguchi
Edward Tantorski
Susan Taves
Mary Templeton
Diane Thomas
Catherine Thompson
David Thompson
Karen Thornton
Suzanne Tinsley
James Tomlinson
Susan Tomlinson
Bette Torrible
Martha Trotter
Dale Turner
Darcy Umphred
Carol Urbanski
Darl VanderLinden
Marianna VanPelt
Ann VanSant
Preeti Verma
Patricia Vine
Nancy Volk
Karen Walker
Gunilla Wannstedt

Nannette Washko	Susan Whitney	Ann Winters	Kay Youens
Deirdre Webster	Lynne Wiesel	Marilyn Woods	Ellen Zambo-Anderson
Mary Wehde	Patricia Wilder	Judith Woronuk	John Zenker
Karen Weller	Betsy Willy	Martha Wroe	Mitzi Zeno
Michelle West	Patricia Winkler	Joy Yakura	Maria Zichettella
Sharon White	Carolee Winstein	Hildred Yost	Lisa Zuber

Index